Infectious Diseases of Wild Mammals SECOND EDITION

Infectious Diseases
of Wild Mammals

SECOND EDITION

EDITED BY   **JOHN W. DAVIS,** D.V.M., M.S., Ph.D.
LARS H. KARSTAD, D.V.M., M.S., Ph.D
DANIEL O. TRAINER, M.S., Ph.D.

The Iowa State University Press, AMES, IOWA, U.S.A.

First edition, 1970

Second printing, 1973

Second edition, 1981

Library of Congress Cataloging in Publication Data
Main entry under title:

Infectious diseases of wild mammals.

    Bibliography: p.
    Includes index.
    1. Wildlife diseases. 2. Mammals—Diseases. 3. Communicable diseases in animals. I. Davis, John William, 1917–   . II. Karstad, Lars H. III. Trainer, Daniel O. [DNLM: 1. Communicable diseases—Veterinary. 2. Mammals. 3. Animal diseases. SF 997 D26311]

SF997.I53 1981	636.089'6959	81–6064
ISBN 0-8138–0445–0		AACR2

Authors

J. FREDERICK BELL, M.D. (retired)
10 Vole Road, S.W., Hamilton, Montana

JAMES L. BITTLE, D.V.M.
President, Pitman-Moore, Inc., Washington Crossing, New Jersey

ERIC BROUGHTON, D.V.M.
Veterinary Pathologist, Pathology and Parasitology Division, National Wildlife Research Centre, Ottawa, Ontario, Canada

JOAN BUDD, D.V.M.
Associate Professor, Department of Pathology (retired), Ontario Veterinary College, Guelph, Ontario, Canada

VICTOR J. CABASSO, Sc.D.
Vice President, Research and Development, Cutter Laboratories, Inc., Berkeley, California

L. P. E. CHOQUETTE, D.V.M.
Chief, Pathology and Parasitology Division, National Wildlife Research Centre, Ottawa, Ontario, Canada

G. E. COSGROVE, M.D.
Pathologist, Zoological Society of San Diego, San Diego, California

JOHN W. DAVIS, D.V.M.
Professor, Veterinary Science, Division of Pathobiology and Public Practice, College of Veterinary Medicine, Virginia Polytechnic Institute and State University, Blacksburg, Virginia

ROELOF G. DIJKSTRA, D.V.Sc.
Animal Health Service and Veterinary Investigation Centre, Leeuwarden, The Netherlands

L. D. FAY, D.V.M.
Pathologist, Rose Lake Wildlife Research Center, Michigan Department of Natural Resources, East Lansing, Michigan

JOHN R. GORHAM, D.V.M.
Science and Education Administration, U.S. Department of Agriculture and College of Veterinary Medicine, Washington State University, Pullman, Washington

J. G. GROOTENHUIS, D.V.M.
Wildlife Disease Section, Veterinary Research Laboratory, Kabete, Kenya, East Africa

R. S. HEDGER, M.R.C.V.S.
Head, Department of Epidemiology, Animal Virus Research Institute, Pirbright Woking, Surrey, England

ELMER M. HIMES, D.V.M.
General Pathology and Parasitology, National Veterinary Services Laboratories, USDA, Ames, Iowa

GERALD L. HOFF, Ph.D.
Kansas City Public Health Department, Epidemiology, Kansas City, Missouri

DUANE L. HOWE, D.V.M.
Practitioner, Dubois, Wyoming

J. O. IVERSEN, D.V.M.
Professor, Department of Veterinary Microbiology, Western College of Veterinary Medicine, University of Saskatchewan, Saskatoon, Saskatchewan, Canada

WILLIAM L. JELLISON, Ph.D.
Parasitologist (retired), Hamilton, Montana

DONALD W. JOHNSON, D.V.M.
Professor, Department of Large Animal Clinical Sciences, College of Veterinary Medicine, University of Minnesota, St. Paul, Minnesota

LARS H. KARSTAD, D.V.M.
Wildlife Disease Section, Veterinary Research Laboratory, Kabete, Kenya, East Africa

NORVAL W. KING, JR., D.V.M.
Associate Professor, Comparative Pathology, and Associate Director, New England Regional Primate Research Center, Harvard Medical School, Southborough, Massachusetts

STUART E. KNAPP, Ph.D.
Vice President for Academic Affairs, Montana State University, Bozeman, Montana

FRANCES M. LOVE, M.D.
Regional Medical Director, Gulf Oil Corporation, Houston, Texas

RAYMOND E. MILLEMANN, Ph.D.
Research Staff Member, Oak Ridge National Laboratory, Oak Ridge, Tennessee

PETER F. OLSEN, Ph.D
Senior Ecologist, Dames and Moore Consulting Engineers, Salt Lake City, Utah

W. PLOWRIGHT, D.V.Sc.
Head, Department of Microbiology, The Royal Veterinary College, London, England

JAMES R. REILLY (deceased)

JOHN L. RICHARD, Ph.D.
Research Microbiologist, Mycology, National Animal Disease Center, Ames, Iowa

R. M. ROBINSON, D.V.M.
Pathologist, Texas Veterinary Medical Diagnostic Laboratory, College of Veterinary Medicine, College Station, Texas

MERTON N. ROSEN, M.A. (deceased)

VANCE L. SANGER, D.V.M.
Head, Department of Pathology, College of Veterinary Medicine, Michigan State University, East Lansing, Michigan

GORDON R. SCOTT, M.R.C.V.S.
Department of Animal Health, Royal School of Veterinary Studies, Veterinary Field Station, Easter Bush, Roslin Midlothian, Scotland

CHARLES SEYMOUR, Ph.D.
Research Associate, Department of Veterinary Science, University of Wisconsin, Madison, Wisconsin

DAVID T. SHEN, Ph.D.
Science and Education Administration, U.S. Department of Agriculture and College of Veterinary Medicine, Washington State University, Pullman, Washington

EMMETT B. SHOTTS, JR., Ph.D.
Professor, Medical Microbiology, College of Veterinary Medicine, University of Georgia, Athens, Georgia

RICHARD D. SHUMAN, D.V.M.
Veterinary Medical Officer (retired), National Animal Disease Center, Ames, Iowa

R. KEITH SIKES, SR., D.V.M.
State Epidemiologist, Georgia Department of Human Resources, Atlanta, Georgia

JOSIP SPALATIN, D.V.M.
Research Associate, Department of Veterinary Science, University of Wisconsin, Madison, Wisconsin

WILLIAM G. STONE, D.V.M.
Media, Pennsylvania

CHARLES O. THOEN, D.V.M.
Professor, Department of Veterinary Microbiology and Preventive Medicine, College of Veterinary Medicine, Iowa State University, Ames, Iowa

DANIEL O. TRAINER, Ph.D.
Acting Vice Provost, College of Natural Resources, University of Wisconsin, Stevens Point, Wisconsin

THEODORE F. WETZLER, Ph.D.
4562 35th West Ave., Seattle, Washington

J. FRANKLIN WITTER, D.V.M. (retired)
Professor Emeritus, Animal Pathology, University of Maine, Orono, Maine

G. WOBESER, D.V.M.
Professor, Department of Veterinary Pathology, Western College of Veterinary Medicine, University of Saskatchewan, Saskatoon, Saskatchewan, Canada

RICHARD L. WOOD, D.V.M.
Veterinary Medical Officer, National Animal Disease Center, Ames, Iowa

E. YOUNG, B.V.Sc.
State Veterinarian, Nature Conservation Division, Kruger National Park, Pretoria, South Africa

THOMAS M. YUILL, Ph.D.
Professor and Chairman, Department of Veterinary Science, University of Wisconsin, Madison, Wisconsin

Contents

Preface

Because of the continuous addition of new material and information to the field of infectious diseases of wild mammals it became essential that we revise and update the first edition. We are very fortunate to have many of the original authors, whose chapters led to the success of the first edition, available to contribute to this revised edition as well as a number of new authors whose names and reputations are well known in the field of wildlife diseases. The second edition of *Infectious Diseases of Wild Mammals* is an extensive revision of the first, published in 1970. The nine new chapters and eighteen new authors reflect the rapid advancement of this area of diseases. After consultation with the respective authors, all chapters except Sylvatic (Wild Rodent) Plague, Pseudotuberculosis, and Epizootic Chlamydiosis of Muskrats and Snowshoe Hares were revised.

Errington's disease is now Tyzzer's disease. The individual chapters on the hemorrhagic diseases have been combined into one. The chapters on Lymphocytic Choriomeningitis, Mink Virus Enteritis, and Effects of Toxic Substances are not included in this book. The chapter on toxic substances is scheduled to appear later in a book on wildlife noninfectious diseases.

Some of the original contributors turned over their chapters to other competent individuals who continued the excellent work demonstrated in the first edition. Attempts were made to reduce the size of chapters for economic sake without reducing the effectiveness of the material presented.

To former and current contributors we give our heartfelt appreciation. We honor those who have passed on and hope to reach the goal of excellence that E. E. Roth and J. R. Reilly achieved. We are very pleased that our first editors Dr. L. Karstad and Dr. D. Trainer could again perform their outstanding work for the second edition. We thank all the people who had a hand in making this second edition a reality.

It is hoped that wildlife biologists, veterinarians, zoo personnel, wildlife students, research workers, animal scientists, public health personnel, and other groups interested in infectious diseases of wild mammals will find this a most helpful and useful reference.

JOHN W. DAVIS

1 *Viral Diseases*

1 Rabies

R. KEITH SIKES, SR.

Synonyms: **Hydrophobia, rage, Tollwut, lyssa, rabbia, rabia, raiva, beshenstvo.**

Rabies is an acute infectious disease of the central nervous system caused by a virus that generally persists in nature as a salivary gland infection of carnivorous animals. The virus is usually transmitted from animal to animal and from animal to man by biting. All warm-blooded animals are susceptible.

Epizootics of rabies in domestic dogs and such wild animals as foxes, skunks, coyotes, jackals, and wolves occur when the population of such susceptible animals becomes dense enough to ensure easy animal-to-animal transmission of infection where rabies is present. Johnson (1965) has postulated that species belonging to the families Viverridae and Mustelidae might be permanent hosts of rabies virus. Pawan (1936a,b) has hypothesized that the vampire bat (*Desmodus rotundus murinus*) may be an asymptomatic carrier of this disease.

Rabies has public health as well as agricultural and economic significance. In 1976–1977 there were 1,069 human deaths from rabies reported to the World Health Organization (WHO); 1,158,078 people throughout the world during 1972–1973 received postexposure antirabies prophylaxis, and 80 paralytic accidents were attributed to vaccine treatment (WHO, 1974, 1978).

The loss of livestock from rabies costs hundreds of millions of dollars annually throughout the world. Virtually all cases of rabies in livestock in the United States can be traced to rabid wild animals, especially foxes and skunks. In Latin America, the disease in cattle (derriengue) is transmitted by vampire bats.

HISTORY. Rabies is one of the oldest recorded infectious diseases; it was known to occur in Europe and Asia in ancient times. Democritus (500 B.C.) and Aristotle (322 B.C.) described rabies in domestic animals. Celsus (A.D. 100) noted the relationship of hydrophobia in man to rabies in animals.

As early as 1271, rabies was present in western Europe, where it was prevalent among wolves in France. Epizootics of fox rabies were recorded in Massachusetts in the first decade of the nineteenth century (Thacker 1812). Skunk rabies was reported in Lower California in 1826 (Nelson 1918) and in Kansas in 1871 (Seton 1925). Fox rabies epizootics occurred in Alabama in 1890 (Wilkinson 1894) and in Alaska in 1915 (Ferenbaugh 1916). Coyote rabies epizootics appeared in California, Oregon, and Nevada in 1915 and 1916 (Geiger 1916; Mallory 1915).

Bat-transmitted rabies in cattle was first diagnosed in Brazil by Carini (1911), although this disease, called "mal de caderas de bovinos," had been recognized there in 1908. The actual transmission of rabies by bats was established in 1916 (Haupt and Rehaag 1921) during an outbreak of paralytic disease of cattle in Brazil. In Trinidad between 1929 and 1935, a disease characterized by an ascending paralysis killed people; Hurst and Pawan (1931, 1932) and Pawan (1936a,b) identified this fatal paralytic disease in man and cattle as rabies caused by the bites of infected bats. The vampire bat was the principal vector; this species is still the most important vector of rabies in many parts of Latin America today. Bat rabies was first reported in the United States in 1953 when the virus was isolated from a yellow bat (*Dasypterus floridanus*) that had bitten a child in Florida (Venters et al. 1954).

Rabies epizootics in foxes occurred in most of the countries of central and western Europe, Canada, and the United States between 1953 and 1974. Skunks, raccoons, and insectivorous bats have been recognized as important reservoir hosts in the United States and Canada since 1955.

Historically, Pasteur's contribution to the development of the first antirabies vaccine in 1885 is of great interest. He accomplished this after demonstrating the concept of attenuating the street (wild) strain of virus by serially passaging it over 100 times in rabbits. This attenuated virus was considered fixed for rabbits and was used in his original vaccine; it is still used in rabies vaccines for man and animals, mostly in the developing countries of the world.

DISTRIBUTION AND HOSTS. Rabies is enzootic

on every continent except Australia and has been reported from 57 countries (WHO 1978). It was not present in the following 30 countries, territories, and islands:

Africa
    Lesotho
America
    Bahamas
    Barbados
    Jamaica
    Surinam
    Uruguay
    West Indies
Asia
    Bahrein
    Brunei
    Hong Kong
    Japan
    Qatar
    Singapore
    United Arab
      Emirates

Europe
    Cyprus
    Finland
    Gibraltar
    Iceland
    Malta
    Norway
    Portugal
    Sweden
    United Kingdom
Oceania
    Australia
    Fiji
    Guam
    New Caledonia
    New Zealand
    Papua, New Guinea

Throughout the world, dogs are the most important vectors of the disease, although in almost every country various species of wildlife are important reservoirs or vectors. Jackals are dangerous reservoirs of infection in at least 30 different countries, mainly in Asia and Africa. Fox rabies is a problem in at least 14 countries, most of which are in North America and Europe. Wolves are important reservoirs or vectors in at least 10 countries, chiefly in the eastern Mediterranean area. Mongooses in South Africa, Cuba, the Dominican Republic, Puerto Rico, India, and northern Nigeria and vampire bats in Mexico, Central America, and South America are important sources of infection.

In the first half of the twentieth century, dogs were the most important animal host of rabies in Canada and the United States, but now skunks, raccoons, bats, and foxes are the species most frequently infected with rabies. Skunks and other terrestrial wild mammals transmit the disease to large numbers of livestock, especially cattle, which is the third most frequently infected species in these countries. The shift in species infected with rabies that took place between 1945 and 1977 is shown in Table 1.1. The relative importance of wildlife and domestic animals in transmitting rabies to man is demonstrated in Table 1.2.

The number of rabies cases reported by each state in 1977 is shown in Figure 1.1. Animal rabies is sometimes a problem in an entire state or region, but quite often it is localized in a county or group of counties only. The distribu-

TABLE 1.1   Cases of Rabies in the United States.

Year	Dogs	Cats	Wild-life	Live-stock	Man	Total
1945	8,505	466	372	585	35	9,963
1957	1,758	382	1,942	714	6	4,802
1967	412	293	3,211	691	2	4,609
1977	120	108	2,736	217	1	3,182

Sources: ARS, USDA; National Center for Disease Control, Public Health Service, USDHEW.

TABLE 1.2   Percentage of 167 Fatal Human Rabies Cases from Exposure to Domestic and Wildlife Species by Four-year Periods, United States, 1946–1977.

Four-year Period	Number of Cases	Dog or Cat Exposure	Wildlife Exposure
		%	%
1946–49	48	100	0
1950–53	54	91	9
1954–57	29	83	17
1958–61	15	53	47
1962–65	5	60	40
1966–69	4	50	50
1970–73	7	28[a]	72
1974–77	5	80[b]	20

[a]Includes 2 people, both exposed outside the United States.
[b]Includes 3 people, all exposed outside the United States.

tion of rabies within the United States in 1977 is shown by county for wildlife hosts as well as dogs, cats, and cattle (Figs. 1.2–1.9).

The annual incidence of rabies in the most frequently infected wildlife hosts is shown in Figures 1.1 through 1.10.

Rabies in skunks in the United States is a problem mainly in the Midwest, the Ohio Valley, Texas, and central California. The large striped skunk (*Mephitis mephitis*) is most frequently reported as rabid, although small spotted skunks (*Spilogale putorius* and *S. gracilis*) are also commonly infected.

Fox rabies has occurred most often in the eastern states, particularly in the Appalachian Mountain area from upstate New York through Tennessee, as well as in the states along the Gulf Coast. Both the red fox (*Vulpes fulva*) and the gray fox (*Urocyon cinereoargenteus*) are frequently infected. Since 1972 there has been a precipitous decline in fox rabies, from 642 cases

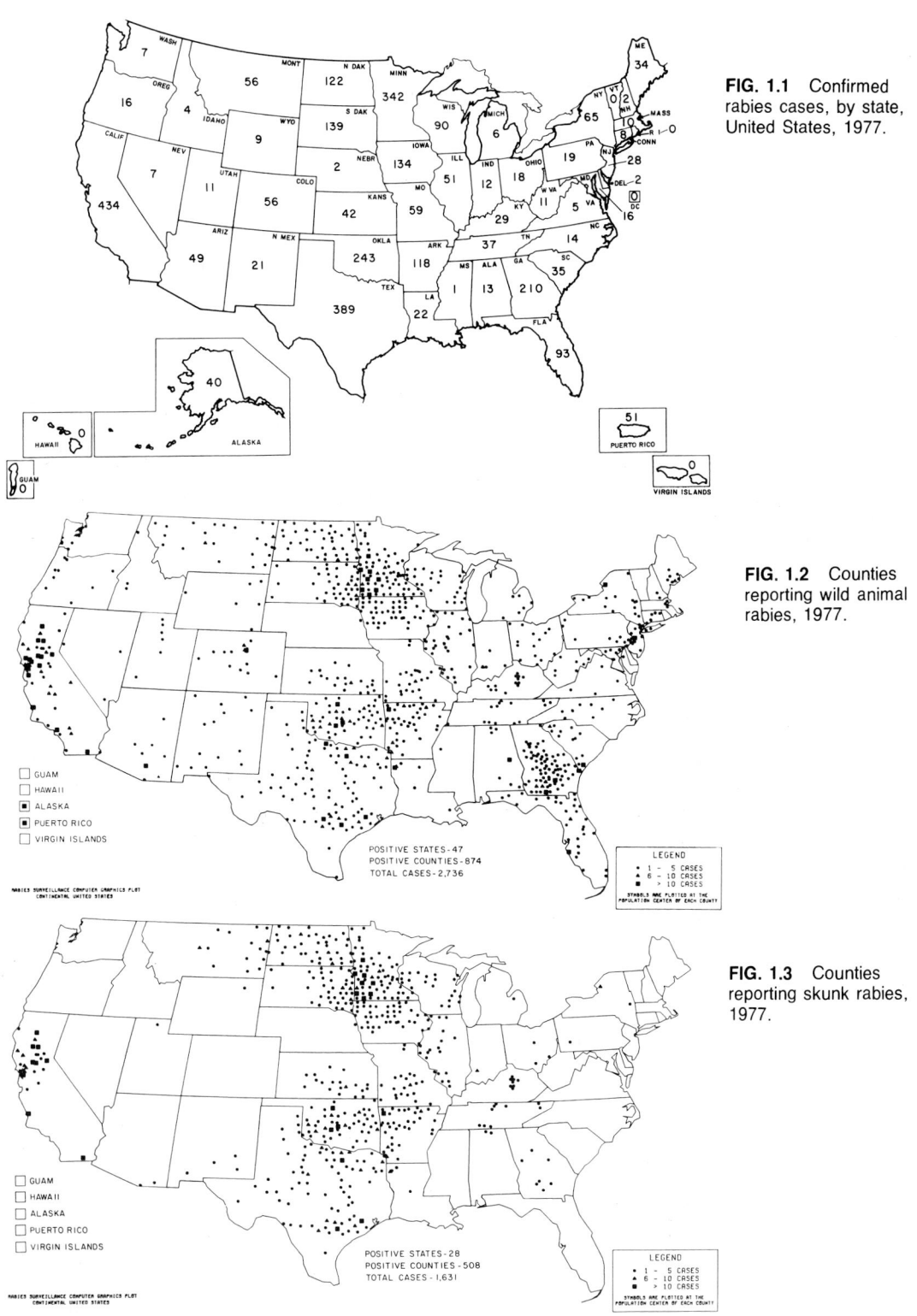

FIG. 1.1 Confirmed rabies cases, by state, United States, 1977.

FIG. 1.2 Counties reporting wild animal rabies, 1977.

FIG. 1.3 Counties reporting skunk rabies, 1977.

FIG. 1.4 Counties reporting fox rabies, 1977.

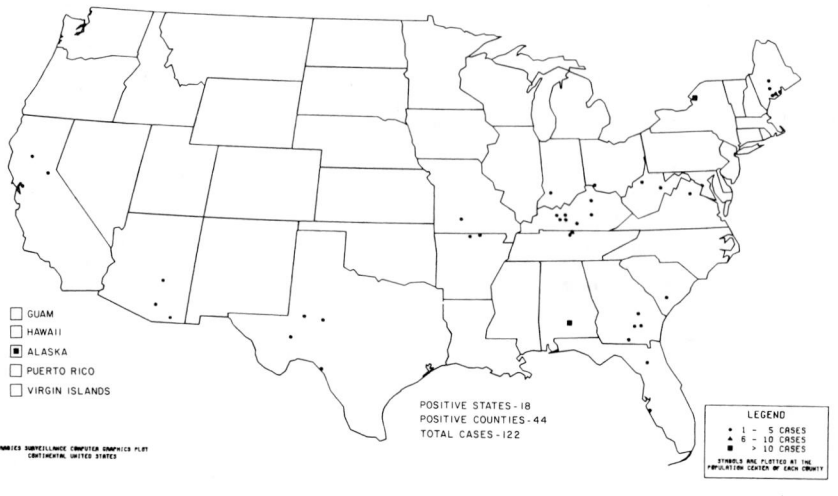

FIG. 1.5 Counties reporting raccoon rabies, 1977.

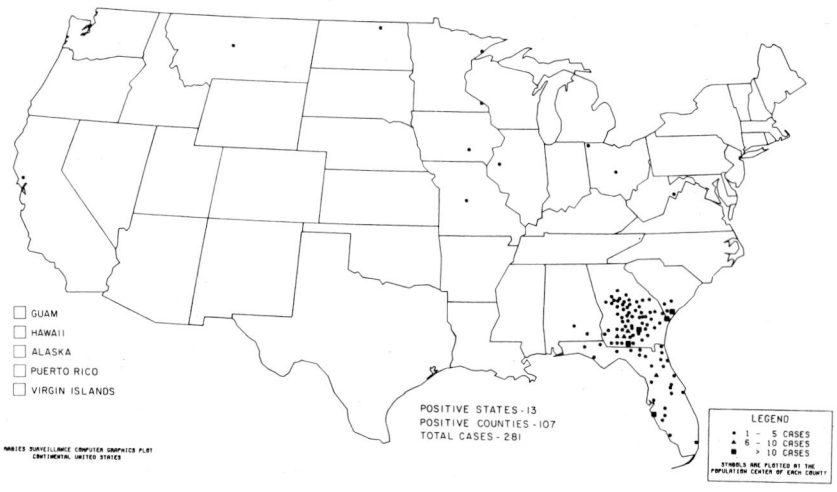

FIG. 1.6 Counties reporting bat rabies, 1977.

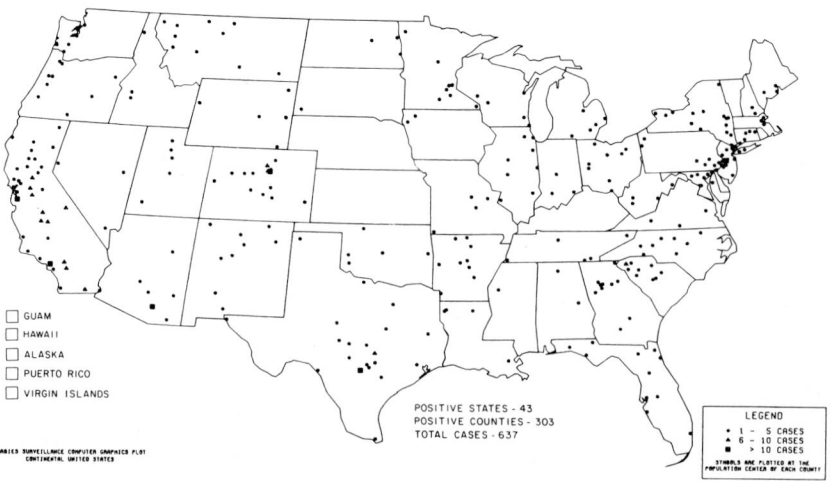

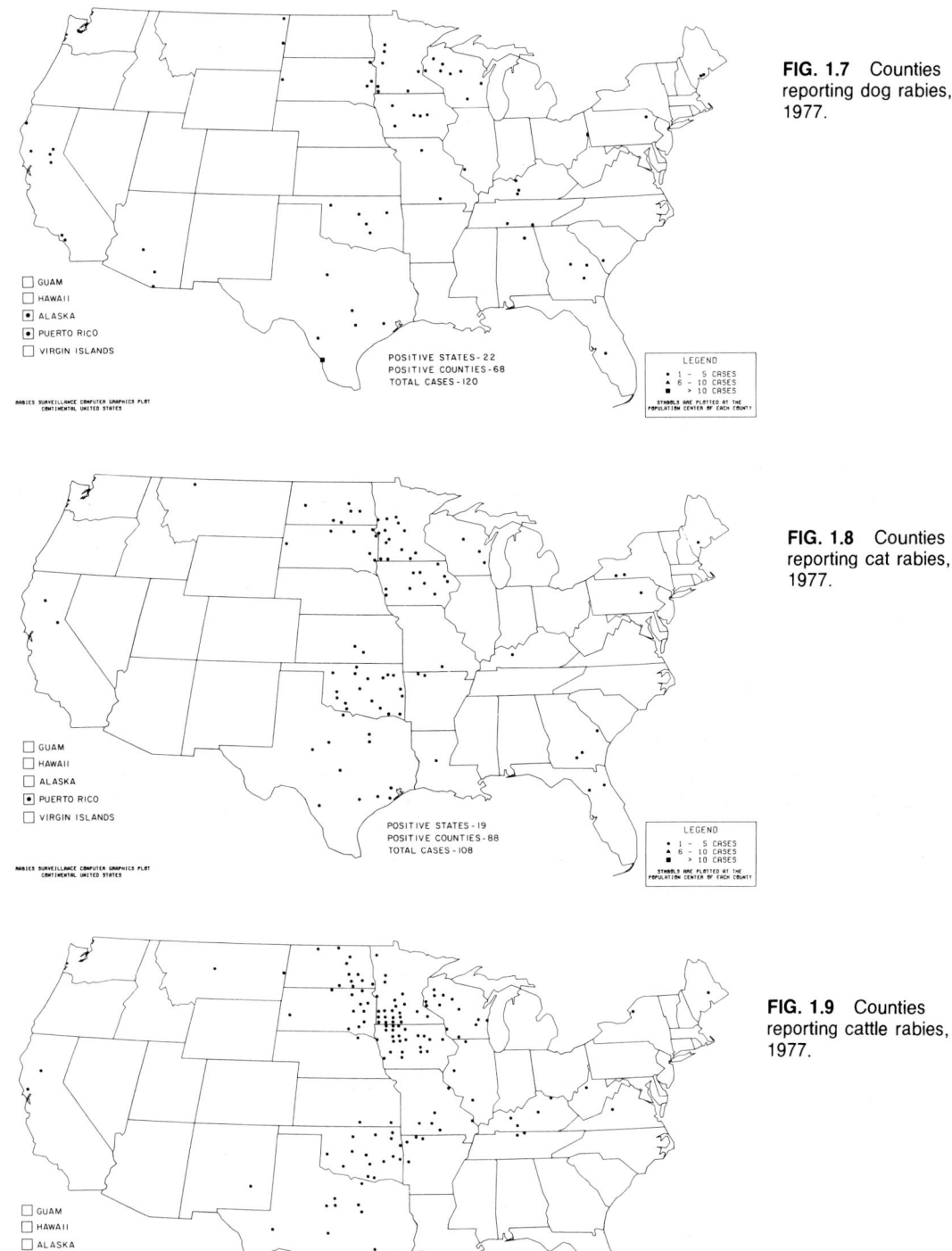

FIG. 1.7 Counties reporting dog rabies, 1977.

FIG. 1.8 Counties reporting cat rabies, 1977.

FIG. 1.9 Counties reporting cattle rabies, 1977.

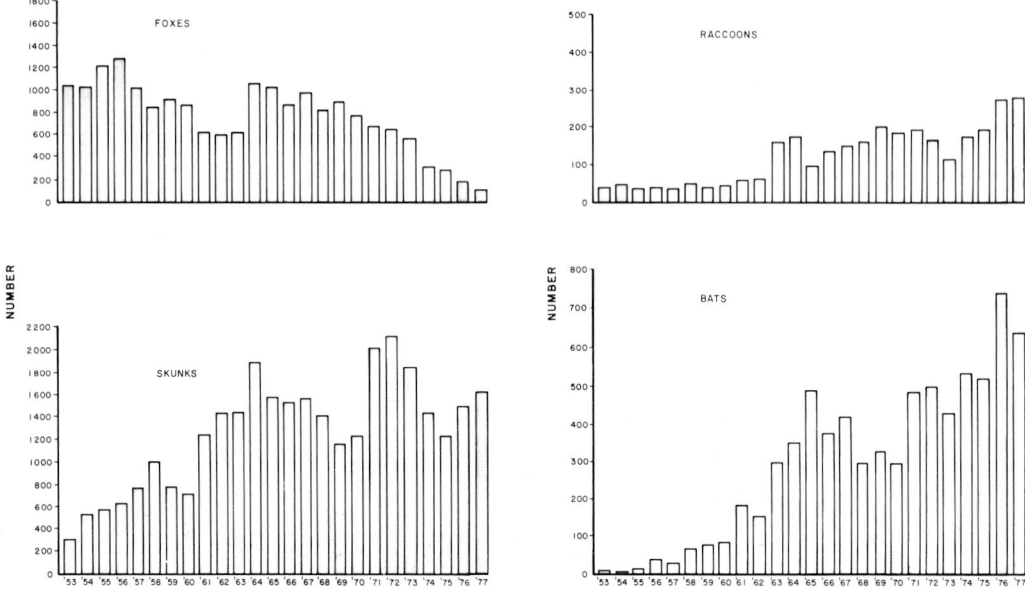

FIG. 1.10   Cases of rabies in wildlife hosts, United States, 1953–1977.

to only 122 in 1977. In Alaska the principal reservoir of infection is the Arctic fox (*Alopex logopus*).

Raccoon rabies is a problem primarily in the Southeast; Florida and Georgia usually report over 70% of the raccoon rabies in the United States annually. In 1978 South Carolina and Alabama reported increased rabies in raccoons.

Since 1953 when the first rabid bat was found in Florida, 48 of the 50 states have reported bat rabies. Rabies virus has been isolated from 26 of the 39 species of insectivorous bats of the United States (Baer and Adams 1970). Although six persons have died from exposure to rabid bats, the importance of bats in the total ecology of rabies has not been determined.

ETIOLOGY. Rabies virus is a rhabdo, RNA type that is sensitive to ether and to a pH lower than 3.0 (Wilner 1965). As seen in an electron microscope it is an elongated rodlike particle (bullet shape) and is approximately 150 nm in length and 75 nm in diameter (Murphy 1975). The filamentous internal component is arranged in the form of double helices with a diameter of 100 Å. Virions have been demonstrated in the Negri body (Miyamoto and Matsumoto 1965).

Sunlight and ultraviolet irradiation destroy rabies virus rapidly. Bichloride of mercu-

ry, strong acids and bases, and formalin inactivate the virus quite readily. Beta propiolactone concentrations of 1:5,000 to 1:10,000 inactivate the virus in suspensions from tissue culture, duck embryo, and purified virus of mouse brain origin (Kissling and Reese 1963; Peck et al. 1956; Sikes and Larghi 1967). Suspensions of virus are inactivated when heated and held at 60°C for 1 hour. Common antibiotics do not inhibit the infectivity of rabies virus.

Virus in infected tissues can be kept alive in 50% glycerol or pure glycerol for weeks at room temperature or for several months at 4°C. Virus infectivity can be preserved for years in 20% infected tissue suspensions containing egg yolk, bovine albumin, or serum when stored in sealed glass ampules at −65°C. Desiccating frozen specimens and storing at 4°C also keeps the virus viable for years.

Purification and concentration of the virus with alcohol precipitation was first reported in 1947 (Cox et al. 1947). The virus from Suckling-mouse brain was partially purified to a high degree by means of a combination of high-speed centrifugation and ECTEOLA-cellulose chromatographic procedures (Sikes and Larghi 1967; Thomas et al. 1963). Tissue culture rabies virus has been purified using chemical purification methods (Sokol 1975).

Unlike most other pathogenic animal

viruses, only one distinct immunologic type or strain of rabies virus has ever been identified. For example, rabies virus isolated from vampire bats in Latin America is immunologically indistinguishable by cross-protection, serum neutralization, or complement fixation tests from virus isolated from rabid dogs, foxes, or skunks in Europe and North America.

TRANSMISSION AND ECOLOGY. Although there is only one strain of virus, two epizootiologic types of rabies exist—one occurs in the wild animal host and the other in dogs and related canines. Both types of disease are perpetuated by bites of infected animals; saliva that contains virus is introduced into the flesh of susceptible animals. The disease frequently is not recognized in wild animals until cases begin to occur in man or domestic animals and the source of infection is sought.

The best examples of the two epizootiologic types of rabies occur in the United States. In 1945 there were 8,505 cases of dog rabies, or 85% of the total 9,963 cases reported in the United States; there were only 372 cases in wildlife species, or 4% of the total. In 1977 only 120 cases of dog rabies, or 4% of the 3,182 total, were reported; wildlife accounted for 2,736, or 86% of the total (Table 1.1).

The sharp decline in the number of cases of canine rabies is due to widespread use of effective rabies vaccines and application of stray-dog control measures. On the other hand, the reported incidence of rabies in skunks, foxes, bats, and raccoons continues to increase despite poor reporting of cases in these species. Most state and federal officials conducting rabies surveillance believe that, at most, only 10% of the rabid wildlife hosts are reported. The increased incidence of rabies in foxes, skunks, and raccoons may be due to population increases that result from a combination of general wildlife conservation practices and the decline in the value of pelts of these animals that began in the mid-1940s (Parker 1961).

In the United States, the ecology of wildlife rabies is peculiar in that areas of fox, skunk, and raccoon rabies have been well defined. Fox rabies has been widespread in the Appalachian Mountain states (until the past 3 years), but few skunk rabies cases have been reported despite large skunk populations in that area. On the other hand, areas of the midwestern United States have a serious skunk rabies problem, but no difficulty with rabies in dense fox populations. In the counties of Florida and Georgia as well as South Carolina (in 1979 also Alabama),

rabies in raccoons is a problem, but virtually no rabies is recognized in the abundant foxes and skunks.

Many ecological factors influence the unique distribution of wildlife rabies in these areas. One explanation is based largely on differences in the quantity of virus emitted in the saliva of skunks and foxes and the susceptibility of the species to infection (Parker and Wilsnack 1966; Sikes 1962).

In experimental studies, foxes proved to be more susceptible to rabies infection than skunks, raccoons, or opossums. Whereas less than 10 mouse LD_{50} were required to infect foxes, 500 to 80,000 were required to infect other species. Foxes that received small doses of virus (between 10 and 1,000 LD_{50}) usually had long incubation periods—more than 30 days—and excreted virus in their saliva, usually 10^2 to 10^5 LD_{50} of rabies virus per 0.03 mL of saliva.

Skunks were shown to be more refractory to rabies infection than foxes. At least 100 times more virus was required to infect skunks than foxes, yet infected skunks usually emitted more virus per volume of saliva than foxes. The quantity of virus emitted in the saliva of skunks was usually optimal for the amount required to infect skunks, but it was an overwhelming amount for foxes.

From these data an explanation of the unique distribution of fox rabies may be hypothesized. Transmission is usually maintained from fox to fox and from skunk to skunk. Occasionally, however, fox-to-skunk transmission would be expected to occur. This, in fact, has happened in a few states that have had an abundance of fox rabies for 10 years or more; new foci of skunk rabies have developed in the areas that previously had reported only rabies in foxes.

Although true reservoirs of rabies may exist among the Viverridae, Mustelidae, and Chiroptera of the United States, sufficient evidence has not been obtained to incriminate them as true carriers of rabies virus. In laboratory studies, all animals of all species that emitted virus in saliva died of rabies a few days after the virus was detected (Baer and Bales 1967; Parker and Wilsnack 1966; Sikes and Tierkel 1960).

Attempts to transmit rabies infection by bloodsucking arthropods have not been successful (Bell et al. 1957).

Rabies is almost always transmitted by the bite of an infected animal; however, transmission of rabies by nonbite routes has been demonstrated in a bat cave (Constantine 1962). Two men who worked in the cave died of rabies without having been bitten by bats at any time during their visits. (*Tadarida brasiliensis mexicana* is the most abundant of the bat species— all insectivorous—found in this cave.) Constantine demonstrated that foxes and coyotes could acquire the infection when left in cages that protected them from being bitten by bats. Because the conditions in this cave are unique, the nonbite route of transmission is not considered of general importance.

The vampire bat is considered by some authorities to be a carrier of rabies. In several transmission experiments in which infected vampire bats were allowed to bite normal terrestrial mammals, Pawan (1936a,b, 1938) concluded that vampire bats are susceptible to rabies virus and may develop either furious or paralytic forms of rabies and are capable of transmitting rabies by their bite while clinically rabid and after recovering from the disease. However, Pawan's most critical experiments did not substantiate his conclusions. In one, a vampire bat with furious rabies bit and transmitted rabies to a calf. This bat recovered; however, no virus was subsequently isolated from it, and it failed to transmit virus to another calf that it bit a few days after its recovery. Pawan described two other bats that had clinical rabies and recovered. Unfortunately, he did not report any attempts to transmit the infection from these bats or to isolate virus from them after their recovery. One might, therefore, question whether vampire bats are actually carriers of rabies—if by *carriers* we mean animals that transmit the disease without showing signs of infection themselves.

Regardless of the exact role of bats in the total ecology of rabies, both the vampire and insectivorous species of bats have been responsible for transmitting rabies to man. Hurst and Pawan (1931, 1932) described an outbreak in Trinidad of an acute myelitis caused by rabies virus that killed 17 people between 1925 and 1931. Vampire bats were considered the vector. In the past 10 years a few people and millions of livestock have died in Latin America of rabies transmitted by vampire bats (P. N. Acha, personal communication, 1966). In the United States since 1951 six human rabies deaths have been attributed to association with bats.

Pawan considered the dog, or canine family, the true host and the appearance of rabies in vampire bats in Brazil in 1908 and in Trinidad in 1925 as a form of aberrant parasitism. Contrary to this, Johnson (1965) thought that "canine rabies is an example of aberrant parasitism" and that the only true hosts are the Mustelidae and Viverridae. It is doubtful whether it will ever be determined which species are true hosts and which are aberrant hosts.

A more practical problem is that of controlling wildlife rabies in the United States, Canada, and certain European countries, where since the 1950s wildlife rabies has increased tremendously, while dog rabies has diminished. In the United States, wildlife rabies has spread over such a large area that the phenomenon must be explained by ecological principles other than those based on aberrant hosts and carriers. Consideration must be given to population fluctuations that occur when disease is enzootic in an area and to the possibility of variable incubation periods—up to 1 year in rabies. Epizootics of fox rabies within a given area have been described as a niche phenomenon within a county or counties (Wood and Davis 1959). Large numbers of susceptible animals, such as foxes, are undoubtedly killed by infection. A large-scale die-off should create a void or vacuum in a given population and thus preclude another epizootic in that area until a new susceptible population is established. Assuming that the food supply and other factors necessary to support a stable population of the species still persist, the population vacuum can be expected to be filled by animals from contiguous, unaffected areas and the offspring of the few animals that survive the infection. During the time required for the buildup of a new population, some of the animals indigenous to the area or migrating from an area of high population density can be expected to be incubating the disease. Then when the ratio of susceptible to infected animals reaches the proper proportion, another rabies epizootic will occur. The disease status of an area may change from enzootic to epizootic according to these shifts of populations and ratios of infected to susceptible hosts.

SIGNS. "The atypical is typical" describes rabies symptomatology in any species of animal.

The incubation period of rabies is extremely variable, but the average is usually 2–12 weeks. It is rarely less than 10 days or more than 6 months in carnivorous animals and bats studied under experimental conditions.

Foxes, skunks, and raccoons inoculated intramuscularly with rabies virus have demonstrated a syndrome similar to that in dogs (Parker and Wilsnack 1966; Sikes 1962; Sikes and Tierkel 1960). The majority of these animals had furious rabies; they exhibited aggressive signs early in the course and then became paralyzed. Some animals had dumb rabies; they simply became paralyzed and died shortly thereafter.

Many caged, rabid wild species, especially foxes, have a detectable change of behavior marking a short prodrome of 1–2 days. In this stage an animal may be anorexic, apprehensive, and nervous or may be more shy and apathetic than usual. Animals with furious rabies have an excitation phase that usually lasts 1–6 days in foxes, raccoons, and skunks. During this time the saliva contains the greatest amount of virus, although virus may be present in the saliva prior to detection of signs and until the day of death. During the excitement phase the animal is restless and soon becomes vicious, biting at sticks, straw, or other objects. Foxes and raccoons often have a characteristic cry or change in bark, believed to be caused by paralysis of laryngeal muscles. Many caged wild animals become so vicious during this furious stage that they break their teeth and cut their mouths biting metal feed dishes, wire, and other objects. Some animals continue to eat and drink, at least for the first 2 or 3 days of the furious stage, although many have difficulty chewing and swallowing. The strong, furious actions slowly subside into weaker, less aggressive behavior, and the animal seems to have used all his energy. Incoordination and muscle tremors are often apparent. Animals in the final stages of furious rabies often act just like those with dumb rabies; their symptoms may include incoordination, often followed by tremors and convulsions, and usually followed by paralysis and prostration before death. Hydrophobia, which is a common symptom of rabies in humans, is not common among animals, although difficulty in swallowing is common, especially in the last stages of the disease. The entire clinical course of the disease in the majority of several hundred foxes observed in the Center for Disease Control laboratory at Atlanta, Georgia, lasted only 2–4 days; in raccoons, 3–5 days and in skunks, 4–9 days.

Bats also show variable signs of rabies. Many vampires have been reported with furious rabies and a few with dumb rabies (Pawan 1936b). Observations of various species of colonial, free-living, and fruit bats are similar (Baer and Bales 1967; Constantine 1966; Stamm et al. 1956). Beamer et al. (1960) and Richards (1963) reported observing signs of rabies in many other species of animals. An important consideration in reaching a clinical diagnosis of rabies in animals, especially wild ones, is that no sign or series of signs is pathognomonic. Signs of other diseases—such as distemper, hepatitis, listeriosis, tetanus, botulism, and some parasite infestations—are similar to those of rabies. Encephalitis syndromes can also be caused by plant or chemical toxins; these clinical signs are so varied and overlapping that limited confidence should be placed on a clinical diagnosis of rabies. The only sure way to diagnose rabies is with laboratory tests.

PATHOGENESIS. Experimental evidence indicates that rabies virus travels centripetally from the site of the bite to the central nervous system via peripheral nerves and then centrifugally to the salivary glands and other tissues of the body. Fixed rabies virus injected into the footpads of rats propagates along nerve pathways (Dean et al. 1963b). Baer et al. (1965), also working with fixed rabies virus injected into rats, confirmed the neural transmission of rabies virus. In their studies, neurectomy of the sciatic and saphenous nerves before challenge proved virtually 100% effective in saving rats from rabies. The nerve fasciculus, which is composed of Schwann cells, endoneurium, and associated tissue spaces, appeared to be the area of the nerve involved in transmitting the virus; neither the axon nor myelin was incriminated as being integrally associated with pathogenesis.

It is possible to obtain virus from the blood of infected animals during the 2 hours following inoculation (Wong and Freund 1951). Large amounts of virus must be given to obtain a viremia in inoculated animals, and no virus can be detected in the blood during the incubation period (Schindler 1961).

Whether the virus multiplies in muscle or connective tissue at the site of exposure and whether invasion of the central nervous system is direct or secondary to the invasion of muscle tissue are still unknown (Johnson 1965). Virus apparently moves to the salivary glands by way of neural pathways after the central nervous system has become infected. Dean et al. (1963b) inhibited transmission of virus to the right salivary gland by removing either a part of the right lingual nerve or the right cranial cervical ganglion or its afferent nerve. The opposite salivary gland contained rabies virus. Salivary glands of several striped skunks and foxes have yielded titers of $10^{6.5}$. Undiluted saliva collected from striped skunks inoculated with pilocarpine had titers as high as $10^{6.0}$. Other tissues of rabid foxes, skunks, and raccoons have been found to contain rabies virus but in smaller quantities than those found in the brain and salivary glands. The adrenal glands and lungs are most frequently infected; occasionally, the kidneys, urinary bladder, ovaries, and testes have traces of virus (Parker and Sikes 1966; Parker and Wilsnack 1966; Sikes 1962; Sikes and Tierkel 1960).

PATHOLOGY. Rabies does not elicit gross pathologic alterations that are evident on postmortem examination. The histopathologic lesions of the central nervous system are inflammatory and are similar to those seen in other viral infections. Usually, there is more damage to the pons, medulla, brainstem, and thalamus than to other parts of the brain. This might be due to the fact that these parts usually contain more virus. Changes that can be seen include nuclear and cytoplasmic degeneration of the neurons, neuronophagia, and diffuse gliosis. Frequently there is evidence of petechial hemorrhage around the blood vessels and perivascular cuffing. Negri bodies, which are cytoplasmic inclusions, in neurons of infected animals are considered positive proof of rabies infection. Without these specific inclusions, a definite diagnosis of rabies cannot be made on the basis of histopathology alone, because lesions produced by other viral encephalitides are similar to those of rabies.

DIAGNOSIS. Every state has one or more laboratories responsible for performing laboratory tests on animals suspected of having rabies. Dogs and cats should be held at least 10 days for observation. An animal with clinical signs of rabies should be killed and its brain examined for Negri bodies. Wild animals that bite humans or domestic animals should be killed immediately and their heads submitted to the laboratory as expeditiously as possible. Attempts to capture and hold wild animals increase the probability that more exposures will occur.

When killing any animal whose head is to be submitted for rabies diagnosis, care must be taken to avoid damaging the brain; otherwise the laboratory cannot perform satisfactory examinations. After decapitation, the head should be cooled promptly, kept cold, and delivered to the laboratory as quickly as possible. The best preservation method is to seal the head in a tin or other suitable watertight metal container and to pack this receptacle with cracked ice in a larger watertight metal container. This cooling method makes it easier for the laboratory to perform direct microscopic (histologic) examination of the brain. Another method is to freeze the specimen in dry ice, but the distortion of brain tissue that occurs when it is thawed makes direct microscopic examination more difficult. Frozen specimens are, however, satisfactory for fluorescent rabies antibody (FRA) and mouse inoculation tests. A third method is to remove the brain carefully and ship it in 50% neutral glycerin. Although glycerinated brain specimens are satisfactory for direct microscopic and mouse inoculation tests, they are not always suitable for the FRA test.

Histologic sections of brain tissue or fresh tissue applied to a slide by the impression or smear technique can be examined microscopically for Negri bodies. Most diagnostic laboratories are not equipped to prepare histologic sections; however, fresh brain tissue impressions, properly applied and stained, are just as good for diagnostic purposes and are much simpler, less expensive, and quicker to prepare.

The three types of tests used for the laboratory diagnosis of rabies are described below.

Direct Microscopic (Histologic) Method. For direct microscopic examination, impressions or smears of the animal's hippocampus, cerebral cortex, and cerebellum are prepared and stained. The stain of choice is Sellers's (1927), which fixes and stains the tissue simultaneously. Visualization of Negri bodies in this test is necessary for rabies diagnosis. A Negri body is well differentiated by Sellers's stain as a magenta (purplish red) round or oval body with blue to black, basophilic, internal bodies. Negri bodies vary in shape, although they are usually round. The size also varies but is usually within the limits of $0.24-27$ μ. Negri bodies are located within the cytoplasm of the neuron. This procedure is not as sensitive or as specific as the FRA and the mouse inoculation method. It has been discontinued in most state and national rabies laboratories.

Fluorescent Rabies Antibody (Immunochemical) Method. The fluorescent antibody technique of Coons and Kaplan (1950) was adapted for rabies diagnosis by Goldwasser and Kissling (1958). The FRA test allows visualization of rabies antigen-antibody reaction by the direct method of staining. Fluorescein-tagged rabies antibody preparation (conjugate) reacts with rabies antigen in a specimen producing a fluorescene that can be seen under a microscope equipped with ultraviolet light.

Mouse Inoculation (Biological) Method. When slides are being prepared for the other tests, portions of the brain (hippocampus, cerebral cortex, and cerebellum) are suspended in a suitable diluent (0.5% bovine albumin, 5–10% rabbit or horse serum, 10% egg yolk) containing penicillin and streptomycin; after centrifugation the supernatant is injected intracerebrally in 3- to 4-week-old Swiss mice. If a virus is demonstrated by mouse deaths, it can be identified as rabies by the FRA, histologic, or virus neutralization test in mice.

IMMUNITY. Antirabies vaccines have been used in domestic animals, primarily before exposure, to prevent infection. In man, however, antirabies vaccines and antisera are used primarily to immunize a person after the exposure. The incubation period will usually be long enough to allow immunization before rabies virus can become established in the nervous system.

Some wild animals maintained in zoos, circuses, or occasionally as pets have been vaccinated against rabies; but it has not been practical in general to consider vaccinating wild animals. As a result only limited information is available about the efficacy of rabies vaccines in wildlife species. Because of the variable susceptibility of different species, the WHO Expert Committee on Rabies (WHO 1971) and the Compendium of Animal Rabies Vaccines in the United States (National Association of State Public Health Veterinarians) do not recommend using live antirabies vaccines without previously determining their safety and efficacy for the species in question. Inactivated antirabies vaccines are considered safe, but the dosage required and the duration of immunity elicited are largely unknown.

VACCINES. In the United States and most other countries of the world, both live and inactivated rabies vaccines are available for use in domesticated animals (Fig. 1.11). Until recently all the inactivated vaccines were prepared from the brains of sheep, goats, or rabbits that had been inoculated with a fixed rabies virus. Following Kissling and Reese's (1963) procedures for adapting fixed rabies virus to a nonnervous cell culture system in hamster kidneys, eight cell culture antirabies vaccines have been developed in the United States and Canada. One of the most immunogenic vaccines for use in animals is a new suckling-mouse brain type that also stimulates a 3-year duration of immunity.

In addition to the inactivated rabies vaccines of tissue culture and nervous tissue origin, live vaccines of tissue culture and chick embryo origin are also available. These are available to veterinarians; care should be used in selecting and administering a safe, effective vaccine for the various species of animals.

In a study reported by Schmidt and Sikes (1968), 50 adult foxes were vaccinated with a single injection of an inactivated, nervous tissue type vaccine; the immunity in half of them was challenged at 6 months and in the other half at 12 months. The immunity of all the foxes vaccinated intramuscularly survived the challenge at 6 and 12 months, but only 13 of 20 foxes vaccinated subcutaneously survived.

There is little doubt that skunks, raccoons, and other species of wildlife can be similarly immunized with inactivated rabies vaccines. Wild animals adopted as pets and carnivorous species in zoos and research work should be vaccinated intramuscularly with an inactivated rabies vaccine.

HUMAN ANTIRABIES TREATMENT. Three types of antirabies treatment are available for use in human beings exposed to rabid animals (WHO, 1973; PHS, 1976):

Local Wound Treatment. Immediate washing and flushing with soap and water, detergent, or water alone have proved most effective in experimental work to prevent rabies infection (Dean et al. 1963a).

Rabies Immune Globulin (Human Origin). This is considered the best specific treatment available for the postexposure prophylaxis of rabies in man. It is recommended in all severe exposures and in all instances of bites by unprovoked wild animals (fox, skunk, wolf, jackal, and bat). Combined globulin plus vaccine gives the best protection obtainable.

Vaccination. When a person needs antirabies treatment, the full dose of globulin plus the full regimen of vaccine doses is required. When the duck embryo vaccine is used, 23 injections are administered. With the newly developed, more antigenic tissue culture (human diploid type), only six doses are currently required.

Once clinical symptoms develop, there is no known treatment for preventing death from rabies.

Preexposure Prophylaxis. The relatively low frequency of systematic reactions to human rabies vaccines has made it more practical to offer preexposure immunization to persons

FIG. 1.11 Vaccines marketed in the United States, 1980. (Courtesy National Association of State Public Health Veterinarians Compendium Committee for 1980.)

Vaccine: Generic Name	Produced By	Marketed By (Product Name)	For Use In	Dosage*	Age at Primary** Vaccination	Booster Recommended
A) MODIFIED LIVE VIRUS						
Canine Cell Line Origin High Egg Passage, Flury Strain	NORDEN License No. 189	Norden (Endurall-R)	Dogs	1 ml	3 mos. & 1 yr. later	Triennially
			Cats	1 ml	3 months	Annually
Porcine Tissue Culture Origin High Cell Passage, SAD Strain	JENSEN-SALSBERY License No. 107	Jensen-Salsbery (ERA Strain Rabies Vaccine)	Dogs	1 ml	3 mos. & 1 yr. later	Triennially
			Cattle	1 ml	4 months	Annually
			Horses	1 ml	4 months	Annually
			Sheep	1 ml	4 months	Annually
			Goats	1 ml	4 months	Annually
Canine Tissue Culture Origin High Cell Passage, SAD Strain	PHILIPS ROXANE License No. 124	Bio-Ceutic (Neurogen-TC)	Dogs	1 ml	3 mos. & 1 yr. later	Triennially
Canine Tissue Culture Origin High Cell Passage, SAD Strain	PHILIPS ROXANE License No. 124	Bio-Ceutic (Unirab)	Dogs	1 ml	3 months	Annually
Canine Tissue Culture Origin High Cell Passage, SAD Strain	PHILIPS ROXANE License No. 124	Pitman-Moore (Rabvax)	Dogs	1 ml	3 mos. & 1 yr. later	Triennially
Bovine Kidney Tissue Culture Origin High Cell Passage, SAD Strain	PITMAN-MOORE License No. 264	Pitman-Moore (Rabies Vaccine)	Dogs	1 ml	3 months	Annually
Hamster Cell Line Origin High Cell Passage, Kissling Strain	BEECHAM License No. 225	Beecham (Rabtect)	Dogs	1 ml	3 months	Annually
B) INACTIVATED VACCINES						
Murine Origin	ROLYNN License No. 266	Ft. Dodge (Trimune)	Dogs	1 ml	3 mos. & 1 yr. later	Triennially
			Cats	1 ml	3 months	Annually
Murine Origin	ROLYNN License No. 266	Ft. Dodge (Annumune)	Dogs	1 ml	3 months	Annually
			Cats	1 ml	3 months	Annually
Murine Origin	DOUGLAS License No. 266	Douglas (SMBV)	Dogs	1 ml	3 months	Annually
			Cats	1 ml	3 months	Annually
***Murine Origin	DOUGLAS License No. 266	Douglas (Pan-Rab)	Cats	1 ml	3 months	Annually
Hamster Cell Line Origin High Cell Passage, Kissling Strain	BEECHAM License No. 225	Beecham (Rabcine)	Dogs	1 ml	3 months	Annually
			Cats	1 ml	3 months	Annually
Hamster Cell Line Origin High Cell Passage, Kissling Strain	BEECHAM License No. 225	Beecham (Rabcine-Feline)	Cats	1 ml	3 months	Annually
Hamster Cell Line Origin	VACCINES, INC. License No. 227	Bandy (Rabies Vacc)	Dogs	1 ml	3 months	Annually

*ALL VACCINE MUST BE ADMINISTERED INTRAMUSCULARLY AT ONE SITE IN THE THIGH.
**Three months is the earliest age recommended. Dogs vaccinated between 3-12 months should be revaccinated one year later.
***Combination vaccine.

in high-risk groups: veterinarians, animal handlers, certain laboratory workers, and personnel stationed in areas of the world where rabies is a constant threat. Others whose vocational or avocational pursuits result in frequent exposures to dogs, cats, foxes, skunks, or bats should also be considered for preexposure prophylaxis.

CONTROL. Rabies in domestic animals can be controlled by vaccinating owned animals and eliminating strays. The ultimate solution to the rabies problem in man and animals depends on the control and eventual elimination of the disease from wildlife reservoir and vector populations in nature. Practical success depends on carefully planned and executed programs, utilizing effective vaccines and control procedures for domestic animal species.

General control procedures that are practiced in the United States and that have been very successful in controlling dog rabies are described below.

Mass Immunization of Dogs and Cats. All owned dogs over 3 months of age should be vaccinated as quickly as possible. In the face of a serious outbreak, at least 70% of the entire dog population of the area should be revaccinated within a 3-week period. Cat owners are encouraged to have their pets immunized.

Elimination of Stray Dogs. Ownerless dogs will not be reached in mass vaccination campaigns and remain a threat in the transmission of rabies. Therefore, these strays should be removed to a local pound or animal shelter. If they are unclaimed at the end of a short period, they should be destroyed.

Rabies Education Programs. A continual and energetic publicity campaign can stimulate local interest in various aspects of a rabies control program.

Control of rabies in wildlife is most difficult; the only available control method is population reduction. There are many techniques of wildlife population reduction, and selection of the proper ones to use depends on local conditions. For maximum effectiveness professional biologists trained in predator control techniques should direct such activities. In the United States the Division of Wildlife Services, Bureau of Sport Fisheries and Wildlife, Department of the Interior, is responsible for population reduction programs to control wildlife rabies. Game and fish commissions are responsible for programs to control densities of wildlife populations in each state.

Poison. When it has been possible to devise bait stations, protected so that children and domestic animals cannot reach them, poisons have been used effectively for foxes and skunks. Strychnine-treated eggs were used in an attempt to control a fox rabies problem in Tennessee (Lewis 1965) and a skunk rabies epizootic in Ohio (Schnurrenberger et al. 1964). Thallium sulfate has been used to control mongoose populations.

Gases. Den gassing is recommended in certain seasons when family groups of vector animals are together. Gases such as cyanide, tear gas, and smoke bombs are available for use by such trained personnel as biologists of state or federal conservation departments. This method is recommended as an adjunct to other methods used to reduce wildlife populations.

Trapping. Although trapping is more expensive than using poisoned baits and not as efficient, it is still the method of choice in most areas because it is safer than poisoning. Usually a urine-scent bait is used to attract foxes, skunks, or other species to the trap; but "cracklings" and other food baits have also been used.

Other Methods. Night hunting by organized groups of citizens or biologists proved to be one of the most selective methods of reducing fox populations in a rabies outbreak in Tennessee (Lewis 1965). Bounty programs—that is, paying for each dead animal of a selected species—are of little value and are not recommended as the best method of accomplishing population reduction programs. Studies on hormonal inhibitors to interrupt the reproduction cycle of wild carnivores as a possible method of controlling population densities have indicated that method as being inadvisable. Automatic vaccinating devices to vaccinate selected wildlife species have also been ruled out as a means of controlling wildlife rabies. However, oral vaccination of wild animals seems to be effective for certain species (Baer et al. 1971). It has been used in a limited manner in Switzerland and might be adopted in a number of countries if the safety of using a modified live virus proves satisfactory.

REFERENCES

Baer, G. M., Abelseth, M. K., and Debbie, J. G. Oral vaccination of foxes against rabbies. *Am. J. Epidemiol.* 93:6, 1971.

Baer, G. M., and Adams, D. B. Rabies in insectivorous bats in the United States, 1953–1965. *Public Health Rep.* 85:7, 637, 1970.

Baer, G. M., and Bales, G. L. Experimental rabies infection in the Mexican free-tail bat. *J. Infect. Dis.* 117:82, 1967.

Baer, G. M., Shanthaveerappa, T. R., and Bourne, G. H. Studies on the pathogenesis of fixed rabies virus in rats. *Bull. WHO* 33:783, 1965.

Beamer, P. D., Mohr, C. O., and Barr, T. R. B. Resistance of the opossum to rabies virus. *Am. J. Vet. Res.* 21:507, 1960.

Bell, J. F., Burdorfer, W., and Moore, G. J. The behavior of rabies virus in ticks. *J. Infect. Dis.* 100:278, 1957.

Carini, A. Sur une grande epizootie de rage. *Ann. Inst. Pasteur* 25:843, 1911.

Carski, T. R., Wilsnack, R. E., and Sikes, R. K. Pathogenesis of rabies in wildlife: II. Fluorescent antibody studies. *Am. J. Vet. Res.* 23:1048, 1962.

Constantine, D. G. Rabies transmission by nonbite routine. *Public Health Rep.* 77:287, 1962.

———. Recent advances in our knowledge of bat rabies. Intern. Symp. Rabies, Talloires, 1965. *Symp. Ser. Immunobiol. Stand.* 1:251, 1966.

Coons, A. H., and Kaplan, M. H. Localization antigen in tissue cells: II. Improvements in a method for the detection of antigens by means of fluorescent antibody. *J. Exp. Med.* 91:1, 1950.

Cox, H. R., Van de Scheer, J., Aiston, S., and Bohnel, E. The purification and concentration of influenza virus by means of alcohol precipitation. *J. Immunol.* 56:149, 1947.

Dean, D. J., Baer, G. M., and Thompson, W. R. Studies on the local treatment of rabies-infected wounds. *Bull. WHO* 28:477, 1963a.

Dean, D. J., Evans, E. M., and McClure, R. C. Pathogenesis of rabies. *Bull. WHO* 29:803, 1963b.

Ferenbaugh, T. L. A note concerning the occurrence of hydrophobia in the foxes of Alaska. *Mil. Surg.* 38:656, 1916.

Fermi, C. Ueber die Immunizierung gegen Wutkrankheit. *Z. Hyg. Infektionskrankh.* 58:232, 1908.

Galtier, V. Etudes sur la rage. *C. R. Acad. Sci.* 89:444, 1879.

Geiger, J. C. Is rabies under control in California? *Calif. State J. Med.* 14:58, 1916.

Goldwasser, R. A., and Kissling, R. E. Fluorescent antibody staining of street and fixed rabies virus antigens. *Proc. Soc. Exp. Biol. Med.* 98:219, 1958.

Haupt, H., and Rehaag, H. Durch Fkedermanuese verbreitete seuchenhafte Tollwut unter Viehbestaenden in Santa Catharina (Sued-Brasilien). *Z. Infektionskrankh. Parasitol. Krankh. Hyg. Haustiere* 22:104, 1921.

Hurst, E. W., and Pawan, J. L. An outbreak of rabies in Trinidad without history of bites and with symptoms of acute ascending myelitis. *Lancet* 221:622, 1931.

———. A further account of the Trinidad outbreak of acute rabies myelitis: histology of the experimental disease. *J. Pathol. Bacteriol.* 35:301, 1932.

Johnson, H. N. Rabies. In Frank L. Horsfall, Jr., and I. Tamm, eds., *Viral and rickettsial infections of man*, 4th ed. Philadelphia/Montreal: Lippincott, 1965.

Kissling, R. E., and Reese, D. R. Anti-rabies vaccine of tissue culture origin. *J. Immunol.* 91:362, 1963.

Lewis, J. C. The fox rabies control program in Tennessee, 1965–66. Paper presented at North Am. Wildlife Conf., Pittsburgh, March 15, 1965.

Mallory, L. B. Campaign against rabies in Modoc and Lassen counties, California. *Calif. State Bd. Health Bull.* 11:273, 1916.

Matsumoto, S. Electron microscopy of nerve cells infected with street rabies virus. *Virology* 17:198, 1962.

Miyamoto, K., and Matsumoto, S. The nature of the Negri body. *J. Cell.* 27:677, 1965.

Murphy, F. A. Morphology and morphogenesis of rabies virus. In G. M. Baer, *Natural history of rabies*, p. 33. New York: Academic Press, 1975.

Negri, A. Beitrag zum Studium der Aetiologie der Tollwuth. *Z. Hyg. Infektionskrankh.* 43:507, 1903.

Nelson, E. W. *Wild animals of North America*. National Geographic Society, Washington, D.C.: Judd & Detweiler, 1918.

Parker, R. L. Rabies in skunks in the north-central states. *Proc. U.S. Livestock Sanit. Assoc.*, Oct. 1961.

Parker, R. L., and Sikes, R. K. Development of rabies-inhibiting substance in skunks infected with rabies virus. *Public Health Rep.* 81:941, 1966.

Parker, R. L., and Wilsnack, R. E. Pathogenesis of skunk rabies virus: Quantitation in skunks and foxes. *Am. J. Vet. Res.* 27:33, 1966.

Pasteur, L. Methode pour prevenir la rage apres morsure. *C. R. Acad. Sci.* 101:765, 1885.

Pasteur, L., Chamberland, C., and Roux, E. Nouvelle communication sur la rage. *C. R. Acad. Sci.* 98:457, 1884.

Pawan, J. L. Rabies in the vampire bat of Trinidad, with special reference to the clinical course and the latency of infection. *Ann. Trop. Med. Parasitol.* 30:401, 1936a.

———. The transmission of paralytic rabies in Trinidad by the vampire bat. *Ann. Trop. Med. Parasitol.* 30:101, 1936b.

———. An unusual strain of rabies virus in a vampire bat. *Ann. Trop. Med. Parasitol.* 32:35, 1938.

Peck, F. B., Jr., and Kohlstaedt, K. C. Pre-exposure rabies prophylaxis problems and procedures. *Indust. Med. Surg.* 33:17, 1964.

Peck, F. B., Jr., Powell, H. M., and Culbertson, C. G. Duck-embryo rabies vaccine-study of fixed virus vaccine grown in embryonated duck eggs and killed with betapropiolactone (BPL). *J. Am. Med. Assoc.* 162:1373, 1956.

Public Health Service, Advisory Committee on Immunization Practices. Rabies prophylaxis. Morbidity and mortality weekly rep., vol. 25, no. 51, week ending Dec. 31, 1976.

Richards, S. H. *A guide for the recognition and control of rabies.* Bismarck: North Dakota Game and Fish Departments, 1963.

Schindler, R. Studies on the pathogenesis of rabies. *Bull. WHO* 25:119, 1961.

Schmidt, R. C., and Sikes, R. K. Immunization of foxes with inactivated-virus rabies vaccine. *Am. J. Vet. Res.* 29:1843, 1968.

Schnurrenberger, P. R., Beck, J. R., and Peden, D. Skunk rabies in Ohio. *Public Health Rep.* 79:161, 1964.

Sellers, T. F. A new method for staining Negri bodies of rabies. *Am. J. Public Health* 17:1080, 1927.

Semple, D. On the nature of rabies and anti-rabic treatment. *Br. Med. J.* 2:333, 1919.

Seton, E. T. *Lives of game animals.* Garden City: Doubleday, vols. 1 and 2, 1925.

Sikes, R. K. Pathogenesis of rabies in wildlife: I. Comparative effect of varying doses of rabies virus inoculated into foxes and skunks. *Am. J. Vet. Res.* 23:1041, 1962.

Sikes, R. K., and Larghi, O. P. Purified rabies vaccine: Development and comparison of potency and safety with two human rabies vaccines. *J. Immunol.* 99:545, 1967.

Sikes, R. K., and Tierkel, E. S. Wildlife rabies studies in the southeast. *65th Ann. Proc. U.S. Livestock Sanit. Assoc.,* Oct. 1960.

Sokol, E. Chemical composition and structure of rabies virus. In G. M. Baer, *Natural history of rabies.* New York: Academic Press, 1975.

Stamm, D. D., Kissling, R. E., and Edison, M. E. Experimental rabies infection in insectivorous bats. *J. Infect. Dis.* 98:10, 1956.

Thacker, J. Observations on hydrophobia. Plymouth, Mass.: Joseph Arey, 1812.

Thomas, J. R., Sikes, R. K., and Ricker, A. S. Evaluation of indirect fluorescent antibody technique for detection of rabies antibody in human sera. *J. Immunol.* 91:721, 1963.

Venters, H. D., Hoffert, W. R., Scatterday, J. E., and Hardy, A. V. Rabies in bats in Florida. *Am. J. Public Health* 44:182, 1954.

Wilkinson, D. L. Rabies and hydrophobia in Alabama. *Alabama Med. Surg. Age* 6:557, 1894.

Wilner, Burton I. A classification of the major groups of human and other animal viruses, 3rd ed. Minneapolis: Burgess, 1965.

Wilsnack, R. E., and Parker, R. L. Pathogenesis of skunk rabies virus. Rabies inhibiting substance as related to rabies diagnosis. *Am. J. Vet. Res.* 27:39, 1966.

Wong, D. H., and Freund, J. Fixed rabies virus in blood following intracerebral inoculation in mice and rabbits. *Proc. Soc. Exp. Biol. Med.* 76:717, 1951.

Wood, J. E., and Davis, D. E. The prevalence of rabies in populations of foxes in the southern states. *J. Am. Vet. Med. Assoc.* 135:121, 1959.

World Health Organization. WHO expert committee on rabies, 5th report. WHO tech. rep. 523, 1973.

———. World Survey of Rabies 9. Geneva, Switzerland: Veterinary Public Health Unit, 1973, 1978.

Zinke, G. G. Neue Ansitchten der Hundswuth, ihrer Ursachen und Folgen, nebst einer sichern Behandlungsart der von tollen Tieren gebissenen Menchen, fuer Aerzte und Nichtaerzte bestimmt. *C. E. Gabler, Jehna* 16:212, 1804.

2 Rinderpest

GORDON R. SCOTT

Synonyms: **Cattle plague, pestis bovina.**

Rinderpest is a viral contagion of the cloven-hoofed artiodactyls characterized by fever, erosive stomatitis, and gastroenteritis.

HISTORY. Rinderpest is an ancient scourge of the livestock of Asia and Europe. In the past, the primary disseminators were military trek oxen. The boom in trade, particularly trade in livestock, that followed the transport revolution of the nineteenth century added significantly to the means of dissemination; for example, the source of a serious outbreak in the Paris Jardin d'Acclimatation in 1865 was traced to two gazelles from the London zoo (Sainte-Hillaire 1865). More recently, an epizootic in the Rome zoo followed the importation of antelope from Somalia (Cilli et al. 1951).

Two important epidemiological events have occurred since 1969. First, rinderpest did not recur in the herds of wildlife that range over the Loita-Mara-Serengeti plains of East Africa (Sinclair 1977). Second, despite modern veterinary infrastructures and the availability of cheap efficient vaccine, a rinderpest panzootic rolled uncontrolled across the Near East from Afghanistan to Turkey (Anon. 1969).

Epizootics in Free Wildlife. Rinderpest commonly attacks domestic cattle (*Bos*) and domestic buffalo (*Bubalus*). On occasion, wildlife suffers. The infamous panzootic that swept through Africa at the end of the nineteenth century killed millions of cattle and countless wild animals. In East Africa the cattle died first, then wild buffalo (*Syncerus*), eland (*Taurotragus*), and warthog (*Phacochoerus*). Later, giraffe (*Giraffa*), kudu (*Strepsiceros*), roan antelope (*Hippotragus*), and bushbuck (*Tragelaphus*) succumbed. Wildebeest (*Connochaetes*) contracted the disease last (Percival 1918). The plains were littered with so many carcasses that the vultures and other scavengers were unable to dispose of the carrion (Simon 1962).

In South Africa the Cape buffalo were hardest hit. Many herds of eland were wiped out. The warthogs and bush pig (*Potamochoerus*) died in large numbers (Stevenson-Hamilton 1911). Many other species were affected: Blesbok (*Damaliscus*), bontebok (*Damaliscus*), bushbuck, duiker (*Cephalophus*), gemsbok (*Oryx*), kudu, reedbuck (*Redunca*), springbok (*Antidorcas*), steinbok (*Raphicerus*), and waterbuck (*Kobus*). Hartebeest (*Alcelaphus*), impala (*Aepyceros*), and wildebeest escaped (Theiler 1897).

Lugard (1892) witnessed the havoc in East Africa and thought that all the buffalo and giraffe had been exterminated, but they and most of the other afflicted species recovered their numbers rapidly (Percival 1918). Nevertheless, many of the current anomalies in the distribution of wildlife in Africa can be attributed to the rinderpest panzootic (Spinage 1962). An unexpected and perhaps tragic sequel was the disappearance of tsetse flies from much of Africa south of the Zambesi River (Stevenson-Hamilton 1957). This phenomenon was often cited to justify wide-scale indiscriminate destruction of wildlife in the name of tsetse-fly control (Glasgow 1963).

The panzootic was so virulent in southern Africa that it burned itself out and no focus of infection remained. In East and West Africa, however, rinderpest lingered on and became enzootic. At intervals, fresh waves of the disease engulfed the wildlife of East Africa and threatened the livestock of central Africa and South Africa (Lobry 1964). An epizootic in 1897 destroyed large numbers of hartebeest and kudu (Simon 1962). A new wave in 1913, fanned later by military campaigns, raged until 1921; in Kenya many eland and giraffe and then buffalo, bushbuck, and reedbuck died (Stordy 1914, 1918). In Uganda buffalo carcasses littered the west bank of the Nile (Hutchins 1918). The disease spread south onto the Kafu Plains—killing bushbuck, duiker, kob (*Adenota*), reedbuck, and warthog (Duke 1919)—and invaded the Parc National Albert in Zaire in 1921 where it devastated the buffalo herds (Bourliere and Verschuren 1960). In the Rukwa Valley of southern Tanzania, the disease destroyed eland, bush pig, and warthog (Gray 1919). Simultaneously, an epizootic swept West Africa killing buffalo, hartebeest, kudu, roan antelope, topi (*Damaliscus*), waterbuck, and warthog; giraffe, gazelle (species not named), oribi (*Ourebia*), and duiker were unaffected (Pecaud 1924).

The next major epizootic followed a similar course, beginning in Uganda in 1929. The first to succumb were buffalo, bushbuck, and warthog. Later, eland and waterbuck were attacked (Allan 1934). For months buffalo lay dying on the shores of Lake George and Lake Edward (Poulton 1933), and kob in the same area were virtually exterminated (Pitman 1942). Again the disease invaded the Parc National Albert, killing topi, forest hog (*Hylochoerus*), and warthog (Jussiant 1933). The wave hit buffalo, giraffe, and wildebeest in Tanzania in 1931 (Hornby 1932). The disease also entered Tanzania from Kenya in Masai cattle (Branagan and Hammond 1965); and from then, if not earlier, a focus of infection smoldered in the wildlife on the Serengeti and Wambiti plains until 1963 (Reid 1950; Atang and Plowright 1969).

A wave in 1937–1941 extended south onto the Mbeya escarpment of Tanzania, where it killed buffalo, eland, and giraffe (Alexander and de Kock 1940). Later the disease entered the Rukwa and Kilambero valleys, destroying buffalo, eland, and kudu (Lowe 1942; Thomas and Reid 1944).

Another wave invaded Uganda from the Sudan in 1942 and again spread slowly southward in buffalo to the shores of Lake George and Lake Edward (Simmons 1943) and from there into Zaire in 1945 where it killed buffalo, bushbuck, bush pig, and forest hog (Guyaux 1951). Further minor epizootics were initiated in Zaire in 1956 and 1960 by infected buffalo and giraffe moving south from the Sudan (Dormal et al. 1961; Els et al. 1957).

In 1949 rinderpest broke out in cattle on the border between Kenya and Tanzania. It spread to wildlife, and infected eland disseminated the disease southward into southern Masailand and Mbulu, where wildebeest suffered severely (Reid 1949).

An epizootic in 1960 swept through the Karamoja district of Uganda and the northern frontier district of Kenya (Sanders 1961; Stewart 1964). Fortunately, it did not penetrate further south. The disease was very virulent, and the local game warden estimated that 60% of the eland, kudu, and warthog; 50% of the buffalo, bushbuck, and giraffe; 40% of the impala; and a considerable number of oryx (*Oryx*) died (Grimwood 1961). Bongo (*Taurotragus*) and bush pig were also affected (Stewart 1964).

Slaughter cattle being trekked south from

Chad in 1968 were believed to be the source of a mild epizootic in wildlife in the Central African Republic (Scott 1968). Clinical disease and death were observed in buffalo, eland, and warthog, but the overall mortality was only 5–10% (Thal 1972). Antibodies were detected in sera from 13 species, 6 being proven host records. A feature of the epizootic was the concurrent presence of bovine virus diarrhea in the buffalo.

Free-living wildlife has also suffered on other continents. Dieckerhoff (1890) blamed rinderpest for the decline of the European bison (*Bison*). Deer (*Cervus*) perished in the epizootic that ravaged Britain in 1865 (Bristowe 1866). Deer (species not named) also died in Brazil in the only outbreak of rinderpest on the American continents (Roberts 1921). In India the disease was observed in deer, wild buffalo, and wild boars (Hallen et al. 1871).

Investigations in India have confirmed the presence of rinderpest in free-living wild bison (species not named) through the isolation of virus (Ramani 1972) and in free-living blue bulls (*Boselaphus*) through the detection of specific antigen (Mathur et al. 1975). In Ceylon wild pigs died after eating the carcasses of infected cattle (Mahamooth 1943). In Southeast Asia rinderpest has been reported in wild pigs, banteng (*Bibos*), buffalo, and gaur (*Bibos*), as well as in smaller ruminants like antelope and deer (Vittoz 1954). The origin of an epizootic in the middle sixties in Laos was attributed to wildlife (Singharaj 1968).

Epizootics in Captive Animals. Rinderpest in captive wildlife is relatively rare. White (1871) reported mortality in deer kept at the Debrooghur jail in India. Sitin (1930) isolated rinderpest virus from a captive wild pig in Russia. Carmichael (1938a) recorded an outbreak in a small zoo in Uganda in which a bushbuck, an oribi, a reedbuck, and two sitatunga (*Strepsiceros*) died. Hilsont and Bourdereau (1954) studied a slow epizootic in captive warthogs at Bamako in West Africa.

Boldrini (1954) related the history of two African buffalo exported to Italy after quarantine in Kenya. One died at sea, and the other was diagnosed as having rinderpest when the ships docked at Trieste. Cattle carried on the same ships from Mogadishu to Suez were considered the source of the infection.

On occasion, animals kept at laboratories engaged in rinderpest research have contracted the disease accidently. Thus a black buck (*Antilope*) died in India (Lingard 1906), and a duiker (*Sylvicapra*) died in Zaire (Caccavella 1936).

Catastrophic episodes have affected four major zoos. In 1865 the livestock in the Paris Jardin d'Acclimatation was devastated. Antelope (*Gazella, Antidorcas*), chevrotain (*Tragulus*), and peccary (*Tayassu*) were wiped out; most of the deer and yak (*Bos*) died; one of the two auroch (*Bos*) died; and losses occurred in the herds of exotic cattle and goats. Sheep and camels were not affected (Sainte-Hillaire 1865). Outbreaks occurred at the Calcutta zoo in 1943 and 1969. Details of the losses in the first outbreak are not available, but in the second outbreak three nilgai (*Boselaphus*), one gayal (*Bibos*), and ten hog deer (*Axis*) died (Ray and Samanta 1974). The infection was contained by instituting quarantine measures and by vaccinating all animals at risk. In the Lucknow zoo in 1948, mortality was very high; all the four-horned antelope (*Tetracerus*), black buck, and a large herd of sambhar (*Cervus*) were wiped out; and most of the barking deer (*Muntiacus*), hog deer, spotted deer (*Axis*), and nilgai died (Gupta and Verma 1949). Similarly serious was the 1950 epizootic in the Rome zoo (Cilli et al. 1951).

DISTRIBUTION AND HOST RANGE. The development of efficient rinderpest vaccines in the thirties led to a dramatic fall in the global incidence of the disease. Success bred complacency, and the panzootic that ravaged the Near East in 1969 surprised everyone. Today, rinderpest remains enzootic in domestic cattle and domestic buffalo in northern equatorial Africa and the subcontinent of India, Pakistan, Bangladesh, and Nepal. Periodically, small epizootics flare up in Near East countries importing live animals from Africa.

The focus once considered permanent in the wildlife on the plains of East Africa has disappeared (Sinclair 1977). This significant achievement has been attributed to intensified campaigns for vaccinating cattle in and around the area.

Reports of natural rinderpest incriminate many species, but few are supported by acceptable proofs (Table 2.1). Some are unbelievable (Table 2.2). Probably most artiodactyls are susceptible. In addition, rinderpest virus has a wide experimental host range that includes species other than artiodactyls (Scott 1964).

Veterinary authorities in the rinderpest-free continents have explored tentatively the susceptibility of some of their fauna. Robertson (1924), for example, injected two Australian opossums (*Trichosurus*) and two kangaroos (*Macropus*); one opossum died 4 days later, but the other animals remained healthy. The cause of death was not ascertained. Workers at Plum Island have shown that American peccaries and white-tailed deer (*Odocoileus*) are highly susceptible to virulent bovine strains of rinderpest (Dardiri et al. 1969; Hamdy et al. 1957b). They

TABLE 2.1   Natural Host Range of Rinderpest.

Scientific Name[a]	Common Name	First Allegation	First Proof
Antilopidae			
Aepyceros	impala	Stevenson-Hamilton 1911	Scott et al. 1960[b]
Antidorcas	springbuck	Sainte-Hillaire 1865	
Antilope	black buck	Lingard 1906	Lingard 1906[c]
Gazella	gazelle	Sainte-Hillaire 1865	Plowright 1963a[d]
Litocranius	gerenuk	Cilli et al. 1951	
Nesotragus	suni	Yedloutschnig and Stone 1974	Yedloutschnig and Stone 1974[d]
Oreotragus	klipspringer	Curasson 1932	
Ourebia	oribi	Poulton 1927	Carmichael 1938a[c]
Raphicerus	steinbok	Theiler 1897	
Bovidae			
Addax	addax	Curasson 1932	
Alcelaphus	hartebeest	Pecaud 1924	Thal 1972[d]
Bison	European bison	Dieckerhoff 1890	
Bos	banteng	Pease 1894	
	gaur	Pease 1894	
	kouprey	Vittoz 1954	
	domestic ox	Dodson 1754	Flemynge 1755[c]
	yak	Sainte-Hillaire 1865	

TABLE 2.1 *(Continued)*

Scientific Name[a]	Common Name	First Allegation	First Proof
Boselaphus	nilgai	Gupta and Verma 1949	Mathur et al. 1975[b]
Bubalus	domestic buffalo	Hallen et al. 1871	Holmes 1911[c]
Syncerus	African buffalo	Lugard 1892	Thomas and Reid 1944[c]
Taurotragus	eland	Lugard 1892	Carmichael 1933[c]
	bongo	Percival 1819	
Tetracerus	four-horned antelope	Gupta and Verma 1949	
Tragelaphus	kudu	Theiler 1897	Thomas and Reid 1944[c]
	sitatunga	Poulton 1927	Carmichael 1938a[c]
	bushbuck	Lugard 1892	Cilli et al. 1951[c]
Camelidae			
Camelus	camel	Pease 1894	Singh and Ata 1967[d]
Capridae			
Ammotragus	arui	Curasson 1932	
Capra	goat	de Sauvages 1746	D'Costa and Singh 1933[d]
Naemorhedus	goral	Pease 1894	
Ovis	sheep	de Sauvages 1746	Roll 1860[c]
Cephalophidae			
Cephalophus	duiker	Theiler 1897	
Sylvicapra	duiker	Caccavella 1936	Thal 1972[d]
Cervidae			
Axis	hog deer	Gupta and Verma 1949	
	spotted deer	Gupta and Verma 1949	
Cervus	red deer	Bristowe 1866	
	sambhar	Gupta and Verma 1949	Gupta and Verma 1949[c]
Muntiacus	barking deer	Sainte-Hillaire 1865	
Capreolus	roe deer	Broudin 1923	
Mazama	brocket	Sainte-Hillaire 1865	
Giraffidae			
Giraffa	giraffe	Lugard 1892	Plowright 1963b[c]
Hippopotamidae			
Hippopotamus	hippopotamus	Plowright et al. 1964	Plowright et al. 1964[d]
Hippotragidae			
Connochaetes	wildebeest	Theiler 1896	Cornell 1934[c]
Damaliscus	topi	Pecaud 1924	Thal 1972[d]
	bontebok	Theiler 1897	
	blesbok	Theiler 1897	
Hippotragus	roan antelope	Stevenson-Hamilton 1911	Thal 1972[d]
	sable antelope	Stevenson-Hamilton 1911	
Kobus	kob	Lugard 1893	Thal 1972[d]
	puku	Sharpe 1893	
	waterbuck	Theiler 1897	Thal 1972[d]
Oryx	oryx	Grimwood 1961	
	gemsbok	Theiler 1897	
Pelea	rhebok	Surmon 1902	
Redunca	reedbuck	Lugard 1893	Carmichael 1938a[c]
Suidae			
Hylochoerus	forest hog	Christy 1924	Thal 1972[d]
Phacochoerus	warthog	Lugard 1892	Hilsont and Bourdereau 1954[c]
Potamochoerus	bush pig	Stevenson-Hamilton 1912	Thal 1972[d]
Sus	domestic pig	Carre and Fraimbault 1898	De Does 1932[c]
Tayassuidae			
Tayassu	peccary	Sainte-Hillaire 1865	
Tragulidae			
Tragulus	chevrotain	Sainte-Hillaire 1865	

[a] According to Crandall 1974.
[b] Antigen detection.
[c] Virus isolation.
[d] Antibody demonstration.

TABLE 2.2 Alleged Rinderpest in Nonartiodactyls.

Common Name	Order	Genus	Reference
Dog	CARNIVORA	*Canis*	Campbell 1869
Elephant	PROBOSCIDAE	*Elephas*	D'Costa 1936
Guinea fowl	GALLIFORMES	*Numida*	Theiler 1897
Hyena	CARNIVORA	*Crocuta*	Scott 1964
Jackal	CARNIVORA	*Canis*	Farrell 1870
Ostrich	STRUTHIONIFORMES	*Struthio*	Pecaud 1924
Tiger	CARNIVORA	*Tigris*	Oxley 1840
Vulture	FALCONIFORMES	*Gyps*	Selous 1899
Zebra	HIPPOMORPHA	*Equus*	Crawshay 1893

also tested the susceptibility of one-toed pigs (species not named) and nine-banded armadillos (*Dasypus*) (Wilder et al. 1974a,b).

ETIOLOGY. The RNA viruses of rinderpest, canine distemper, and human measles are linked antigenically (Breese and de Boer 1973) and are therefore classified together in the morbillivirus group of the family Paramyxoviridae (Fenner 1976). A newly recognized member of the group is the virus of peste des petits ruminants, which induces a rinderpestlike syndrome in goats and sheep (Hamdy et al. 1975a). The morbilliviruses have similar morphologies, densities, and polypeptides (Underwood and Brown 1974). They differ in their specific natural host ranges (Imagawa 1968). Although the only member of the group that hemagglutinates is measles, the reaction is inhibited not only by human measles convalescent serum but by bovine rinderpest convalescent serum, by caprine peste des petits ruminants convalescent serum, and, sometimes, by canine distemper convalescent serum (Ramachandran 1970).

Rinderpest virus is fragile and sensitive to the effects of putrefaction (Curasson 1932). Consequently, in the tropics infected carcasses are rendered harmless within a few hours.

Strains of rinderpest virus differ markedly in invasiveness, virulence, and host preference, but fortunately, there is only one immunologic type. Rinderpest vaccines, irrespective of their origin, protect against all known strains of the virus (Scott 1964).

TRANSMISSION. Transmission requires close contact between sick and healthy animals (Hornby 1926). The virus is spread in relatively large airborne droplets; hence, windborne dispersion over long distances occurs very rarely (Hyslop 1972). The longevity of airborne rinderpest virus is greatest at low relative humidities (Hyslop 1972). Pigs may become infected

also through eating infected carcasses (Molinie 1931). Claims that bloodsucking insects, leeches, vultures, and other carrion feeders spread rinderpest were investigated by Minett (1954) who concluded that their role as vectors was minimal.

The dissemination of epizootic rinderpest in African wildlife is largely blamed on buffalo; often the route of dissemination is a clearly defined tract blazed by dead buffalo. En route the buffalo infect warthog and bushbuck, which spread the disease locally in other directions (Allan 1934).

SIGNS. Incubation periods in cattle and domestic buffalo range from 3 to 15 days, being longest in animals possessing a high innate resistance. Incubation periods in domestic pigs appear to be shorter (Scott et al. 1962). Incubation periods in experimentally infected wildlife are similar to those expected in domestic animals; 2 days in deer injected with virulent bovine virus (Jacotot 1927; Hamdy et al. 1975b); 3–4 days in peccaries injected with virulent virus (Dardiri et al. 1969); and 7 days in reedbuck and bush pig injected with an attenuated strain of virus that induced incubation periods in cattle of 4–6 days (Daubney 1942).

The clinical response of different species varies widely, even in virgin epizootics, and ranges from inapparent infections to peracute reactions that terminate fatally (Table 2.3). A few species like Uganda kob and waterbuck sometimes failed to react, but at other times they reacted acutely and died (Carmichael 1938a). Similarly, hartebeest in East Africa and South Africa rarely sickened (Duke 1919; Theiler 1897), but in West Africa they were severely affected (Pecaud 1924).

The onset of peracute and acute reactions is a sudden high fever that persists for several days. In bush pig the fever may be diphasic (Wilde 1948). Bushbuck and duiker have been

TABLE 2.3 Clinical Response of Wildlife Species to Rinderpest.

Subacute	Acute	Peracute
Gazelle	banteng	buffalo
Hartebeest	black buck	eland
Hippopotamus	bongo	kudu
Impala	bushbuck	warthog
Kob	bush pig	
Oribi	chevrotain	
Oryx	deer	
Reedbuck	dik-dik	
Roan antelope	duiker	
Sable antelope	forest hog	
Topi	gaur	
Waterbuck	giraffe	
	nilgai	
	peccary	
	sambhar	
	sitatunga	
	wildebeest	

known to die without developing fevers (Caccavella 1936). Most affected animals appear normal at first despite the high fever, but within a day or two they are sick, depressed, and restless and many die within the next 48 hours (Carmichael 1938a). Many buffalo become dangerously aggressive and stampede in search of water to allay thirst (Branagan 1966). Other buffalo stand immobile, backs arched, in the same spot for days, dying where they stand (Thal 1972). Sick eland leave the herd and travel long distances (McCall 1923). Sick kudu also segregate (Thomas and Reid 1944).

Nasal and lacrimal discharges become profuse and later mucopurulent. At first, respiration is shallow and rapid, becoming in the terminal stages labored and painful. Blindness from bilateral corneal opacities has been observed in eland (Thomas and Reid 1944) and giraffe (Grimwood 1961).

Three to 4 days after the onset of fever, shallow erosions develop and coalesce in the mucosae of the vagina and mouth, particularly inside the lower lips, in the adjacent gum, and in the soft palate. Salivation is excessive and the breath is fetid. In addition, excoriation of the skin has been observed in buffalo (Thomas and Reid 1944). Sitatunga, on the other hand, have died without developing mucosal lesions (Carmichael 1938b).

Purging begins within 2–3 days of the appearance of the mucosal erosions, and its onset coincides with the regression of the fever. The fluid feces are fetid and often bloodstained. The resulting dehydration causes rapid emaciation. Nevertheless, in wildebeest vigor and power of flight are maintained until the terminal collapse (Cornell 1934).

Most peracute and many acute reactions are fatal, death following prostration and occurring 1–2 weeks after the illness is evident. Warthogs often die quickly while still in good bodily condition (Thal 1972). Convalescence in surviving animals is prolonged, the return to full health taking weeks. Pregnant animals abort in 3–4 weeks.

The signs in subacute reactions vary; minor transient illnesses have been observed in deer (Jacotot 1927), and the absence of purging has been noted in sick impala (Brown and Scott 1960). Most animals undergoing subacute reactions survive, and their convalescence is short.

Inapparent infections have been reported; gazelles are seldom observed sick, yet they sero-convert (Plowright 1963a). Similarly, rinderpest has never been recognized in the hippopotamus, although specific antibodies have been detected in the sera of aged animals culled in Uganda (Plowright et al. 1964).

Rinderpest virus selectively destroys lymphocytes suppressing both the humoral antibody response and cell-mediated immunity (Yamanouchi et al. 1974). The sequel is a high incidence of activated latent infections that complicate the clinical picture, many pathogens, particularly protozoa, being implicated (Curasson 1932).

PATHOGENESIS. Although the pathogenesis of rinderpest infections in wildlife has not been studied, the clinical signs and the postmortem findings mimic those in cattle, and it is reasonable to assume that the pathogenesis is also similar. Moreover, the most thorough studies in cattle were carried out with a strain of virus isolated from a reticulated giraffe (Liess and Plowright 1964; Plowright 1964; Taylor et al. 1965).

The virus enters the body through the mucosa of the upper respiratory tract (Taylor et al. 1965) and disappears for several hours (Todd and White 1914). Primary multiplication occurs in the pharyngeal and submaxillary lymph nodes and in the tonsils (Taylor et al. 1965), where high titers are attained before viremia is apparent (Scott 1955). The onset of viremia and the resulting generalization precede the onset of fever (Plowright 1964). The virus is disseminated by mononuclear leukocytes (Plowright 1968) to which it is so firmly attached that it is seldom found free in plasma (Todd and White

1914). Multiplication of the virus in epithelial cells follows. The virus is excreted first from the lungs and later in the fluid feces (Plowright 1964). High titers of virus persist during the fever and thereafter decline. The development of a persistent carrier state, if it ever occurs, is rare (Jacotot 1931).

PATHOGENICITY. Strains of rinderpest vary widely in their pathogenicity for different species. Lingard (1906) was the first to allege attenuation of rinderpest virus for cattle after passage through wildlife. Caccavella (1936) drew a similar conclusion from experimental studies using antelopes. Carmichael (1938a) claimed that cattle infected directly from wild buffalo or wild pig rarely died, but as the disease spread through cattle, the number of deaths increased. The Masai held similar beliefs and immunized their cattle by mingling them with sick buffalo (Beaton 1954). Subsequent virus isolations from sick cattle, eland, and buffalo in Masailand showed that the virus

responsible was attenuated and virtually nonlethal for cattle (Lowe et al. 1947; Plowright 1962; Robson et al. 1959). In contrast, the virus responsible for the 1960 epizootic in the wildlife of northern Kenya proved to be highly virulent for cattle (Liess and Plowright 1964).

PATHOLOGY. Several descriptions of the pathology of rinderpest in wild animals have been published (Table 2.4). Some are detailed but most are not; all emphasize the similarity of the findings with those encountered in domestic animals.

Clinical Pathology. The prominent feature in cattle is the profound lymphocytopenia that develops at the onset of illness (Maurer et al. 1956). The loss of body water from purging causes a hemoconcentration that is reflected in an increased packed cell volume (Heuschele and Barber 1966). In addition, the diarrhea induces a terminal fall in serum chloride levels (Heuschele and Barber 1966) and in total serum pro-

TABLE 2.4 Reports on the Gross Pathology of Rinderpest in Wildlife.

Scientific Name	Common Name	References
Antilopidae		
Aepyceros	impala	Scott et al. 1960
Gazella	Grant's gazelle	Brown and Scott 1960
Ourebia	oribi	Carmichael 1938a
Bovidae		
Strepsiceros	kudu	Thomas and Reid 1944
Syncerus	African buffalo	Els 1930; Thomas and Reid 1944; Guyaux 1951; Thal 1972
Taurotragus	eland	Thomas and Reid 1944
Tragelaphus	bushbuck	Caccavella 1936
Cephalopidae		
Sylvicapra	duiker	Caccavella 1936
Cervidae		
Cervus	deer	Bristowe 1866
	sambhar	Gupta and Verma 1949
Odocoileus	white-tailed deer	Hamdy et al. 1975b
Hippotragidae		
Connochaetes	wildebeest	Cornell 1934; Brown and Scott 1960
Redunca	reedbuck	Carmichael 1938a; Wilde 1948
Suidae		
Phacochoerus	warthog	Thal 1972
Potamochoerus	bush pig	Wilde 1948; Brown and Scott 1960
Sus	wild pig	Sitin 1930
Tayassuidae		
Tayassu	peccary	Dardiri et al. 1969

teins (French 1936). High serum bilirubin levels have been detected in the terminal stages of peracute infections (Heuschele and Barber 1966).

Gross Pathology. Carcasses are emaciated, soiled, and fetid. The striking lesions occur in the alimentary tract. The mucosa of the oral and pharyngeal structures is eroded and that of the abomasum is congested and eroded. Peyer's patches are swollen, hemorrhagic, and necrotic. The cecal and colonic mucosa is striped longitudinally by congested capillaries that resemble petechiae, and its surface is often ulcerated and bleeding. Similar gross changes affect the urogenital tract.

The nasal passages are coated with a thick mucopurulent discharge, and the lungs are often emphysematous. Subendocardial hemorrhages may be present in the left cardiac ventricle.

Histopathology. Thomas and Reid (1944) carried out one of the few histopathologic studies of rinderpest in wildlife when they examined tissues from buffalo, eland, and kudu. There are degeneration and necrosis of the lymphoid follicles leading to severe depletion of lymphocytes, reticular cell hyperplasia, and formation of multinucleate giant cells (Tajima and Ushijima 1971). The erosive mucosal lesions are also associated with giant cells. They start as necrotic foci in the prickle cell layer and extend toward the surface where the necrotic debris is shed leaving a shallow erosion (Maurer et al. 1956).

DIAGNOSIS. The diagnosis of rinderpest in wildlife is usually based on the clinical signs and necropsy findings. Unfortunately, confirmation is seldom sought (Table 2.1). A field diagnosis is probably reliable when the species attacked are buffalo, eland, kudu, and warthog. A field diagnosis, however, is difficult and may be impossible when the species involved react less acutely.

Confirmation requires either isolation and identification of the virus or detection of specific antigens. The specimens required are blood in anticoagulant, lymph node, spleen, and tonsil; and they are best collected from animals shot in the early erosive phase of the disease. Soiled, emaciated animals are not good donors. Specimens from dead animals, however, are worth examining for antigen but not for infective virus (Scott 1967).

The preferred method for seeking virus is to inoculate rolled primary cultures of calf kidney cells with washed leukocytes from the blood specimens (Plowright and Ferris 1962). If virus is present, cytopathic changes are visible 3–12 days later. Serologic identification may be obtained simultaneously by incorporating rinderpest antiserum in the maintenance medium of some of the cultures.

Virus can also be sought and identified by injecting blood or tissue suspensions into rinderpest-susceptible and immune cattle or goats. The immunity of survivors is challenged 2–3 weeks later with stock virus (Scott and Brown 1961).

Complement fixation, conglutinating complement absorption, and immunodiffusion tests identify specific rinderpest antigens in lymph node tissue (Nakamura 1958; Singh 1970; White 1958). Immunofluorescence also detects rinderpest virus in lymph node cells, but background fluorescence renders interpretation difficult (Provost 1970). All these procedures require rinderpest hyperimmune antiserum as a stock reagent.

Two as yet unappraised techniques for detecting rinderpest antigens have been published. Ishii and Watanabe (1971) reported that boiled suspensions of lymph nodes from rinderpest-infected cattle yielded antigens detectable by an indirect or passive hemagglutination inhibition test in which specific antigen was coupled to tannic acid–treated erythrocytes. Singh and his colleagues (1972) favored the simpler passive hemagglutination test using formalinized sheep erythrocytes coated with hyperimmune antiserum.

The demonstration of a rising antibody titer in paired serum samples is not a practical method for confirming a presumptive diagnosis of rinderpest in wildlife. Nevertheless, the detection of antibody in single serum samples reveals past experience to the infection (Table 2.1). Antibody surveys, for example, have been used to monitor the disease status of the herds of wildlife on the plains of East Africa; surveys during the years 1959–1961 revealed that 65% of Serengeti wildebeest had rinderpest antibodies (Plowright 1963a), whereas later surveys clearly indicated that there was no evidence of infection in any wild species after 1962 (Atang and Plowright 1969).

The commonest procedure for detecting antibodies to rinderpest is a neutralization test using cell culture–adapted virus (Plowright and Ferris 1961). Antibodies can also be detected by measles hemagglutination inhibition (Bogel et al. 1964), conglutinating complement absorption (Singh and Gulrajani 1968), and indirect immunodiffusion tests (Yedloutschnig and Stone 1974). Antibodies are rarely demonstrated in the sera of convalescent animals by complement fixation, direct immunodiffusion, or passive hemagglutination (Ishii and Watanabe 1971; Yedloutschnig and Stone 1974).

Differential Diagnosis. Several diseases known to afflict wildlife have clinical manifestations that mimic rinderpest, but only two—bovine virus diarrhea and peste des petits ruminants—are clinically and pathologically indistinguishable from rinderpest. Bovine virus diarrhea has a worldwide distribution in domestic and wild ruminants. Fortunately, the viruses, antigens, and antibodies of rinderpest and bovine virus diarrhea are readily differentiated in the laboratory. In contrast, peste des petits ruminants is recognized only in sheep and goats in West Africa and is difficult, even in the laboratory, to differentiate from rinderpest.

PROGNOSIS. The prognosis for wild animals bred, reared, and infected in enzootic areas is favorable because they possess a high innate resistance through a long ancestral association with the disease. Elsewhere, the prognosis is poor. Fortunately, following an epizootic most species regain their former numbers within a few years (Spinage 1962).

IMMUNITY. Immunologically, rinderpest is a simple disease, an attack conferring a lifelong active resistance to reinfection in animals that survive. A quantal, but not infallible, measure of this active resistance is the presence of humoral neutralizing antibodies. Newborn animals acquire a passive protection through the ingestion of antibodies in the colostrum; the duration of the passive protection ranges from 4 to 10 months in cattle (Brown 1958) and from 3 to 5 months in wildebeest (Plowright 1963a). Consequently, the only animals at risk in enzootic areas are the weaned immatures. A vivid example was the yearling disease of wildebeest that formerly devastated the annual calf crop of the Serengeti herds (Talbot and Talbot 1963).

TREATMENT AND CONTROL. Attempted treatment of established cases of rinderpest in wild animals is not justified because of the stress attendant on capture. The provision of ample supplies of clean drinking water, however, relieves distress and counteracts the tendency of some species such as buffalo and eland to stampede (Branagan 1966).

If legally permitted, treatment of captive

animals is worthwhile. It is largely symptomatic, the objectives being to counteract the depletion of essential electrolytes and to control the diarrhea (Heuschele and Barber 1966). Antibiotics and sulfonamides have no effect on the course of the disease (Brown 1965a,b). Antiserum given in massive doses during the incubation period or prodromal fever will save lives, but it is useless once the disease is overt (Curasson 1932).

Rinderpest, theoretically, is one of the easiest diseases to control; there is one serotype and the available vaccines are safe and efficient; the period during which the virus is shed is short; and transmission normally requires close contact among animals. Moreover, the discovery that intensive vaccination of domestic livestock protects in-contact wildlife (Sinclair 1977) opens the door to complete eradication. The disease in Africa remains enzootic because of nomadism and civil strife. In Asia it is enzootic because of civic ignorance and, perhaps, irresponsibility together with weak or nonexistent legislation for the control of animal diseases.

Enzootics. The only practical control procedure in countries where rinderpest is enzootic is routine vaccination of domestic cattle; a sound regimen is vaccination of calves with revaccination at 9 months and 15 months. Domestic sheep, goats, and pigs are rarely vaccinated. Efficient attenuated and inactivated vaccines are available, the most widely used being Plowright's attenuated cell-cultured virus vaccine (Plowright 1963c).

Vaccines developed to protect cattle have been tested experimentally in various species of wildlife with results that confirm field observations on variable innate resistances. Bushbuck, duiker, reedbuck, and oryx injected with goat-adapted virus vaccine reacted clinically, and the reedbuck died (Daubney 1943). The others proved to be immune when challenged later with virulent virus. The response of vaccinated warthogs was much milder (Daubney 1944). On the other hand, buffalo and giraffe proved difficult to vaccinate (Daubney 1942). Wilde (1950) induced postvaccinal febrile reactions in dik-dik (*Rhynchotragus*) and Thomson's gazelle. Brown and Scott (1960) vaccinated 72 newly captured wild animals from 12 species with rabbit-adapted virus; 28 reacted clinically and 14 (19%) died. In other words, vaccination of wildlife with vaccines developed for cattle is not without hazard.

There is also the problem of administering vaccines in the field. Results of trials with cattle hold little promise for the administration of vaccines in food, water, or salt (Scott 1976). The only vaccination of free-living wildlife so far recorded was carried out by Harthoorn and Lock (1960) who first immobilized buffalo with drugs delivered by darts and then injected them with rabbit-adapted virus. The vaccinated buffalo were kept under observation for 3 months, and no untoward effects were detected. Harthoorn and Lock calculated that 20–30 buffalo could be vaccinated daily by a team of four people.

Epizootics. The control of epizootics in wildlife necessitates prompt and drastic action to limit dissemination of the disease. Practical and effective control procedures were formulated during the 1913–1921 and 1937–1941 threats to southern Africa. The former wave was stopped by establishing a *cordon sanitaire* along the border between Zambia and Malawi within which all cattle were immunized and all game destroyed (Gray 1919).

Similar measures in the 1937–1941 epizootic were supplemented by the erection of game-proof fences between Lake Tanganyika and Lake Malawi (Lowe 1942). Wire fencing was useless, but fences constructed with local timber and bush stopped everything except elephants. All game for 40.2 km on each side of the fences was exterminated and every 9.7 km of fence was patrolled daily by a team of three men. The fences were finally abandoned in the 1960s.

The handling of epizootics of rinderpest in captive wildlife has depended on the disease status of the country involved. In the Rome zoo, for example, all the ungulates and pigs were destroyed (Cilli et al. 1951), whereas in the Calcutta zoo goat-adapted virus vaccine was administered to the species at risk (Ray and Samanta 1974).

REFERENCES

Alexander, R. A., and de Kock, G. Rinderpest in southern Africa. *Farm. S. Afr.* 15:173, 1940.

Allan, W. A. *Rept. Vet. Dept., Uganda, 1933.* Government Printing, Entebbe: 1934.

Anon. Consultative sub-regional meeting on rinderpest with participation of F.A.O. and O.I.E. *Bull. Off. Int. Epizoot.* 71:1365, 1969.

Atang, P. G., and Plowright, W. Extension of the JP-15 Rinderpest Control Campaign to eastern Africa: The epizootiological background. *Bull. Epizoot. Dis. Afr.* 17:161, 1969.

Beaton, W. G. Le role des animaux sauvages dans la transmission des maladies animales contagieuses autre que la rage. *Bull. Off. Int. Epizoot.* 42:223, 1954.

Bogel, K., Enders-Ruckle, G., and Provost, A. Une reaction serologiquerapide de mesure des anticorps antibovipestiques. *C. R. Acad. Sci.* 259:482, 1964.

Boldrini, G. Un episodio di peste bovina su una nave del Lloyd Triestino. *Vet. Ital.* 5:1182, 1954.

Bourliere, F., and Verschuren, J. *Introduction a l'ecologie des ongules du Parc National Albert.* Brussels: Inst. Parcs Nat. Congo Belge, 1960.

Branagan, D. Behaviour of buffalo infected with rinderpest. *Bull. Epizoot. Dis. Afr.* 14:341, 1966.

Branagan, D., and Hammond, J. A. Rinderpest in Tanganyika: A review. *Bull. Epizoot. Dis. Afr.* 13:225, 1965.

Breese, S. S., and de Boer, C. J. Ferritin-tagged antibody cross-reactions among rinderpest, canine distemper, and measles viruses. *J. Gen. Virol.* 20:121, 1973.

Bristowe, J. S. Supplementary report on the morbid anatomy of the cattle plague, as it occurs in sheep, goats, and deer. *Third Report of the Commissioners Appointed to Inquire into the Origin and Nature, etc. of the Cattle Plague.* London: H. M. Stationary Office, 1866.

Broudin, L. Notes d'epidemiologie animal en Cochinchine. *Bull. Soc. Pathol. Exotique* 16:425, 1923.

Brown, R. D. Rinderpest immunity in calves: I. The acquisition and persistence of maternally derived antibody. *J. Hyg.* 56:427, 1958.

———. The effect of oxytetracycline hydrochloride on rinderpest in cattle. *Bull. Epizoot. Dis. Afr.* 13:247, 1965a.

———. The effect of sulphapyridine and sulphadimidine on rinderpest in cattle. *Bull. Epizoot. Dis. Afr.* 13:317, 1965b.

Brown, R. H., and Scott, G. R. Vaccination of game with lapinised rinderpest virus. *Vet. Rec.* 72:1232, 1960.

Caccavella, A. E. Observations sur la transmission de la peste bovine chez les antilopes pongo (*Tragelaphus scriptus*) et isha (*Sylvicapra grimmi*). Serotherapie et virus de passage sur les bovides. *Ann. Soc. Belge Med. Trop.* 16:309, 1936.

Campbell, J., 1869. Cited by J. H. B. Hallen, K. McLeod, J. G. Charles, H. C. Kerr, and M. M. A. Jan. *Report of the Indian Cattle Plague Commission with appendices.* Calcutta: Government Printing, 1871.

Carmichael, J. The virus of rinderpest and its relation to *Glossina morsitans* Westw. *Bull. Entomol. Res.* 24:337, 1933.

———. Rinderpest in African game. *J. Comp. Pathol.* 51:264, 1938a.

———. *Rept. Vet. Dept., Uganda, 1937.* Entebbe: Government Printing, 1938b.

Carre, H., and Fraimbault, [?]. Note sur la contagiosite de la peste bovine au porc. *Ann. Inst. Pasteur* 12:848, 1898.

Christy, C. *Big game and pygmies.* London: Macmillan, 1924.

Cilli, V., Mazzaracchio, V., and Roetti, C. Le foyer de peste bovine au Jardin Zoologique de Rome. *Bull. Off. Int. Epizoot.* 35:444, 1951.

Cornell, R. L. *Rept. Vet. Dept. Tanganyika, 1933.* Dar

es Salaam: Government Printing, 1934.

Crandall, Lee S. *The management of wild mammals in captivity*. Chicago: University of Chicago Press, 1964.

Crawshay, [?], 1893. Cited by F. D. Lugard. *The rise of our eastern African empire*. Edinburgh: Blackwood, 1893.

Curasson, G. *La peste bovine*. Paris: Vigot Freres, 1932.

Dardiri, A. H., Yedloutschnig, R. J., and Taylor, W. D. Clinical and serologic response of American white-collared peccaries to African swine fever, foot-and-mouth disease, vesicular stomatitis, vesicular exanthema of swine, hog cholera, and rinderpest viruses. *Proc. U.S. Anim. Health Assoc.* 73:437, 1969.

Daubney, R. *Rept. Vet. Dept., Kenya, 1941*. Nairobi: Government Printing, 1942.

——. *Rept. Vet. Dept., Kenya, 1942*. Nairobi: Government Printing, 1943.

——. *Rept. Vet. Dept., Kenya, 1943*. Nairobi: Government Printing, 1944.

D'Costa, J., and Singh, B. Rinderpest clinical syndrome in goats in India. *Indian J. Vet. Sci.* 3:122, 1933.

——. Rinderpest: Its symptoms. *Indian Vet. J.* 13:7, 1936.

De Does, J. K. F., 1909. Cited in G. Curasson. *La peste bovine*. Paris: Vigot Freres, 1932.

De Sauvages, [?], 1746. Cited in W. Dieckerhoff. *Geschichter der Rinderpest und ihrer Literatur*. Berlin: Enslin, 1890.

Dieckerhoff, W. *Geschichter der Rinderpest und ihrer Literatur*. Berlin: Enslin, 1890.

Dodson, [?], 1754. Cited in J. Gamgee. *The cattle plague*. London: Hardwicke, 1866.

Dormal, R., Herin, V., and Bugyaki, L. Relation concernant le foyer de peste bovine identifie dans les elevages du nord de la province de l'equateur de la Republique du Congo. *Bull. Epizoot. Dis. Afr.* 9:127, 1961.

Duke, H. L. An enquiry into the relation of *Glossina morsitans* and ungulate game, with special reference to rinderpest. *Bull. Entomol. Res.* 10:7, 1919.

Els, T. La peste bovine a la frontiere orientale du Congo Belge. *Bull. Agr. Congo Belge* 1:1029, 1930.

Els, T., Jezierski, A., Pojer, J., Scott, G. R., and Wiktor, T. J. La campagne contre la peste bovine en Ituri en 1954. *Bull. Agr. Congo Belge* 48:947, 1957.

Farrell, H., 1870. Cited in J. H. B. Hallen, K. McLeod, J. G. Charles, H. C. Kerr, and M. M. A. Jan. *Report of the Indian Cattle Plague Commission with Appendices*. Calcutta: Government Printing, 1871.

Fenner, F. J. The classification and nomenclature of viruses. Summary of the results of meetings of the International Committee on Taxonomy of Viruses in Madrid, Sept. 1974. *Intervirology.* 7:1, 1976.

Flemynge, M., 1755. Cited in J. Gamgee. *The cattle plague*. London: Hardwicke, 1866.

French, M. H. The serum protein changes induced by rinderpest virus. *J. Comp. Pathol. Ther.* 49:118, 1936.

Glasgow, J. P. *The distribution and abundance of tsetse*. Oxford: Pergamon, 1963.

Gray, C. E. *Rinderpest campaign in East Africa. Final Report, Rinderpest Commission*. London: Colonial Office, 1919.

Grimwood, I. R. *Rept. Game Dept., Kenya, 1960*. Nairobi, Government Printing, 1961.

Gupta, K. C. S., and Verma, N. S. Rinderpest in wild ruminants. *Indian J. Vet. Sci.* 19:219, 1949.

Guyaux, R. Gibier et peste bovine: Cas de transmission de la peste bovine du buffle au betail bovin. *Bull. Agr. Congo Belge* 42:123, 1951.

Hallen, J. H. B., McLeod, K., Charles, J. G., Kerr, H. C., and Jan, M. M. A. *Report of the Indian Cattle Plague Commission with Appendices*. Calcutta: Government Printing, 1871.

Hamdy, F. M., Dardiri, A. H., Breese, S. S., and de Boer, C. J. Immunologic relationships between rinderpest and peste des petits ruminants viruses. *Proc. U.S. Anim. Health Assoc.* 79:168, 1975a.

Hamdy, F. M., Dardiri, A. H., Ferris, D. H., and Breese, S. S. Experimental infection of white-tailed deer with rinderpest virus. *J. Wildl. Dis.* 11:508, 1975b.

Harthoorn, A. M., and Lock, J. A. A note on the prophylactic vaccination of wild animals. *Brt. Vet. J.* 116:252, 1960.

Heuschele, W. P., and Barber, T. L. Changes in certain blood components of rinderpest-infected cattle. *Am. J. Vet. Res.* 27:1001, 1966.

Hilsont, P., and Bourdereau, C. Une enzootie pestique cryptogenetique sur des phacocheres en captivite a Bamako (Soudan Francais). *Rev. Elev. Med. Vet. Pays Trop.* 7:79, 1954.

Holmes, J. D. E. Rinderpest: Experiments carried out to test the susceptibility to rinderpest of cattle from several districts in India and on improved methods of rinderpest serum preparation. *Mem. Indian Civil Vet. Dept.* 3:98, 1911.

Hornby, H. E. Studies in rinderpest immunity: II. Methods of infection. *Vet. J.* 82:348, 1926.

——. *Rept. Vet. Dept., Tanganyika, 1931*. Dar es Salaam: Government Printing, 1932.

Hutchins, E. *Rept. Chief Vet. Off. Dept. Agr., Uganda, 1917–18*. Entebbe: Government Printing, 1918.

Hyslop, N. St. G. Observations on pathogenic organisms in the airborne state. *Trop. Anim. Health Prod.* 4:28, 1972.

Imagawa, D. T. Relationships among measles, canine distemper, and rinderpest viruses. *Prog. Med. Virol.* 10:160, 1968.

Ishii, S., and Watanabe, M. An indirect hemagglutination test of rinderpest virus. *Natl. Inst. Anim. Health Q.* 11:55, 1971.

Jacotot, H. Transmission experimentale de la peste bovine a *Cervus aristotelis*. *C. R. Soc. Biol.* 96:1134, 1927.

——. Existe-t-il en Indo-Chine des porteurs de virus pestique? *Bull. Soc. Pathol. Exot.* 24:51, 1931.

Jussiant, A. Rapport annuel sur la situation de l'agriculture de la province du Katanga (annee

1932): IV. Service veterinaire. *Bull. Agr. Congo Belge* 24:329, 1933.

Liess, B., and Plowright, W. Studies in tissue culture on the pH-stability of rinderpest virus. *J. Hyg.* 61:205, 1963.

———. Studies on the pathogenesis of rinderpest in experimental cattle. I. correlation of clinical signs, viraemia, and virus excretion by various routes. *J. Hyg.* 62:81, 1964.

Lingard, A. *Rept. Imp. Bacteriologist, 1905–1906.* Calcutta: Government Printing, 1906.

Lobry, M. A. Existence chez les animaux sauvages en Afrique de cas de maladies infectieuses des animaux domestiques. *Bull. Epizoot. Dis. Afr.* 12:43, 1964.

Lowe, H. J. Rinderpest in Tanganyika territory. *Emp. J. Exp. Agr.* 10:189, 1942.

Lowe, H. J., Wilde, J. K. H., Lee, R. P., and Stuchbery, H. M. An outbreak of an aberrant type of rinderpest in Tanganyika Territory. *J. Comp. Pathol. Ther.* 57:175, 1947.

Lugard, F. D. Travels from the east coast to Uganda, Lake Albert Edward, and Lake Albert. *Proc. R. Geogr. Soc.* 14:817, 1892.

———. *The rise of our Eastern African empire.* Edinburgh: Blackwood, 1893.

McCall, F. J. *Rept. Vet. Dept., Tanganyika, 1922.* Dar es Salaam: Government Printing, 1923.

Mahamooth, T. M. Z. Rinderpest. *Trop. Agr.* 99:20, 1943.

Mathur, S. C., Majumdar, S. S., and Jain, V. K. Suspect rinderpest in a blue bull (*Boselaphus tragocamelus*). *Indian Vet. J.* 52:412, 1975.

Maurer, F. D., Jones, T. C., Easterday, B., and DeTray, D. E. The pathology of rinderpest. *Proc. 92nd Ann. Meeting Am. Vet. Med. Assoc. Minneapolis, 1955*, p. 201, 1956.

Minett, F. C. Dissemination of animal disease in India: Role of man and carrion feeders. *Br. Vet. J.* 110:19, 1954.

Molinie, J. P. La peste bovine. Contamination a l'espece porcine. *Rec. Med. Vet. Exot.* 4:5, 1931.

Nakamura, J. *Complement-fixation reaction in rinderpest study: Guide for technique and application.* Paris: Off. Int. Epizoot., 1958.

Oxley, T., 1840. Cited in J. H. B. Hallen, K. McLeod, J. G. Charles, H. C. Kerr, and M. M. A. Jan. *Report of the Indian Cattle Plague Commission with appendices.* Calcutta: Government Printing, 1871.

Pease, H. T., 1894. Cited by D. Hutcheon. Rinderpest in South Africa. *J. Comp. Pathol. Ther.* 15:300, 1902.

Pecaud, G. Contribution a l'etude de la pathologie veterinaire de la colonie du Tchad. *Bull. Soc. Pathol. Exot.* 17:196, 1924.

Percival, A. B. Game and disease. *J. East Afr. Uganda Nat. Hist. Soc.* 13:302, 1918.

Pitman, C. R. S. *A game warden takes stock.* London: Nisbet, 1942.

Plowright, W. Rinderpest virus. *Ann. N.Y. Acad. Sci.* 101:327, 1962.

———. The role of game animals in the epizootiology of rinderpest and malignant catarrhal fever in East Africa. *Bull. Epizoot. Dis. Afr.* 11:149, 1963a.

———. Some properties of strains of rinderpest virus recently isolated in E. Africa. *Res. Vet. Sci.* 4:96, 1963b.

———. The production and use of culture-attenuated rinderpest vaccine. *Proc. 17th World Vet. Congr., Hannover, 1963.* 1:679, 1963c.

———. Studies on the pathogenesis of rinderpest in experimental cattle: II. Proliferation of the virus in different tissues following intranasal infection. *H. Hyg.* 62:257, 1964.

———. Rinderpest virus. *Virol. Monogr.* 3:25, 1968.

Plowright, W., and Ferris, R. D. Studies with rinderpest virus in tissue culture: III. The stability of cultured virus and its use in virus neutralization tests. *Arch. Ges. Virusforsch.* 11:516, 1961.

———. Studies with rinderpest virus in tissue culture: A technique for the detection and titration of virulent virus in cattle tissues. *Res. Vet. Sci.* 3:94, 1962.

Plowright, W., Laws, R. M., and Rampton, C. S. Serological evidence for the susceptibility of the hippopotamus (*Hippopotamus amphibius* Linnaeus) to natural infection with rinderpest virus. *J. Hyg.* 62:329, 1964.

Poulton, W. F. *Game preservation and economic development.* Entebbe: Government Printing, 1927.

———. *Rept. Vet. Dept., Uganda, 1932.* Entebbe: Government Printing, 1933.

Provost, A. Peste bovine et immunofluorescence. Application au diagnostic differentiel de l'infection bovipestique. *Bull. Off. Int. Epizoot.* 73:915, 1970.

Ramachandran, S. *Aspects of the serological relationships between measles, rinderpest, and canine distemper.* Edinburgh: Thesis, 1970.

Ramani, K., 1972. Cited in D. K. Ray and D. P. Samanta, *Indian Vet. J.* 51:199, 1974.

Ray, D. K., and Samanta, D. P. A syndrome simulating rinderpest among captive wild animals at Calcutta zoo. *Indian Vet. J.* 51:199, 1974.

Reid, N. R. *Rept. Vet. Dept., Tanganyika, 1947.* Dar es Salaam: Government Printing, 1949.

———. *Rept. Vet. Dept., Tanganyika, 1948.* Dar es Salaam: Government Printing, 1950.

Roberts, G. A. Rinderpest (peste bovina) in Brazil. *J. Am. Vet. Med. Assoc.* 13:177, 1921.

Robertson, W. A. M. *Rinderpest in western Australia 1923.* Melbourne: Government Printing, 1924.

Robson, J., Arnold, R. M., Plowright, W., and Scott, G. R. The isolation from an eland of a strain of rinderpest virus attenuated for cattle. *Bull. Epizoot. Dis. Afr.* 7:97, 1959.

Roll, M. F. *Lehrbuch der Pathologie und Therapie der Haustiere.* Vienna: Braumueller, 1860.

Sainte-Hillaire, M. A. G. Note sur le typhus contagieux au Jardin d'Acclimatation. *Bull. Soc. Imp. Zool. Acclim.* 2:685, 1865.

Sanders, R. N. *Rept. Vet. Dept., Uganda, 1960.* Entebbe: Government Printing, 1961.

Scott, G. R. Life expectancy of rinderpest virus. *Bull. Epizoot. Dis. Afr.* 3:19, 1955.

———. Rinderpest. *Adv. Vet. Sci.* 9:113, 1964.

———. *Diagnosis of rinderpest.* Rome: FAO, 1967.

————. *Report of the UNDP (Special Fund) Mission to the Central African Republic on an epizootic disease of wildlife*. Rome: FAO, 1968.

————. Oral vaccination against rinderpest. *Trans. R. Soc. Trop. Med. Hyg.* 70:287, 1976.

Scott, G. R., and Brown, R. D. Rinderpest diagnosis with special reference to the agar gel double diffusion test. *Bull. Epizoot. Dis. Afr.* 9:83, 1961.

Scott, G. R., Cowan, K. M., and Elliott, R. T. Rinderpest in impala. *Vet. Rec.* 72:787, 1960.

Scott, G. R., DeTray, D. E., and White, G. Rinderpest in pigs of European origin. *Am. J. Vet. Res.* 23:452, 1962.

Selous, F. C. *Great and small game in Africa*. London: Rowland Ward, 1899.

Sharpe, A. A journey from the Shire River to Lake Nweru and the Upper Luapula, *Geog. J. London* 1:524, 1893.

Simmons, R. J. *Rept. Vet. Dept., Uganda, 1942*. Entebbe: Government Printing, 1943.

Simon, N. *Between the sunlight and the thunder: The wild life of Kenya*. London: Collins, 1962.

Sinclair, A. R. E. *The African buffalo: A study of resource limitation of populations*. Chicago: University of Chicago Press, 1977.

Singh, G. Conglutinating complement absorption test in rinderpest: II. Rinderpest antigen—some observations. *Indian J. Anim. Health* 9:7, 1970.

Singh, G., and Gulrajani, T. S. A note on the application of the conglutinating complement absorption test for the detection of rinderpest antibodies. *Curr. Sci.* 37:203, 1968.

Singh, K. V., and Ata, F. Experimental rinderpest in camels: A preliminary report. *Bull. Epizoot. Dis. Afr.* 15:19, 1967.

Singh, S. N., Tanwani, S. K., Singh, R., and Kangude, C. M. Detection of rinderpest virus by an indirect haemagglutination test. *Indian Vet. J.* 49:355, 1972.

Singharaj, K. La peste bovine au Laos. *Bull. Off. Int. Epizoot.* 69:21, 1968.

Sitin, S. P. The infections of wild swine by the horned cattle plague. *Vestn. Sovremennoi Vet.* (11): 348, 1928. Abstr. *Biol. Abstr.* 4:2684, 1930.

Spinage, C. A. Rinderpest and faunal distribution patterns. *Afr. Life* 16:55, 1962.

Stevenson-Hamilton, J. The relation between game and tsetse flies. *Bull. Entomol. Res.* 2:113, 1911.

————. *Animal life in Africa*. London: Heinemann, 1912.

————. Tsetse fly and the rinderpest epidemic of 1896. *S. Afr. J. Sci.* 58:216, 1957.

Stewart, D. R. M. Rinderpest among wild animals in Kenya, 1960-62. *Bull. Epizoot. Dis. Africa* 12:39, 1964.

Stordy, R. J. *Rept. Chief Vet. Off. Dept. Agr., Br. East Afr., 1913–14*. Nairobi: Government Printing, 1914.

Stordy, R. I. *Rept. Chief Vet. Off. Dept. Agr., Br. East Afr., 1916–17*. Nairobi: Government Printing, 1918.

Surmon, [?], 1902. Cited in D. Hutcheon, Rinderpest in South Africa. *J. Comp. Pathol.* 15:300, 1902.

Tajima, M., and Ushijima, T. The pathogenesis of rinderpest in the lymph nodes of cattle. *Am. J. Path.* 62:221, 1971.

Talbot, L. M., and Talbot, M. H. *The wildebeest in western Masailand, East Africa*. Washington, D.C.: Wildlife Society, 1963.

Taylor, W. P., Plowright, W., Pillinger, R., Rampton, C. S., and Staple, R. F. Studies on the pathogenesis of rinderpest in experimental cattle: IV. Proliferation of virus following contact infection. *J. Hyg.* 63:497, 1965.

Thal, J. A. *Les maladies similaries a la peste bovine: Etudes et Lutte, Ndele, Republique Centrafricaine*. Rome: FAO, 1972.

Theiler, A., 1896. Cited in H. H. Curson. Theiler and the rinderpest epizootic of 1896–1903. *J. S. Afr. Vet. Med. Assoc.* 7:187, 1936.

————. Rinderpest in Sud-Afrika. *Schweiz. Arch. Tierheilkd.*, 39:49, 1897.

Thomas, A. D., and Reid, N. R. Rinderpest in game: A description of an outbreak and an attempt at limiting its spread by means of a bush fence. *Onderstepoort J. Vet. Res.* 20:7, 1944.

Todd, C., and White, R. G. *Experiments on cattle plague*. Cairo: Government Press, 1914.

Underwood, B., and Brown, F. Physico-chemical characterisation of rinderpest virus. *Med. Microbiol. Immunol.* 160:125, 1974.

Vittoz, R. Considerations pratiques sur le role des animaux sauvages dans la transmission des maladies contagieuses et la prophylaxie de celles-ci dans le Sud-Est Asiatique. *Bull. Off. Int. Epizoot.* 42:206, 1954.

White, G. A specific diffusible antigen of rinderpest virus demonstrated by the agar double-diffusion precipitation reaction. *Nature* 181:1409, 1958.

White, J. B., 1870. Cited by J. H. B. Hallen, K. McLeod, J. G. Charles, H. C. Kerr, and M. M. A. Jan. *Report of the Indian Cattle Plague Commission with appendices*. Calcutta: Government Printing, 1871.

Wilde, J. K. H. Rinderpest in some African wild mammals. *J. Comp. Pathol. Ther.* 58:64, 1948.

————. *Rept. Vet. Dept., Tanganyika, 1948*. Dar es Salaam: Government Printing, 1950.

Wilder, F. W., Dardiri, A. H., Gay, J. G., Beasley, H. C., Heflin, A. A., and Acree, J. A. Susceptibility of one-toed pigs to certain diseases exotic to the United States. *Proc. U.S. Anim. Health Assoc.* 78:195, 1974a.

Wilder, F. W., Dardiri, A. H., and Yedloutschnig, R. J. Clinical and serologic response of the nine-banded armadillo (*Dasypus novemcinctus*) to viruses of African swine fever, hog cholera, rinderpest, vesicular exanthema of swine, vesicular stomatitis and foot-and-mouth disease. *Proc. U.S. Anim. Health Assoc.* 78:188, 1974b.

Yamanouchi, K., Fukuda, A., Kobane, F., Yoshikawa, Y., and Chino, F. Pathogenesis of rinderpest virus infection in rabbits: II. Effect of rinderpest virus on the immune functions of rabbits. *Infect. Immun.* 9:206, 1974.

Yedloutschnig, R. J., and Stone, S. S. An indirect agar gel diffusion precipitation test for detecting rinderpest nonprecipitating antibody in cattle and zoological ruminant sera. *Proc. Am. Assoc. Vet. Lab. Diag.* 17:189, 1974.

3 *Distemper*

JOAN BUDD

Synonyms: **La maladie de Carre.**

Distemper is an acute or subacute febrile disease of many species of the order Carnivora. It may be manifested by signs of generalized infection, hyperkeratosis, central nervous system disturbance, or any combination of these. Morbidity and mortality rates vary among species but may be high in susceptible populations.

HISTORY. The early history of distemper in the dog indicates its presence in Europe in the mid-sixteenth century (Kirk 1922). Although uncontrolled dogs undoubtedly had contact with susceptible wild species, there is scant reference to distemper in wildlife. Until 1955 reports of distemper in species other than the domestic dog (Table 3.1) were confined to captive species on fur farms or in zoological collections, and in some of these the diagnosis is suspect, having been made on clinical signs without reference to histopathologic examination or animal transmission.

It is generally assumed that all members of the Canidae and Mustelidae are susceptible, but an acceptable diagnosis is lacking for many species. Distemper occurs in the free-living raccoon and in some other members of the Procyanidae, but the authenticity of reports of distemper in the Viverridae has been questioned (Cabasso 1966). Experimental infection of cats with distemper virus and resulting inapparent infection (Appel et al. 1974) suggests that infection without clinical signs of disease may occur in other species including those in the family Felidae. Further research, serologic surveys, and accurate, well-documented reports of distemper in both free-living and confined wildlife are required to complete the list of susceptible species.

DISTRIBUTION. Distemper in the dog is a world problem. From reports of distemper in sled dogs in Alaska (Gorham 1966) and from the various zoological collections indicating the susceptibility of tropic- or subtropic-inhabiting Canidae, one may assume that the occurrence of distemper in wildlife in any temperature zone is limited only by the species composition, density of the wildlife population, and the availability of infective virus.

ETIOLOGY. Distemper is caused by a single antigenic type virus (Ott 1966) known as the virus of Carre (Carre 1905). Distemper and the

TABLE 3.1 Species Reported to Be Susceptible to Distemper.

Scientific Name	Common Name	References
Canidae		
Canis spp.	wolf	Dobrich 1904; Parent 1906; Blair 1916; Fox 1923; Hamerton 1937; Sedgwick and Young 1968; Monson and Stone 1976
Canis adustus	jackal	Hobley 1932; Hamerton 1937
Canis dingo	Australian dingo	Hamerton 1937; Armstrong and Anthony 1942; Grunberg 1959
Canis latrans	coyote	Blair 1916, 1921, 1922; Rewell 1947; Gier and Ameel 1959; Monson and Stone 1976[a]; Anon. 1968
Canis mesomelas	black-backed jackal	Goss 1942; Rewell 1947
Chrysocyon brachyurus	maned wolf	Cabasso et al. 1956; Sedgwick and Young 1968
Cynalopex chama	silver jackal	Blair 1907; Martinaglia 1937; Hofmeyer 1956
Dusicyon spp.	Chilean wild dog	Goss 1942
	South American foxes	Armstrong and Anthony 1942
	South American fox dog	Sedgwick and Young 1968
Dusicyon gymnocercus	azaras dog	Blair 1907

TABLE 3.1 *(Continued)*

Scientific Name	Common Name	References
Lycaon pictus	Cape hunting dog	Hofmeyer 1956; Crandall 1964
Nycterentes procyonoides	raccoon dog	Armstrong and Anthony 1942; Sedgwick and Young 1968
Alopex lagopus	Arctic fox	Hamerton 1945
Otocyon spp.	big-eared fox	Goss 1942; Karstad 1978[a]
Otocyon megalotus	long-eared fox	Hofmeyer 1956
Urocyon cinereoargenteus	gray fox	Armstrong and Anthony 1942; Helmboldt and Jungherr 1955[a]; Jakowski and Wyand 1971; Hoff et al. 1974[a]; Monson and Stone 1976[a]
Vulpes fulva	red fox	Blair 1921; Armstrong and Anthony, 1942; Helmboldt and Jungherr 1955; Haberman et al. 1958[a]; Monson and Stone 1976[a]
Vulpes fulva	silver fox[b]	Green 1925; Allen and McLure 1926
Vulpes karagon	karagon fox	Hamerton 1937
Vulpes macrotus macrotus	kit fox	Armstrong and Anthony 1942
Hyaenidae		
Hyaena spp.	hyena	Blair 1909; Rewell 1947
Mustelidae		
Grison spp.	grison	Sedgwick and Young 1968
Martes fiona	stone marten	Ulbrich 1972[a]
Martes pennanti	fisher	Monson and Stone 1976[a]
Meles meles	Eurasian (Old World) badger	Armstrong and Anthony 1942; Fischer 1965; Goss 1948; Helmboldt and Jungherr 1955[a]; Wade-Smith and Richmond 1975; Monson and Stone 1976[a]; Diters and Nielsen 1978[a]
Mustela spp.	weasel	Goss 1948
Mustela erminea	ermine (stoat)	Keymer and Epps 1969
Mustela nigripes	black-footed ferret	Carpenter et al. 1976
Mustela nivalis	least weasel	Keymer and Epps 1969
Mustela putorius furo	ferret (polecat)	Fox 1923; Dunkin and Laidlaw 1926; Dalling 1931
Mustela rixosa	dwarf weasel	Keymer and Epps 1969
Mustela vison	mink	Rudolph 1930; Shaw 1932[b]; Monson and Stone 1976[a]
Mustela zibellina	sable	Pankov and Sytaya 1963
Taxidea taxus	American badger	Armstrong 1942; Farrel 1957
Procyonidae		
Ailurus fulgens	lesser panda	Anon. 1960, Fiennes 1961; Von Mickwitz and Schroder 1967; Von Mickwitz 1968; Erken and Jacobi 1972; Bush et al. 1976
Nasau spp.	coati	Blair 1907; Noback 1929; Muller 1962; Risser 1963; Sedgwick and Young 1968
Potos flavus	kinkajou	Von Mickwitz 1968
Procyon lotor	raccoon	Blair 1907; Noback 1929; Helmboldt and Jungherr 1955[a]; Kilham et al. 1956[a]; Robinson et al. 1957[a]; Karstad and Budd 1964[a]; Hoff et al. 1974[a]; Monson and Stone 1976[a]
Viverridae		
Arctitis binturong	binturong	Hamerton 1945; Goss 1942, 1948; Crandall 1964
Genetta spp.	spotted genet	Goss 1942
Viverra spp.	civet	Blair 1907

Note: Scientific names were lacking in several reports.
[a] Studies of free-living species.
[b] Reports from ranch-raised species.

closely related measles and rinderpest viruses are classified in the family Paramyxoviridae, genus *Morbillivirus* (Andrewes et al. 1978).

Differing biological reactions in the host and variation in form have been reported for some strains of distemper virus (Confer et al. 1975a,b; Reculard and Guillon 1972). Distemper virions are 120–300 nm in diameter, helical in form, and composed of single-stranded RNA (Andrewes et al. 1978). Tubular structures resembling nucleocapsids may be seen in the nucleus and cytoplasm of distemper-virus-infected cells. The virus is inactivated within a few hours by 0.1% formaldehyde, 0.75% phenol, and 0.2% roccal at 4°C. It is unstable under some conditions at room temperature, and it is light sensitive. Lyophilized virus may be stored in sealed vials for long periods at 5°–7°C. Spleens stored at −65°C contained viable virus for 7 years (Appel and Gillespie 1972).

TRANSMISSION. Aerosol or direct contact are the presumed methods of natural transmission. Transplacental infection has been reported in the dog (Krakowka et al. 1977), but an attenuated strain of virus failed to cross the placental barrier in experimentally exposed pregnant mink and ferrets (Hagen et al. 1970). Nasal and conjunctival exudates, urine, and feces contain virus. After artificial aerosol infection, mink and ferrets shed distemper virus in nasal exudate from 5 days postinfection for up to 46 days, or until death (Crook et al. 1958). Airborne infection of ferrets occurred over a distance of 1.5 m (Gorham and Brandly 1953).

In captive animals the possibility exists of transmission via fomites because distemper-virus-contaminated gloves retained infectivity for mink for 20 minutes (Gorham and Brandly 1953). Because viremia persists, bloodsucking arthropods have been suggested as vectors of the virus. Inapparent infections and carrier animals are suggested by the experimental studies of Appel et al. (1974) and serologic surveys of dogs (Ott et al. 1955) and wildlife populations (Choquette and Kuyt 1974; Jamison et al. 1973; Parker et al. 1961; Trainer and Knowlton 1968). Little is known of the epizootiology of distemper in wildlife populations.

SIGNS. In young mink experimentally infected with distemper, the first signs include erythema of the skin on the chin, around the eyes, and on the ears and footpads. This progresses to swelling of these areas and erythema and swelling of the muzzle and the area around the

anus. Papules form on the lips. Serous exudate from the affected areas of the skin becomes dry and scurfy in appearance. A watery lacrimal exudate becomes purulent, which, combined with swollen eyelids, prevents the animal from seeing. A hairless encrusted area develops around the eyes and on the muzzle. The feet become markedly swollen, and the skin is thickened and covered with dried exudate giving the characteristic snowshoe-foot appearance. Dermatitis, which may extend over most of the body, results in thickening of the skin in folds, particularly ventrally. The ventral surface may become wet from dribbled urine. Until the mink is moribund and unable to see or reach food, the appetite remains normal and loss of condition is gradual. Diarrhea may occur in advanced cases. Neurological signs including screaming, frothing at the mouth, grasping the wire with the teeth, and epileptiform seizures may be the only signs, or they may appear with generalized infection.

Signs of distemper in the laboratory ferret are similar to those of mink distemper. In ferrets conditioned to handling, normal rectal temperatures range from 37.7° to 39.1°C. Distemper-infected ferrets occasionally have had a rise in temperature to 41°C as early as the 3rd day postinoculation (PI) and frequently by the 5th day. Temperatures may remain high for 3 days or more. Early signs of hyperemia may be observed in some by the 5th day PI (Belcher 1951) but may not occur until the 8th–10th day or later in others (Crook et al. 1958). The duration of illness varies. Ferrets may be moribund by the 10th or 11th day in an acute infection, but the time may be extended to the 22nd day or longer (L. Karstad, personal communication, 1961; Reculard and Guillon 1972). Temperature drops to subnormal before death. In recently captured black-footed ferrets, signs of distemper were similar. The ferrets died within a couple of days after nervous signs were observed (Carpenter et al. 1976).

Signs of distemper in ranch-raised foxes (Allen and McLure 1926; Gorham 1956; Shillinger 1942) are similar to those seen in mink but with modified dermatitis mainly confined to skin of the head. Thirst and a hot, dry nose accompanied the early hyperemia of lips and skin around the eyes. Swollen eyelids and a purulent lacrimal exudate caused loss of vision. Listlessness and anorexia resulted in emaciation. Diarrhea, unkempt appearance of the fur, dyspnea, and a cough were seen in some cases. Affected foxes may succumb at the height of clinical signs; others recover only to die later barking and in convulsions. The variation in signs among individuals and from one outbreak to another makes clinical diagnosis difficult (Allen and McLure 1926). In some epizootics, visible signs of disease were confined to convulsions and death (Green 1925; Heath and Plummer 1943).

Wild red and gray foxes with distemper had signs similar to those described in captive foxes, including dyspnea, anorexia, emaciation, ascending paralysis, ataxia, terminal convulsions, and coma. Some were blind, and most displayed a lack of fear of man and other abnormal behavior, including aimless wandering and circling suggestive of rabies (Helmboldt and Jungherr 1955; Monson and Stone 1976).

Distemper in free-ranging raccoons resembled the disease in wild foxes. Signs included purulent conjunctivitis, nasal discharge, and variable neurological disturbances including aggressiveness. Emaciation and weakness were occasionally seen (Haberman et al. 1958; Hoff et al. 1974; Karstad and Budd 1964; Monson and Stone 1976; Robinson et al. 1957).

Hyperemia and edema of anal, gingival, and buccal mucosa and jaundice were seen in experimentally infected raccoons. The incubation period in raccoons inoculated with ferret and raccoon strains of distemper virus was 8–20 days; duration of illness was 2–10 days with 50% recovery (Kilham and Herman 1954; Kilham et al. 1956). Signs of distemper were seen in two raccoons 11 and 30 days after inoculation with brain and spleen suspensions from distemper-infected raccoons. These animals survived 5 and 9 days after signs of overt disease (Hoff et al. 1974).

Skin lesions in wild skunks and raccoons were mainly on the face, chest, limbs, and anal areas. Skunks had blistering of the skin on the face, nose, and lips (Monson and Stone 1976). One skunk with multiple infections including distemper had a slight ocular discharge (Diters and Nielsen 1978). Skunks observed in captivity developed skin and eye lesions as noted in wild skunks and became listless and disoriented. Breathing was labored. Convulsive movements of head and paws terminated in convulsions and death. Signs of illness were observed from 2 to 10 days before death (Wade-Smith and Richmond 1975). Distemper in the lesser panda (Erkin and Jacobi 1972; Bush et al. 1976) was manifested clinically by a rise in temperature to 39.5°C, anorexia, respiratory distress, purulent ocular and nasal discharge, epileptic seizures, and coma before death in 4–7 days.

Four American badgers were experimentally infected by subcutaneous injection of fer-ret-passaged virus from a dog (Armstrong 1942) and another badger by facial spraying of distemperoid virus (Farrel 1957). Incubation periods ranged from 8 to 12 days. Clinical signs were similar to those described for the fox. Death occurred on the 12th–18th day PI.

Keymer and Epps (1969) described distemper in a colony of weasels and stoats (Table 3.1) characterized by reduced activity, photophobia, watery ocular discharge, hyperemic footpads, typical lesions around the nose and lip, and muscular spasms. The duration of illness was up to 12 weeks.

PATHOGENESIS. The spread of distemper virus in the host has been studied in the ferret, mink, and dog. Liu and Coffin (1957), using fluorescein-labeled antibody, traced the spread of the virus in ferrets after intranasal exposure to virulent virus. On the 2nd day PI, viral antigen was present in reticular cells of cervical lymph nodes. By the 3rd or 4th day, most of the cells of those lymph nodes contained antigen, as did the lymphoid tissue in other nodes and the spleen and mononuclear cells in peripheral blood smears. It was not until the 9th day PI that antigen appeared in epithelial cells of the respiratory, gastrointestinal, and urinary systems and in cutaneous tissue. Antigen appeared only in vascular endothelial cells of the brain in the two ferrets which survived to the 14th and 15th day.

Crook et al. (1958) and Crook and McNutt (1959) used ferrets to titrate virus from aerosol-infected mink and ferrets. Infective virus was present in nasal tissues, lung, spleen, and blood of ferrets on the 2nd day PI, and viremia continued until death on the 12th day PI. Viremia occurred in mink on the 3rd day and continued until after the 12th day, but virus titer fell rapidly after the 16th day. Crook and coworkers concluded that the respiratory epithelium was the primary site of multiplication of the virus but that all tissues eventually contained virus. Since virus appeared also in the liver, kidney, bladder, and brain soon after it appeared in the blood, they suggested that the virus was spread via the blood.

Appel (1969, 1970), using the direct fluorescent antibody (FA) technique, followed the development of distemper viral antigen in dogs. After aerosol exposure, antigen appeared in mononuclear cells of the bronchial lymph nodes at 2 days PI. Between the 2nd and 5th day PI viral antigen spread in blood leukocytes and appeared in most lymphatic tissues. By the 9th day PI reticuloendothelial type cells in connective tissue contained antigen, but only single epithelial cells were infected. Serum neutralizing antibody was present by the 8th or 9th day, and about 50% of dogs had rapid production of antibody. If the dog developed an antibody titer of 1:100 or greater early in the course of the disease, the virus could no longer be detected in tissues and clinical signs were usually lacking. If high serum neutralizing titer was not attained by the 14th day, the virus continued to spread, heavy viral infection was seen in epithelial cells, and the dog usually succumbed.

Because dogs with demyelinating encephalitis have higher serum and cerebrospinal fluid neutralizing antibodies than dogs that die early in the disease, Storts et al. (1974) postulated that virus invaded the brain early before antibody was present to prevent spread of virus. McMartin et al. (1972a,b) demonstrated enzyme activity associated with demyelination in the encephalitic form of distemper in dogs. Koestner et al. (1974) concluded that mutant forms of canine distemper virus were responsible for demyelination.

PATHOLOGY

Gross Pathology. With the exception of the skin, eye, and footpad lesions seen clinically, there are no pathognomonic gross lesions in distemper.

An enlarged spleen is common in distemper-infected mink and ferrets and was noted in all species examined by Monson and Stone (1976). Pinkerton et al. (1945) described lung lesions in mink ranging from congestion to consolidation either in patches or affecting whole lobes. Similar lesions were seen in ferrets (Dunkin and Laidlaw 1926; Sawada 1965). Reported also were lung congestion in skunks (Wade-Smith and Richmond 1975) and lung consolidation in weasels (Keymer and Epps 1969).

In ranch-raised foxes, jaundice, ulceration of mouth and tongue, lung consolidation, and enlarged spleens were mentioned (Allen and McLure 1926). Helmboldt and Jungherr (1955) noted pneumonia in wild foxes with distemper. Icterus of mucous membranes was seen in raccoon dogs (Sedgwick and Young 1968), in raccoons (Kilham and Herman 1954; Kilham et al. 1956), and in red foxes (Monson and Stone 1976). Wild raccoons with distemper had enlarged lymph nodes and pale, patchy consolidation of the lung (Karstad and Budd 1964). Black-footed ferrets had focal abscesses; areas of congestion, hemorrhage, and consolidation in the lung; inflammation of the trachea; subcap-

sular renal hemorrhages; hyperemia of kidney and bladder mucosa; and hemorrhage of the epicardium (Carpenter et al. 1976).

In the lesser panda, Bush et al. (1976) described depressed, grayish, firm areas in the lung and atrophy of lymph nodes. Pankov and Sytaya (1963) observed hyperemia and hemorrhage in the mucosa of the gastrointestinal and urinary system, necrotic foci on the heart, and splenic infarcts in distemper-infected sables.

Histopathology. Histopathologic lesions of distemper in the dog, fox, mink, and ferret are comparable. In mink focal pneumonitis was present with hyperplastic, often multinucleated histiocytes in alveolar walls. Giant cells containing both intranuclear and intracytoplasmic inclusion bodies were present in the lumen of alveoli and in bronchiolar epithelium (Pinkerton 1940; Pinkerton et al. 1945). Tajima et al. (1971) noted degeneration and necrosis of lymphoid cells and hyperplasia of reticular cells in lymph nodes of mink.

Inclusion bodies in fox, mink, and ferret have been described as variable in size, and as eosinophilic, spherical, or ovoid bodies that occasionally contain refractile particles. They are usually intracytoplasmic but may be intranuclear. They may be present in epithelial cells of the skin and the lining of the bronchial, gastrointestinal, biliary, and urinary tracts; in salivary and adrenal glands; in astrocytes of the central nervous system; and in the reticuloendothelial cells of lymph nodes and spleen (Crook and McNutt 1959, Green and Evans 1939b; Watson and Plummer 1942; Wisnicky and Wipf 1942).

Intranuclear inclusion bodies were seen in lymph nodes of infected wild foxes, skunks, and raccoons (Helmboldt and Jungherr 1955). Intranuclear inclusions were prominent in lymphoid follicles in the spleen of a wild bat-eared fox in Kenya (L. Karstad, personal communication, 1978). Crook and McNutt (1959) found necrosis in the spleen and lymph nodes in experimentally infected ferrets and in the spleen of mink. They postulated that destruction of lymphoid elements was responsible for the lethal effect of distemper virus.

In experimentally infected raccoons, Hoff et al. (1974) observed that germinal centers in the spleen lacked mature lymphocytes. In the black-footed ferret, there was lymphoid depletion in the spleen and necrosis of malpighian corpuscles and lymph sheaths surrounding arterioles. In one ferret there was myocardial degeneration and necrosis (Carpenter et al. 1976).

Several authors describing distemper in raccoons have noted lesions in the central nervous system, including a diffuse purulent encephalitis with intranuclear acidophilic inclusions in glial cells and histiocytes of the brain. Hoff et al. (1974) found diffuse focal areas of demyelination and malacia in the cerebrum and midbrain. Large gitter cells were seen in some sections and giant cells were present in areas of malacia. Eosinophilic intranuclear inclusions were found in glial cells in foci of demyelination and malacia. Pinkerton (1940) noted rare instances of focal collections of neuroglial cells and some demyelination in mink.

Bush et al. (1976) described interstitial pneumonia characterized by numerous syncytial giant cells containing intracytoplasmic eosinophilic inclusion bodies in a lesser panda, similar to the lesions reported in raccoons (Karstad and Budd 1964).

DIAGNOSIS. Clinical signs of distemper in species such as the mink, fox, and highly susceptible ferret may be sufficiently characteristic that a tentative diagnosis can be made; however, even in these cases the use of laboratory methods is essential for a confirmed diagnosis. Often gross signs of disease are lacking or nonspecific: sudden death with no previously recognized signs of illness are recorded in ranch-raised mink and foxes; mild signs of illness may remain unnoticed; and, especially in free-living wildlife, signs are variable and may resemble those seen in other diseases, for example, rabies in several species (Helmboldt and Jungherr 1955) and feline panleukopenia in the raccoon (Fowler and Theobald 1978). Shen and Gorham (1977) described a disease in ranch-raised mink that clinically resembled mink distemper but that failed to satisfy the usual criteria for confirmed diagnosis of mink distemper. Intracytoplasmic and less frequently intranuclear eosinophilic inclusion bodies in circulating leukocytes and in epithelial cells are considered to be pathognomonic for distemper. Stained smears from circulating blood or mucous membranes of conjunctiva, nasal mucosa, tongue, vagina, prepuce, and urethra have been used to attempt diagnosis in the living animal (Appel and Gillespie 1972), but the lack of inclusions in such samples does not necessarily rule out distemper infection. Inclusions may be present in small numbers in the early stages of distemper, and the success of the method may vary depending on the time postinfection and the antibody titer of the individual animal (Appel 1970).

The FA test was used by Liu and Coffin (1957) to demonstrate viral antigen in peripheral blood leukocytes of infected ferrets. Blood smears were positive if they were made even before the onset of fever and persisted until the ferret died. This was considered a simple, rapid diagnostic test for distemper. Appel (1969), using blood and conjunctival smears and cerebrospinal fluid from dogs, considered that success in diagnosing distemper using the FA test was related to antibody production by the animal. Antigen could be detected in circulating leukocytes at 2 days PI, but if the dog developed measurable antibody by the 9th day, viral antigen could no longer be detected. Viral antigen appeared in conjunctival and cerebrospinal fluid cells later than in leukocytes. Von Mickwitz and Schroder (1967) judged the FA test to be of greater value for distemper diagnosis than the finding of inclusion bodies, but inclusion bodies persisted longer than the fluorescence in cell culture, underlining the importance of timing.

Serum from infected mink and ferrets and egg-adapted distemper virus have been used in virus-neutralizing tests on the chorioallantoic membrane (CAM) of embryonating eggs (Baker et al. 1954). The paper disk method (Adams and Hanson 1956) for collecting sera for the virus neutralization test in embryonating eggs was utilized by Choquette and Kuyt (1974). Hansen (1971) used the virus neutralization test in cell-culture- and tissue-culture-adapted distemper virus to test the antibody response in vaccine trials in mink. Jamison et al. (1973) used embryonating eggs in virus neutralization tests in their serologic survey of wild raccoons and skunks for presence of distemper antibodies. A microneutralization test developed by Appel and Robson (1973) is as sensitive as the virus neutralization test on CAM and has the advantage of rapid results. Appel and Robson used cell culture attenuated virus and microtitration plates. Complement fixation tests using fox, ferret, raccoon, or skunk spleen as antigen have been utilized (Gorham 1960), but this test requires standardization before it can be used with confidence as a diagnostic tool in all wildlife.

Generally the ferret is used as a test animal. Conjunctival and nasal secretions or blood are inoculated into susceptible ferrets. If the test ferrets show the usual signs of distemper and histologic examination of ferret tissues reveals typical inclusions in epithelial cells, the diagnosis is confirmed. This is not a rapid test as it takes at least 10 days before a diagnosis can be made and isolation facilities are required for the test animals.

Ferret kidney cell cultures were used for virus isolation by Vantsis (1959) and Cornwell et al. (1965a,b), but the latter considered the living ferret to be more sensitive for detection of virus. Alveolar macrophage cultures from dogs and ferrets were shown to be susceptible to distemper virus (Appel and Jones 1967; Poste 1971). Intracytoplasmic inclusions appeared within 1–2 days, and giant cells were formed within 2 days.

The use of various cell cultures for the isolation of virulent distemper virus and a description of the cytopathogenic effect was reviewed by Appel and Gillespie (1972); those laboratory methods considered to be most practical for diagnosing distemper in the dog were reviewed by Wright et al. (1974). The success of the method employed depends largely on the time postinfection at which tests are attempted.

If death occurs, clinical diagnosis should be confirmed by histologic examination and detection of distemper inclusions in stained tissue sections and by reproduction of the disease in test animals or by the observation of a typical response in cell cultures with virus-containing tissue suspensions. The FA test may also be used. The use of cryostat sections may speed diagnosis. Kristensen and Vandevelde (1978) used cryostat sections as well as cold alcohol fixation on dog brains for the FA technique in diagnosing distemper. Phase microscopy was used to identify distemper inclusions in unstained sections (Angulo et al. 1949).

In diagnosing distemper in a free-living wild species, the ferret as test animal is particularly useful. Ground lung, spleen, or other suitable tissues from frozen or partly decomposed specimens, which are unfit for histopathologic examination because inclusion bodies cannot be identified in the fragmented cells, may be suspended in antibiotic-treated saline as the inoculum. Under these circumstances, inoculated ferrets should be kept under observation for an extended period of time. Ferrets injected with tissues from distemper-suspect wolves and coyotes did not show gross signs of distemper, confirmed by histologic examination, until 30 or more days after exposure (L. Karstad, personal communication, 1961).

Stains used for identification of distemper inclusion bodies in smears or tissue sections include hematoxylin and eosin (Green and Evans 1939a), Shorr's S_3 modified stain (Page and Green 1942), or Pollak's trichrome method (Gorham 1948). Inclusion bodies may be small,

sparse, and poorly stained in tissues from animals in the early stages of distemper. Generally, if the animal is moribund and sufficient tissues are examined, typical inclusion bodies will be found. In foxes, mink, and ferrets, inclusion bodies are present in the transitional epithelium of the urinary tract in a high percentage of fatal cases. In raccoons, Karstad and Budd (1964) found inclusion bodies most frequently in bronchial epithelium and in the multinucleate giant cells of the lungs. Similar findings in mink were reported by Pinkerton (1940). For routine diagnosis in the dog, Dobos-Kovacs (1975) recommended examination of sections from urinary bladder, lung, the third eyelid, stomach, cerebellum, and Ammon's horn.

Differential Diagnosis. Eosinophilic bodies resembling distemper inclusions have been reported in normal animals (Watson and Plummer 1942), in foxes with bladder trouble (Wisnicky and Wipf 1942), and in mink with plasmacytosis. Karstad (1964) differentiated such inclusions in mink with plasmacytosis from distemper inclusions by the periodic acid-Schiff (PAS) staining technique. Distemper inclusion bodies did not stain by this method, but the nonspecific inclusions were PAS positive.

In fox encephalitis, clinical signs resemble those of the nervous form of distemper, although fox encephalitis is generally more acute. The inclusion bodies of fox encephalitis are always intranuclear and are found in endothelial cells, particularly in the meninges of the brain and in the liver where they occur also in hepatic and Kupffer cells but not in bile duct epithelium (Green and Evans 1939b). Hunt et al. (1963) found that the inclusion bodies of infectious canine hepatitis were DNA positive, but distemper inclusions were not.

Wild animals exhibiting abnormal behavior, if found to be free of rabies, should be examined for the inclusion bodies characteristic of distemper (Haberman et al. 1958; Helmboldt and Jungherr 1955; Hoff et al. 1974).

Toxoplasmosis in mink may be manifested by signs similar to those of the nervous form of distemper (Pridham and Belcher 1958). Concurrent distemper and toxoplasma infections, which have been reported in mink (Innes and Saunders 1962; Momberg-Jorgensen 1956); fox, raccoon, and skunk (Diters and Nielsen 1978; Moller and Nielsen 1964; Robinson et al. 1957); and Cape hunting dog (Hofmeyer 1956) present a problem in clinical diagnosis.

Other diseases in wildlife in which the

clinical signs may resemble distemper include tularemia and listeriosis (Jakowski and Wyand 1971), Chastek's paralysis in the captive mink and fox, and histoplasmosis in raccoons (Menges et al. 1955).

PROGNOSIS. Prognosis is generally poor for distemper-infected animals. In susceptible mink populations, mortality ranges from 20% to 90%. Pastel mink, thought to have higher mortality from distemper, were tested by Hansen et al. (1973) and were found to be similar to dark mink in their immunologic capabilities. Distemper in the ferret is usually fatal. The mortality in ranch-raised foxes is similar to that in mink (Watson et al. 1933). The mortality in experimentally infected raccoons was 50% (Kilham and Herman 1954).

IMMUNITY. The history of early vaccine production, the modification of the distemper virus by serial passage in various hosts, and the use of these modified strains as immunizing agents have been reviewed by Gorham (1960) and Appel and Gillespie (1972).

The age at which young animals should be vaccinated to produce an immunity to distemper depends on the immune status of the dam, the passive transfer of immunity to the offspring, and the length of time that this immunity persists in the offspring.

Ferrets. From the work of Ott and Gorham (1955) and Ott et al. (1965), it appears that ferrets from nonimmune dams are capable of producing distemper virus-neutralizing antibody as early as 8 days after birth. Because passive immunity conferred by the dam apparently inhibits this capability for a period of up to 6 weeks, it is evident also that young ferrets from immune dams should not be vaccinated before they are about 6 weeks of age. When ferret-tissue-origin killed virus vaccines were used, resistance to challenge could not be detected until at least 7 days after vaccination, and the protection was only about 75% effective (Ott et al. 1959). In comparison, chicken-embryo-adapted live virus distemper vaccines attenuated for ferrets have protected them from challenge with an infective dose of virulent virus within 48 hours after vaccination (Baker et al. 1952). Effective immunity is produced in a high percentage of ferrets and lasts for the life of the animal (Burger and Gorham 1964). Some modified live virus vaccines used for immunizing dogs are virulent for ferrets (AVMA 1966); therefore, only an egg-adapted or tissue-cul-

ture-origin vaccine that has been shown to be avirulent for ferrets should be used. Vaccines of this type produced for immunizing mink have been used successfully for immunizing ferrets.

Live virus vaccines are effective immunizing agents only when stored and handled according to the manufacturer's directions.

Mink. Attenuated live virus vaccines, either chicken embryo or tissue culture origin, are produced for immunizing mink. These have replaced the killed virus vaccines formerly in use. To ensure that passive immunity acquired from the mother does not interfere with antibody production, mink kits from immune dams should not be vaccinated until 8–10 days after they are weaned. Gorham et al. (1962) found that mink kits from hyperimmune dams failed to produce effective immunity until they were 10–12 weeks of age. They did not state whether these kits were weaned. On some establishments, mink kits are weaned 5–6 weeks after birth and should be protected from distemper soon after weaning. Ideally, mink retained for breeding stock should be revaccinated during the early months of the year (January or February) to boost the immune status of the dams. Pregnant female mink and ferrets have been vaccinated with egg-adapted live virus vaccines without detrimental effect on the offspring (Hagen et al. 1970). This procedure is not recommended unless it is necessary in the event of an epizootic of distemper.

Fox. Fox pups from immune dams should be immunized at a time comparable to that recommended for dogs (AVMA 1966, 1970) or mink, that is, after weaning. Although the ferret-adapted live virus vaccine of Green (1939) has been used widely to immunize ranch-raised foxes, there is evidence that some clinical signs of disease may follow its use; therefore it may be wise to adopt the recommendation suggested for the dog and use attenuated live virus vaccine of chicken embryo or tissue culture origin. Gorham (1957) found that the duration of immunity in the fox was 2 years after the use of egg-propagated virus vaccine. An annual booster should be given to breeding stock or display animals, as recommended for mink and dogs.

Application of the aerosol technique for the vaccination of ranch-raised mink, ferrets, and foxes (Ackerman and Kruger 1971; Hagen and Gorham 1970; Kull et al. 1970) is widely accepted. This method avoids the handling of individual animals, an advantage especially when distemper virus is present on the premises; it also speeds the operation. Its use could be adapted to other captive species that are housed in family units.

Other Wildlife. Some of the recommendations adopted by the panel of the symposium on canine distemper immunization as guidelines for vaccination of dogs (AVMA 1970) and the review of prevention by Appel and Gillespie (1972) may be useful as a guide for immunization of closely related species of wildlife. Sedgwick and Young (1968) recommended live virus vaccine to protect susceptible animals in zoological collections. They report the use of a tissue-culture-origin, modified live canine distemper vaccine, without producing clinical signs in species from each of the Canidae, Mustelidae, Procyanidae, and Viverridae families. Miller (1971) noted the successful use of tissue-culture-origin live virus distemper vaccines on several raccoons, two coatis, and one kinkajou. K. Mehrin, (personal communication, 1978) reported the routine use of modified live virus distemper vaccine, canine cell culture origin, for Canidae, Mustelidae, and Viverridae, beginning at 7−8 weeks and repeated every 2 weeks until the young are 12 weeks of age. Thereafter annual boosters are given. Fowler and Theobold (1978) stated that modified live virus vaccines have been used on most of the carnivores commonly exhibited. They recommended distemper immunization for Canidae, Procyonidae, and Hyaenidae but qualified this for Mustelidae and Viverridae. Caution should be observed in the use of live virus vaccines. The recent accounts of distemper in the black-footed ferret (Carpenter et al. 1976) and in the lesser panda (Bush et al. 1976) following the use of live virus distemper vaccine emphasize the dangers inherent in its use for some species. Rosendal and Rasmussen (1970) tested various vaccines and found that the ability of a vaccine to produce a serologic response varied with the property of the vaccine and the animal species. Reculard and Guillon (1972) emphasized the variation in biological behavior of strains of distemper virus. Erken and Jacobi (1972) suggested that killed distemper vaccine or measles vaccine be used to protect the lesser panda instead of live virus vaccines; however, neither has been shown to provide protection in the panda. Fisher (1971) recommended the use of killed distemper vaccines for skunks. Sedgwick (1971) suggested caution in the use of inactivated distemper vaccines for exotic pets as they may fail to provide protection.

Adams and Imagawa (1957), using measles virus in ferrets, noted some immunity, but Gorski (1973) reported that measles virus failed to provide protection from challenge in polecat ferrets, mink, and foxes. Gorham et al. (1957) demonstrated the multiplication of virus in ferret, mink, and fox following vaccination with egg-adapted virus. Obviously there is no absolute rule concerning the vaccination of captive wildlife either in zoological collections or as single individuals. If there is no precedent for use of live virus vaccines in the broad guidelines supplied by those with experience, the use of inactivated virus vaccine should be considered (if such is available), and the decision to vaccinate should be weighed in terms of the risk of exposure.

TREATMENT. Treatment is not recommended in ranch-raised mink or ferrets. In the face of an outbreak of distemper, ideally all animals showing signs of illness should be destroyed. Immediate vaccination of all apparently unaffected animals, using a modified live virus vaccine, egg-adapted or tissue culture origin, suitable for the species often will control the disease (Hartsough and Gorham 1953). The use of aerosol vaccination in these outbreaks is recommended (Hagen et al. 1970; Hansen and Lund 1976; Kull et al. 1970). However, it is impossible to detect those animals which are in the early incubation stages of distemper, and although experimentally Burger and Gorham (1964) were able to show some protection when attenuated virus vaccine was administered 2 days after challenge with virulent virus, they did note variation in results depending on the ratio of the number of immunizing doses to lethal doses administered. In an outbreak it may be 8 or 10 days before clinical signs are evident; therefore, it is impossible to estimate the number of animals infected, and vaccination after infection generally fails to alter the course of the disease (Farrell et al. 1958). Green and Stulberg (1946) reported protection in foxes when the ferret-passaged virus was administered as late as 12 days after virulent virus, but one must be cautious in anticipating this effect.

There is no known cure for distemper. Canine antiserum (or globulin) has been used in the treatment of dogs but is thought to be of little value if there are clinical signs of distemper (AVMA 1966, 1970). There are reports of its use to protect unvaccinated animals in zoological collections and on fox ranches, but experimental data on its efficacy are lacking.

The use of diethyl ether as a therapeutic measure in distemper-infected dogs was reviewed by Womer (1973). Isoprinosine failed to alter the course of distemper in ferrets (Glasgow and Galasso 1972). Stalling (1974) suggested that therapy for distemper-infected dogs should attempt to control secondary bacterial infections and generally improve the health of the animal.

CONTROL. In a collection of distemper-susceptible animals, control of distemper may be achieved by:

1. Preventing contact with the virus. All animals to be added to the collection should be quarantined before they contact the resident population. Vaccination of the new resident should be achieved during this quarantine period. All equipment capable of carrying virus should be cleaned and disinfected before reuse. Distemper virus was inactivated by heat, formalin, and roccal in tests by Dickson et al. (1955).
2. Protection by immunization. The importance of implementing a suitable immunization program, as outlined above, should be stressed.

Control in free-living, distemper-susceptible wild animals is achieved naturally when the opportunity for transmission of the virus is limited. This may occur during an epizootic when the lethal effect of the virus results in a lowered population density.

REFERENCES

Ackerman, O., and Kruger, A. The application and testing of Candur D. distemper aerosol vaccine for mink under practical conditions. *Vet. Blue Book* 19:8, 1971.

Adams, E., and Hanson, R. P. A procedure for adsorbing virus neutralizing antibodies on paper discs. *J. Bacteriol.* 72:572, 1956.

Adams, J. M., and Imagawa, D. T. Immunological relationship between measles and distemper virus. *Proc. Soc. Exp. Biol. Med.* 96:240, 1957.

Allen, J. A., and McLure, W. C. S. *Theory and practice of fox ranching.* Charlottetown, PEI: Irwin Printing Co., 1926.

American Veterinary Medical Association. Conclusions and recommendations of the panel of the symposium on canine distemper immunization. *J. Am. Vet. Med. Assoc.* 149:714, 1966.

———. Symposium on immunity to selected canine infectious diseases. *J. Am. Vet. Med. Assoc.* 156:175, 1970.

Andrews, C., Pereira, H. G., and Wildy, P. *Viruses of vertebrates.* London: Bailliere, Tindall, 1978.

Angulo, J. J., Richards, O. W., and Roque, A. L. Demonstration of viral inclusion bodies in unstained tissue sections with the aid of the phase microscope. *J. Bacteriol.* 57:297, 1949.

Anon. Susceptibility of the lesser panda to canine distemper: Veterinary work and zoological research. *Int. Zoo Year Book,* 2:107, 1960.

Anon. Canine distemper prophylaxis. In Smithsonian Institute National Zoological Park Report for the year ending June 30, 1968, p. xix. Washington, D.C. Smithsonian Institute, 1968.

Appel, M. J. G. Pathogenesis of canine distemper. *Am. J. Vet. Res.* 30:1167, 1969.

———. Distemper pathogenesis in dogs. *J. Am. Vet. Med. Assoc.* 156:1681, 1970.

Appel, M. J. G., and Gillespie, J. H. Canine distemper virus. In *Virology Monographs,* vol. 11. New York: Springer-Verlag, 1972.

Appel, M. J. G., and Jones, O. R. Use of alveolar macrophages for cultivation of canine distemper virus. *Proc. Soc. Exp. Biol. Med.* 126:571, 1967.

Appel, M. J. G., and Robson, D. S. A microneutralization test for canine distemper virus. *Am. J. Vet. Res.* 34:1459, 1973.

Appel, M., Sheffy, B. E., Percy, D. H., and Gaskin, J. M. Canine distemper virus in domesticated cats and pigs. *Am. J. Vet. Res.* 35:803, 1974.

Armstrong, W. H. Canine distemper in the American badger. *Cornell Vet.* 32:447, 1942.

Armstrong, W. H., and Anthony, C. G. An epizootic of canine distemper in a zoological park. *Cornell Vet.* 32:286, 1942.

Baker, G. A., Gorham, J. R., and Leader, R. W. Studies on an *in ovo* neutralization test for distemper. *Am. J. Vet. Res.* 15:102, 1954.

Baker, G. A., Leader, R. W., and Gorham, J. R. Immune reponse of ferrets to vaccination with egg-adapted distemper virus: I. Time of development of resistance to virulent distemper virus. *Vet. Med.* 47:463, 1952.

Belcher, J. Certain characteristics of egg-adapted strains of distemper virus. M. S. thesis, University of Wisconsin, 1951.

Blair, W. R. Report of the veterinarian. 12th Ann. Rep. N.Y. Zool. Soc. p. 119, Bronx, N.Y.: New York Zoological Society, 1907.

———. Report of the veterinarian. 14th Ann. Rep. N.Y. Zool. Soc. p. 89, Bronx, N.Y.: New York Zoological Society, 1909.

———. Report of the veterinarian. 21st Ann. Rep. N.Y. Zool. Soc. p. 79, Bronx, N.Y.: New York Zoological Society, 1916.

———. Report of the veterinarian. 26th Ann. Rep. N.Y. Zool. Soc. p. 80, Bronx, N.Y.: New York Zoological Society, 1921.

———. Report of the veterinarian. 27th Ann. Rep. N.Y. Zool. Soc. p. 53, Bronx, N.Y.: New York Zoological Society, 1922.

Burger, D., and Gorham, J. R. Response of ferrets and mink to vaccination with chicken embryo adapted distemper virus: II. Interference phenomenon and duration of resistance. *Arch. Ges. Virusforsch.* 14:449, 1964.

Bush, M., Montali, R. J., Brownstein, D., James A. E., Jr., and Appel, M. J. G. Vaccine-induced canine distemper in a lesser panda. *J. Am. Vet. Med. Assoc.* 169:959, 1976.

Cabasso, V. J. Discussion: The epizootiology of distemper. *J. Am. Vet. Med. Assoc.* 149:618, 1966.

Cabasso, V. J., Schroeder, C. R., and Stebbins, M. R. Isolation of distemper virus from the South American maned wolf (*Chrysocyon jubatus*). *Vet. Med.* 51:330, 1956.

Carpenter, J. W., Appel, M. J. G., Ericson, R. C., and Novilla, M. N. Fatal vaccine-induced canine distemper virus infection in black-footed ferrets. *J. Am. Vet. Med. Assoc.* 69:961, 1976.

Carre, H. Sur la maladie des jeunes chiens. *C. R. Acad. Sci.* 140:689, 1489, 1905. Cited by J. R. Gorham. Canine distemper (la maladie de Carre). *Ad. Vet. Sci.* 6:287, 1960.

Choquette, L. P. E.., and Kuyt, E. Serological indication of canine distemper and of infectious canine hepatitis in wolves (*Canis lupus* L.) in northern Canada. *J. Wild. Dis.* 10:321, 1974.

Confer, A. W., Kahn, D. E., Koestner, A., and Krakowka, S. Properties of a canine distemper virus isolate associated with demyelinating encephalitis. *Infec. Immun.* 11:835, 1975a.

———. Comparison of canine distemper viral strains. An electron microscopic study. *Am. J. Vet. Res.* 36:741, 1975b.

Cornwell, H. J. C., Campbell, R. S. F., Vantsis, S. T., and Penny, W. Studies on experimental canine distemper: I. Clinico-pathological findings. *J. Comp. Pathol. Ther.* 75:3, 1965a.

———. Studies in experimental canine distemper: II. Virology, inclusion body studies and hematology. *J. Comp. Pathol. Ther.* 75:19, 1965b.

Crandall, L. S. *Management of wild mammals in captivity.* Chicago: University of Chicago Press, 1964.

Crook, E., Gorham, J. R., and McNutt, S. H. Experimental distemper in mink and ferrets: I. Pathogenesis. *Am. J. Vet. Res.* 19:955, 1958.

Crook, E., and McNutt, S. H. Experimental distemper in mink and ferrets: III. Appearance and significance of histopathological changes. *Am. J. Vet. Res.* 20:378, 1959.

Dalling, T. Distemper in the fitch. *Vet. Rec.* 2:1051, 1931.

Dickson, M. E., Dickson, W. M., and Gorham, J. R. The pH stability of the Wisconsin FXNO strain of egg-adapted distemper virus. *Am. J. Vet. Res.* 16:616, 1955.

Diters, R. W., and Nielsen, S. W. Toxoplasmosis, distemper and herpes virus infection in a skunk (*Mephitis mephitis*). *J. Wild. Dis.* 14:132, 1978.

Dobos-Kovacs, M. Studies on the diagnostic value of cell inclusions in canine distemper. *Acta Vet. Acad. Sci. Hung.* 25:185, 1975.

Dobrich, D. Staupe beim Wolf. *Tieraerztl. Zentr.* 12:83, 1904. Cited in P. O. C. Halloran. A bibliography of references to diseases of wild mammals and birds. *Am. J. Vet. Res.* 16(pt. 2): 139. 1955.

Dunkin, G. W., and Laidlaw, P. P. I. Dog distemper in the ferret. II. Experimental distemper in the dog. *J. Comp. Pathol. Ther.* 39:201, 1926.

Erken, A. H. M., and Jacobi, E. F. Successful breeding of lesser panda (*Ailurus fulgens* F. Cuvier, 1825) and loss through inoculation. *Bijdr. Dierko.* 42:92, 1972.

Farrell, R. K. The susceptibility of the American badger to Green's distemperoid vaccine. *West. Vet.* 4:61, 1957.

Farrell, R. K., Ott, R. L., and Gorham, J. R. The failure of egg-propagated distemper virus to interfere with experimental neurotopic distemper in mink. *J. Am. Vet. Med. Assoc.* 133:269, 1958.

Fiennes, R. N. T. W. Report of the pathologist for the year 1960. *Proc. Zool. Soc. London* 137:179, 1961.

Fischer, K. Staupe-Encephalitis bei Dachsen. *Schweiz. Arch. Tierheilkd.* 107:87, 1965. Cited in M. J. G. Appel and J. H. Gillespie. Canine distemper virus. *Virology Monographs,* vol. 2. New York: Springer-Verlag, 1972.

Fisher, L. E. Skunks. In R. W. Kirk, ed. *Current veterinary therapy small animal practice,* vol. 4. Toronto: W. B. Saunders, p. 456, 1971.

Fowler, M. E., and Theobold, J. Immunizing procedures. In M. E. Fowler, ed. *Zoo and wild animal medicine,* p. 63. Toronto: W. B. Saunders, 1978.

Fox, H. *Disease in captive wild mammals and birds.* Philadelphia: Lippincott, 1923.

Gier, H. T., and Ameel, D. J. Parasites and diseases of Kansas coyotes. *Kan. Agr. Station Tech. Bull.* 91:27, 1959.

Glasgow, L. A., and Galasso, G. J. Isoprinosine: Lack of antiviral activity in experimental model infections. *J. Infec. Dis.* 126:162, 1972.

Gorham, J. R. Pollack's trichrome stain for demonstrating distemper inclusion bodies in tissue sections. *Science* 107:175, 1948.

———. Diseases and parasites of foxes. In *Yearbook of agriculture.* Washington, D.C.: USDA, 1956.

———. Egg propagated distemper virus. *Vet. Med.* 52:33, 1957.

———. Canine distemper (La maladie de Carre). *Adv. Vet. Sci.* 6:287, 1960.

———. The epizootiology of distemper. *J. Am. Vet. Med. Assoc.* 149:610, 1966.

Gorham, J. R., and Brandly, C. A. The transmission of distemper among ferrets and mink. *Proc. 90th Ann. Meeting Am. Vet. Med. Assoc.,* p. 129. Chicago: American Veterinary Medical Association, 1953.

Gorham, J. R., Farrell, R., and Lauerman, L. Immunologic response of young mink. *Vet. Med.* 57:896, 1962.

Gorham, J. R., Farrell, R. K., Ott, R. L., and Parisot, T. Multiplication of attenuated egg-adapted distemper virus in the vaccinated host. *Vet. Med.* 52:289, 1957.

Gorski, J. Attempts at obtaining an assessment of the efficacy of a heterologous (measles) vaccine against distemper. *Polarch. Weter.* 16:121, 1973.

Goss, L. J. Mammals: Hospital and laboratory. *47th Ann. Rept. N.Y. Zool. Soc.,* p. 10. Bronx, N.Y.:

New York Zoological Society, 1942.

———. Species susceptibility to the viruses of Carre and feline enteritis. *Am. J. Vet. Res.* 9:65, 1948.

Green, R. G. Distemper in the silver fox (*Vulpes vulpes*). *Proc. Soc. Exp. Biol. Med.* 22:546, 23:677, 1925.

———. Modification of distemper virus. *J. Am. Vet. Med. Assoc.* 95:465, 1939.

Green, R. G., and Evans, C. A. Rapid diagnosis of canine distemper. *Cornell Vet.* 29:35, 1939a.

———. A comparative study of distemper inclusions. *Am. J. Hyg.* 29:73, 1939b.

Green, R. G., and Stulberg, C. S. Cell blockade in canine distemper. *Proc. Soc. Exp. Biol. Med.* 61:117, 1946.

Grunberg, W. Zur staupe bei Polarhund und Dingo. *Dtsch. tierarztl. Wschr.* 66:444, 1959. Cited in M. J. G. Appel and J. H. Gillespie. Canine distemper virus. *Virology Monographs*, vol. 2. New York: Springer-Verlag, 1972.

Haberman, R. T., Herman, C. M., and Williams, F. P. Distemper in raccoons and foxes suspected of having rabies. *J. Am. Vet. Med. Assoc.* 132:31, 1958.

Hagen, K., and Gorham, J. Distemper control by aerosol vaccination. *U.S. Fur Rancher* 49:15, 1970.

Hagen, K. W., Goto, H., and Gorham, J. R. Distemper vaccine in pregnant ferrets and mink. *Res. Vet. Sci.* 11:458, 1970.

Hamerton, A. E. Diseases due to infection. *Proc. Zool. Soc. Lond.* 107(B):443, 1937.

———. Report on deaths occurring in the society's gardens during 1944. *Proc. Zool. Soc. Lond.* 115:371, 1945.

Hansen, M. The antibody response and the protection obtained by using different types of (distemper) vaccines in two genotypes of mink. *Nord. Vet. Med.* 23:374, 1971.

Hansen, M., Jacobsen, P., and Lund, E. Comparative distemper vaccine titrations in ferrets and minks. *Nord. Vet. Med.* 25:1, 1973.

Hansen, M., and Lund, E. Prophylactic, postinfectious and neonatal vaccination against canine distemper in mink. *Nord. Vet. Med.* 28:585, 1976.

Hartsough, G. R., and Gorham, J. R. Control of distemper in mink. *J. Am. Vet. Med. Assoc.* 122:383, 1953.

Heath, L. M., and Plummer, P. J. G. Distemper studies in foxes: Maintenance of virulence of distemper virus for foxes. *Can. J. Comp. Med. Vet. Sci.* 7:306, 1943.

Helmboldt, C. F., and Jungherr, E. L. Distemper complex in wild carnivores simulating rabies. *Am. J. Vet. Res.* 16:463, 1955.

Hobley, C. W. Wildlife and disease. *J. Soc. Preserv. Fauna Emp.* 16:16, 1932. Cited P. O'C. Halloran. A bibliography of references to diseases of wild mammals and birds. *Am. J. Vet. Res.* 16:2, 1955.

Hoff, G. L., Bigler, W. J., Proctor, S. J., and Stalling, L. P. Epizootic of canine distemper virus infection among urban raccoons and gray foxes. *J. Wild. Dis.* 10:423, 1974.

Hofmeyer, C. F. B. 284 autopsies at the National Zoological Gardens, Pretoria. *J. S. Afr. Vet. Med. Assoc.* 27:263, 1956.

Hunt, R. D., Farrell, J. F., Thompson, S. W., and Walton, G. A histochemical comparison of the inclusion bodies of canine distemper and infectious canine hepatitis. *Am. J. Vet. Res.* 24:1248, 1963.

Innes, J. R. M., and Saunders, L. Z. *Comparative neuropathology*. New York: Academic Press, 1962.

Jamison, R. K., Lazar, E. C., Binn, L. N., and Alexander, A. D. Survey for antibodies to canine viruses in selected wild mammals. *J. Wild. Dis.* 9:2, 1973.

Jakowski, R. M., and Wyand, D. S. Listeriosis associated with canine distemper in a gray fox. *J. Am. Vet. Med. Assoc.* 159:626, 1971.

———. Viral plasmacytosis (Aleutian disease) in mink: IV. Cytoplasmic glycoprotein inclusions and their differentiation from the viral inclusions of distemper. *Can. J. Comp. Med. Vet. Sci.* 28:143, 1964.

Karstad, L., and Budd, J. Distemper in raccoons characterized by giant cell pneumonitis. *Can. Vet. J.* 5:326, 1964.

Keymer, I. F., and Epps, H. B. G. Canine distemper in the family Mustelidae. *Vet. Rec.* 85:204, 1969.

Kilham, L., Habermann, R. T., and Herman, C. M. Jaundice and bilirubinemia as manifestations of canine distemper in raccoons and ferrets. *Am. J. Vet. Res.* 17:144, 1956.

Kilham, L., and Herman, C. M. Isolation of an agent causing bilirubinemia and jaundice in raccoons. *Proc. Soc. Exp. Biol. Med.* 85:272, 1954.

Kirk, H. *Canine distemper: Its complications sequelae and treatment*. London: Bailliere, Tyndall and Cox, 1922.

Koestner, A., McCullough, B., Krakowka, G. S., Long, J. F., and Olsen, R. G. Canine distemper: A virus-induced demyelinating encephalomyelitis. In W. Zeman and E. H. Lennette, eds. *Slow virus diseases*. Baltimore: Williams and Wilkins, p. 86, 1974.

Krakowka, S., Hoover, E. A., Koestner, A., and Ketring, K. Transplacental infection with C.D.V. in the dog: Experimental and naturally occurring transplacental transmission of canine distemper virus. *Am. J. Vet. Res.* 38:919, 1977.

Kristensen, B., and Vandevelde, M. Immunofluorescence studies of canine distemper encephalitis on paraffin-embedded tissue. *Am. J. Vet. Res.* 39:1017, 1978.

Kull, K-E., Svensson, T., and Ackerman, O. Immunization trials with aerosol vaccine against distemper in mink in Sweden. *Nord. Vet. Med.* 22:13, 1970.

Liu, C., and Coffin, D. L. Studies on canine distemper infection by means of fluorescein-labelled antibody: I. The pathogenesis, pathology and diagnosis of the disease in experimentally infected ferrets. *Virology* 3:115, 1957.

McMartin, D. N., Horrocks, L. A., and Koestner, A.

Enzyme activities associated with the demyelinating phase of canine distemper: II. Plasmalogenase. *Acta Neuropathol.* 22:288, 1972b.

McMartin, D. N., Koestner, A., and Lond, J. F. Enzyme activities associated with the demyelinating phase of canine distemper: I. Beta-glucuronidase acid and neutral proteinases. *Acta Neuropathol.* 22:275, 1972a.

Martinaglia, G. Some considerations regarding the health of wild animals in captivity. *S. Afr. J. Sci.* 33:833, 1937. Cited in W. H. Armstrong and C. G. Anthony, an epizootic of canine distemper in a zoological park. *Cornell Vet.* 32:286, 1942.

Menges, R. W., Habermann, R. T., and Stains, H. J. A distemper-like disease in raccoons and isolation of *Histoplasma capsulatum* and *Haplosporangium parvum. Trans. Kans. Acad. Sci.* 58:1, 1955.

Miller, R. M. Raccoons, kinkajous and coatis. In R. W. Kirk, ed. *Current veterinary therapy:* IV. *Small animal practice.* Toronto: W. B. Saunders, p. 457, 1971.

Moller, T., and Nielsen, S. W. Toxoplasmosis in distemper susceptible carnivora. *Pathol. Vet.* 1:189, 1964.

Momberg-Jorgensen, H. C. Simultaneous infection: Distemper-toxoplasmosis in mink. *Nord. Vet. Med.* 8:239, 1956.

Monson, R. A. and Stone, W. B. Canine distemper in wild carnivores in New York. *N.Y. Fish Game J.* 23:149, 1976.

Muller, R. M. Modern veterinary practice reference and data service H-2-64 1962. Cited in M. J. G. Appel and J. H. Gillespie, Canine distemper virus. *Virology Monographs,* vol. 11. New York: Springer-Verlag, 1972.

Noback, C. V. Report of the veterinarian. *33rd Ann. Rept. N.Y. Zool. Soc.* p. 43. Bronx, N.Y.: New York Zoological Society, 1929.

Ott, R. L. Introduction to the symposium on canine distemper immunization. *J. Am. Vet. Med. Assoc.* 149:607, 1966.

Ott, R. L., and Gorham, J. R. The response of newborn and young ferrets to intranasal administration with egg-adapted distemper virus. *Am. J. Vet. Res.* 16:571, 1955.

Ott, R. L., Gorham, J. R., and Farrell, R. K. A note on the use of adjuvated vaccines in ferrets. *Can. J. Comp. Med. Vet. Sci.* 29:214, 1965.

Ott, R. L., Gorham, J. R., and Gutierrez, J. C. Distemper in dogs: I. Virus neutralizing antibodies in serum collected from healthy dogs. *J. Am. Vet. Med. Assoc.* 126:299, 1955.

Ott, R. L., Svehag, S. E., and Burger, D. Resistance to experimental distemper in ferrets following the use of killed tissue vaccine. *West. Vet.* 6:107, 1959.

Page, W. G., and Green, R. G. An improved diagnostic stain for distemper inclusions. *Cornell Vet.* 32:265, 1942.

Pankov, C. A., and Sytaya, A. S. Distemper in sables (Chuma u sobolei). *Krolikovod. Zverovod.* 6:28, 1963. Abstr. *Biol. Abstr.* 45:29794, 1964.

Parent, A. Ueber Stauepe bei Jungen Woelfen. *Rev. Vet.* 1908:307, 1906. Cited in P. O'C. Haloran. A bibliography of references to diseases of wild mammals and birds. *Am. J. Vet. Res.* 16(pt.2):139, 1955.

Parker, R. L., Cabasso, V. J., Dean, D. J., and Cheatum, E. L. Serologic evidence of certain virus infections in wild animals. *J. Am. Vet. Med. Assoc.* 138:437, 1961.

Pinkerton, H. Immunological and histological studies on mink distemper. *J. Am. Vet. Med. Assoc.* 96:347, 1940.

Pinkerton, H., Smiley, W. L., and Anderson, W. A. D. Giant cell pneumonia: A lesion common to Hecht's disease, distemper and measles. *Am. J. Pathol.* 21:1, 1945.

Poste, H. The growth and cytopathogenicity of virulent and attenuated strains of canine distemper in dog and ferret macrophages. *J. Comp. Pathol.* 81:49, 1971.

Pridham, T. J., and Belcher, J. Toxoplasmosis in mink. *Can. J. Comp. Med. Vet. Sci.* 22:99, 1958.

Reculard, P., and Guillon, J. C. Experimental study of individual strains of dog distemper virus: Identification and definition of variant strains. *Ann. Inst. Pasteur* 123:477, 1972.

Rewell, R. E. Report of the pathologist for the year 1947. *Proc. Zool. Soc. London* 118:501, 1947.

Risser, A. C., Jr. A study of the coati mundi *Nasua narica* in southern Arizona. Master's thesis, University of Arizona, 1963. Cited in J. H. Kaufman, D. V. Lanning, and S. E. Poole, Current status and distribution of the coati in the United States. *J. Mammal.* 57:621, 1976.

Robinson, V. B., Newberne, J. W., and Brooks, D. M. Distemper in the American raccoon (*Procyon lotor*). *J. Am. Vet. Med. Assoc.* 131:276, 1957.

Rosendal, S., and Rasmussen, P. G. Antibody response in mink, ferret and dog with different distemper vaccines. *Nord. Vet. Med.* 22:329, 1970.

Rudolph, S. Bietrag zur staupe beim Silberfuchs, nerz und Waschbaren. *Dtsch. Tierarztl. Wschr.* 38:728, 1930. Cited in M. J. G. Appel and J. H. Gillespie, Canine distemper virus. *Virology Monographs,* vol. 11. New York: Springer-Verlag, 1972.

Sawada, M. Pathological studies on canine distemper: I. Histopathological changes in ferrets infected with experimental canine distemper. *Jap. J. Vet. Sci.* 27:121, 1965.

Sedgwick, C. J. A clinical view of exotic pet practice. *J. Zool. Anim. Med.* 2:5, 1971.

Sedgwick, C. J., and Young, W. A. Distemper outbreak in a zoo. *Mod. Vet. Prac.* 49:39, 1968.

Shaw, R. N. Distemper in minks. *Vet. Med.* 27:511, 1932.

Shen, D. T., and Gorham, J. R. A disease resembling mink distemper. *Vet. Med. Small Anim. Clin.* 72:935, 1977.

Shillinger, J. E. *Diseases of fur animals.* U.S. Dept. Int. Fish and Wildlife Serv. Conserv. Bull. 20. Washington, D.C.: U.S. Government Printing Office, 1942.

Stalling, E. P. Canine distemper therapy. In R. W. Kirk, ed., *Current veterinary therapy*, 5th ed. Toronto: W. B. Saunders, 1974.

Storts, R. W., Boenig, D. M., and Johnson, W. D. Canine distemper: The present status of the disease including some new considerations concerning its pathogenesis. *Southwest. Vet.* 27:37, 1974.

Tajima, M., Itabashi, M., and Motohashi, T. Light and electron microscopic studies of lymph node of mink exposed to canine distemper virus. *Am. J. Vet. Res.* 32:913, 1971.

Trainer, D. O., and Knowlton, F. F. Serologic evidence of diseases in Texas coyotes. *J. Wild. Manage.* 32:981, 1968.

Ulbrich, F. Distemper virus infections in wild beech martens (*Martes fiona Erxleben*). In *Diseases of zoo animals*. Fourteenth Int. Symp. 1972, Wroclaw. Berlin: Akademie Verlag, p. 327, 1972.

Vantsis, J. T. Preliminary note on the propagation of canine distemper virus in different tissue culture systems. *Vet. Rec.* 71:99, 1959.

Von Mickwitz, C. V. Zur Staupe der Kleinbaren (Procyoniden). *Kleinter Prax.* 13:80, 1968. Cited in M. J. G. Appel and J. H. Gillespie. Canine distemper virus. *Virology Monographs*, vol. 11. New York: Springer-Verlag, 1972.

Von Mickwitz, C. V., and Schroder, H. D. Staupeinfektion beim katzenbar (*Ailurus fulgens*). Verh.-Ber.: IX Internationales symposium uber Erkrankungen der zootiere, Prag. Berlin: Akad. Verlag, 1967. Cited in M. J. G. Appel and J. H. Gillespie, Canine distemper virus. *Virology Monographs*, vol. 11. New York: Springer-Verlag, 1972.

Wade-Smith, J., and Richmond, M. E. Care management and biology of captive striped skunks (*Mephitis mephitis*). *Lab. Anim. Sci.* 25:575, 1975.

Watson, E. A., and Plummer, P. J. G. Distemper inclusion bodies. *Am. J. Vet. Res.* 3:350, 1942.

Watson, E., Plummer, P., and West, J. *Distemper studies: Distemper of foxes, mink and other fur animals.* In Report of the Veterinary Director General, p. 42. Can. Dept. Agric., Ottawa: Queen's Printer, 1933.

Wisnicky, W., and Wipf, L. Significance of inclusion bodies in distemper. *Am. J. Vet. Res.* 3:285, 1942.

Womer, R. A study on the efficacy of diethyl ether inhalation in the treatment of canine distemper. *Auburn. Vet.* 29:52, 1973.

Wright, N. G., Cornwell, H. J. C., Thompson, H., and Lander, I. M. Canine distemper: Current concepts in laboratory and clinical diagnosis. *Vet. Rec.* 94:86, 1974.

4 Hemorrhagic Diseases of Wild Ruminants

GERALD L. HOFF   DANIEL O. TRAINER

Synonyms: **Blacktongue, hemorrhagic septicemia, soremuzzle.**

Bluetongue (BLU) and epizootic hemorrhagic disease (EHD) are closely related infectious, often fatal, viral diseases of wild ruminants. Clinical disease may occur in domestic ruminants following BLU or EHD virus infection. Both diseases are transmitted by *Culicoides* midges. Extensive hemorrhaging is characteristic of both maladies. Significant epizootics have occurred among white-tailed deer (*Odocoileus virginianus*) and pronghorn antelope (*Antilocapra americana*).

HISTORY AND DISTRIBUTION. BLU was first recognized in South Africa during the 1870s as a serious febrile disease, resulting in high morbidity and mortality among introduced European breeds of sheep. Clinical disease was observed also among cattle but not to the extent that occurred among sheep. Wild ruminants were suspected as the reservoir host with arthropod transmission as the mechanism of spread. It was not until 1944 that arthropods were definitely incriminated in the BLU transmission cycle. BLU currently has a wide distribution, part of which may be the result of international trade in cattle, which can be inapparent carriers of the virus. Reports include most of Africa, the Middle East, the Mediterranean countries, the Indian subcontinent, Australia, the Virgin Islands, Canada, and the United States (Goltz, 1978; Howell and Verwoerd 1971; St. George et al. 1978; Thomas and Prestwood 1976). The only documented die-offs of wildlife due to BLU have come from the United States (C. Hibler, personal communication, 1978; Hoff and Hoff 1976; Thomas and Prestwood 1976).

Outbreaks of a hemorrhagic disease syndrome have occurred among white-tailed deer in the United States since the 1890s. However, it was not until 1955 that a causative agent was recovered from deer afflicted with the syndrome. From die-offs in Michigan and New Jersey, the virus of EHD was isolated (Fay et al. 1956; Shope et al. 1955). Subsequently, EHD virus has been isolated in many parts of the United States, in western Canada, and in Nigeria (Hoff and Trainer 1978). Serologic evidence indicates EHD virus may also occur in the Virgin Islands (Thomas and Prestwood 1976). Although recently detected in Africa, EHD virus has not been associated with disease in wildlife or livestock (Moore and Kemp 1974).

The exact distribution of BLU and EHD in wildlife populations in the United States is difficult to determine. BLU had been considered primarily a disease of domestic livestock and wild ruminants west of the Mississippi River. However, scattered outbreaks have occurred in the eastern states, and the virus is probably endemic in the southeastern states. EHD virus has been found to parallel the distribution of the white-tailed deer. Outbreaks, documented or suspected, have been reported for all parts of the deer range, with the noticeable exception of the southwestern and extreme northeastern states. Some of the earlier die-offs in the Midwest, which were attributed to EHD on the basis of only clinical signs or pathologic lesions, also may have involved BLU. Both diseases in white-tailed deer present almost identical signs and lesions, and both viruses can be active concurrently in the same deer population.

HOST RANGE. Studies on BLU and EHD viruses in wildlife have been largely restricted to those species native to North America or Africa. The majority of the studies in Africa and the Middle East have been serologic to detect antibody prevalence, to ascertain host range, and to collect geographic data. In North America, emphasis on both viruses has been toward the documentation of die-offs and definition of clinical signs and pathologic changes in experimental animals.

BLU virus has been isolated from clinically normal, free-ranging mountain gazelle (*Gazella gazella*), from dead kudu (*Tragelaphus strepsiceros*), bighorn sheep (*Ovis canadensis*), white-tailed deer, mule deer (*O. hemionus*), elk (*Cervus canadensis*), muntjak (*Muntiacus reevesi*), and pronghorn antelope (Hoff and Trainer 1978). BLU virus has been isolated repeatedly from nonartiodactyls in Africa—the striped field mouse (*Rhabdomys pumilio*), the water rat (*Obomys irroradus*), and the shrew (*Crocidura* spp.) (Hoff and Trainer 1978).

Serologic studies have detected BLU virus antibodies in gazelle (*G. gazella, G. grantii, G. thomsonii*), eland (*Taurotragus oryx*), reedbuck (*Redunca fulvorufula*), sitatunga (*Tragelaphus spekei*), hartebeest (*Alcelaphus buselaphus*), wildebeest (*Connochaetes taurinus*), topi (*Damaliscus korrigum*), impala (*Aepyceros melampus*), waterbuck (*Kobus ellipsiprymnus*), oryx (*Oryx beisa*), oribi (*Ourebia ourebia*), bontebok (*Damaliscus dorcas*), elephant (*Loxodonta africana*), buffalo (*Syncerus caffer*), camel (*Camelus dromedarius*), yak (*Poephagus grunniens*), reindeer (*Rangifer tarandus*), fallow deer (*Dama dama*), white-tailed deer, mule deer, elk, pronghorn antelope, moose (*Alces alces*), bison (*Bison bison*), barbary sheep (*Ammatragus lervia*), and bighorn sheep (Hoff and Trainer 1978). Serologic surveys on other mammals, birds, and reptiles in Africa and North America have been negative for BLU virus antibodies.

The impact of BLU on free-ranging artiodactyl populations is not totally known, but it is an ecological factor to be recognized and considered in wildlife management plans. In Africa, the virus appears to have little effect on native animals, mortality having been suspected only in topi (Wells 1962). Experimentally, white-tailed deer, pronghorn antelope, and African buffalo calves have succumbed to BLU infection; blesbok (*Damaliscus albifrons*), mountain gazelle, elk, and hog deer (*Axis procinus*) experienced subclinical infections, developing viremias sufficient to infect *Culicoides* vectors (Hoff and Trainer 1978).

In North America, BLU has caused mortality in white-tailed deer, mule deer, pronghorn antelope, bighorn sheep, and zoo animals. It has been postulated that BLU was the major factor in the disappearance of bighorn sheep from west Texas, because bighorn sheep populations declined appreciably at the time BLU was a rampant disease among domestic sheep on the same range. Bighorn sheep are extremely susceptible to the disease, and BLU has hampered efforts aimed at restocking bighorn sheep on their former ranges (Marburger et al. 1970). Significant die-offs in wildlife were not documented until 1971, when both BLU and EHD were incriminated in white-tailed deer mortality in the southeastern United States. This was followed by dramatic epizootics in the western states during the mid-1970s involving mule deer, bighorn sheep, and pronghorn antelope (Kistner et al. 1975; Trainer 1978).

Perhaps more important than the spectacular epizootics of BLU is its role as a mortality factor among white-tailed and mule deer fawns (Anderson 1973; Hoff et al. 1974b; Marburger et al. 1970). In south Texas, 89% of the adult white-tailed deer had BLU antibody, as did 36% of the juvenile deer (Hoff et al. 1974b). Approximately 93% of neonatal fawns had BLU antibody. This maternal antibody declined after 3 months and resulted in fawns that either lacked detectable antibodies to BLU virus or had very low antibody titers at the time when virus transmission occurred in late summer to early fall. At this time fawns were susceptible to BLU infection, and mortality has been documented.

Additional losses may occur in utero when BLU transmission and the gestation period overlap. Experimentally induced BLU virus infection during the first trimester of gestation in white-tailed deer resulted in early absorption or uncomplicated abortion (Thomas and Trainer 1970b). Field evidence supporting these studies is lacking. Does that survive infection with BLU or EHD viruses during the fall may succumb to the stress of pregnancy as a result of their earlier infection (Roughton 1975).

In Africa, the history of BLU suggests that it was a viral disease of wildlife that was capable of exploiting the introduced, susceptible population of European livestock. In North America, however, available data suggest that the opposite may be true. Although viremic titers in wildlife are sufficient to infect *Culicoides* vectors and thereby maintain an epizootic, all evidence for transpecies spread of the disease has been from domestic livestock to wildlife (Hoff and Trainer 1978). The devastation of the bighorn sheep population in Texas coincided with a period of rampant BLU among domestic sheep. In Oregon and California, mortality from BLU among mule deer, pronghorn antelope, and bighorn sheep followed an outbreak of the disease in cattle and sheep. BLU occurred in zoo animals in California after an outbreak on a neighboring sheep ranch. A similar situation occurred in Texas, where captive white-tailed deer developed BLU after infected sheep were introduced to the area.

In contrast to BLU virus, the virus of EHD has a more limited host range. Naturally occurring mortality from EHD has been reported for white-tailed deer, mule deer, and pronghorn antelope. White-tailed deer are highly susceptible to experimental EHD infection, whereas elk develop only mild signs of disease (Hoff and Trainer 1973; Thomas and Trainer 1970a). Mule deer, fallow deer, muntjak (*Muntiacus muntjac*), red deer (*Cervus elaphus*), and roe deer (*Capreolus capreolus*) did not develop overt clinical signs when experimentally infected with EHD virus but did respond with pyrexia, viremia, and development of virus-specific antibody (Gibbs and Lawman 1977; Stauber et al. 1977). Moose and nonruminant wildlife species have not succumbed to infection (Hoff and Trainer 1978).

BLU is recognized as an important disease to the sheep and cattle industry, but the role of EHD remains unclear. Antibodies to EHD have been detected in pigs, sheep, and cattle (Parikh 1968; Thomas and Prestwood 1976), and the virus has been isolated from cattle in Colorado and New Jersey. Clinical illness was observed in a cow from New Jersey, and experimentally, viremia without pyrexia and antibody response have been elicited in sheep and cattle (Gibbs and Lawman 1977; McConnell et al. 1977).

In North America, the impact of EHD virus on free-ranging artiodactyls has been more overt than that of BLU virus. Usually the disease has manifested itself through sporadic, locally severe die-offs among white-tailed deer. Field and experimental studies indicate that the case fatality rate approaches 90%. Although occasional mortality has been reported in mule deer and pronghorn antelope, this loss has been insignificant compared with that sustained by white-tailed deer. Following epizootics, antibody prevalence is high among mule deer, indicating that most infected animals survive the infection, a fact supported by experimental studies. Carcass counts during epizootics involving mule and white-tailed deer suggest a differential mortality rate of white-tailed to mule deer of approximately 23:1. Mortality among white-tailed deer populations can be severe, involving hundreds or even thousands of animals. An outbreak in South Dakota in 1952, where EHD is considered to be the most important disease affecting white-tailed deer, was estimated to have killed 60% of the West River prairie herd (Richardson and Petersen 1974). White-tailed deer herds in southwest North Dakota were reduced drastically by a 1962 EHD epizootic to a number that required 8 years for recovery; these herds were again devastated by EHD in 1970 and 1971 (Hoff et al. 1973b). Major epizootics have been sporadic and in many cases do not recur in the same geographic areas. Small enzootic die-offs do occur, and their significance has not been established.

The role of nonartiodactyl wildlife in the epizootiology of EHD virus has not been determined (Hoff and Trainer 1978).

ETIOLOGY. The closely related viruses of BLU and EHD are classified as members of the bluetongue subgroup of the orbiviruses, which itself is considered a subgroup of the reoviruses. Also included are Eubenangee and several un-named viruses. These viruses possess no common antigen but are grouped together on the basis of individual cross-reactions as determined by complement fixation tests. They are distinguished from the reoviruses by physical properties, acid lability, slight sensitivity to lipid solvents or sodium deoxycholate, and lack of serologic relationship.

BLU virus and EHD virus each possess a double-stranded RNA genome, cubic symmetry, no envelope, a single capsid with 32 capsomeres, and a virion diameter of 50–65 nm. The genome of BLU virus and of EHD virus may or may not be segmented. Earlier studies indicated 5–10 segments in the genome; however, more recent work suggests that the segments are artifacts caused by laboratory procedures (Foster et al. 1978). More detailed information concerning the physiochemical properties of the viruses can be found in Borden et al. (1971) and Konter and Welch (1976).

Plaque-reduction neutralization assays have revealed the existence of at least 16 distinct serotypes of BLU (Howell 1970). Each serotype produces a solid and durable immunity against itself, but only a variable degree of protection to challenge by heterologous serotypes. With the same techniques, two serotypes of EHD virus have been recognized (Barber and Jochim 1975).

TRANSMISSION. Epizootics of BLU and EHD have generally occurred in the late summer and early fall, although early summer transmission has been reported. Both diseases are associated with wet weather, and most epizootics have been in moist, low-lying areas.

Although arthropod transmission of BLU virus was suspected in the early 1900s, it was not until 1944 that BLU virus was isolated from wild-caught *Culicoides pallidepennis* in South Africa (DuToit 1944). Subsequent isolations came from *C. milnei*, *C. tororoensis*, and *C. pallidepennis* in Kenya (Walker and Davises 1971), *C. variipennis* in Texas (Price and Hardy 1954), and *Culicoides* spp. in Australia (St. George et al. 1978). Experimental studies further demonstrated that *C. variipennis* can serve as a biological vector of BLU virus (Luedke et al. 1976) and that *C. actoni* and *C. brevitarsis* may also act as biological vectors (Standfast et al. 1978). BLU virus has also been isolated from naturally infected cattle lice, *Haematopinus eurysternus* (J. F. Anderson, personal communication, 1971).

On the basis of epizootiologic observations, arthropod transmission also was considered for EHD virus. In 1967, EHD virus was isolated from *C. schultzei* in Nigeria (Moore and Lee 1972). Subsequent laboratory studies by Boorman and Gibbs (1973) demonstrated that *C. variipennis* could be infected with EHD virus via the oral route, and that a variety of European species could be infected following intrathoracic inoculation. These investigations suggested that *Culicoides* spp. of the *nebeculosis* group had the potential of being EHD virus vectors in Europe and Russia. In 1971, the virus was isolated from naturally infected *C. variipennis* during an epizootic of EHD involving white-tailed deer in Kentucky (Jones et al. 1977), and biological transmission of the virus among deer by the midge was demonstrated (Foster et al. 1977).

Based on experimental data, following oral infection of *C. variipennis* with either virus, an incubation period of 10–20 days is required before transmission can take place. The susceptibility rate for the midges to infection is variable and is believed to be a function of the genetic makeup of the vector population. In the insect, the most rapid increase in viral concentration occurred within 48–72 hours postinfection. After 5–8 days of incubation, the average viral titer increase was of the order of 10,000-fold for BLU virus and 1,000-fold for EHD virus, with replication occurring in the salivary glands. Viral titers in midges have been reported as approximately 4.7 $\log_{10}$ $TCID_{50}$ EHD (Boorman and Gibbs 1973) and 5.0 $\log_{10}$ $TCID_{50}$ BLU (Jochim and Jones 1966). Transovarian transmission of BLU virus does not occur in *C. variipennis* (Jones and Foster 1971); there are no comparable reports for EHD virus.

Much attention has been given to the role of the insect vector in the transmission of these viruses, and other routes of transmission have generally been disregarded. Domestic sheep can be infected by repeated oral administration of BLU virus, thus suggesting the possibility of infection during confined, continuous contact, as has occurred experimentally among white-tailed deer (Thomas and Trainer 1970a). Following oral inoculation of white-tailed deer with EHD virus, a febrile response existed on postinoculation days 5–7, but the deer were not clinically ill (Ditchfield et al. 1964). The infection was primarily enteric, and the virus was shed in the feces; however, attempts to transmit the virus by pen contact with orally infected deer have been reported as negative for both morbidity and development of immunity.

SIGNS. In white-tailed deer, clinical signs and lesions resulting from BLU and EHD virus infection are similar, and their severities are directly proportional to the period of morbidity. Both diseases are characterized by sudden onset, and the first sign of disease is pyrexia (41°C). As the disease progresses, animals lose their appetite and wariness; edema of the head and neck may occur; animals become dehydrated and progressively weaker, have increased respiration and heartbeat, and often salivate excessively. Hyperemia of the mucosa of the orbital and oral regions results in a rosy or blue appearance. In prolonged cases, ulceration of the dental pad, the hard palate, and the tongue can occur, with severe necrotizing glossitis. The feces and urine may show blood flecks, and in severe cases, blood diarrhea may develop. Lameness and lines of hemorrhage at the coronary band of the hooves have been observed in prolonged cases of BLU, with the sloughing of hooves in some animals. Infected deer avoid and appear hypersensitive to sunlight. Many animals are found in or near water, probably an attempt by the deer to lower the body temperature. EHD is fatal to approximately 90% of the infected deer within 8–36 hours after onset of overt signs. BLU, in contrast, is not as lethal, and the case fatality rate and duration of morbidity is variable.

Although EHD can cause mortality among mule deer, experimental studies have reported that mule deer, red deer, roe deer, fallow deer, and muntjac remain free of clinical signs of disease, except for a febrile response (Gibbs and Lawman 1977; Stauber et al. 1977).

Anorexia, ataxia, dyspnea, and central nervous system depression were observed in pronghorn antelope following experimental infection with BLU virus (Hoff and Trainer 1972). The clinical signs developed 6 days postinoculation, and death ensued within the next 48 hours. Antelope with naturally acquired EHD had convulsions, "running fits," and ataxia; death was caused by cardiac failure during a convulsion (Richards 1963).

Elk infected with BLU virus developed mild pyrexia, conjunctivitis, leukopenia, and diarrhea containing small amounts of blood and mucus on postinoculation days 9 and 10 (Murray and Trainer 1970). Experimental infection with EHD virus did not induce overt signs of disease in elk, but a slight febrile response was detected (Hoff and Trainer 1973).

African buffalo inoculated with BLU virus developed ulceration of the lips and palate, hyperemia of the mucosal surfaces, and swollen and cyanotic tongues (Young 1969). One animal became paralyzed and died.

PATHOGENESIS. After BLU or EHD virus is introduced into the peripheral circulation of a susceptible animal, localized multiplication takes place in the cytoplasm of vascular endothelial cells. Viral replication results in the development of cytoplasmic inclusion bodies. With BLU virus, infection of the cells results in very rapid onset of inhibition of cellular protein and DNA synthesis by some inactivating effect of the viral protein coat on existing cellular polyribosomes. Transcription of the virus genome has been shown to be by an RNA-dependent RNA polymerase present in the viral capsid. Mature viral particles of EHD and BLU are released through cytocidal reactions.

A cell-associated, primarily erythrocytic viremia follows, which in some species may persist during and after the development of viral-specific antibodies. As the viremic titers increase, the body temperature rises, with peak titer and highest temperature generally coinciding. The duration of BLU viremia in the blesbok is 17 days; white-tailed deer, 16 days; elk, 10 days; pronghorn antelope, 3 days; and mountain gazelle, 35 days (Hoff and Trainer 1978). With EHD, viremias are recorded for white-tailed deer as 6 days; red deer, 14 days; fallow deer, 14 days; roe deer, 11 days; and elk, 30 days (Gibbs and Lawman 1977; Hoff and Trainer 1978).

The prime pathogenic mechanism of BLU and EHD seems to be disseminated intravascular coagulation associated with degenerative changes and necrosis of the blood vessel walls as the result of viral injury to endothelial cells during viral replication. The inciting mechanism for disseminated intravascular coagulation has not been determined. The virus causes damage to the vascular endothelial cells, thus predisposing to platelet aggregation and breakdown and release of thromboplastin. Late in EHD viral infection, there is a decrease in fibrinogen and in activity of factor VIII, the result of their utilization in clotting (Debbie and Abelseth 1971). The thrombocyte count may fall from a normal number of 600,000/mm³ to 60,000 or even 20,000/mm³ just before death. As the coagulation factors are rapidly depleted, hemorrhages occur both from thrombosed vessels and widespread diapedesis. In spite of the hemorrhages that develop, examination of the blood just before death reveals above normal packed cell volumes, which is evidence of hemoconcentration resulting from the acute edema. Increased pericardial fluids, pleural and pulmonary edema, and edema generally distributed throughout the retroperitoneal and connective tissues of the subcutaneous and intermuscular areas consistently occur. These changes reflect the widespread interference with the normal blood circulation. The most significant hematologic finding in the two diseases is leukopenia, resulting from lymphopenia and eosinopenia.

PATHOLOGY. The gross and microscopic lesions of BLU and EHD have been characterized as those of extensive hemorrhaging (Hoff and Trainer 1978). The hemorrhages, although variable in size and extent, can occur in any organ, with the heart, liver, spleen, kidney, lung, and intestinal tract being the most regularly involved. Hemorrhages also occur in the striated musculature, particularly the muscles of the tongue. The liver, spleen, and lymph nodes may be enlarged and congested. Edema is generally widespread throughout the body. Erosion of portions of the epithelium of the lips, tongue, and buccal surfaces may occur, as can enteritis and typhilitis. White-tailed deer, mule deer, pronghorn antelope, and bighorn sheep have all been reported to have these lesions in varying degrees. The primary lesions of BLU in pronghorn antelope and bighorn sheep are those associated with acute pneumonia.

IMMUNITY. BLU and EHD are not uniformly fatal diseases, although the mortality rate for EHD in white-tailed deer epizootics approaches 90%. In an enzootic situation, BLU-virus-specific antibodies have been detected in 89% of adult white-tailed deer in the population studied (Hoff et al. 1974b). Similar antibody rates for BLU virus have been reported in Kenyan wildlife species (Davies and Walker 1974; Walker and Davies 1971).

Many strains of BLU may be active in a geographic area over a period of a few years. Nineteen strains were recorded in a sentinel cattle herd in Kenya (Davies 1978). Continuous challenge by multiple virus strains that have varying degrees of protection against one another in the laboratory failed to cause clinical illness or reproductive problems among the cattle. Other examples of BLU virus plurality in parts of Africa exist (Owen et al. 1965). Since the known *Culicoides* vectors of BLU in Africa feed almost entirely on Bovidae (Walker and Boreham 1976), many wildlife species would be subjected to the same situation described above for cattle. This may explain the lack of reports on mortality among African species in their native environment and high antibody prevalence. Removed from that environment, animals have been susceptible to clinical BLU (Hoff et al. 1973a). The plurality of strains is believed to reflect a function of the genetic makeup of the vector population; consequently, the occurrence of strain changes is in response to changes in the oral infection rates of the midges (Jones and Foster 1978). However, recombinant viruses of related orbiviruses have been isolated in the laboratory, and this may occur in nature. Such changes could affect the epizootiologic patterns in an area (Gorman et al. 1978).

Vosdingh et al. (1968) reported that white-tailed deer that were immune to EHD virus withstood challenge with BLU virus, based on clinical signs and mortality, suggesting that the two viruses cross-protect. Subsequent expanded studies reported the lack of cross-protection, although the incubation period in deer challenged with the heterologous virus was prolonged in comparison to that among the nonimmune control deer (Hoff and Trainer 1974; Thomas 1970). Roughton (1975) provided field evidence that tends to support these experimental findings. In 1971, an epizootic of hemorrhagic disease occurred among white-tailed deer in Mammoth Cave National Park, Kentucky. The epizootic was bimodal and was later shown to be caused by EHD and BLU viruses, apparently moving through the herd together or in separate waves. Deer died during a 36-day period, and 62% of the herd succumbed. The duration of clinical signs before death averaged 24 hours or less during the first 15 days of the outbreak, and the case fatality rate was 97–100%. The duration of clinical signs before death during the second half of the outbreak averaged 5 days (range 1–13 days), and 27 deer that recovered had signs for an average of 10.5 days (range 6–18 days). The case fatality rate was 58%. Unfortunately, there was no way to determine the sequence of viral infection in each deer or if each deer was infected with both viruses, although both EHD and BLU viruses were isolated from a single animal that died during the epizootic. Thirteen percent of the survivors of the outbreak died during the winter and spring following a brief clinical illness and, at necropsy, had lesions suggestive of BLU/EHD. This may represent recrudescence of a chronic infection.

BLU virus is an exceptionally potent inducer of interferon in mice and tissue culture (Huismans 1969), but this aspect of the immune response has not been studied in livestock or wildlife. No reports on interferon induction by EHD virus have been published.

DIAGNOSIS. A diagnosis of BLU or EHD is based upon the clinical signs and lesions, confirmed by the isolation and identification of the causative virus. BLU and EHD cannot be differentiated on the basis of gross or histopathologic lesions alone. Dual infections of BLU and EHD viruses may occur in an individual animal (Thomas et al. 1974). In addition, the lesions are similar to the lesions caused by malignant catarrhal fever and mucosal disease of deer.

BLU and EHD viruses can be recovered from a variety of tissues in animals that die of infection, with the liver being a very good source, especially for EHD virus. In light of recent discoveries concerning the cell-associated viremia of both diseases, the cellular fractions, after disruption of the cells, should be tested when possible. Virus can be recovered from the cellular fractions, especially the erythrocytes, if attempts with whole blood are unsuccessful. It is not known if the viruses are adsorbed to the erythrocytic membrane or have an intraerythrocytic location as does Colorado tick fever virus, another member of the orbivirus group. Quantitative assay of virus in the plasma, buffy coat, and erythrocytic fractions showed that there was 10–100 times the concentration of virus in the erythrocytic fraction than in the buffy coat fraction and 1,000–1,000,000 times the concentration than in the plasma fraction. Viremia in white-tailed deer became undetectable in all fractions within 2–8 days after the development of virus-specific neutralizing antibodies (Hoff and Trainer 1974). In cattle, viremia can persist for over 4.5 years with subsequent transmissions via *C. variipennis* (Luedke et al. 1977). It is not known if a similar situation exists for BLU or EHD viruses in wildlife species.

The most rapid and reliable method for field isolation of BLU and EHD viruses has been inoculation of susceptible domestic sheep and white-tailed deer, respectively. Embryonating chicken eggs can be used to isolate BLU virus; consistent results are more dependent on an incubation temperature of 33.5°C than embryo age or route of inoculation. The intravenous route of inoculation is believed to be more sensitive than the chorioallantoic membrane or yolk sac routes in isolating from samples with low viral titers. EHD cannot be isolated in eggs (Hoff et al. 1974a). Both viruses can be isolated by intracerebral inoculation of suckling mice, but the technique is not sensitive to samples with low virus titers. A variety of tissue culture systems, particularly baby hamster kidney (BHK-21) cultures, can be used to isolate either virus. These systems and embryonating eggs have become the techniques of choice for attempted isolation of BLU and EHD viruses. Viral plaque neutralization tests are the best procedures for identification and serotyping of isolates (Jochim and Jones 1976).

Antibody studies should utilize the plaque-reduction neutralization procedures in order to avoid the cross-reactivity problems between BLU and EHD viruses encountered with the complement fixation and gel diffusion procedures.

TREATMENT AND CONTROL. An effective treatment for animals clinically ill with BLU or EHD does not exist. In captive situations, preexposure vaccination programs can be employed for white-tailed deer and bighorn sheep (Hoff and Trainer 1974; Robinson et al. 1974); however, the results might not extrapolate to other species. Injectable vaccines, although suitable for many captive situations, are not yet applicable to field situations. Oral vaccines and methodologies for distributing the vaccines to free-ranging animals have potential but do not exist at the present time. Although polyvalent vaccines exist, they do not include all known serotypes. The value of vaccination has been questioned, especially in Africa where multiple BLU virus serotypes occur in the same geographic area.

It is doubtful, with current knowledge and resources, that vertebrate carriers of BLU or EHD can be eliminated. Cattle are recognized long-term carriers, and the status of other species, particularly wildlife, remains to be determined. The hunting of animals during an epizootic is of questionable value in its influence on the course and duration of the outbreak. At present there is no established public health risk associated with handling or eating infected animals, or exposure to infected midges. It should be pointed out that appropriate studies to assess any human risk have not been published. The value of allowing hunting of infected deer is basically a sociological and public relations decision (McConnell et al. 1977).

REFERENCES

Anderson, C. K. Comments on bluetongue in cattle, *J. Am. Vet. Med. Assoc.* 163:194, 1973.

Barber, T. L., and Jochim, M. M. Serotyping bluetongue and epizootic hemorrhagic disease virus strains. *Proc. Annu. Meet. Am. Assoc. Vet. Lab. Diag.* 18:149–162, 1975.

Boorman, J., and Gibbs, R. P. J. Multiplication of the virus of epizootic hemorrhagic disease of deer in *Culicoides* species (Diptera, Ceratopogonidae). *Arch. Gesamte Virusforsch.* 41:259–266, 1973.

Borden, E. C., Shope, R. E., and Murphy, F. A. Physicochemical and morphological relationships of some arthropod-borne viruses to bluetongue virus: A new taxonomic group. Physicochemical and serological studies. *J. Gen. Virol.* 13:261–271, 1971.

Davies, F. G. Bluetongue studies with sentinel cattle in Kenya. *J. Hyg.* 80:197–204, 1978.

Davies, F. G., and Walker, A. R. The distribution in Kenya of bluetongue disease and antibody and the *Culicoides* vector. *J. Hyg.* 72:265–272, 1974.

Debbie, J. G., and Abelseth, M. K. Pathogenesis of epizootic hemorrhagic disease: I. Blood coagulation during viral infection. *J. Infect. Dis.* 124:217–222, 1971.

Ditchfield, J., Debbie, J. G., and Karstad, L. H. The virus of epizootic hemorrhagic disease of deer. *Trans. North Am. Wildl. Nat. Res. Conf.* 29:196–199, 1964.

DuToit, R. M. The transmission of bluetongue and African horse-sickness by Culicoides. *Onderstepoort J. Vet. Sci. Anim. Ind.* 19:7–26, 1944.

Fay, L. D., Boyce, A. P., and Youatt, W. G. An epizootic of deer in Michigan. *Trans. North Am. Wildl. Nat. Res. Conf.* 21:173–184, 1956.

Foster, N. M., Alders, M. A., and Walton, T. E. Continuity of the dsRNA genome of bluetongue virus. *Curr. Microbiol.* 1:171–174, 1978.

Foster, N. M., Breckton, R. D., Luedke, A. J., Jones, R. H., and Metcalf, H. E. Transmission of two strains of epizootic hemorrhagic disease virus in deer by *Culicoides variipennis*. *J. Wildl. Dis.* 13:9–16, 1977.

Gibbs, E. P. J., and Lawman, M. J. P. Infection of British deer and farm animals with epizootic hemorrhagic disease of deer virus. *J. Comp. Pathol.* 87:335–343, 1977.

Goltz, J. Bluetongue in cattle: A review. *Can. Vet. J.* 19:95–98, 1978.

Gorman, B. M., Taylor, J., Walker, P. J., and Young, P. R. The isolation of recombinants between related orbiviruses. *J. Gen. Virol.* 41:333–342, 1978.

Hoff, G. L., Griner, L. A., and Trainer, D. O. Bluetongue virus in exotic ruminants. *J. Am. Vet. Med. Assoc.* 163:565–567, 1973a.

Hoff, G. L., and Hoff, D. M. Bluetongue and epizootic hemorrhagic disease: A review of these diseases in non-domesticated artiodactyls. *J. Zoo. Anim. Med.* 7:26–30, 1976.

Hoff, G. L., Richards, S. H., and Trainer, D. O. Epizootic hemorrhagic disease in North Dakota deer. *J. Wildl. Manage.* 37:331–335, 1973b.

Hoff, G. L., Spalatin, J., and Trainer, D. O. Attempts to propagate EHD in avian host systems. *Am. J. Vet. Res.* 35:817–819, 1974a.

Hoff, G. L., and Trainer, D. O. Bluetongue virus in pronghorn antelope. *Am. J. Vet. Res.* 33:1013–1016, 1972.

———. Experimental infection in North American

elk with epizootic hemorrhagic disease virus. *J. Wildl. Dis.* 9:129–132, 1973.

———. Observations on bluetongue and epizootic hemorrhagic disease viruses in white-tailed deer: (1) Distribution of the virus in the blood; (2) cross-challenge. *J. Wildl. Dis.* 10:25–31, 1974.

———. Bluetongue and epizootic hemorrhagic disease viruses: Their relationship to wildlife species. *Adv. Vet. Sci. Comp. Med.* 22:111–132, 1978.

Hoff, G. L., Trainer, D. O., and Jochim, M. M. Bluetongue virus and white-tailed deer in an enzootic area of Texas. *J. Wildl. Dis.* 10:158–163, 1974b.

Howell, P. G. The antigenic classification and distribution of naturally occurring strains of bluetongue virus. *J. South Afr. Vet. Med. Assoc.* 41:215–223, 1970.

Howell, P. G., and Verwoerd, D. W. Bluetongue virus. *Virol. Monogr.* 9:37–94, 1971.

Huismans, H. Bluetongue virus induced interferon synthesis. *Ondersterpoort J. Vet. Res.* 36:181–186, 1969.

Jochim, M. M., and Jones, R. H. Multiplication of bluetongue virus in *Culicoides variipennis* following artificial infection. *Am. J. Epidemiol.* 84:241–246, 1966.

———. Plaque neutralization of bluetongue virus and epizootic hemorrhagic disease virus in BHK-21 cells. *Am. J. Vet. Res.* 37:1345–1347, 1976.

Jones, R. H., and Foster, N. M. Transovarian transmission of bluetongue virus unlikely for *Culicoides variipennis*. *Mosquito News* 31:434–437, 1971.

———. Oral infection of *Culicoides variipennis* with bluetongue virus: Development of susceptible and resistant lines from a colony population. *J. Med. Entomol.* 11:316–323, 1974.

———. Heterogeneity of *Culicoides variipennis* field populations to oral infection with bluetongue virus. *Am. J. Trop. Med. Hyg.* 27:178–183, 1978.

Jones, R. H., Roughton, R. D., Foster, N. M., and Bando, B. M. *Culicoides*, the vector of epizootic hemorrhagic disease in white-tailed deer in Kentucky in 1971. *J. Wildl. Dis.* 13:2–8, 1977.

Kistner, T. P., Reynolds, G. E., Koller, L. D., Trainer, C. E., and Eastman, D. L. Clinical and serological findings on the distribution of bluetongue and epizootic hemorrhagic disease viruses in Oregon. *Proc. Annu. Meet. Am. Assoc. Vet. Lab. Diag.* 18:135–148, 1975.

Kontor, E. J., and Welch, A. B. Characterization of an epizootic hemorrhagic disease virus. *Res. Vet. Sci.* 21:190–196, 1976.

Leudke, A. J., Jones, R. H., and Walton, T. E. Overwintering mechanism for bluetongue virus: Biological recovery of latent virus from a bovine by bites of *Culicoides variipennis*. *Am. J. Trop. Med. Hyg.* 26:313–325, 1977.

McConnell, P. A., Lund, R. C., and Boss, N. R. The 1975 outbreak of hemorrhagic disease among white-tailed deer in northwestern New Jersey. *Trans. Northeast Sect. Wildl. Soc.* 33:35–44, 1977.

Marburger, R. G., Robinson, R. M., Thomas, J. W., and Clark, K. A. Management implications of disease of big game animals in Texas. *Proc. Annu. Conf. Southeast Assoc. Fish Game Comm.* 24:46–50, 1970.

Moore, D. L., and Kemp, G. E. Bluetongue and related viruses in Ibadan, Nigeria: Serologic studies of domesticated and wild animals. *Am. J. Vet. Res.* 35:1115–1120, 1974.

Moore, D. L., and Lee, V. H. Antigenic relationship between the virus of epizootic hemorrhagic disease of deer and bluetongue virus. *Arch. Gesamte Virusforsch.* 37:282–284, 1972.

Murray, J. O., and Trainer, D. O. Bluetongue virus in North American elk. *J. Wildl. Dis.* 6:144–148, 1970.

Owen, N. C., DuToit, R. M., and Howell, P. G. Bluetongue in cattle: Typing of virus isolated from cattle exposed to natural infections. *Onderstepoort J. Vet. Sci.* 32:3–6, 1965.

Parikh, G. C. Epizootic hemorrhagic disease study. South Dakota Pittman-Robertson Project. W-75-R-9, 1968.

Price, D. A., and Hardy, W. T. Isolation of the bluetongue virus from Texas sheep: *Culicoides* shown to be the vector. *J. Am. Vet. Med. Assoc.* 124:255–258, 1954.

Richards, S. H. Deer and antelope epizootic in the North Dakota badlands. *Proc. North Dakota Acad. Sci.* 17:70–71, 1963.

Richardson, A. H., and Petersen, L. E. History and management of South Dakota deer. *S. Dakota Dept. Game Fish Parks Bull.* 1974.

Robinson, R. M., Marburger, R. G., and Wishuhn, L. Vaccination trials in desert bighorn sheep against bluetongue virus. *J. Wildl. Dis.* 10:228–231, 1974.

Roughton, R. D. An outbreak of a hemorrhagic disease in white-tailed deer in Kentucky. *J. Wildl. Dis.* 11:177–186, 1975.

St. George, T. D., Standfast, H. A., Cybinski, D. H., Dyce, A. L., Muller, M. J., Doherty, R. L., and Carley, J. G. The isolation of a bluetongue virus from *Culicoides* collected in the Northern Territory of Australia. *Aust. Vet. J.* 54:153–154, 1978.

Shope, R. E., MacNamara, L. G., and Mangold, R. Report on the deer mortality: Epizootic hemorrhagic disease of deer. *N. J. Outdoors* 6:16–21, 1955.

Standfast, H. A., St. George, T. D., Cybinski, D. H., Dyce, A. L., and McCaughan, C. A. Experimental infection of *Culicoides* with a bluetongue virus isolated in Australia. *Aust. Vet. J.* 54:457–458, 1978.

Stauber, E. H., Rarrell, R. K., and Spencer, G. R. Nonlethal experimental inoculation of Columbian black-tailed deer (*Odocoileus hemionus columbianus* with virus of epizootic hemorrhagic deer disease. *Am. J. Vet. Res.* 38:411–412, 1977.

Thomas, F. C. Bluetongue virus. Ph.D. thesis. University Wisconsin, 1970.

Thomas, F. C., and Prestwood, A. K. Plaque neutralization test reactors to bluetongue and EHD viruses in the southeastern U.S.A. In L. A. Page, ed., *Wildlife Diseases*. New York: Plenum Press, 1976.

Thomas, F. C., and Trainer, D. O. Bluetongue virus in white-tailed deer. *Am. J. Vet. Res.* 31:271–278, 1970a.

———. Bluetongue virus: (1) In pregnant white-tailed deer, (2) a plaque reduction neutralization test. *J. Wildl. Dis.* 6:384-388, 1970b.

Thomas, F. C., Willis, N., and Rucherbauer, G. Identification of viruses involved in the 1971 outbreak of hemorrhagic disease in southeastern United States white-tailed deer. *J. Wildl. Dis.* 10:187–189, 1974.

Trainer, D. O. Wildlife disease: A profession. *J. Wildl. Dis.* 14:152–156, 1978.

Vosdingh, R. A., Trainer, D. O., and Easterday, B. C. Experimental bluetongue disease in white-tailed deer. *Can. J. Comp. Med. Vet. Sci.* 32:382–387, 1968.

Walker, A. R., and Boreham, P. F. L. Blood feeding of *Culicoides* (Diptera, Ceratopogonidae) in Kenya in relation to the epidemiology of bluetongue and ephemeral fever. *Bull. Entomol. Res.* 66:181–188, 1976.

Walker, A. R., and Davies, F. G. A preliminary survey of the epidemiology of bluetongue in Kenya. *J. Hyg.* 69:47–60, 1971.

Wells, E. A. A disease resembling bluetongue occurring in topi in Queen Elizabeth National Park, Uganda. *Vet. Rec.* 74:1372–1373, 1962.

Young E. The significance of infectious diseases in African game populations. *Zool. Afr.* 4:275–281, 1969.

5 *Arboviruses*

CHARLES SEYMOUR   THOMAS M. YUILL

The term *arbovirus* is an acronym for arthropod-borne virus. It refers to any virus that infects and multiplies in a hematophagous arthropod vector and is then transmitted by bite to a susceptible vertebrate host and produces an infective viremia for new arthropod vectors. This definition excludes mechanically transmitted agents such as myxomatosis virus (see chapter 12). There are more than 300 agents that are either proven arboviruses or known to be antigenically and morphologically related to them (Berge 1975). Hematophagous arthropod vectors include ticks, mosquitoes, phlebotomine and *Culicoides* sandflies, and cimicid bugs. The importance of mites, tabanids, and black flies is unclear.

All known arboviruses fall into one of four major morphological taxa: togaviruses (including alphaviruses and flaviviruses), bunyaviruses, rhabdoviruses, and orbiviruses. (The orbiviruses, including the agents of bluetongue and epizootic hemorrhagic disease of deer, are discussed in other chapters.) Arboviruses are also classified into more than 40 antigenic groups by complement fixation (CF), hemagglutination inhibition (HI), and neutralization (N) tests. CF and HI cross-reactions within a given group are usually resolved by the more specific N test; but serologic surveys and serologic diagnosis using paired sera must be interpreted with consideration of viruses antigenically related to the agent in question.

We present detailed discussions only of those arboviruses known to cause naturally acquired disease in wild mammals. We will not consider viruses that are morphologic and antigenic relatives of arboviruses and not biologically transmitted by arthropods. These agents include, for instance, Montana myotis leukoencephalitis virus, a natural pathogen of wild bats. We will also not consider arboviruses that cause experimental disease in wild mammals in the absence of any field evidence of natural infection.

Finally, we will consider only in passing those arboviruses that cause no known disease in wild mammals but that naturally infect them. The natural cycles of some of these viruses may depend, in our judgment, on wild mammals as principal vertebrate hosts (Table 5.1) or may involve wild mammals only tangentially (Table 5.2). Table 5.2 also includes viruses known to infect wild mammals but with poorly understood natural cycles. Agents of significant human and domestic animal disease are found in both groups.

Yellow Fever

Synonyms: **Yellow jack, fiebre amarilla.**

HISTORY. Yellow fever virus (YFV) has caused devastating epidemics in the tropical Americas since the 1600s (Warren 1951; Clarke and Casals 1965; Johnson 1975). The disease was periodically introduced into coastal cities of North America, and even Europe, during the summer season. Thousands of cases occurred in New Orleans as recently as 1905. The seriousness of this disease led to the establishment of the Yellow Fever Commission in 1900, and to the classic work of Walter Reed and his colleagues demonstrating that the disease was transmitted between humans in urban settings by *Aedes aegypti* mosquitoes and was caused by a filterable virus. Elucidation of sylvan (jungle) zoonotic YFV cycles of transmission was begun in the early 1930s by Soper and colleagues. The disease remains a real, although much reduced, problem up to the present in the tropical countries of the Americas and of Africa. Tropical Asia has remained strangely free of the disease, despite the abundance of *A. aegypti* in much of the area.

ETIOLOGY. YFV is the prototype flavivirus (antigenic group B), of the Togaviridae. The virus is approximately 38 nm in diameter and is enveloped (Bergold and Weibel 1962). Although some antigenic differences have been demonstrated between American and African strains of YFV (Clarke 1960), this virus is considered a single serotype. Its structure is typical of the other flaviviruses discussed in this chapter.

TRANSMISSION. YFV has both urban and sylvan cycles in tropical America and in Africa,

TABLE 5.1 Arboviruses Not Known to Cause Natural Disease in Wild Mammals but Which Are Maintained in Wild Mammal Populations.

Virus	Wild Mammal Species: (Evidence of Natural Infection)[a]	Natural Disease	Reference
Acara	*Nectomys squamipes*: (A, V) *Didelphis marsupialis*, *Marmosa* spp., *Proechimys semispinosus*: (A)	unknown	Berge 1975; Theiler and Downs 1973
African swine fever	*Phacochoerus aethiopicus, Potamochoerus porco, Hylochoerus meinhertzageni*: (V)	swine	Berge 1975
Apeu	*Caluromys* spp., *Marmosa* spp.: (A, V) *Metachirus* spp., *Proechimys* spp., *Oryzomys* spp.: (A)	human	Berge 1975
Arumowot	*Tatera kempii, Arvicanthis niloticus, Thamnomys macmillani, Crocidura* spp., *Lemnyscomys striatus*: (V)	unknown	Berge 1975
Bimiti	*Heteromys anomalus, Oryzomys* spp., *Zygodontomys brevicauda, Proechimys guyannensis*: (V)	unknown	Berge 1975
Bujaru	*Proechimys guyannensis*: (A, V) *Oryzomys* spp., *Nectomys* spp., *Didelphis* spp., *Marmosa* spp., *Metachirus* spp.: (A)	unknown	Woodall 1967
Bussuquara	*Proechimys guyannensis*: (A, V) sentinel *Alouatta*: (V)	sentinel *Alouatta*	Woodall 1967 Berge 1975
Buttonwillow	*Sylvilagus audubonii, Lepus californicus*: (A, V) *Lepus americanus, Ammospermophilus nelsoni, Citellus beecheyi*: (A)	unknown	Berge 1975
California encephalitis	*Lepus californicus*: (A)	human	Hardy et al. 1977
Capim	*Proechimys guyannensis*: (A, V) *Caluromys philander*: (V) *Oryzomys* spp.: (A)	unknown	Woodall 1967
Caraparu	*Oryzomys capito, O. laticeps, Proechimys guyannensis, Nectomys squamipes, Zygodontomys brevicauda, Heteromys anomalus, Marmosa* spp.: (A, V) *Artibeus* spp.: (A)	human	Berge 1975
Carey Island	*Macroglossus lagochilus, Cynopterus brachyotis*: (V)	unknown	Berge 1975
Catu	*Proechimys guyannensis, Nectomys squamipes, Oryzomys laticeps, O. capito, Didelphis marsupialis*: (A, V) *Molossus obscurus, Oecomys* spp.: (V) *Philander* spp., *Marmosa* spp., *Caluromys* spp., *Metachirus* spp.: (A)	human	Berge 1975
Changuinola	*Choloepus hoffmanni, Bradypus variegatus*: (A, V) *Didelphis marsupialis*: (A)	human	Berge 1975; Gorgas Memorial Laboratory 1977
Colorado tick fever	*Citellus lateralis, Erythizon dorsatum*: (A, V) *Citellus columbianus, Eutamias minimus, Tamiasciurus hudsonicus, Peromyscus maniculatus*: (V)	human	Berge 1975
Everglades	*Sigmodon hispidus, Didelphis marsupialis*: (A, V) *Peromyscus gossypinus, Procyon lotor, Oryzomys palustris, Odocoileus virginianus, Lynx rufus*: (A)	human	Berge 1975
Germiston	*Arvicanthis niloticus, Rattus rattus, Lophuromys flavipunctatus, L. sikapusi*: (A, V) *Lophuromys striatus, Otomys tropicalis, Tatera valida*: (A)	unknown	Henderson et al. 1972

[a]V=virus isolated; A=antibody detected.

TABLE 5.1 *(Continued)*

Virus	Wild Mamal Species (Evidence of Natural Infection)[a]	Natural Disease	Reference
Guajara	*Proechimys guyannensis*: (A, V) *Didelphis marsupialis*, *Marmosa* spp., *Metachirus nudicaudatus*: (A)	unknown	Berge 1975
Guama	*Oryzomys* spp., *Proechimys guyannensis*, *Nectomys squamipes*, *Caluromys* spp., *Marmosa* spp., *Didelphis marsupialis*, *Metachirus* spp.: (A, V) *Heteromys anomalus*, *Zygodontomys brevicauda*, *Coendou* spp., "bat": (V) *Philander opossum*: (A)	human	Woodall 1967; Berge 1975
Gumbo Limbo	*Sigmodon hispidus*: (V)	unknown	Henderson et al. 1969
Icoaraci	*Proechimys guyannensis*: (A, V) *Nectomys aquaticus*, *Oryzomys goeldi*, unspecified marsupials: (A)	unknown	Berge 1975
Inkoo	*Lepus timidus*, *Vulpes vulpes*, *Alces alces*: (A)	human	Brummer-Korvenkontio 1973
Issyk-Kul	*Nyctalus noctula*, *Vespertilio serotinus*, *Myotis blythi*: (V)	unknown	Lvov et al. 1973
Itaqui	*Metachirus opossum*, *Marmosa murina*, *Proechimys guyannensis*, *Oryzomys capito*, *Nectomys squamipes*: (A, V) *Caluromys* spp., *Didelphis marsupialis*: (A)	human	Berge 1975; Woodall 1967
Jamestown Canyon/Jerry Slough	*Odocoileus virginianus*: (A, V)	unknown	Berge 1975
Kaeng Khoi	*Tadarida plicata*, *Taphozous theobaldi*: (A, V) *Rattus rattus*: (A)	unknown	Berge 1975
Keterah	*Scotophilus temmenckii*: (V) *Cynopterus brachyotis*, *Tadarida plicata*: (A)	unknown	Berge 1975
Keystone	*Sigmodon hispidus*: (A, V) *Oryzomys palustris*, *Sylvilagus* spp., *Odocoileus virginianus*: (A)	unknown	Berge 1975
Koutango	*Tatera kempi*, *Mastomys* spp., *Lemnyscomys* spp.: (V)	unknown	Berge 1975
La Crosse	*Tamias striatus*, *Sciurus carolinensis*: (A, V) *Sciurus niger*, *Sylvilagus floridanus*, *Glaucomys volans*: (A)	human	Moulton and Thompson 1971; Ksiazek and Yuill 1978
Lokern	*Lepus californicus*, *Sylvilagus audubonii*: (A, V) *Ammospermophilus nelsoni*, *Citellus beecheyi*, *Sciurus griseus*, *Neotoma* spp.: (A)	unknown	Berge 1975
Madrid	*Proechimys semispinosus*: (V)	human	Berge 1975
Mahogany Hammock	*Sigmodon hispidus*: (V)	unknown	Coleman et al. 1969
Main Drain	*Lepus californicus*: (A, V) *Sylvilagus audubonii*, *Ammospermophilus nelsoni*, *Citellus beecheyi*, *Sciurus griseus*, *Neotoma* spp.: (A)	unknown	Berge 1975
Marituba	*Didelphis marsupialis*: (V) *Caluromys* spp. and *Marmosa* spp.: (A)	human	Berge 1975
Mayaro/Uruma	*Tamarin* spp., *Pitheca* spp., *Cebus* spp., Opossums incl. *Marmosa* spp., *Bradypus tridactylus*: (A)	human	Berge 1975

TABLE 5.1 *(Continued)*

Virus	Wild Mamal Species (Evidence of Natural Infection)[a]	Natural Disease	Reference
Moju	*Oryzomys* (2 spp.), *Proechimys guyannensis, Didelphis marsupialis, Nectomys squamipes:* (A, V) *Oecomys* spp.: (V) *Marmosa* spp., *Caluromys* spp.: (A)	unknown	Berge 1975
Mucambo	*Oryzomys laticeps, Oryzomys capito, Proechimys guyannensis, Nectomys squamipes, Zygodontomys brevicauda, Heteromys anomalus, Philander opossum, Marmosa mitis, Metachirus nudicaudatus, Metachirops opossum:* (A, V) *Bradypus tridactylus:* (V)	human	Berge 1975; Woodall 1967; Theiler and Downs 1973
Murutucu	*Nectomys squamipes, Oryzomys* spp., *Proechimys guyannensis, Didelphis marsupialis, Marmosa* spp., *Metachirus nudicaudatus:* (A, V) *Bradypus tridactylus:* (V) *Caluromys philander:* (A)	human	Berge 1975
Nepuyo	*Proechimys guyannensis, Nectomys* spp.: (A, V) *Artibeus jamaicensis, A. lituratus:* (V) *Oryzomys* spp.: (A)	human	Woodall 1967; Berge 1975
Oriboca	*Proechimys guyannensis, Oryzomys capito, Didelphis marsupialis:* (A, V) *Marmosa* spp., *Metachirus* spp., *Caluromys* spp.: (A)	human	Woodall 1967; Berge 1975
Ossa	*Proechimys semispinosus:* (V)	human	Berge 1975
Pacui	*Zygodontomys brevicauda, Oryzomys capito:* (V, A) *Proechimys guyannensis, Nectomys squamipes, Didelphis marsupialis, Metachirus nudicaudatus, Philander opossum, Caluromys philander, Marmosa* spp.: (A)	unknown	Berge 1975
Patois	*Sigmodon hispidus, Proechimys semispinosus:* (A, V)	unknown	Berge 1975
Pixuna	*Proechimys guyannensis:* (V) *Didelphis marsupialis:* (A)	unknown	Berge 1975; Gard et al. 1973
Ross River	*Wallabia agilis:* (V) *Pteropus poliocephalus, Pteropus scapulatus, Pseudomys novaehollandiae, Antechinus stuartii, Rattus lutreolus, Trichosurus vulpecula, Petaurus breviceps:* (A)	human	Berge 1975
Saboya	*Tatera kempi:* (V)	unknown	Berge 1975
Shark River	*Sigmodon hispidus:* (V)	unknown	Berge 1975
Silverwater	*Lepus americanus:* (A, V)	unknown	Berge 1975
Tahyna	*Lepus europaeus, Oryctolagus* spp., *Vulpes vulpes, Erinaceus* spp., *Capreolus capreolus, Sus scrofa:* (A)	human	Berge 1975
Tick-borne encephalitis (Central European encephalitis, including Kumlinge and Hypr strains)	*Sciurus vulgaris, Lepus timidus:* (A, V) *Apodemus sylvaticus, Talpa europaea, Erinaceus roumanicus, Sorex araneus, Microtus agrestis, Clethrionomys glareolus,* bat: (V)	human	Berge 1975

TABLE 5.1 *(Continued)*

Virus	Wild Mamal Species (Evidence of Natural Infection)[a]	Natural Disease	Reference
Tick-borne encephalitis (Russian spring-summer encephalitis)	At least 10 species of forest rodents: (A, V) *Erinaceus roumanicus*: (A)	human	Berge 1975
Trivittatus	*Sigmodon hispidus*: (A, V) *Sylvilagus floridanus, Odocoileus virginianus*: (A)	unknown	Berge 1975; Pinger et al. 1975
Utinga	*Bradypus tridactylus*: (V)	unknown	Theiler and Downs 1973
Witwatersrand	*Lophuromys flavopunctatus, Arvicanthis niloticus*: (A, V) *Arvicanthis kaiseri, Dasymus incomtus, Lophuromys striatus, L. sikapusi, Otomys tropicalis*: (A)	unknown	Henderson et al. 1972
Zegla	*Sigmodon hispidus*: (A, V) *Proechimys semispinosus*: (A)	unknown	Berge 1975

TABLE 5.2 Arboviruses Not Known to Cause Natural Disease in Wild Mammals and for Which Wild Mammals Play Partial, Minor, or Unclear Roles in Maintenance.

Virus	Wild Mammal Species: (Evidence of Natural Infection)[a]	Natural Disease	Reference
Anhanga	*Choloepus brasiliensis*: (V)	unknown	Woodall 1967
Anhembi	*Proechimys inheringi*: (V)	unknown	Berge 1975
Bandia	*Muridae*: (A, V)	unknown	Berge 1975
Barur	*Rattus rattus wroughtoni*: (V)	unknown	Berge 1975
Batai/Calovo	*Mus cervicolor, Rattus exulans, R. rattus, Bandicota indica, Cynopterus sphinx, Capreolus capreolus, Sus scrofa*: (A)	human	Berge 1975
Belmont	*Macropus giganteus, Megaleia rufa, Wallabeia rufogrisea, W. dorsalis, W. agilis*: (A)	unknown	Doherty et al. 1972
Bhanja	*Atelerix albiventris, Xerus erythropus*: (V)	unknown	Berge 1975
Bouboui	*Papio papio*: (V)	unknown	Berge 1975
Bunyamwera	*Pan troglodites*: (A)	human	Osterieth and Deleplanque-Liegeois
Cache Valley	*Rattus norvegicus, Microtus pennsylvanicus, Marmota monax, Odocoileus virginianus, Procyon lotor, Urocyon argenteocinereus*: (A)	unknown	Buescher et al. 1970
Chandipura	*Atelerix spiculus, Atelerix albiventris*: (V) *Macaca rhesus*: (A)	human	Berge 1975
Chikungunya	*Scotophilus* spp.: (V) *Pan troglodites, Colobus* spp.: (A)	human	Berge 1975
Cocal	*Heteromys anomalus*: (A, V) *Oryzomys* spp., *Zygodontomys brevicauda*: (A)	horse	Berge 1975
D'Aguilar	*Macropus giganteus/Megaleia rufa*: (A)	unknown	Doherty et al. 1972
Dengue-1, 2	*Presbytis* spp. sentinel: (V) *Presbytis* spp.: (A)	human	Berge 1975

[a]V-virus isolated; A-antibody detected.

TABLE 5.2 *(Continued)*

Virus	Wild Mammal Species: (Evidence of Natural Infection)[a]	Natural Disease	Reference
Dugbe	*Cricetomys gambianus*: (A, V)	human	Berge 1975
Edge Hill	*Perameles nasutus, Isoodon macrourus, Wallabeia rufogrisea, W. elegans,* bandicoots: (A)	unknown	Berge 1975
Eubenangee	*Wallabeia* spp., *Macropus*: (A)	unknown	Berge 1975
Ganjam/Nairobi sheep disease	*Connochaetes taurinis, Alcelaphus buselaphus, Gazella thompsoni, G. granti, Aepyceros melampus*: (A)	human, sheep	Davies 1978
Gordil	*Lemnyscomys striatus, Tatera* spp.: (V)	unknown	Berge 1975
Ilheus	*Tamarin* spp., *Bradypus tridactylus,* rodents, marsupials: (A)	human	Woodall 1967
Irituia	*Oryzomys* spp.	unknown	Woodall 1967
Itaporanga	*Caluromys* spp.: (V) *Marmosa* spp., *Didelphis marsupialis,* bats (4 species): (A)	unknown	Woodall 1967; Berge 1975
Japanaut	*Syconycteris crassa*: (V)	unknown	Berge 1975
Japanese encephalitis	*Hipposideros a. terasensis, Miniopterus schreiberi*: (V)	human, horse	Berge 1975
Jugra	*Cynopterus brachyotis*: (V)	unknown	Berge 1975
Jutiapa	*Sigmodon hispidus*: (V)	unknown	Berge 1975
Kairi	*Saimiri* spp., *Oecomys* spp.: (V)	unknown	Woodall 1967
Kemerovo	*Clethrionomys rutillus, C. glareolus*: (A)	human	Berge 1975
Keuraliba	*Tatera kempi, Mastomys* spp., *Taterillus* spp.: (V)	unknown	Berge 1975
Kookaburra	wallabies, *Macropus major, M. rufus*: (A)	unknown	Doherty et al. 1970
Koongol	wallabies: (A)	unknown	Doherty et al. 1970
Kowanyama	kangaroo, wallaby, rat, bandicoot: (A)	unknown	Doherty et al. 1970
Langat	*Rattus bowersi, R. mulleri, R. sabanus, R. rajah, R. annandeli*: (A)	unknown	Berge 1975
Lanjan	*Rattus sabanus, R. surifer*: (A)	unknown	Berge 1975
Lebombo	*Thryonomys swinderianus*: (V)	human	Berge 1975
Lone Star	*Procyon lotor*: (A)	unknown	Kokernot et al. 1969a
Maguari	*Alouatta seniculus*: (A)	unknown	Theiler and Downs 1973
Manzanilla	*Alouatta seniculus*: (V)	unknown	Anderson et al. 1960
Mirim	*Proechimys, Nectomys, Caluromys, Marmosa* spp.: (A)	unknown	Berge 1975
Mitchell River	*Macropus agilis, Macropus giganteus/Megaleia rufa*: (A)	unknown	Doherty et al. 1973
Mossuril	*Papio cynocephalus*: (A)	unknown	Berge 1975
Murray Valley encephalitis	opossum: (A)	human	Berge 1975
Ngaingan	*Macropus agilis, Macropus giganteus/Megaleia rufa*: (A)	unknown	Doherty et al. 1973
Northway	*Ursus americanus, Alces alces, Ovis canadensis, Rangifer caribou, Lepus americanus*: (A)	unknown	Zarnke 1978
Oropouche	*Bradypus tridactylus*: (V) *Cebus, Alouatta, Ateles* spp.: (A)	human	Woodall 1967; Berge 1975

TABLE 5.2 *(Continued)*

Virus	Wild Mammal Species: (Evidence of Natural Infection)[a]	Natural Disease	Reference
Piry	*Philander opossum*: (V) *Oryzomys capito, Proechimys* spp., *Caluromys* spp., *Didelphis marsupialis*: (A)	unknown	Theiler and Downs 1973
Potiskum	*Cricetomys gambianus*: (V)	unknown	Theiler and Downs 1973
St. Floris	*Tatera* spp.: (V)	unknown	Berge 1975
San Angelo	*Canis latrans, Procyon lotor, Didelphis marsupialis, Odocoileus virginianus*: (A)	unknown	Berge 1975
Semliki Forest	*Atelerix albiventris*: (V) *Pan troglodites,* rodents: (A)	unknown	Berge 1975; Theiler and Downs 1973
Tacaiuma	bats, *Nectomys* spp., *Oryzomys* spp.: (A)	human	Berge 1975
Tanjong Rabok	*Macaca nemestrina*: (V) *Macaca fascicularis, Presbytis cristata, P. melalophos, Nycticebus coucang, Iomys horsfieldi,* rodent and bat spp.: (A)	possible human	Berge 1975
Thottapalayam	*Suncus murinus*: (V)	unknown	Berge 1975
Toure	*Tatera kempi*: (V)	unknown	Berge 1975
Tribec	*Clethrionomys glareolus, Pitimys subterraneus*: (V)	unknown	Berge 1975
Trubanam	kangaroos, wallabies: (A)	unknown	Doherty et al. 1970
Turlock	*Lepus californicus*: (V)	unknown	Berge 1975
Tyuleniy	*Callorhinus arsinus*: (A)	unknown	Lvov et al. 1972
Upolu	kangaroo: (A)	unknown	Doherty et al. 1970
Uukuniemi	*Apodemus flavicollis*: (A, V)	unknown	Berge 1975
Wallal	*Macropus rufogrisea/dorsalis, M. agilis, M. gigantea/Megaleia rufa*: (A)	unknown	Doherty et al. 1970
Warrego	*Macropus rufogrisea/dorsalis, M. agilis, M. gigantea/Megaleia rufa*: (A)	unknown	Doherty et al. 1970
West Nile	*Arvicanthis niloticus,* bats: (A, V) *Pan troglodites, Cercopithecus* spp., *Rattus rattus, R. norwegicus, Acomys cahirinus*: (A)	human	Berge 1975
Whataroa	*Trichosurus vulpecula*: (A)	unknown	Berge 1975
Wongorr	*Macropus rufogrisea/dorsalis, M. agilis*: (A)	unknown	Doherty et al. 1970
Yogue	*Rousettus aegyptiacus*: (V)	unknown	Berge 1975
Zika	*Pan troglodites, Colobus* spp.: (A)	human	Theiler and Downs 1973
Zinga	monkey spp., rodent spp. *Syncerus caffer, Loxodonta africana, Alcelaphus buselaphus, Phacochoerus aethiopicus,* other big mammals: (A)	human	Berge 1975

TABLE 5.3 Mortality and Probable Host Status of Wild Mammals for Epidemic VEEV.

Mammal (Binomial)	Isolations from Field	Maximum Viremia Titer[a]	Estimated Host Potential
No Mortality			
Blacktail jackrabbit (*Lepus californicus*)[b]	0	5.4	moderate
Eastern cottontail rabbit (*Sylvilagus floridanus*)[b]	0	4.7	moderate
Cotton rat (*Sigmodon hispidus*)[b]	0	9.0	minor
Opossum (*Didelphis marsupialis*)[b]	8	4.5	unknown
Raccoon (*Procyon lotor*)[b]			
Adult	0	<4.5	insignificant
Juvenile	0	5.2	insignificant
Striped skunk (*Mephitis mephitis*)[b]	0	4.6–5.5	unknown
Big brown bat (*Eptesicus fuscus*)[b]	0	5.5–6.4	unknown
Little brown bat (*Myotis lucifugus*)[b]	0	5.5–6.4	unknown
Jamaican fruit-eating bat (*Artibeus jamaicensis*)[c]	0	7.4	unknown
Big fruit-eating bat (*Artibeus lituratus*)[c]	1[d]	7.2	unknown
Pale spear-nosed bat (*Phyllostomus discolor*)[c]	0	4.5	insignificant
High (over 50%) Mortality			
Mexican ground squirrel (*Spermophilus mexicanus*)[b]	0	9.1	minor
Southern plains wood rat (*Neotoma micropus*)[b]			
Adult	0	7.7	minor
Juvenile	0	9.5	minor
Northern grasshopper mouse (*Onychomys leukogaster*)[b]	0	10.4	minor
Mexican pocket mouse (*Liomys irroratus*)[b]	0	11.5	minor
White-footed mouse (*Peromyscus leucopus*)[b]	0	9.0	minor
Low (under 50%) Mortality			
Coyote (*Canis latrans*)[b]			
Adult	0	5.5–6.4	minor
Juvenile	0	6.5–8.5	insignificant
Gray squirrel (*Sciurus carolinensis*)[b]	0	6.5–8.5	unknown
Deer mouse (*Peromyscus maniculatus*)[b]	0	<4.6	unknown
Mortality Unreported			
Rats (*Rattus* spp.)[b]	11	unknown	unknown
House mouse (*Mus musculus*)[b]	3	unknown	unknown
Gray fox (*Urocyon cinereoargenteus*)[b]	1	unknown	unknown

[a]Mean or median peak viremia titer of group expressed as $\log_{10}$ infectious units.
[b]As summarized in Sudia and Newhouse 1975; Bowen 1976.
[c]Seymour et al. 1978.
[d]Sanmartin et al. 1973.

but the wild vertebrate host and mosquito vector species are different. In the Americas, the virus is transmitted in the forest canopy between monkeys by *Haemagogus* spp. and *Sabethes chloropterus* mosquitoes. The main monkey YFV hosts include several marmosets and tamarins, howlers (*Alouatta* spp.), the squirrel monkey (*Saimiri sciureus*), the night monkey (*Aotus trivirgatus*), spider monkeys (*Ateles* spp.) and cebus monkeys (*Cebus* spp.) (Johnson 1975). In the classic neotropical "woodcutter's disease" cycle, tree cutting brings the mosquitoes to ground level, where forest workers are bitten. Infected individuals then transport the virus to populated areas where *A. aegypti* are abundant, initiating the urban cycle of transmission. Sylvan YF is most prevalent among the adult male cohort of the human population because they are most likely to be exposed in the forest. However, on occasion, *Haemogogus* spp. will come to ground level in small agricultural clearings in the forest. They have been collected in and around houses, thus infecting women and children (Clarke and Casals 1965).

Aedes africanus transmits YFV to wild primates in the African forest canopy. In more brushy areas, the vector is *A. luteocephalus*. The principal African primate YFV hosts are green monkeys (*Cercopithecus* spp.), red monkeys (*Erythrocebus patas*), baboons (*Papio* spp.), leaf-eating monkeys (*Colobus* spp., especially *C. abyssinicus*), and bush babies (*Galago* spp.) (Taufflieb et al. 1971). Infected monkeys such as *Cercopithecus aethiops* and *C. nictitans* come into agricultural areas that adjoin the forest, where they are bitten by *A. simpsoni*, an efficient monkey-human vector. This mosquito breeds in leaf axils of banana and other plants around human dwellings and may also transmit YFV from human to human (Johnson 1975).

In Africa or the Americas, monkey populations within a limited area are not large enough to sustain enzootic virus maintenance for a long period. Areas of virus transmission move as wandering foci, sometimes over great distances. Often, the only indication of recent passage of the virus through an area is the presence of dead and dying monkeys, especially howlers (in the Americas), or a sudden decline in their populations. However, it has not been proved that these moving foci can persist indefinitely, and there is some evidence to suggest that some species of neotropical arboreal marsupials (*Metachirus* spp., *Caluromys* spp., and *Marmosa* spp.) may contribute to YFV maintenance (Johnson 1975). YFV was isolated from an epaulette bat (*Epomophorus* sp.) in Africa, but the role of bats in virus maintenance and dissemination is unknown (Andral et al. 1968). Experimental inoculation of hedgehogs (*Erinaceus europaeus*), rodents (*Steatomys opimus*), and genets (*Genetta tigrina*) with YFV resulted in viremia high enough to infect mosquito vectors (Taufflieb et al. 1971). However, the role of these mammals in YFV maintenance in nature has not been established.

PATHOLOGY. Neotropical monkeys are more susceptible to severe disease and mortality from YFV infection than are African primates. However, the bush baby (*Galago crassicaudatus*) suffers significant mortality from experimental YFV infection. An African macaque, *Macacus sylvanus*, is as susceptible to YFV as the rhesus monkey. Populations of *M. sylvanus* living on Gibraltar were decimated during a YF epidemic in 1828, presumably by YFV (Taufflieb 1971). In contrast, several New World monkeys die from YFV infection, including the howlers, the night monkey, and marmosets.

Signs of disease in humans and in monkeys are similar (Bearcroft 1957). After a 3–6-day incubation period, there is sudden onset of fever and depression, with headache, nausea, vomiting, and myalgia in humans (Burgher 1951; Clarke and Casals 1965; Johnson 1975). Recovery may begin at this time, or there may be a biphasic course with a toxic phase of returning fever and bradycardia (Faget's sign). In severe cases, there is marked hemorrhage (gastrointestinal and uterine, with epistaxis and melena), jaundice (usually not intense), and renal failure leading to death. In fatal human cases, hemorrhage in the gastrointestinal tract and in other tissues is seen. The stomach and intestines may contain substantial amounts of blood. Microscopically, degeneration and necrosis of the kidney and midzonal areas of the liver occur without inflammation. The necrotic liver cells affected contain hyaline intracytoplasmic (Councilman) bodies. In the kidneys the tubule epithelium is affected, and cellular debris and casts are found within the tubules.

DIAGNOSIS. Timely and accurate YF diagnosis is of paramount importance in surveillance and control of the disease (World Health Organization 1971). Clinical and epidemiological observations are helpful in establishing a tentative, working diagnosis of YF. Definitive diagnosis is made on the basis of isolation of the virus, demonstration of a significant rise in specific YF antibodies, or in observation of characteristic liver lesions in fatal cases. YFV can be isolated from blood early in the course of disease or from liver suspensions from fatal cases. The virus can be isolated in suckling mice (Berge 1975) or in a mosquito (*A. pseudoscutellaris*) cell line reported to be more sensitive than suckling mice for recovery of field strains of YFV (Varma et al. 1976). Standard serologic tests can be used to demonstrate YFV antibody. However, YFV occurs in areas where other flaviviruses frequently infect people and wild mammals, and the possibility of significant cross-reaction may complicate interpretation. Although examination of liver tissue may not be as reliable for establishing a diagnosis as are virus isolation or even serologic tests, histologic examination of the tissue may be the only practical diagnostic method in many remote areas where sylvan YF occurs (Clarke and Casals 1965).

TREATMENT. No specific treatment is available. Fluid and blood replacement is indicated in patients with significant vomiting or hemorrhage (Clarke and Casals 1965).

CONTROL. Human disease can be effectively prevented by application of the highly effective 17D or French neurotropic vaccines. The vaccine elicits antibody titers that persist at least 17–19 years (Clarke and Casals 1965). Vaccination programs must be continuous enough to maintain a high proportion of immunity in the population. There have been several YF outbreaks in Africa after mass vaccination programs were discontinued in 1960 (Hamon and Brown 1972). Control of YFV vectors in Africa is difficult because, unlike *A. aegypti* in other parts of the world, the mosquito species involved do not breed in easily observed and treated containers. Control of the urban YF cycle in the Americas can be accomplished by reduction of *A. aegypti* populations. In recent years, the *A. aegypti* control program has stalled in Central and South America; 34 of 51 countries were infested in 1975 (Center for Disease Control 1976). Control campaigns are costly to maintain effectively and often compete unsuccessfully with high priority social and economic programs in developing countries (Schliessmann and Calheiros 1974). *Aedes aegypti* populations are abundant and extensive enough to support sustained epidemics of dengue fever (World Health Organization 1976, 1977), another flavivirus transmitted from person to person by this vector. Therefore, it seems probable that massive YF epidemics could be spread similarly in human populations, many of which are not adequately vaccinated in the neotropics. Elimination of the sylvan cycle is not feasible. The remoteness from medical attention of people at risk to sylvan YF and the rapidity with which human populations are expanding into forested areas suggest that occurrence of sylvan YF will continue (Johnson 1975).

St. Louis Encephalitis

Synonyms: **None.**

HISTORY. St. Louis encephalitis virus (SLEV), a mosquito-borne flavivirus, causes sporadic but extensive human epidemics in North America. First isolated from a fatal human case in St. Louis (Muckenfuss et al. 1933), it has since been found from Canada to Argentina. It has been isolated from diseased California gray foxes (*Urocyon argenteocinereus*) (Emmons and Lennette 1967).

TRANSMISSION AND HOST RANGE. *Culex* mosquitoes transmit SLEV in North America; *C. tarsalis* is the generally acknowledged vector in the West, *C. pipiens* in the East, and *C. nigripalpus* in Florida. Numerous virus isolations and serologic surveys have shown that birds are the chief amplifying hosts throughout North America. However, in the southeastern United States, wild mammals may play more than just a tangential role in the transmission cycle. In Florida and Mississippi, SLEV has been isolated from a raccoon (*Procyon lotor*) (Wellings et al. 1972), an opossum (*Didelphis marsupialis*), a cotton rat (*Sigmodon hispidus*), and an impala (*Aepyceros melampus*) (F. M. Wellings, cited in McLean and Bowen 1980). Neutralizing (N) antibody has been found in Florida in raccoons, opossums, an armadillo (*Dasypus novemcinctus*), and a cotton mouse (*Peromyscus gossypinus*) (Bigler and Hoff 1975). Elsewhere in North America, wild mammals are probably insignificant compared with birds as SLEV hosts.

On the Pacific coast, aside from Emmons and Lennette's (1967) gray fox isolate, evidence for SLEV infection of wild mammals is only serologic. From Kern County, California, to 52°N in British Columbia, N or monotypic HI antibodies have been detected in blacktail jackrabbits (*Lepus californicus*), snowshoe hares (*L. americanus*), Nuttall's cottontails (*Sylvilagus nuttallii*), Fresno and Heermann's kangaroo rats (*Dipodomys nitratoides* and *D. heermanni*), southern grasshopper mice (*Onychomys torridus*), deer mice (*Peromyscus maniculatus*), harvest mice (*Reithrodontomys megalotis*), antelope ground squirrels (*Ammospermophilus nelsoni*), California ground squirrels (*Citellus beecheyi*), marmots (*Marmota flaviventris*), woodrats (*Neotoma fuscipes*), pocket gophers (*Thomomys talpoides*), house mice (*Mus musculus*), and rats (*Rattus rattus* and *R. norvegicus*) (Hammon et al. 1942; Hardy et al. 1974; Howitt and Van Herrick 1942; McLean et al. 1970, 1971). In Texas, SLEV has been isolated from Mexican free-tailed bats (*Tadarida brasiliensis*), and Allen et al. (1970) suggested that hibernating bats serve as overwintering hosts for the virus. SLEV N antibodies occur in this bat species (Allen et al. 1970) and in Texas white-tailed deer (*Odocoileus virginianus*) (Trainer and Hanson 1969). In north-central North America (Wisconsin, Wyoming, North Dakota, and Alberta), SLEV N antibodies have been detected in snowshoe hares, moose (*Alces alces*), a pronghorn (*Antilocapra americana*), and both white-tailed and mule deer (*Odocoileus hemionus*) (Hoff et al. 1970, 1973; Trainer and Hanson 1969; Trainer and Hoff 1971).

In the tropics the cycle of SLEV remains unclear. At least 15 tropical mosquito species of 7 genera have yielded SLEV (Berge 1975). As in temperate North America, in the tropics most of the vertebrate isolates and serologic positives have been from birds. However, in Argentina SLEV has been isolated from a vesper mouse (*Calomys musculinus*) and a house mouse (*Mus musculus*) (Sabattini, cited in McLean and Bowen 1979). In Brazil SLEV was isolated from the grass mouse (*Akodon arviculoides*), a rice rat (*Oryzomys nigripes*), *Gigantolaelaps* mites combed from another rice rat (*Oryzomys macconnelli*), and from the blood of a roof rat (*Rattus rattus*), opossums (*Didelphis marsupialis*), a howler monkey (*Alouatta nigerrina*), a spider monkey (*Ateles paniscus chamek*), and a three-toed sloth (*Bradypus tridactylus*) (F. Pinheiro and O. de Sousa Lopez, cited in McLean and Bowen 1980; Woodall 1967). The sloth isolate is of special interest because sloths (*Bradypus variegatus* and *Choloepus hoffmanni*) in Panama have the highest prevalence of SLEV N antibody of any forest birds and mammals tested (Gorgas Memorial Laboratory 1977). Panamanian spiny rats (*Proechimys semispinosus*) also have SLEV N antibody (de Rodaniche and Galindo 1961).

PATHOLOGY. SLEV was isolated in 1957 by Emmons and Lennette (1967) from the brain of an Amador City, California, gray fox suspected of rabies. Although the animal was obviously ill, it did not run or attack. Unpublished data of R. W. Emmons include a second isolation under similar circumstances from a Madera, California, gray fox. No histologic studies were made of either fox.

Experimental SLEV inoculation by peripheral routes has not caused disease in any wild mammals. Of those species discussed above that are known to be naturally infected by SLEV, subcutaneous inoculation has consistently produced experimental viremia and antibody in opossums, a single gray fox (Kokernot et al. 1969b), antelope ground squirrels, and Fresno kangaroo rats (J. L. Hardy and W. C. Reeves, cited in McLean and Bowen 1979), and both types of sloth (Gorgas Memorial Laboratory 1977). Variable results in which some but not all animals became viremic or developed antibodies have been reported for Mexican free-tailed bats (Sulkin et al. 1963), cotton rats (McLean and Bowen 1980), and black-tailed jackrabbits (J. L. Hardy and W. C. Reeves, cited in McLean and Bowen 1980). Raccoons did not develop detectable viremia, but were not tested for antibody development (Kokernot et al. 1969b). Species that were entirely refractory to peripheral SLEV inoculation are roof rats (Kissling 1958) and deer mice (J. L. Hardy and W. C. Reeves, cited in McLean and Bowen 1980). Western harvest mice became infected but showed no signs of disease when inoculated intracerebrally with large doses of laboratory mouse-virulent SLEV (Greutter et al. 1940). Of these species, the longest and among the most intense experimental viremias occurred in sloths and free-tailed bats, particularly in hibernating bats.

In humans, disease ranges from inapparent infection through mild febrile illness to coma and fatal encephalitis. Disease is usually more severe in elderly people than in young and can leave neurological sequelae such as slowness of movement and speech. Histologic changes include perivascular cuffing, glial nodules, and marked reduction of Purkinje cells (Shinner 1963).

DIAGNOSIS. Because the symptoms of SLEV infection resemble those of many other viral diseases, diagnosis depends on virus isolation or on a fourfold or greater increase in antibody titer in paired sera. SLEV is most easily isolated by intracranial inoculation of suckling mice; it is identified using specific antisera in N, HI, and CF tests. The same tests are used to detect antibody increase in paired sera.

TREATMENT AND CONTROL. There is presently no licensed vaccine, in spite of research to develop one (Darwish and Hammon 1966). The most effective prevention methods are elimination of mosquito breeding sites and spraying to control mosquito vector populations, either by widespread application of insecticides (Hopkins et al. 1975; Mitchell et al. 1979) or by hand-spraying special localized urban mosquito habitats (Steelman et al. 1967). The appearance of SLEV antibodies in the sera of juvenile birds is a useful early indicator of virus activity. A high prevalence of antibodies in young house sparrows has been a signal to begin intensive mosquito control measures (Lord et al. 1974). However, extensive SLEV outbreaks continue to occur in spite of control efforts.

Omsk Hemorrhagic Fever

Synonyms: **None.**

HISTORY. Omsk hemorrhagic fever virus (OHFV), a flavivirus, occurs in the lake belt of the forest-steppe zone of western Siberia (Ravdonikas et al. 1968). It causes outbreaks of severe hemorrhagic disease in both humans and muskrats (*Ondatra zibethica*) in Omsk, Novosibirsk, Kurgan, and Tyumen oblasts. It was first isolated in 1947 by Chumakov (1948).

ETIOLOGY. OHFV is a member of the tick-borne encephalitis complex of flaviviruses and so is closely related to Powassan, louping-ill, and Kyasanur Forest disease viruses. Clarke (1964) has described two antigenic varieties; Kornilova et al. (1970) have detected both antigenic and growth curve differences between selected strains of OHFV.

TRANSMISSION. The ticks *Dermacentor pictus*, and to a lesser extent *D. marginatus* and *Ixodes persulcatus*, are strongly implicated by virus isolations and by ecology as the vectors of OHFV to humans (Gagarina 1965; Vorob'eva et al. 1971). However, the circulation of virus at times and in areas where *D. pictus* is not active suggests an alternate transmission in moist areas by the tick *I. apronophorus*, from which OHFV has been isolated (Ravdonikas et al. 1971). Probably neither *D. pictus* nor *I. apronophorus* is the vector of muskrat epizootics,

because muskrats are rarely infested with them or with any other ticks (Alifanov 1966). In moist areas, OHFV may be transmitted through rodent urine. Kharitonova and Leonov (1971) isolated OHFV from the urine of wild-caught muskrats and water voles (*Arvicola terrestris*) that use muskrat burrows and from the urine of experimentally infected muskrats, water voles, root voles (*Microtus oeconomus*), and red-cheeked suslik (*Citellus erythrogenus*). They have shown that muskrats and root voles become infected by the oral route. Nonarthropod transmission is also a factor in OHFV cases in hunters and trappers who handle infected wild muskrats (Fedorova and Sizemova 1964). The significance of reported isolates from mosquitoes, mites, and fleas is not clear (Kukharchuk et al. 1974; Tarasevich et al. 1969, 1974).

HOST RANGE. Hemorrhagic disease and frequent virus isolation, summarized by Fedorova (1966a), have shown that muskrats are infected in nature. However, the true maintenance hosts of this virus are probably small rodents and insectivores. Water voles, root voles, and shrews (*Sorex araneus*) have yielded isolates (Leonov et al. 1969). Sera from 14 species of rodents and shrews have reacted positively against OHF antigen in the HI test (Kharitonova 1969; Leonov and Fedorova 1966, 1969; Ravdonikas et al. 1971). The species that have reacted positively by HI most frequently and most consistently from year to year and from area to area are shrews (*S. araneus*), water and root voles, muskrats, northern red-backed voles (*Clethrionomys rutilis*), and red-cheeked susliks. These results were not confirmed by neutralization tests. N antibody has been detected in muskrats and humans (Gavrilovskaya and Chumakov 1964). Reports of HI antibody in birds (Danilov et al. 1969) are inconclusive because Eurasian birds have frequently been infected by other flaviviruses, antibodies to which would cross-react in the HI test with OHFV antigen. Reports of HI antibody in frogs and fish (Leonov and Kharitonova 1969) and of OHF virus isolation from frogs (Rad'kova and Vorob'eva 1971) await confirmation. Sera from heterothermic vertebrates may contain nonspecific HI factors, and OHFV and other tick-borne encephalitis complex viruses are notorious laboratory contaminants.

PATHOLOGY. Subcutaneous inoculation of $10-100$ mouse LD_{50} of OHFV into muskrats produces severe hemorrhagic disease with blood vessel changes. The changes include swelling of the vessel walls and perivascular edema. Small blood vessel endothelial cells become swollen and pycnotic and slough. Widespread hemorrhage and degeneration occur, with accompanying generalized acute lymphadenitis and focal necrosis in the brain. Coinfection with tularemia increases the severity of the disease. Viremia lasts until death, up to 23 days after inoculation, with maximum concentrations of up to $10^{7.5}$ adult mouse intracerebral LD_{50} per ml (Marenko et al. 1974). In another study, 90% of 50 inoculated animals died with clinical signs of asthenia, depression, and lethargy. Only 7 animals developed paresis or paralysis, and hemorrhage was reported for a single muskrat (Fedorova 1966b).

Both subcutaneous and intranasal infection of red-cheeked susliks produced a transient asthenia and lethargy, followed by a detectable antibody response and no pathologic changes after recovery (Kharitonova and Leonov 1969). Narrow-skulled voles (*Microtus gregalis*) experimentally infected by tick bite developed lethargy, asthenia, and spasms, and OHFV was isolated from their brains (Gagarina 1965). Water voles became ill from mixed infection with tularemia and OHFV, but not from OHFV alone (Dunaev 1976).

Human OHFV disease ranges from a mild febrile illness to fatal hemorrhaging. Infection is typically marked by leukopenia with a pronounced shift to mononuclears, low blood pressure, respiratory illness, a biphasic fever curve, and often hemorrhaging at any of several sites (Sizemova 1968). Long-lasting sequelae include limb pains, headache, weakened memory and hearing, hair loss, a tendency toward bleeding, and limited work capacity (Tatarintsev 1968).

DIAGNOSIS. Clinical symptoms and epidemiology may be helpful in differential diagnosis of some human cases. However, the most accurate and dependable method is virus isolation in suckling mice or cell cultures and identification using specific antisera in the N, agar gel precipitation, and fluorescent antibody tests (Vorob'eva et al. 1971). Convalescent sera react with OHFV antigen in CF and HI tests (Sizemova 1968).

TREATMENT AND CONTROL. Tick avoidance measures by forest workers and sanitary precautions by muskrat trappers may help reduce human infection rates. Field tests of an inactivated virus vaccine developed soon after the initial virus isolation yielded no clinical cases in vaccinated humans and numerous cases in unvaccinated controls (Chumakov 1949).

Louping-Ill

Synonyms: None.

HISTORY AND ETIOLOGY. Louping-ill virus (LIV), a flavivirus, was first isolated by Pool et al. (1930). It is the cause of an often fatal encephalitis in sheep. It also causes occasional natural disease in horses, humans, pigs, and cattle (Timoney et al. 1976; West 1975; Williams and Thorburn 1962). LIV is a member of the tick-borne encephalitis complex of flaviviruses, which also includes Omsk hemorrhagic fever, Powassan, and Kyasanur Forest disease viruses. It has been found only in the United Kingdom and Ireland.

TRANSMISSION AND HOST RANGE. LIV is transmitted by the tick *Ixodes ricinus*. The wild vertebrates from which the virus has been isolated include grouse (*Lagopus lagopus*) (Williams et al. 1963), mice (*Apodemus sylvaticus*), and shrews (*Sorex araneus*) (Smith et al. 1964). The virus was also isolated from the brain of a dead roe deer *Capreolus capreolus* (Reid et al. 1976). In Scotland, antibody was detected in all of 9 hares (*Lepus* spp.) (Berge 1975) and in 30% of 324 roe deer, red deer (*Cervus elaphus*), and Sika deer (*C. nippon*) (Adam et al. 1977).

PATHOLOGY. Reid et al. (1976) studied a roe deer fawn dead from natural causes in a Scottish wildlife park. The brain contained high concentrations of LIV (8.4 $\log_{10}$ plaque-forming units per gram of tissue), strongly suggesting that louping-ill encephalitis was the cause of death. Pathologic lesions in the deer brain included mild, widespread tigrolysis involving Purkinje cells and brainstem neurons, accompanied by granular disintegration of neurofibrils. The inflammatory response was minimal, consisting of activated pericytes around small arteries and internal adherence of lymphocytes to small veins and arteries. There was some swelling of astrocytes and oligodendroglia, but the perivascular cuffing and microglial proliferation typical of LIV-infected sheep were absent. The changes observed in the deer were interpreted as an early, very acute response to viral infection.

DIAGNOSIS. Definitive diagnosis is made by virus isolation from blood or tissues by intracerebral inoculation of suckling mice, and subsequent identification with specific antisera in neutralization, HI, CF, and agar gel precipitation tests. Louping-ill may also be diagnosed by a rise in titer of paired sera tested by these serologic procedures. For sheep, diagnosis is sometimes aided by the distinctive encephalitic jumping movements (termed *louping* in Scotland) and by typical brain lesions.

TREATMENT AND CONTROL. Postexposure treatment is limited to injection of immune serum as soon as possible following known exposure. Since exposure may not be obvious, serum treatment is of limited practical value, and prevention may be the only feasible approach. An inactivated virus vaccine from Moredun Institute is available for use in animals (Brotherston and Boyce 1970). Otherwise, control is limited to tick reduction in infested pastures and to prophylactic sheep dipping against ticks. In the absence of vaccine, sheep on farms where LIV is enzootic are generally bound to those farms, that is, they are not sold or replaced by new nonimmune animals (Pool et al. 1930). Rams introduced for breeding are carefully tended and are often not allowed into infested pastures during louping-ill seasons in spring and fall.

Powassan

Synonyms: **None.**

HISTORY AND ETIOLOGY. Powassan virus (POWV) was first isolated in 1958 from a fatal human encephalitis case in Ontario (McLean and Donahue 1959). Like louping-ill, Omsk hemorrhagic fever, and Kyasanur Forest disease viruses, POWV is a member of the tick-borne encephalitis antigenic complex of flaviviruses. It is distributed across northern North America from California and British Columbia to New York and has been reported from eastern Siberia. POWV occasionally causes human encephalitis and was the apparent cause of natural encephalitis and death in a wild-caught gray fox (*Urocyon argenteocinereus*) (Whitney and Jamnback 1965).

TRANSMISSION AND HOST RANGE. POWV is transmitted by hard ticks. It has been isolated from *Dermacentor andersoni* both in Colorado (Thomas et al. 1960) and in South Dakota (C. M. Eklund, personal communication, cited in

Berge 1975). Lvov et al. (1974) reported the isolation of Powassan virus from *Haemaphysalis neumanni* ticks in the southern Primorye region of the far eastern Soviet Union. The majority of tick isolates have been from various species of *Ixodes*. In studies in Ontario (McLean et al. 1964a, b, 1966, 1967; McLean and Larke 1963), POWV was isolated from 18 pools of *Ixodes cookei*, each pool collected from a different woodchuck (*Marmota monax*). Circulating POWV was also found in two other woodchucks. Similarly, isolates were made once from a pool of *I. marxi* collected from a red squirrel (*Tamiasciurus hudsonicus*) and once from the blood of another red squirrel. In Ontario, antibody against POWV was found to be more prevalent in woodchucks and red squirrels than in any other species tested. However, gray squirrels (*Sciurus carolinensis*), chipmunks (*Tamias striatus*), snowshoe hares (*Lepus americanus*), porcupines (*Erethizon dorsatum*), and skunks (*Mephitis mephitis*) were also positive.

Studies in New York State (Whitney 1963; Whitney and Jamnback 1965) have also incriminated woodchucks as POWV hosts by virus isolation from the tissues of two animals. *Ixodes cookei* collected from these two woodchucks also contained POWV. Antibody was found in foxes (species not designated) and raccoons (*Procyon lotor*). Finally, POWV was isolated from the brain of a fatally ill gray fox.

In South Dakota, Eklund (1963) recovered POWV from the blood of *Peromyscus* spp. mice, as well as from *I. spinipalpus* ticks collected from *Peromyscus*. Antibody was detected principally in *Peromyscus*, but also in meadow mice (*Microtus* spp.) and chipmunks (*Eutamias* spp.). In British Columbia, McLean et al. (1968, 1970) detected POWV antibody in ground squirrels (*Spermophilus columbianus* and *S. lateralis*), chipmunks (*Eutamias amoenus*), red squirrels, and marmots (*Marmota flaviventris*). In California, Johnson isolated POWV from a spotted skunk (*Spilogale gracilis*) (Berge 1975).

PATHOLOGY. POWV was isolated from the brain of a wild gray fox that had been suspected of rabies. The animal exhibited choreiform movements when captured and died 48 hours later (Whitney and Jamnback 1965). Parenteral inoculation of skunks, red foxes, gray foxes, and woodchucks results in a symptomless viremia (Kokernot et al. 1969b). Inoculation of gray squirrels produces viremia in adult animals and death in neonates (Timoney 1971). No histologic studies of POWV-infected wild mammals have been published. However, histologic changes in fatal POWV human cases are indistinguishable from those in other fatal flavivirus encephalitides (McLean and Donohue 1959). Inflammation occurs throughout the brain, with perivascular cuffing predominantly by lymphocytes and monocytes and focal infiltration in the brain parenchyma by macrophages and microglia.

DIAGNOSIS. Diagnosis requires virus isolation by intracerebral inoculation of suckling mice, followed by identification using specific antisera and the agar gel precipitation, HI, CF, or N tests. A fourfold rise in paired sera titers by any of these serologic tests is also diagnostic of POWV infection.

TREATMENT AND CONTROL. There is no vaccine against POWV. The only possible treatment is administration of immune serum in cases of known exposure. Control of either vector ticks or wild vertebrate host populations is impractical.

Kyasanur Forest Disease

Synonyms: **None.**

HISTORY AND ETIOLOGY. In 1956 an epidemic of fatal illness in humans and monkeys was first noticed in areas near Kyasanur Forest, Shimoga District, Mysore State, southern India. In 1957, the etiological agent was isolated from sick humans and monkeys and was named Kyasanur Forest disease virus (KFDV) (Work and Trapido 1957). Human and monkey disease continues to the present time. The virus has been isolated only within a restricted area in Mysore State. The disease typically appears in early spring and lasts until midsummer (Work et al. 1959), although virus has been recovered from ticks in all months of the year (Boshell-M. et al. 1968c). The prevalence of disease and location of foci of transmission vary from season to season and year to year within a 2,500 sq km area; mortality in langurs (*Presbytis entellus*) and bonnet monkeys (*Macaca radiata*) is highest from February to April (Goverdhan et al. 1974). KFDV is a flavivirus; antigenically it is a member of the tick-borne encephalitis virus complex and so is closely related to Omsk hemorrhagic fever, louping-ill, and Powassan viruses.

TRANSMISSION. The principal vectors of KFDV are *Haemaphysalis* ticks; nine species of this genus have yielded KFDV isolates (Boshell-M. et al. 1968c). From data on natural and experimental infestations and virus isolations from ticks attached to diseased hosts, the principal KFDV vectors to monkeys are *H. spinigera* and *H. turturis* (Boshell-M. and Rajagopalan 1968a; Boshell-M. et al. 1968c; Trapido et al. 1964). KFDV was also occasionally isolated from *Ixodes petauristae*. Experimentally both *I. petauristae* and *H. spinigera* are able to transmit KFDV transovarially to progeny ticks (Singh et al. 1968a). These two tick species, as well as four other *Haemaphysalis* species found infected in nature can transmit KFDV to vertebrates experimentally (Bhat et al. 1975; Singh et al. 1968b; Varma et al. 1960). Bat ticks (*Ornithodoros* spp.) collected during an epidemic from the roosts of naturally infected bats yielded KFDV (Rajagopalan et al. 1969a); the related tick species *O. crossi* transmitted KFDV experimentally (Bhat and Goverdhan 1973). Although the virus appears in the milk of experimentally infected monkeys, it is not readily transmitted to nursing young (Shah 1965).

HOST RANGE. Langur and bonnet monkeys are frequently infected in nature as evidenced by disease, virus isolations, and antibodies (Goverdhan et al. 1974). Roving monkey bands may be important in the expansion of old KFDV foci of transmission and in initiating new foci. However, the natural histories of closely related viruses, combined with slow monkey population turnover rates, suggest that monkeys are not the primary vertebrate hosts of KFDV.

Small rodents and shrews are thought to be the probable maintenance hosts. KFDV has been isolated from the forest rats *Rattus rattus wroughtoni* and *R. blanfordi* (3 and 11 isolates, respectively) and twice from shrews (*Suncus murinus*) (Boshell-M. et al. 1968a; Rajagopalan et al. 1969a). Naturally acquired antibodies against KFDV have been found in these three species as well as in palm squirrels (*Funambulus tristriatus*), gerbils (*Tatera indica*), and forest mice (*Mus budooga*) (Berge 1975). Laboratory experiments (Singh et al. 1968b) have shown that viremic palm squirrels, shrews, and *R. blanfordi* are infective for ticks. Virus isolations, population densities (Boshell-M. and Rajagopalan 1968b), and experimental viremia levels (Boshell-M. et al. 1968b; Webb 1965) point to shrews and *R. blanfordi* as particularly efficient virus maintenance hosts. The other rodent species are also potentially efficient hosts, with the exception of *R. rattus wrought-oni*, which, though abundant, circulates KFDV briefly and only at low levels.

The role of other vertebrates in the KFDV transmission cycle has been relatively little studied. KFDV has been isolated four times from insectivorous bats (*Rhinolophus rouxi*) and once from their ticks (Rajagopalan et al. 1969b). Antibody against KFDV has been detected in frugivorous bats (*Rousettus leschenaulti* and *Cynopterus sphinx*) (Pavri and Singh 1965; Theiler and Downs 1973), although subsequent laboratory inoculations showed that they could circulate KFDV only at low levels (Pavri and Singh 1968; Theiler and Downs 1973). N antibody has been detected in wild birds, which are important hosts for tick vector species, but KFDV has never been isolated from birds (Theiler and Downs 1973).

PATHOLOGY. Epizootic KFDV disease is typically hemorrhagic in monkeys and humans. Iyer et al. (1960) have described changes in recently dead langurs and bonnet monkeys during epizootics. Grossly, they found anal blood clots and swelling and pallor of the adrenal cortex. In the liver, microscopic changes seen were focal necrosis, degeneration and pigment in central and midzonal cells and parenchymal cells, prominent Kupffer cells, and eosinophil cytoplasmic inclusions. Kidneys had tubular degeneration. Patchy neuronal degeneration, clusters of microglia, and moderate perivascular cuffing were seen in the brain, but without obvious encephalitis. Hemorrhages were seen in lungs, kidneys, brain, or adrenals in 14 of 22 animals, and virus was isolated from a variety of tissues.

Experimental infections of bonnet monkeys by Webb and Chatterjea (1962) produced diarrhea, bradycardia, hypotension, and death. They noted marked leukopenia, lowered hematocrit, and thrombocytopenia and suggested that these changes may have been caused by the marked phagocytosis in peripheral blood of white cells, erythrocytes, and platelets, perhaps mediated immunologically. Further studies (Webb and Burston 1966) showed spinal cord lesions. The infrequency of hemorrhages in these monkeys may have been caused by the use of a mouse-adapted strain. Encephalitis in one monkey may have been a late disease manifestation in a survivor of the hemorrhagic phase.

In humans, three fatal cases were marked by fever, myalgia, toxemia, and widespread hemorrhage (Iyer et al. 1959); pathology was essentially similar to that in monkeys. Disease

is sometimes biphasic, with late central nervous system symptoms (Webb and Rao 1961).

Inoculation of KFDV into *Rattus blanfordi*, *R. rattus wroughtoni*, *Suncus murinus*, and *Mus* spp. produced a symptomless viremia; infection of palm squirrels (*Funambulus tristriatus*) caused high viremia and was frequently fatal (Boshell-M. et al. 1968a; Webb 1965). Inoculation of KFDV into frugivorous bats *Cynopterus sphinx* can cause viremia, weakness, paralysis, and death; high virus concentrations may be found in salivary glands (Pavri and Singh 1968).

DIAGNOSIS. The combined seasonality, restricted distribution, and hemorrhagic symptoms of Kyasanur Forest disease make this a distinctive illness. Diagnosis is confirmed by virus isolation and identification using specific antisera and the N, CF, HI, and agar gel diffusion techniques. For diagnostic studies of paired sera, especially in cases where virus was not isolated, CF and HI tests are recommended (Webb and Chatterjea 1962).

TREATMENT AND CONTROL. An unsuccessful early attempt to protect humans used an inactivated virus vaccine against Russian spring-summer encephalitis virus, a close antigenic relative of KFDV (Shah et al. 1962). Research is now aimed at developing both live attenuated virus and inactivated viral subparticle vaccines (Indian Council of Medical Research 1977).

Tensaw

Synonyms: **None.**

HISTORY AND ETIOLOGY. Tensaw virus (TENV) is a bunyavirus, belonging to the Bunyamwera antigenic group of the Bunyamwera supergroup. TENV was first isolated in 1960 from *Anopheles crucians* mosquitoes caught near the Tensaw River, Alabama (Chamberlain et al. 1969a), and is apparently restricted to the southeastern United States. TENV is not a common cause of animal or human illness but was isolated from a sick Florida gray fox (*Urocyon cinereoargenteus*) (Bigler and Hoff 1975) and from one sick human (McGowan et al. 1973).

TRANSMISSION AND HOST RANGE. Although TENV has been found in a wide variety of mosquito species, the great majority of isolates have been from *A. crucians* (Chamberlain et al. 1969a; Wellings et al. 1972). Sudia et al. (1969) have shown experimentally that other colonized *Anopheles* species can be biological vectors. In addition to the Florida gray fox, wild mammals from which TENV has been isolated are two marsh rabbits (*Sylvilagus palustris*) and a sentinel cotton rat (*Sigmodon hispidus*), all from Florida (Wellings et al. 1972). Antibody has been found in Georgia and Florida raccoons (*Procyon lotor*), and in marsh rabbits, as well as in humans, cattle, and dogs (Bigler and Hoff 1975; Chamberlain et al. 1969a).

PATHOLOGY. Bigler and Hoff (1975) isolated TENV from the brain of a Marion County, Florida, rabies-suspect gray fox with central nervous system symptoms. They reported no histologic studies. Subcutaneous inoculation of dogs, cottontail rabbits (*Sylvilagus transitionalis*), raccoons, and cotton rats produces a symptomless viremia and an antibody response (Sudia et al. 1969). Gray squirrels (*Sciurus carolinensis*), chipmunks (*Tamias striatus*), and opossums (*Didelphis marsupialis*) did not become viremic, and some did not develop antibody. TENV has caused a single reported case of human encephalitis (McGowan et al. 1973).

DIAGNOSIS. As with most other arboviruses, diagnosis depends on virus isolation in suckling mice and identification by N, HI, and CF tests using group and monotypic reagent antisera. A rise in antibody titer of at least fourfold in paired sera is also diagnostic.

TREATMENT AND CONTROL. TENV is not known to be a major human or animal pathogen. Consequently there are no vaccines, vector control measures, or specific treatment procedures.

Snowshoe Hare

HISTORY AND ETIOLOGY. Snowshoe hare virus (SSHV) is a bunyavirus. Antigenically it is a member of the California encephalitis complex of the Bunyamwera supergroup. It was first isolated in Montana in 1959 from a sick snowshoe hare (*Lepus americanus*) (Burgdorfer et al. 1961) and has since been found across northern North America from Alaska to upper New York State (Iversen et al. 1969, 1973; McKiel et al. 1966; McLean et al. 1970, 1975,

1977c; Newhouse et al. 1967; Ritter and Feltz 1974; Whitney et al. 1969). SSHV is not known to cause human or domestic animal disease.

TRANSMISSION. SSHV is mosquito-borne. Isolates from adult mosquitoes have come from 2 species of the genus *Culiseta* and from at least 10 different *Aedes* species (Iversen et al. 1969, 1973; McLean et al. 1970, 1974, 1975, 1977b; Newhouse et al. 1967; Ritter and Feltz 1974). Of these, *A. cinereus* has yielded isolates from the greatest geographic range: Alaska, Yukon, and upper New York State (McLean et al. 1975; Ritter and Feltz 1974; Whitney et al. 1969). In northwestern North America (Alaska, Yukon and Northwest Territories, and Alberta), SSHV has consistently been isolated from wild adult *A. communis* or *communis* group (Hoff et al. 1971; Iversen et al. 1969; McLean et al. 1973, 1975, 1977c; Ritter and Feltz 1974). Experimentally, *A. communis* is also an efficient experimental vector (McLean et al. 1977a). SSHV probably passes to progeny mosquitoes through the overwintering egg, as indicated by isolations from *A. implicatus* and *Aedes* spp. larvae (McLean et al. 1977b; McLintock et al. 1976). Three isolates from ticks are considered unimportant because these arthropods are experimentally resistant to infection and unable to transmit SSHV (Newhouse et al. 1963). The significance of a single black fly isolate is unclear (Ritter and Feltz 1974).

VERTEBRATE HOST RANGE. Both virus isolation and antibody detection indicate that snowshoe hares are the principal vertebrate hosts of SSHV. In addition to the original Montana isolate, snowshoe hares have yielded 22 SSHV isolates in Alaska (Ritter and Feltz 1974) and 1 in Alberta (Hoff et al. 1971). In Alaska, SSHV has been isolated once from a red-backed vole (*Clethrionomys rutilus*) and once from a lemming (*Dicrostomyx rubicans*) (Ritter and Feltz 1974). Neutralizing antibodies have been detected in snowshoe hares from British Columbia (McLean et al. 1971), Yukon Territory (McLean et al. 1975), Alberta (Yuill et al. 1969; Zarnke 1978), Northwest Territories (Gaunt et al. 1974), Montana (Newhouse et al. 1967), northern Michigan (Newhouse et al. 1963), and upper New York State (Whitney et al. 1969).

SSHV antibodies are less prevalent in other wild mammal species than in snowshoe hares and are absent in birds. Ground squirrels (*Spermophilus undulatus* and *S. lateralis*) have been seropositive in British Columbia and Montana, respectively (McLean et al. 1975;

Newhouse et al. 1967). In British Columbia, N antibodies have also been detected in marmots (*Marmota flaviventris*) and chipmunks (*Eutamias amoenus*) (McLean et al. 1970). In the Yukon Territory, red squirrels (*Tamiasciurus hudsonicus*) have N antibodies (McLean et al. 1975). Zarnke (1978) detected SSHV N antibody in Alberta black bears (*Ursus americanus*), moose (*Alces alces*), and bighorn sheep (*Ovis canadensis*). In northern New York State, Whitney et al. (1969) reported N antibodies against a local SSHV strain in cottontail rabbits (*Sylvilagus floridanus*), woodchucks (*Marmota monax*), raccoons (*Procyon lotor*), red foxes (*Vulpes vulpes*), a skunk (*Mephitis mephitis*), a porcupine (*Erethizon dorsatum*), a Norway rat (*Rattus norvegicus*), and deer (*Odocoileus virginianus*).

PATHOLOGY. No gross or microscopic changes were reported for the "emaciated, rather sluggish" Montana hare from which the first isolate originated (Burgdorfer et al. 1961). Subsequent experimental inoculation of the natural SSHV hosts, snowshoe hares and ground squirrels, resulted in a symptomless viremia (Newhouse et al. 1971). These experiments suggest that SSHV infection was simply coincidental with the emaciation and lethargy of the original Montana hare. However, Yuill et al. (1969) found that wild Alberta hares convalescent from SSHV infection experienced higher mortality than did those which had not been infected. Disease has not been reported in humans or cattle, although N antibodies have been detected in both (Iversen et al. 1971; Kettyls et al. 1972).

TREATMENT AND CONTROL. Neither vaccines nor vector controls exist to date, because SSHV disease is unknown in humans and domestic animals and probably not widespread in wild vertebrates. The concept of control of the hordes of arctic and boreal *Aedes* vector mosquitoes is impractical.

Western Equine Encephalitis

Synonyms: **Western encephalitis, western equine encephalomyelitis.**

HISTORY AND ETIOLOGY. Western equine encephalitis virus (WEEV) was first isolated from horses in California (Meyer et al. 1931). Although the virus is distributed across the United States, northward into western Canada and southward into South America, it causes epizootics only in far western North America and in the prairie states and provinces.

WEEV is an alphavirus (group A) of the Togaviridae. It is related to eastern and Venezuelan equine encephalitis viruses (Berge 1975).

TRANSMISSION AND HOST RANGE. The transmission cycles of WEEV vary in far western North America, the eastern United States, and in South America. In the West, *Culex tarsalis* is the principal vector, although its capacity to transmit varies from place to place (Hardy et al. 1976). *Aedes melanimon*, a mammal feeder, is also a WEEV vector (Hardy et al. 1974). Although birds have long been recognized as important hosts of WEEV (Holden et al. 1973), the role of wild mammals as WEEV hosts has recently received more attention. *Culex tarsalis*, usually a bird feeder, does feed preponderantly on jackrabbits (*Lepus californicus*) in some localities (Nelson et al. 1976; Tempelis and Washino 1967), and antibody prevalence rates in these mammals are high. Jackrabbits infected with some strains of WEEV develop viremias sufficient to infect mosquitoes (Hardy et al. 1974). WEEV has been isolated periodically over several years from California tree squirrels (*Sciurus grisius*) and ground squirrels (*Spermophilus beecheyi*) (Berge 1975), and once from an opossum (*Didelphis marsupialis*) (Emmons and Lennette 1969). Several of the squirrels exhibited excitable, aggressive behavior and had bitten people. The role that these mammals play (if any) in the maintenance of WEEV in the West is not clear.

In the prairies and transitional aspen parklands of western Canada, *C. tarsalis*, *A. melanimon*, and *Culiseta inornata* are WEEV vectors (Burton and McLintock 1970; Hayles et al. 1972). Wild mammals may also be important WEEV hosts in the North. Snowshoe hares (*Lepus americanus*) (Kiorpes and Yuill 1975; Yuill and Hanson 1964) and Richardson's ground squirrels (*Spermophilus richardsonii*) (Leung et al. 1975, 1976) are naturally infected and develop significant viremias. Richardson's ground squirrels were infected experimentally by intranasal exposure to WEEV, and transmission without arthropod vectors, by cannibalism or via contaminated urine, has been suggested (Leung et al. 1977).

WEEV is enzootic in swamp foci along the East Coast of the United States but is not responsible for equine or human disease (Hayes and Wallis 1977). The vector mosquito, *Culiseta melanura*, transmits the virus to wild birds (Dalrymple et al. 1972). Mammals do not appear to play a role in the maintenance of WEEV in the East.

The mechanisms for overwintering of WEEV throughout the temperate zone have not been established. The virus has been isolated from hibernating snakes and frogs in the West (Burton et al. 1966; Gebhardt et al. 1973). However, the timing of the posthibernation viremia would have to coincide with spring emergence of blood-seeking mosquitoes. Tortoises (*Gopherus berlandieri*) infected with WEEV in Texas developed high-titered viremias of 105 days, a time sufficient to accomplish overwintering in warmer, southern areas (Bowen 1977). Virus overwintering might also be accomplished by hibernation of infected mosquitoes, reintroduction of the virus by migrating birds or bats, or persistent infections of warm-blooded vertebrates (Hayes and Wallis 1977).

Sporadic WEE cases have occurred in equines but not in man in South America (Theiler and Downs 1973). The mosquito vectors and important vertebrate hosts have not been determined. Antibody prevalence is high in forest birds of the Amazon Basin.

PATHOLOGY. Richardson's ground squirrels infected with WEEV via the subcutaneous or intranasal routes became ill and died (Leung et al. 1976, 1977). The ground squirrels were weak and depressed and developed ataxia as the limbs became paralyzed. A few individuals became hyperexcitable. Grossly, the livers were tan with white focal to diffuse mottling. Vascular congestion and petechial hemorrhaging in the cerebral hemispheres was seen in the brain. Histologic changes were seen most frequently in the olfactory bulbs, cerebral cortex, and leptomeninges. In the first 3 days of infection, focal mononuclear cell infiltration of the meninges and pyknosis of neurons occurred. Marked meningitis was seen beginning on the 4th day, with neural degeneration, neuronophages, perivascular cuffing, gliosis, vasculitis, and parenchymal hemorrhage in the cerebral cortex and brainstem. These lesions persisted until death. On the 5th day hemorrhage became more extensive and perivascular edema occurred in the brainstem and cerebrum. Liver degeneration and necrosis of brown fat were observed also.

DIAGNOSIS AND TREATMENT. Diagnosis is established by isolation of the virus or demonstration of the development of specific neutralizing antibodies in animals that survive. Isolation can be accomplished from brain tissue in a variety of cell cultures, laboratory mice, or embryonating chicken eggs. Attempts at isolation of the virus are frequently unsuccessful from animals with lingering illness (encephalitis for more than a week). These animals may have significant antibody titers at death that interfere with recovery of infectious virus from tissue suspensions. Serologic diagnosis is based on a fourfold or greater rise of antibody titer in convalescent phase sera compared to sera taken during acute illness. Standard serologic tests are employed (N, CF, and HI tests). Demonstration of specific early antibody (immunoglobulin M or its equivalent) within a month of illness can also be used to establish serologic diagnosis of WEEV infection. However, with any of the serologic tests, care must be taken to establish the specificity of the reaction. Serologic cross-reaction can occur between WEEV and its alphavirus relatives, eastern and Venezuelan equine encephalitis viruses. The illness produced by these three viruses in equines is indistinguishable.

Effective vaccines are available for preventive use. Epizootic spread may be prevented or controlled by timely vector control. No specific treatment is available, but symptomatic supportive therapy may be helpful.

Eastern Equine Encephalitis

Synonyms: **Eastern encephalitis, eastern equine encephalomyelitis.**

HISTORY. Fatal encephalitis compatible with that produced by eastern equine encephalitis virus (EEEV) occurred among horses on the eastern coast of the United States in the mid-1800s (Hanson 1973). The virus was first isolated from fatal encephalitis in Maryland horses in 1933 (Giltner and Shahan 1933). EEEV is enzootic in eastern North America and has caused epizootics in horses in the Caribbean Islands and scattered epizootics and cases in Central America, Panama, and throughout

South America (Hanson 1973). The virus is classified as an alphavirus (group A) of the Togaviridae. Interestingly, the North and South American EEEV strains can be differentiated serologically (Casals 1964).

HOST RANGE AND PATHOLOGY. In the temperate zone, the EEEV warm weather maintenance cycle involves wild birds and *Culiseta melanura* mosquitoes (Chamberlain 1968). Many workers have reported antibodies in wild mammals (Berge 1975), but only Goldfield et al. (1969) reported frequent EEEV isolations from a mammal, the white-footed mouse (*Peromyscus leucopus*), throughout the year. However, this observation was not confirmed in white-footed mice from an enzootic focus on the eastern shore of Maryland (T. M. Yuill et al., unpublished data). Experimental infection of eight midwestern rodent species produced no mortality following peripheral inoculation and caused encephalitis and death in gray squirrels (*S. carolinensis*) and in *P. leucopus* inoculated intracerebrally. Signs of encephalitis were supported by histologic changes. *Peromyscus leucopus* from the enzootic focus in Maryland inoculated subcutaneously with 10^6 or more infectious units of low passage EEEV from that area developed encephalitis and died. Inoculation of lesser amounts did not cause mortality (T. M. Yuill, unpublished data). Thus, wild rodents do not appear to play a significant role in EEEV maintenance in the North, and it is unlikely that this virus causes significant mortality in wild mammal populations. The overwintering mechanism for EEEV is unknown.

In the neotropical rainforests, EEEV infects both birds and mammals (Theiler and Downs 1973). The virus and antibodies have been found frequently in a wide variety of bird species in both enzootic and epizootic situations. However, the antigenic differences between North and South American EEEV strains indicate that migrating birds do not cause mixing of the virus between the Northern and Southern hemispheres. The virus also has been isolated from sentinel mice and hamsters and from a sentinel *Cebus* sp. monkey. EEEV also has been isolated from wild-caught rodents (*Proechimys* spp. and *Oryzomys* spp.), and from an opossum (*Marmosa* sp.). EEEV has been isolated most frequently from *Culex* (*Melanoconion*) *taeniopus* in the tropics. However, until the virus-vector-mammal relationships are tested in the laboratory and confirmed in the field, the role of wild mammals in EEEV maintenance and am-

plification or the impact of EEEV on wild mammal populations will remain unknown.

DIAGNOSIS AND TREATMENT. As with WEEV, EEEV diagnosis is established by isolation of the virus or by serologic methods. Care must be taken to differentiate EEEV from WEE or Venezuelan equine encephalitis viruses, especially in tropical areas where all three may occur.

An inactivated virus vaccine is available for administration to equines. Vector control for EEEV is not routinely practiced to the degree that it is for WEEV. Symptomatic treatment may be helpful for affected animals.

Venezuelan Equine Encephalitis

Synonyms: **Peste loca, Venezuelan encephalitis.**

HISTORY AND ETIOLOGY. Periodic outbreaks of encephalitis among equine animals and people have been recognized in northern South America, especially the coastal lowlands of Colombia and Venezuela, since the early 1930s (Groot 1972). The etiologic agent, Venezuelan equine encephalitis virus (VEEV), was isolated from the brain of a sick horse in 1939 (Kubes and Rios 1939). Epidemics occurred as far south as Peru. An epizootic among horses on the cool, high (3,000 m altitude) Bogota altiplano gave one of the first hints of the ecological versatility of VEEV. The sudden appearance of VEE in Guatemala, possibly spread from an outbreak in Ecuador and Peru, signaled the beginning of an epidemic that spread over a 4,000 km area from 1969 to 1971. This outbreak extended northward through Mexico to the lower Rio Grande Valley of Texas, and southward through Central America to Costa Rica. Encephalitis occurred in several thousand humans, and equine mortality exceeded 44,000 animals (Groot 1972), establishing VEE as one of the major arbovirus problems in the Western Hemisphere.

Enzootic or sylvan equine avirulent forms of VEEV were recognized in the neotropics and subtropics. Viral subtypes designated Mucambo, Pixuna, and Everglades were shown to be closely related to VEEV (Berge 1975; Young and Johnson 1969). These subtypes and VEEV are alphaviruses of the Togaviridae.

HOST RANGE AND TRANSMISSION. Epizootic VEEV has equines as the main vertebrate host and a variety of mosquitoes as vectors. The virus has been isolated over 1,000 times from a total of 33 mosquito species in 8 genera (Sudia and Newhouse 1975; Sudia et al. 1975). The majority of the isolations came from *Psorophora confinnis*, *P. discolor*, and *Aedes sollicitans*. *Aedes aegypti* has been implicated in human-to-human spread, in the absence of infected equines, in Venezuela (Suarez and Bergold 1968). The role of wild mammals in the maintenance of epidemic VEEV, if any, is clearly secondary to equines in importance. Many reports have documented VEEV infection of wild mammals during outbreaks. VEEV has been isolated from several mammalian species; some of these, and others from which VEEV has not been isolated, have been shown to be susceptible to experimental infection and to develop viremia (Table 5.3). Several tropical and temperate zone rodents develop high-titered, sustained viremia, and a large proportion die (Bowen 1976). Direct rodent-to-rodent transmission, without arthropod vectors, has been shown experimentally. Cotton rats (*Sigmodon hispidus*) had virus in throat secretions following inoculation with an epidemic VEEV strain, and the virus was transmitted to uninoculated animals housed in the same cage (Howard 1974). The viremias of lagomorphs are of lesser magnitude and shorter duration than those of rodents. Although VEEV has been isolated from opossums (*Didelphis marsupialis* and *Caluromys derbianus*), viremia is low. The role of these marsupials as VEEV reservoir or amplifying hosts is not clear. Canids are susceptible to VEEV infection and develop viremias that appear to be sufficient to infect mosquitoes. However, populations of foxes and coyotes are relatively low, and they may play a more important role as disseminators of the virus than as amplifiers. Bats may play an important part in VEEV epidemiology, as they are susceptible to infection, abundant, and highly mobile (Bowen 1976; Seymour et al. 1978b). VEEV was isolated from a bat (*Artibeus lituratus*) during an outbreak in equines in Colombia (Sanmartin et al. 1973). However, their involvement in the field awaits clarification. VEEV has been isolated from naturally infected vampire bats (*Desmodus rotundus*) in Ecuador (Gutierrez 1972) and Mexico (Correa-G. et al. 1972), and Sanmartin showed that vampires have the virus in their saliva

following inoculation and are capable of transmitting the virus to equines by bite (Seymour and Dickerman 1978). The role of wild birds in VEEV maintenance and spread is unclear (Bowen and McLean 1977; Dickerman et al. 1976), but avian species appear to be far less important in VEEV epizootiology than in EEEV or WEEV. However, birds, mobile wild mammals, or transported domestic animals (equines and dogs) may account for the sudden appearance of VEEV in new locales over long distances.

Although wild mammals may contribute to transmission of VEEV during an outbreak, they do not appear to be able to sustain or maintain virus transmission in the absence of equine populations. There is no evidence that epidemic VEEV persists in wild mammal populations after the virus has disappeared from equine populations in the area. It appears that intense epidemics of VEEV have considerable potential for causing direct mortality among some wild mammalian species, especially among the younger cohorts.

In contrast to epidemic VEEV, the sylvan strains of this virus are maintained in wild mammals, and not in equines, and are associated with a more limited group of arthropod vectors. The maintenance of sylvan VEEV strains has been associated mainly with species of *Melanoconion* subgenus of *Culex* mosquitoes from northern South America (Galindo and Grayson 1971; Woodall 1972) to Mexico (Scherer et al. 1976) and Florida (Chamberlain et al. 1969b; Sudia et al. 1969). Rodents are important vertebrate hosts, including *Oryzomys capito*, *Proechimys guyannensis*, and *Sigmodon hispidus* in the neotropics (Mackenzie, 1972; Shope and Woodall 1973; Zarate and Scherer 1968) and cotton rats, cotton mice (*Peromyscus gossypinus*), opossums, and raccoons in subtropical Florida (Bigler et al. 1974; Lord et al. 1973). Sylvan VEEV was isolated from several sentinel and naturally infected opossums (*Didelphis marsupialis*, *Philander opossum*, and *Marmosa mitis*) (Grayson 1972; Scherer et al. 1972) and bats (*Artibeus phaeotis* (*turpis*), *Carollia subrufa*, and *Uroderma bilobatum*) (Scherer et al. 1972; Seymour et al. 1978a). These more mobile mammals may serve to disseminate the sylvan strains to new forest or swampy areas where foci are established. Birds do not appear to be involved in maintenance or spread of sylvan VEEV; antibody prevalence in and around endemic foci have been low or nil (Dickerman et al. 1972; Scherer et al. 1976). The impact that sylvan VEEV may have on wild mammal populations is unassessed.

PATHOLOGY. The pathologic changes caused by VEEV infection have not been studied in wild mammals. VEEV infection may cause either encephalitis or only an undifferentiated fever, or may be asymptomatic in equines and in humans. The pathologic changes observed in experimental infections varies with the animal species infected (Gochenour 1972). VEEV infection of guinea pigs results in prostrating, febrile disease with death 2–4 days after inoculation. Encephalitis does not occur; rather, there is massive necrosis of lymphocytes in the spleen and lymph nodes and bone marrow depletion. The course of infection in laboratory mice is longer than in guinea pigs. The mice survive the lymphocyte destruction and bone marrow depletion and develop extensive encephalitis involving the entire brain, cord (with marked necrosis of the motor neurons), and meninges. Death occurred in a few dogs receiving high doses of VEEV. The animals had minimal central nervous system involvement (mild perivascular cuffing, congestion of meningeal and cerebral vessels, and slight neuronal degeneration), and the cause of death was not clear.

Disease in experimentally infected equines is similar to that of naturally infected ones. Disease can be mild, limited to fever and leukopenia, through severe leukopenia with marked destruction of lymphocytes in lymph nodes and depletion of myeloid elements of the bone marrow, to severe, diffuse necrotizing meningoencephalitis and vasculitis terminating in death. The sylvan strains do not cause disease in equines. The disease produced in rhesus monkeys was dependent on the VEEV strain used. The Trinidad strain produced a benign, febrile illness. A Colombian strain, in contrast, produced a disease more like severe infections in equines with central nervous system involvement. In the Texas outbreak, 88 human cases were studied (Bowen et al. 1976). Usual signs and symptoms included headache, myalgia, chills, vomiting, sore throat, and diarrhea. Central nervous system signs were observed in 36% of the individuals under 17 years of age and in 11% of those 17 years old or older. Transplacental human infection has been documented with resulting microencephaly, massive brain necrosis and hemorrhage, and other fetal damage leading to neonatal death (Wenger 1977). Similar congenital defects have been observed following experimental infection of pregnant rhesus monkeys with VEEV (London et al. 1977). Colombian children had neurological sequelae 1–4 years after VEEV infection (Leon et al. 1975).

The pathologic changes reported for VEEV infection in equines are similar to those described for EEEV and WEEV. Case fatality ranges from 38% to 83% (Groot 1972). Sequelae are common in surviving animals, often rendering them unfit for work.

DIAGNOSIS. As with EEEV and WEEV, VEEV diagnosis is established by isolation of the virus or demonstration of a significant rise in antibody to the virus. It is often difficult to isolate the virus from brain tissues of fatal cases, probably because of the presence of antibody. Success in demonstrating the presence of the virus in the herd may be enhanced by taking the temperatures of the other horses not yet showing central nervous system signs, and attempting virus isolation from the blood of febrile animals in cell cultures or in suckling mice. Considerable caution must be exercised in handling materials containing virus, as the potential for aerosol infection of laboratory personnel is extremely high.

TREATMENT AND CONTROL. Prevention of epidemic VEEV has been accomplished by vaccination of equine animals. Both live attenuated (TC-83) and inactivated vaccines are currently being employed, but their comparative safety and potency are disputed. Although originally developed for human use, the live vaccine was used extensively (over 10 million doses administered to equines) during the 1969–1971 outbreak. A single dose has been shown to be safe and effective (McKinney 1972). Mosquito control was carried out in Texas, where over 51,000 km² were sprayed with dibrom and malathion (Center for Disease Control 1972). Prevention of human cases is best achieved by control of the infection in equine populations through vaccination. Avoidance of mosquito bites is recommended during an outbreak or to prevent infection with the sylvan strains of the virus. Symptomatic treatment is the only therapeutic approach currently available.

Vesicular Stomatitis

Synonyms: **Erosive stomatitis, stomatatis contagiosa of horses, aphthous stomatitis, mal de tierra, and pseudo aftosa.**

HISTORY. Disease comparable to vesicular stomatitis (VS) was reported in horses during the

Civil War in the United States, in South African horses in the late 1800s, in cattle in a series of outbreaks in the United States in the early 1900s, and in France in horses arriving from the United States in 1915. Two serologically distinct VS viruses were isolated from infected cattle in 1925 and 1926 and were designated VS-Indiana (VSVI) and VS-New Jersey (VSVNJ) (Hanson 1952; Yuill 1979). Enzootic VSI and VSNJ were recognized in horses, cattle, and swine in South and Central America (Hanson 1975). Since the initial recognition of VSVI and VSVNJ, related viruses of the VS complex have been isolated from domesticated animals, wild mammals, and insects around the world (Yuill 1979). Cocal virus (COCV) was isolated from *Gigantolaelaps* sp. mites from Trinidadian rodents and from horses with vesicular disease in Argentina. Alagoas virus (ALAV) was recovered from infected Brazilian horses. Piry virus (PIRV) was isolated from an opossum captured in Brazil. Chandipura virus (CHPV) was isolated from humans and sandflies in India, and later from two species of Nigerian hedgehogs. Isfahan virus (ISFV) was isolated from sandflies in Iran.

ETIOLOGY. VS complex viruses are rhabdoviruses (Rhabdoviridae) (Knudson 1973).

TRANSMISSION. Despite decades of study, the epizootiology of VS viruses is incompletely understood. Both VSVNJ and VSVI cause periodic epizootics in livestock. The mechanisms by which these viruses persist during interepizootic periods is not known. Although the viruses may be spread mechanically within milking herds by virus-contaminated milking machines or milker's hands (Ellis and Kendall 1964) or among swine with lacerated feet (Patterson et al. 1955), there is no evidence for direct animal-to-animal transmission among domestic stock on pasture. The role of wild vertebrates in VS transmission is not clear. Many species are infected in nature, yet very few have been shown to develop viremias sufficient to infect biting arthropods. It has been proposed that VSVI and VSVNJ are plant viruses that become infectious for wild or domesticated vertebrates following passage through arthropods (Hanson 1968; Johnson et al. 1969). In the southeastern United States, where VSVNJ is enzootic, antibody prevalence among wild mammals is highest among deer, feral swine, and raccoons (Karstad and Hanson 1957) especially from low-lying areas, suggesting that omnivores may acquire their infection from other forms of an-

imal life on which they feed (Hanson and Karstad 1958). VSVNJ antibody prevalence rates in the neotropics were highest among several species of rodents, bats, and carnivores (Tesh et al. 1969). However, it is not known if these animals contribute to virus maintenance or are dead-end hosts. Sudden outbreaks, seasonal occurrence, and movements of VSNJ outbreaks in North American livestock suggest arthropod spread of the virus. However, isolation of the virus is less frequent than would be expected if arthropod transmission were occurring.

The wildlife hosts of VSVI in North America are not known. In the tropics, antibody prevalence rates were highest in arboreal and semiarboreal mammals, including two-toed sloths (*Choloepus hoffmani*), spider monkeys (*Ateles* spp.), and a porcupine (*Coendou rothschildi*) (Srihongse 1969). Sandflies, principally *Lutzomyia trapidoi*, are naturally infected in the American tropics; they transovarially transmit the virus to their progeny (Tesh et al. 1972) and experimentally by bite to laboratory mice (Tesh et al. 1971). VSVI has also been isolated from blackflies during an outbreak in dairy cattle in Colombia, South America, but it is not known if these arthropods are vectors (Theiler and Downs 1973).

COCV epizootiology also is unclear. Isolation of this virus from small tropical rodents, their ectoparasitic mites, and *Culex* spp. mosquitoes suggests a rodent-arthropod transmission cycle (Jonkers et al. 1965). However, the viremia in experimental infections of rodents was too low for efficient virus transmission by mites or mosquitoes (Jonkers et al. 1964). In contrast, viremia in experimentally infected bats (*Myotis lucifugus*) have been of relatively high titer, sufficient to permit transmission of the virus by *Aedes aegypti* to suckling mice (Donaldson 1970). The role of bats in natural COCV transmission is unknown.

PIRV has been associated with small mammals also. The virus was isolated from an opossum, and antibodies have been found in sera from several species of marsupials, rodents, bats, primates, edentates, pigs, and water buffalo (Theiler and Downs 1973). Experimentally infected marsupials (*Didelphis marsupialis* and *Philander* spp.) developed viremia and some died. Although PIRV has not been associated with arthropods in nature, the virus did replicate in inoculated *A. aegypti* (Theiler and Downs 1973).

It is not clear if the epizootiologies of CHPV in India and in Africa are similar. In India, the virus has been isolated from man and from

Phlebotomus spp. sandflies (Dhanda et al. 1970). In Africa, the virus was isolated from hedgehogs (*Atelerix spiculatus* and *A. albiventris*) (Berge 1975). Several domesticated animal species had antibodies in nature, and mice and langur monkeys were susceptible to experimental infection (Dhanda et al. 1970).

ISFV has been isolated from sandflies (*P. papatasi*), and serologic surveys indicated that two gerbil species (*Rhombomys opimus* and *Tatera indica*) and people are infected naturally (Tesh et al. 1977). The role of wild vertebrates or arthropods in ALAV transmission is unknown.

SIGNS. The incubation period of VSI and VSNJ in cattle, swine, horses, and deer varies from 24 hours to several days, terminating with the onset of fever. The fever may be biphasic, especially in older calves. Large vesicles may form in the mouth and on the nose, lips, muzzle, coronary band, and teats. During the vesicular stage, animals are often anorexic and depressed. Cattle may salivate copiously and make a characteristic sucking noise; horses grind their teeth. The thin tissue overlying the vesicle breaks, leaving a raw erosion. The erosions heal within a few days, barring secondary bacterial or mycotic infection. Animals may become lame. Teat lesions frequently make it impossible for the dam to be milked or suckled, and mastitis may result, with loss of quarters. Although the signs of VS in naturally infected domesticated animals and experimentally infected deer have been well described (Brandley et al. 1951; Chow and McNutt 1953; Karstad and Hanson 1957), the signs of natural and experimental VS infection in other wild vertebrates have not been documented.

VSI and VSNJ viruses produce an acute influenzalike febrile disease in humans. Chills and fever occur 1–2 days following exposure to the virus from infected animals or in the laboratory. The febrile response may be biphasic, last up to 6 days, and reach 40°C. Fever is accompanied by general malaise, myalgia, headache, and, sometimes, eye and chest pain and vomiting. Occasionally, vesicles may form in the mouth or on the lips and nose. Human infection with ALAV, PIRV, and CHPV also causes acute, febrile disease in man (Yuill 1979). Laboratory infections of PIRV are particularly prevalent.

PATHOLOGY. Virus replication begins in the prickle cells of the stratum malpighii of the epithelium. The virus particles mature and bud off the cell surface and intracytoplasmic vacuo-lar membranes, accumulating in the intercellular spaces and infecting adjoining cells. Infected cells contain desmosomes and cytoplasmic vacuoles, plasma membranes become thickened, and the tonofibrils are scattered. The cytoplasm shrinks, and intercytoplasmic bridges are conspicuous. The epithelium becomes edematous, and a papule forms. The area may be erythematous. Transudates and polymorphonuclear cells accumulate in lacunae and form vesicles under the stratum corneum. The dermis breaks, leaving an erosion, which is quickly repaired by proliferation of fibrous tissue and the epithelium (Proctor and Sherman 1975; Ribelin 1958; Seibold and Sharp 1960; Murphy 1973).

DIAGNOSIS. The signs of lesions of VS are not pathognomonic. VS cannot be distinguished from foot-and-mouth disease in cattle and swine, and the differential diagnosis must be made in the laboratory. Laboratory diagnosis is based on isolation of the virus or demonstration of the development of specific antibodies. The virus can be isolated from the epithelium of ruptured vesicles, fluid from intact vesicles, throat swabs in experimental animals, embryonated chicken eggs, or a variety of cell cultures (Rosenthal and Shechmeister 1971; Valle 1971).

Although serologic diagnosis can be made on the basis of significant rise of VSV antibody, greater caution in interpretation must be exercised than with other groups of arboviruses. VSV-neutralizing antibody titers fluctuate widely (Geleta and Holbrook 1961), and an increasing titer could be due to recent infection or to one of the fluctuations that occur many months after the original exposure to the virus. Complement-fixing antibodies fluctuate less and are a more reliable indicator of recent infection (Holbrook 1962).

The population at risk to VSV infection cannot be assessed by presence or absence of antibodies, as it can with other arboviruses. Animals convalescent from VSV infection may again become susceptible to infection with the homologous virus, despite the presence of neutralizing antibody (Casteneda et al. 1964). The serum protection test in the mouse appears to be the best in vitro indicator of immunity to reinfection (Casteneda et al. 1964).

CONTROL. Control in livestock or in wildlife is difficult without a clearer understanding of the epizootiology of the disease. Livestock can be vaccinated with attenuated or inactivated

VSVNJ or VSVI vaccines (Correa 1964; Lauerman and Hanson 1963). Antibiotics may be
useful to treat secondary infection from erosions.

REFERENCES

Adam, K. M. G., Beasley, S. J., and Blewitt, D. A. The
    occurrence of antibody to *Babesia* and to the
    virus of louping-ill in deer in Scotland. *Res. Vet.
    Sci.* 23:133–38, 1977.
Alifanov, V. I. [Study data on the ectoparasite fauna
    of muskrats in Omsk oblast. In A. A. Maksimov
    and G. I. Netsky, eds. *The muskrat of western
    Siberia (biocenotic relations, parasite fauna,
    epizootics, and measures of prophylaxis)*], pp.
    66–71. Novosibirsk: Biol. Inst. Akad. Nauk
    SSSR, Sibirsk. Otd., 1966.
Allen, R., Taylor, S. K., and Sulkin, S. E. Studies of
    arthropod-borne virus infections in Chiroptera:
    VIII. Evidence of natural St. Louis encephalitis
    virus infection in bats. *Am. J. Trop. Med. Hyg.*
    19:851–859, 1970.
Anderson, C. R., Spencer, L. P., Downs, W. G., and
    Aitken, T. H. G. Manzanilla virus: A new virus
    from the blood of a howler monkey in Trinidad,
    W. I. *Am J. Trop. Med. Hyg.* 9:78–80, 1960.
Andral, L., Bres, P., Serie, C., Casals, J., and Panth-
    ier, R. Etudes sur la fievre jaune en Ethiopie: 3.
    Etude serologique et virologique de la faune syl-
    vatique. *Bull. WHO* 38:855–861, 1968.
Bearcroft, W. G. C. The histopathology of the liver of
    yellow fever-infected rhesus monkeys. *J. Pathol.
    Bacteriol.* 74:295–303, 1957.
Berge, T. O., ed. *International catalogue of arbo-
    viruses including certain other viruses of verte-
    brates*, 2d ed. USDHEW publ. no. (CDC)
    75–8301, 1975.
Bergold, G. H., and Weibel, J. Demonstration of yel-
    low fever virus with the electron microscope.
    Virology 17:554–562, 1962.
Bhat, H. R., Sreenivasan, M. A., Goverdhan, M. K.,
    and Naik, S. V. Transmission of Kyasanur
    Forest disease virus by *Haemaphysalis kyasan-
    urensis* Trapido, Hoogstraal, and Rajagopalan,
    1964 (Acarina: Ixodidae). *Indian J. Med. Res.*
    63:879–887, 1975.
Bhat, U. K. M., and Goverdhan, M. K. Transmission
    of Kyasanur Forest disease by the soft tick *Or-
    nithodorus crossi. Acta Virol.* 17:337–342, 1973.
Bigler, W. J., and Hoff, G. L. Arbovirus surveillance
    in Florida: wild vertebrate studies, 1965–1974.
    J. Wildl. Dis. 11:348–356, 1975.
Bigler, W. J., Ventura, A. K., Lewis, A. L., Wellings,
    F. M., and Ehrenkranz, N. J. Venezuelan equine
    encephalomyelitis in Florida: Endemic virus cir-
    culation in native rodent populations of Ever-
    glades hammocks. *Am. J. Trop. Med. Hyg.*
    23:513–521, 1974.
Boshell-M., J., Goverdhan, M. K., and Rajagopalan, P.
    K. Preliminary studies on the susceptibility of

wild rodents and shrews to KFD virus. *Indian J.
    Med. Res.* 56:614-627, 1968a.
———. Preliminary studies on the susceptibility of
    wild rodents and shrews to KFD virus. *Indian J.
    Med. Res.* 56:614–627, 1968b.
Boshell-M., J., and Rajagopalan, P. K. Observation on
    the experimental exposure of monkeys, rodents,
    and shrews to infestations of ticks in forest in
    Kyasanur Forest disease area. *Indian J. Med.
    Res.* 56:573–588, 1968a.
———. Small rodents and shrews in the Sagar-Sorab
    area, Mysore State, India: population studies,
    1961–1964. *Indian J. Med. Res.* 56:527–540,
    1968b.
Boshell-M., J., Rajagopalan, P. K., Patil, A. P., and
    Pavri, K. M. Isolation of Kyasanur Forest dis-
    ease virus from *Ixodid* ticks: 1961–1964. *Indian
    J. Med. Res.* 56:541–568, 1968c.
Bowen, G. S. Experimental infection of North Ameri-
    can mammals with epidemic Venezuelan en-
    cephalitis virus. *Am. J. Trop. Med. Hyg.*
    25:891–899, 1976.
———. Prolonged western equine encephalitis vire-
    mia in the Texas tortoise (*Gopherus berlandieri*).
    Am. J. Trop. Med. Hyg. 26:171–175, 1977.
Bowen, G. S., Fashinell, T. R., Dean, P. B., and Gregg,
    M. B. Clinical aspects of human Venezuelan
    equine encephalitis in Texas. *Bull. Pan Am.
    Health Org.* 10:46–57, 1976.
Bowen, G. S., and McLean, R. G. Experimental infec-
    tion of birds with epidemic Venezuelan encepha-
    litis virus. *Am. J. Trop. Med. Hyg.* 26:808–814,
    1977.
Brandley, C. A., Hanson, R. P., and Chow, I. I. Ve-
    sicular stomatitis with particular reference to
    the 1949 Wisconsin epizootic. *Proc. 88th Ann.
    Meeting Am. Vet. Med. Assoc.*, p. 61, 1951.
Brotherston, J. G., and Boyce, J. B. Development of a
    non-infective protective antigen against loup-
    ing-ill (arbovirus group B). *J. Comp. Pathol.*
    80:377–388, 1970.
Brummer-Korvenkontio, M. Arboviruses in Finland:
    V. Serological survey of antibodies against Inkoo
    virus in human, cow, reindeer, and wildlife sera.
    Am. J. Trop. Med. Hyg. 22:654–661, 1973.
Buescher, E. L., Byrne, R. J., Clarke, G. C., Gould, D.
    J., Russell, P. K., Scheider, F. G., and Yuill, T. M.
    Cache Valley virus in the Del Mar, Va. penin-
    sula: I. Virologic and serologic evidence of infec-
    tion. *Am. J. Trop. Med. Hyg.* 19:493-502, 1970.
Burgdorfer, W., Newhouse, V. F., and Thomas, L. A.
    Isolation of California encephalitis virus from
    the blood of a snowshoe hare (*Lepus americanus*)
    in Western Montana. *Am. J. Hyg.* 73:344–349,
    1961.
Burgher, J. C. The pathology of yellow fever. In G. K.
    Strode, ed. *Yellow fever*, pp. 137–163. New
    York: McGraw-Hill, 1951.
Burton, A. N., and McLintock, J. Further evidence of
    western encephalitis infection in Saskatchewan
    mammals and birds and in reindeer in northern
    Canada. *Can. Vet. J.* 11:232–235, 1970.
Burton, A. N., McLintock, J., and Rempel, J. G. 1966.

Western equine encephalitis virus in Saskatchewan garter snakes and leopard frogs. *Science* 154:1029–1031, 1966.

Casals, J. Antigenic variants of eastern equine encephalitis virus. *J. Exp. Med.* 119:547–565, 1964.

Casteneda, G. J., Lauerman, L. H. J., and Hanson, R. P. Evaluation of virus neutralization tests and association of indices to cattle resistance. *Proc. U.S. Livestock Sanit. Assoc.* 68:455–468, 1964.

Center for Disease Control. *Venezuelan equine encephalitis annual summary.* Atlanta: U.S. Department of Health, Education and Welfare, Public Health Service, 1972.

———. Yellow fever in 1975. *Wkly. Epidemiol. Rec.* 51:301–305, 1976.

Chamberlain, R. W. Arboviruses, the arthropod-borne animal viruses. In *Current topics in microbiology and immunology*, vol. 42, pp. 35–58. Berlin: Springer, 1968.

Chamberlain, R. W., Sudia, W. D., and Coleman, P. H. Isolations of an arbovirus of the Bunyamwera group (Tensaw virus) from mosquitoes in the southeastern United States. *Am. J. Trop. Med. Hyg.* 18:92–97, 1969a.

Chamberlain, R. W., Sudia, W. D., Work, T. H., Coleman, P. H., Newhouse, V. F., and Johnston, J. G., Jr. Arbovirus studies in south Florida, with emphasis on Venezuelan equine encephalomyelitis virus. *Am. J. Epidemiol.* 89:197–210, 1969b.

Chow, T. L., and McNutt, S. H. Pathological changes of experimental vesicular stomatitis of swine. *Am. J. Vet. Res.* 14:420, 1953.

Chumakov, M. P. [Etiology, epidemiology, and prevention of hemorrhagic fever.] In *Tezisy Dokl. 4. Nauch. Sess. Pozvyashch. Probl. Kraev. Neiroinfekts. Patol.*, pp. 40–43. Moscow: 1949.

———. [Results of the study made on Omsk hemorrhagic fever (OHF) by an expedition of the Institute of Neurology.] *Vestn. Akad. Nauk SSSR* 2:19–28, 1948.

Clarke, D. H. Antigenic analysis of certain Group B arthropod-borne viruses by antibody absorption. *J. Exp. Med.* 111:21–32, 1960.

———. Further studies on antigenic relationships among the viruses of the group B tick-borne complex. *Bull. WHO* 31:45–56, 1964.

Clarke, D. H., and Casals, J. Arboviruses: Group B. In F. L. Horsfall and I. Tamm, eds. *Viral and rickettsial infections of man*, pp. 606–658. Philadelphia: Lippincott, 1965.

Coleman, P. H., Ryder, S., and Work, T. H. Mahogany Hammock virus: A new Guama group arbovirus from the Florida Everglades. *Am. J. Epidemiol.* 89:217–221, 1969.

Correa, W. M. Prophylaxis of vesicular stomatitis: A field trial in Guatemalan dairy cattle. *Am. J. Vet. Res.* 25:1300–1302, 1964.

Correa-G., P., Calisher, C. H., and Baer, G. M. Epidemic strain of Venezuelan equine encephalomyelitis virus from a vampire bat captured in Oaxaca, Mexico, 1970. *Science* 175:546–547, 1972.

Dalrymple, J. M., Young, O. P., Eldridge, B. F., and Russell, P. K. Ecology of arboviruses in a Maryland freshwater swamp: III. Vertebrate hosts. *Am. J. Epidemiol.* 96:129–140, 1972.

Danilov, O. N., Fedorova, T. N., and Matyukhin, V. N. [Results of bird examination for the presence of antibodies to Omsk hemorrhagic fever virus in northern Kulunda. In A. I. Cherepanov et al., eds. *Migratory birds and their role in the transport of arboviruses*], pp. 333–338. Novosibirsk: Sibirsk. Otd. Akad. Nauk SSSR, Biol. Inst., Akad. Med. Nauk SSSR, Inst. Polio. Entsef., Minist. Zdravookhr. RSFSR, Omsk. Inst. Prirod.-Ochag. Infekts., 1969.

Darwish, M. A., and Hammon, W. McD. Preparation of inactivated St. Louis encephalitis virus vaccine from hamster kidney cell cultures. *Proc. Soc. Exp. Biol. Med.* 123:242–246, 1966.

Davies, F. G. A survey of Nairobi sheep disease antibody in sheep and goats, wild ruminants, and rodents within Kenya. *J. Hyg., Camb.* 81:251–258, 1978.

de Rodaniche, E., and Galindo, P. St. Louis encephalitis in Panama: III. Investigation of local mammals and birds as possible reservoir host. *Am. J. Trop. Med. Hyg.* 10:390–392, 1961.

Dhanda, V., Rodrigues, F. M., and Gosh, S. N. Isolation of Chandipura virus from sandflies in Aurangabad. *Indian J. Med. Res.* 58:179, 1970.

Dickerman, R. W., Bonacorsa, C. M., and Scherer, W. F. Viremia in young herons and ibis infected with Venezuelan encephalitis virus. *Am. J. Epidemiol.* 104:678–683, 1976.

Dickerman, R. W., Scherer, W. F., Moorhouse, A. S., Toaz, E., Essex, M. E., and Steele, R. E. Ecologic studies of Venezuelan encephalitis virus in southeastern Mexico: VI. Infection of wild birds. *Am. J. Trop. Med. Hyg.* 21:66–78, 1972.

Doherty, R. L., Carley, J. G., Standfast, H. A., Dyce, A. L., Kay, B. H., and Snowdon, W. A. Isolation of arboviruses from mosquitoes, midges, sandflies, and vertebrates collected in Queensland, 1969 and 1970. *Trans. R. Soc. Trop. Med. Hyg.* 67:536–543, 1973.

Doherty, R. L., Carley, J. G., Standfast, H. A., Dyce, A. L., and Snowdon, W. A. Virus strains isolated from arthropods during an epizootic of bovine ephemeral fever in Queensland. *Aust. Vet. J.* 48:81–86, 1972.

Doherty, R. L., Whitehead, R. H., Wetters, E. J., Gorman, B. M., and Carley, J. G. A survey of antibody to 10 arboviruses (Koongol group, Mapputta group and ungrouped) isolated in Queensland. *Trans. R. Soc. Trop. Med. Hyg.* 65:748–753, 1970.

Donaldson, A. I. Bats as possible maintenance hosts for vesicular stomatitis virus. *Am. J. Epidemiol.* 92:132–136, 1970.

Dunaev, N. B. [Mixed infection: tularemia and Omsk hemorrhagic fever in an experiment on *Arvicola terrestris* L.] *Zh. Mikrobiol. Epidemiol. Immunobiol.* 8:118–122, 1976.

Eklund, C. M. Role of mammals in maintenance of

arboviruses. *An. Microbiol.* 11:99–105, 1963.

Ellis, E. M., and Kendall, H. E. The public health and economic effects of vesicular stomatitis in a herd of dairy cattle. *J. Am. Vet. Med. Assoc.* 144:377, 1964.

Emmons, R. W., and Lennette, E. H. Isolation of St. Louis encephalitis from a naturally infected gray fox *Urocyon cinereoargenteus. Proc. Soc. Exp. Biol. Med.* 125:443–447, 1967.

———. Isolation of western equine encephalomyelitis virus from an opossum. *Science* 163:945–946, 1969.

Fedorova, T. N. [Results of virological study of Omsk hemorrhagic fever (OHF) in muskrats in western Siberia. In A. A. Maksimov and G. I. Netsky, eds. *The muskrat of western Siberia (biocenotic relations, parasite fauna, epizootics, and measures of prophylaxis)*], pp. 136–140. Novosibirsk: Biol. Inst., Akad. Nauk SSSR, Sibirsk. Otd., 1966a.

———. [Susceptibility and sensibility in muskrats to Omsk hemorrhagic fever virus. In A. A. Maksimov and G. I. Netsky, eds. *The muskrat of western Siberia (biocenotic relations, parasite fauna, epizootics, and measures of prophylaxis)*], pp. 131–135. Novosibirsk: Biol. Inst., Akad. Nauk SSSR, Sibirsk. Otd., 1966b.

Fedorova, T. N., and Sizemova, G. A. [Incidence of Omsk hemorrhagic fever in man and the muskrat during winter.] *Zh. Mikrobiol. Epidemiol. Immunobiol.* 41:134–136, 1964.

Gagarina, A. V. [Transmission of Omsk hemorrhagic fever by ticks. In M. P. Chumakov, ed. *Endemic viral infections (hemorrhagic fever with renal syndrome, Crimean hemorrhagic fever, Omsk hemorrhagic fever, and Astrakhan virus from Hyalomma pl. plumbeum tick.*] *Sborn. Trudy Inst. Polio. Virus. Entsef. Akad. Med. Nauk SSSR* 7:422–429, 1965.

Galindo, P., and Grayson, M. A. *Culex (Melanoconion) aikenii*: Natural vector in Panama of endemic Venezuelan encephalitis. *Science* 172:594–559, 1971.

Gaunt, R. A., Stowe, P. C., and Watson, C. G. Antibody to human pathogens in the wildlife of the Yellowknife, N.W.T., area. *Can. J. Public Health* 65:61, 1974.

Gavrilovskaya, I. N., and Chumakov, M. P. [Application of the neutralization test in tissue culture for serological investigations of Omsk hemorrhagic fever.] *Mater. 11. Nauch. Sess. Inst. Polio. Virus. Entsef.*, pp. 314–315. Moscow: 1964.

Gebhardt, L. P., St. Jeor, S. C., Stanton, G. J., and Stringfellow, D. A. Ecology of western encephalitis virus. *Proc. Soc. Exp. Biol. Med.* 142:731–733, 1973.

Geleta, J. N., and Holbrook, A. A. Vesicular stomatitis: Patterns of complement-fixing and serum-neutralizing antibody in serum of convalescent cattle and horses. *Am. J. Vet. Res.* 22:713, 1961.

Giltner, L. T., and Shahan, M. S. The 1933 outbreak of infectious equine encephalomyelitis in the eastern states. *North Am. Vet.* 14:25–27, 1933.

Gochenour, W. S., Jr. The comparative pathology of

Venezuelan equine encephalitis virus infection in selected animal hosts. In *Venezuelan encephalitis*. Pan Am. Health Org. sci. publ. no. 243, pp. 113–117, 1972.

Goldfield, M., Sussman, M. S., Altman, R., and Kandle, R. P. Eastern equine encephalitis in New Jersey during 1968. *Proc. N.J. Mosq. Exterm. Assoc.* 56:56–63, 1969.

Gorgas Memorial Laboratory. *48th Annual Report, Fiscal Year 1976.* 95th Congress, 1st Session, House Document No. 95–39. Washington, D.C.: U.S. Government Printing Office, 1977.

Goverdhan, M. K., Rajagopalan, P. K., Narasima Marthy, D. P., Upadhaya, S., Boshell-M., J., Trapido, H., and Ramachandra, T. Epizootiology of Kyasanur Forest Disease in wild monkeys of Shimoga District, Mysore State (1957–1964). *Indian J. Med. Res.* 62:497–510, 1974.

Grayson, M. A. Discussion on mammalian hosts of VEE. In *Venezuelan encephalitis*. Pan Am. Health Org. publ. 243, pp. 276–277, 1972.

Greutter, J. E., Fulton, J. D., Meuther, R. O., Hanss, E. V., and Broun, G. O. Susceptibility of field mice and meadow mice to St. Louis encephalitis. *Proc. Soc. Exp. Biol. Med.* 44:253–254, 1940.

Groot, H. The health and economic impact of Venezuelan equine encephalitis (VEE). In *Venezuelan encephalitis*. Pan Am. Health Org. sci. publ. no. 243, pp. 7–16, 1972.

Gutierrez, E. Discussion of human cases, Ecuador. In *Venezuelan encephalitis*. Pan Am. Health Org. sci. publ. no. 243, pp. 195–201, 1972.

Hammon, W. McD., Lundy, H. W., Gray, J. A., Evans, F. C., Bang, F., and Izumi, E. M. A large-scale serum-neutralization survey of certain vertebrates as part of an epidemiological study of encephalitis of western equine and St. Louis types. *J. Immunol.* 44:75–86, 1942.

Hamon, J., and Brown, A. W. A. [Introduction to the conference on yellow fever in tropical Africa, Bobo-Dioulasso, Upper Volta, 20–23 March, 1971.] *Cah. Off. Rech. Sci. Tech. Outre-Mer Entomol. Med. Parasit.* 10:87, 1972.

Hanson, R. P. Discussion of the natural history of vesicular stomatitis. *Am. J. Epidemiol.* 87:264, 1968.

———. The natural history of vesicular stomatitis virus. *Bacteriol. Rev.* 16:179, 1952.

———. Vesicular stomatitis. In H. W. Dunne and A. D. Leman, eds. *Diseases of swine*, p. 308. Ames: Iowa State University Press, 1975.

———. Virology and epidemiology of eastern and western arboviral encephalomyelitis of horses. In II. *American arboviral encephalomyelitides of Equidae*, pp. 200–214. Proc. 3rd Int. Conf. Eq. Inf. Dis. Basel: Karger, 1973.

Hanson, R. P., and Karstad, L. Further studies on vesicular stomatitis. *Proc. U.S. Livestock Sanit. Assoc.* 61:300, 1958.

Hardy, J. L., Milby, M. M., Wright, M. E., Beck, A. J., and Bruen, J. B. Natural and experimental arboviral infections in a population of blacktail jackrabbits along the Sacramento River in Butte

County, California (1971–1974). *J. Wildl. Dis.* 13:383–392, 1977.

Hardy, S., Milby, M. M., Wright, M. E., Beck, A. J., Presser, S. B., and Bruen, J. B. Natural and experimental arboviral infections in a population of blacktail jackrabbits along the Sacramento River in Butte County, California (1971–1974). *J. Wildl. Dis.* 13:373–392, 1977.

Hardy, J. L., Reeves, W. C., Scrivani, R. P., and Roberts, D. R. Wild mammals as hosts of Group A and Group B arboviruses in Kern County, California. *Am. J. Trop. Med. Hyg.* 23:1165–1177, 1974.

Hardy, J. L., Reeves, W. C., and Sjogren, R. D. Variations in the susceptibility of field and laboratory populations of *Culex tarsalis* to experimental infection with western equine encephalomyelitis virus. *Am. J. Epidemiol.* 103:498–505, 1976.

Hayes, C. G., and Wallis, R. C. Ecology of western equine encephalomyelitis in the eastern United States. *Adv. Vir. Res.* 21:37–83, 1977.

Hayles, L. B., McLintock, J., and Saunders, J. R. Laboratory studies on the transmission of western equine encephalitis virus by Saskatchewan mosquitoes: I. *Culex tarsalis. Can. J. Comp. Med.* 36:83–88, 1972.

Henderson, B. E., Calisher, C. H., Coleman, P. H., Fields, B. N., and Work, T. H. Gumbo Limbo: A new group C arbovirus from the Florida Everglades. *Am J. Epidemiol.* 89:227–231, 1969.

Henderson, B. E., McCrae, A. W. R., Kirya, B. G., Ssenkubuge, Y., and Sempala, S. D. K. Arbovirus epizootics involving man, mosquitoes and vertebrates at Lunyo, Uganda, 1968. *Ann. Trop. Med. Parasitol.* 66:343–355, 1972.

Hoff, G. L., Anslow, R. O., Spalatin, J., and Hanson, R. P. Isolation of Montana snowshoe hare serotype of California encephalitis virus group from a snowshoe hare and *Aedes* mosquitoes. *J. Wildl. Dis.* 7:28–34, 1971.

Hoff, G. L., Issel, G. J., Trainer, D. O., and Richard, S. H. Arbovirus serology in North Dakota mule and white-tailed deer. *J. Wildl. Dis.* 9:291–295, 1973.

Hoff, G. L., Yuill, T. M., Iversen, J. O., and Hanson, R. P. Selected microbial agents in snowshoe hares and other vertebrates of Alberta. *J. Wildl. Dis.* 6:472–478, 1970.

Holbrook, A. A. Duration of immunity and serologic patterns in swine convalescing from vesicular stomatitis. *J. Am. Vet. Med. Assoc.* 141:1463, 1962.

Holden, P., Hayes, R. O., Mitchell, C. J., Francy, D. B., Lazuick, J. S., and Hughes, T. B. House sparrows, *Passer domesticus* (L.) as hosts of arboviruses in Hale County, Texas: I. Field studies, 1965–1969. *Am. J. Trop. Med. Hyg.* 22:244–253, 1973.

Hopkins, C. C., Hollinger, F. B., Johnson, R. F., Dewlett, H. J., Newhouse, V. F., and Chamberlain, R. W. The epidemiology of St. Louis encephalitis virus in Dallas, Texas, 1966. *Am. J. Epidemiol.* 102:1–15, 1975.

Howard, A. T. Experimental infection and intracage transmission of Venezuelan equine encephalitis virus (subtype IB) among cotton rats, *Sigmodon hispidus* (Say and Ord). *Am J. Trop. Med. Hyg.* 23:1178–1184, 1974.

Howitt, B. F., and Van Herrick, V. Relationship of the St. Louis and the western equine encephalitis viruses to fowl and mammals in California. *J. Infect. Dis.* 71:171–191, 1942.

Indian Council of Medical Research. Report of the Director-general. New Delhi, 1977.

Iversen, J. O., Hanson, R. P., Papadopoulos, O., Morris, C. V., and de Foliart, G. R. Isolation of viruses of the California encephalitis virus group from boreal *Aedes* mosquitoes. *Am. J. Trop. Med. Hyg.* 18:735–742, 1969.

Iversen, J. O., Seawright, G., and Hanson, R. P. Serologic survey for arboviruses in Central Alberta. *Can. J. Public Health* 62:125–132, 1971.

Iversen, J. O., Wagner, R. J., Dejong, C., and McLintock, J. California encephalitis virus in Saskatchewan: Isolation from boreal *Aedes* mosquitoes. *Can. J. Public Health* 64:590–594, 1973.

Iyer, C. G. S., Rao, R. L., Work, T. H., and Murthy, D. P. N. Kyasanur Forest disease: IV. Pathological findings in three fatal human cases of Kyasanur Forest disease. *Indian J. Med. Sci.* 13:1011–1022, 1959.

Iyer, C. G. S., Work, T. H., Murthy, D. P. N., Trapido, H., and Rajagopalan, P. K. Kyasanur Forest disease: VII. Pathological findings in monkeys, *Presbytis entellus* and *Macaca radiata*, found dead in the forest. *Indian J. Med. Res.* 48:276–286, 1960.

Johnson, K. M. Yellow fever. In W. T. Hubbert, W. F. McCulloch, and P. R. Schnurrenberger, eds., *Diseases transmitted from animals to man*, pp. 929–938. Springfield: Thomas, 1975.

Johnson, K. M., Tesh, R. B., and Peralta, P. H. Epidemiology of vesicular stomatitis virus: Some new data and a hypothesis for transmission of the Indiana serotype. *J. Am. Vet. Med. Assoc.* 155:2133, 1969.

Jonkers, A. H., Spence, L., and Aitken, T. H. G. Cocal virus epizootiology in Bush Bush forest and the Nariva swamp, Trinidad, W. I.: Further studies. *Am. J. Vet. Res.* 26:758, 1965.

Jonkers, A. H., Spence, L., Coakwell, C. A., and Thornton, J. J. Laboratory studies with wild rodents and viruses native to Trinidad. *Am. J. Trop. Med. Hyg.* 13:613, 1964.

Karstad, L., and Hanson, R. P. Vesicular stomatitis in deer. *Am. J. Vet. Res.* 18:162–166, 1957.

Kettyls, G. D., Verrall, V. M., Wilton, L. D., Clapp, J. B., Clarke, D. A., and Rublee, J. D. Arbovirus infections in man in British Columbia. *Can. Med. Assoc. J.* 106:1175–1179, 1972.

Kharitonova, N. N. [Results of serological investigation of blood from wild and domestic animals in the Omsk hemorrhagic fever focus of northern Kulunda. In A. I. Cherepanov et al., eds., *Migratory birds and their role in the disperson of arboviruses*], pp. 317–321. Novosibirsk: Sibirsk. Otd. Akad. Nauk SSSR, Biol. Inst., Akad. Med.

Nauk SSSR, Inst. Polio. Entsef., Minist. Zdravookhr. RSFSR, Omsk. Inst. Prirod.-Ochag. Infekts., 1969.

Kharitonova, N. N., and Leonov, Yu. A. [Infection of
mammals and birds with Omsk hemorrhagic
fever virus by the alimentary route.] *Mater. 6
Simp. Izuch. Virus. Ekol. Svyazan. Ptits.*, pp.
31–32. Omsk: 1971.

_____. [On the role of the red-cheeked suslik in the
Omsk hemorrhagic fever (OHF) focus in northern Kulunda. In A. I. Cherepanov et al., eds.,
*Migratory birds and their role in the disperson of
arboviruses*], pp. 349–351. Novosibirsk: Sibirsk.
Otd. Akad. Nauk SSSR, Biol. Inst., Akad. Med.
Nauk SSSR, Inst. Polio. Entsef., Minist. Zdravookhr. RSFSR, Omsk. Inst. Prirod.-Ochag. Infekts., 1969.

Kiorpes, A. L., and Yuill, T. M. Environmental modification of western equine encephalomyelitis infection in the snowshoe hare (*Lepus americanus*). *Inf. Imm.* 11:986–990.

Kissling, R. E. Host relationship of the arthropod-
borne encephalitides. *Ann. N.Y. Acad. Sci.*
70:320–327, 1958.

Knudson, D. L. Rhabdoviruses. *J. Gen. Virol.* 20:105,
1973.

Kokernot, R. H., Calisher, C. H., Stannard, L. J., and
Hayes, J. Arbovirus studies in the Ohio-Missis-
sippi basin, 1964–1967: VII. Lone Star virus: A
hitherto unknown agent isolated from the tick
Amblyomma americanum (Linn.). *Am. J. Trop.
Med. Hyg.* 18:789–795, 1969a.

Kokernot, R. H., Radivojevic, B., and Anderson, R. J.
Susceptibility of wild and domesticated animals
to four arboviruses. *Am. J. Vet. Res.*
30:2197–2203, 1969b.

Kornilova, E. A., Gagarina, A. V., and Chumakov, M.
P. [Comparative characteristics of Omsk hemorrhagic fever virus isolated from different objects in a natural focus.] *Vopr. Virusol.*
2:232–236, 1970.

Ksiazek, T. G., and Yuill, T. M. Viremia and antibody
responses to La Crosse virus in sentinel gray
squirrels (*Sciurus carolinensis*) and chipmunks
(*Tamias striatus*). *Am. J. Trop. Med. Hyg.*
26:815–821, 1978.

Kubes, V., and Rios, F. A. The causative agent of
infectious equine encephalomyelitis in Venezuela. *Science* 90:20–21, 1939.

Kukharchuk, L. P., Strizhak, M. V., and Karavaev, V.
S. [The role of mosquitoes in Omsk hemorrhagic
fever (OHF) virus circulation in ornithocenoses
of western Siberia. In A. I. Cherepanov, ed.,
Questions of entomology in Siberia], pp.
145–146. Novosibirsk: Akad. Nauk SSSR, Sibirsk. Otd. Biol. Inst. Vses. Ent. Obshch., 1974.

Lauerman, L. H., and Hanson, R. P. Field trial vaccination against vesicular stomatitis in Panama.
Proc. U.S. Livestock Sanit. Assoc. 67:483, 1963.

Leon, C. A., Jaramillo, R., Martinez, S., Fernandez,
F., Tellez, H., Lasso, B., and de Guzman, R.
Sequelae of Venezuelan equine encephalitis in
humans: A four year follow-up. *Int. J. Epidemiol.*
4:131–140, 1975.

Leonov, Yu. A., Barbash, L. A., and Kharitonova, N.
N. [The significance of mass small mammal species in the epizootiology of Omsk hemorrhagic
fever in northern Kulunda. In A. I. Cherepanov
et al., eds., *Migratory birds and their role in the
transport of arboviruses*], pp. 322–327. Novosibirsk: Sibirsk. Otd. Akad. Nauk SSSR, Biol.
Inst., Akad. Med. Nauk SSSR, Inst. Polio. Entsef., Minist. Zdravookhr. RSFSR, Omsk. Inst.
Prirod.-Ochag. Infekts., 1969.

Leonov, Yu. A., and Fedorova, T. N. [The role of
rodents and shrews in OHF foci of northern
Kulunda. In G. I. Netsky, A. A. Maksimov, and
K. T. Yurlov, eds., *The role of migrating birds in
the distribution of arboviruses.*] *Mater. 2. Mez-
hinst. Simp.*, Novosibirsk, April 26–27, pp.
31–33. Novosibirsk: 1966.

_____. [Immunological activity to Omsk hemorrhagic
fever (OHF) of small mammals in northern Kulunda. In A. I. Cherepanov et al., eds., *Migratory
birds and their role in the dispersion of arboviruses*], pp. 344–348. Novosibirsk: Sibirsk. Otd.
Akad. Nauk SSSR, Biol. Inst., Akad. Med. Nauk
SSSR, Inst. Polio. Entsef., Minist. Zdravookhr.
RSFSR, Omsk. Inst. Prirod.-Ochag. Infekts.,
1969.

Leonov, Yu. A., and Kharitonova, N. N. [The role of
heterothermic animals in the circulation of
Omsk hemorrhagic fever virus. In A. I. Chere-
panov et al., eds., *Migratory birds and their role
in the transport of arboviruses*], pp. 339–343.
Novosibirsk: Sibirsk. Otd. Akad. Nauk SSSR,
Biol. Inst., Akad. Med. Nauk SSSR, Inst. Polio.
Entsef., Minist. Zdravookhr. RSFSR, Omsk. Inst.
Prirod.-Ochag. Infekts., 1969.

Leung, M. K., Burton, A., Iversen, J., and McLintock,
J. Natural infections of Richardson's ground
squirrels with western equine encephalomyelitis
virus, Saskatchewan, Canada, 1964–1973. *Can.
J. Microbiol.* 21:954–958, 1975.

Leung, M. K., Iversen, J., McLintock, J., and
Saunders, J. R. Subcutaneous exposure of the
Richardson's ground squirrel (*Spermophilus richardsonii* Sabine) to western equine encephalomyelitis virus. *J. Wildl. Dis.* 12:237–246, 1976.

Leung, M. K., McLintock, J., and Iversen, J. Intranasal exposure of the Richardson's ground
squirrel to western equine encephalomyelitis
virus. *Can. J. Comp. Med.* 42:184–191, 1977.

London, W. T., Levitt, N. H., Kent, S. G., Wong, V. G.,
and Sever, J. L. Congenital cerebral and ocular
malformations induced in rhesus monkeys by
Venezuelan equine encephalitis virus. *Teratology* 16:285–296, 1977.

Lord, R. D., Calisher, C. H., Chappell, W. A., Metzger,
W. R., and Fisher, G. W. Urban St. Louis en-
cephalitis surveillance through wild birds. *Am.
J. Epidemiol.* 99:360–363, 1974.

Lord, R. D., Calisher, C. H., Sudia, W. D., and Work,
T. H. Ecological investigations of vertebrate
hosts of Venezuelan equine encephalomyelitis
virus in south Florida. *Am. J. Trop. Med. Hyg.*
22:116–123, 1973.

Lvov, D. K., Chervonski, V. I., Gostinshchikova, I. N.,

Zemit, A. S., Gromashevski, V. L., Tsyrkin, Yu. M., and Veselovskaya, O. V. Isolation of Tyuleniy virus from ticks *Ixodes (Ceratixodes) putus* Pick-Camb. 1878 collected on Commodore Islands. *Arch. Ges. Virusforsch.* 38:139–142, 1972.

Lvov, D. K., Leonova, G. N., Gromashevski, V. L., Belikova, N. P., Berezina, L. K., Safronov, A. V., Veselovskaya, O. V., Gofman, Yu. P., and Klimenko, S. M. Isolation of Powassan virus from *Haemaphysalis neumanni*, Donitz 1905, ticks in Primorye. *Vopr. Virusol.* 5:538–541, 1974.

Lvov, D. K., Karas, F. R., Timofeev, E. M., Tsyrkin, Yu. M., Vargina, S. G., Veselovskaya, O. V., Osipova, N. Z., Grebenyuk, Yu. I., Gromashevski, V. L., Steblyanko, S. N., and Fomina, K. B. "Issyk-kul" virus, a new arbovirus isolated from bats and *Argas (Carios) vespertilionis* (Latr., 1802) in the Kirghiz S.S.R. *Arch. Ges. Virusforsch.* 42:207–209, 1973.

McGowan, J. E. Jr., Bryan, J. A., and Gregg, M. B. Surveillance of arboviral encephalitis in the United States, 1955–1971. *Am. J. Epidemiol.* 97:199–207, 1973.

Mackenzie, R. B. The role of silent vertebrate hosts in epidemics of Venezuelan encephalitis. In *Venezuelan encephalitis.* Pan Am. Health Org. sci. publ. no. 243, pp. 239–243, 1972.

McKiel, J. A., Hall, R. R., and Newhouse, V. F. Viruses of the California encephalitis complex in indicator rabbits. *Am. J. Trop. Med. Hyg.* 15:98–102, 1966.

McKinney, R. W. Inactivated and live VEE vaccines: A review. In *Venezuelan encephalitis.* Pan Am. Health Org. sci. publ. no. 243, pp. 369–376, 1972.

McLean, D. M., Bergman, S. K. A., Goddard, E. J., Graham, E. A., and Purvin-Good, K. W. Northsouth distribution of arbovirus reservoirs in British Columbia, 1970. *Can. J. Public Health* 62:120–124, 1971.

McLean, D. M., Bergman, S. K. A., Gould, A. P., Grass, P. N., Miller, M. A., and Spratt, E. E. California encephalitis virus prevalence throughout the Yukon Territory, 1971–1974. *Am. J. Trop. Med. Hyg.* 24:676–684, 1975.

McLean, D. M., Bergman, S. K. A., Graham, E. A., Greenfield, G. P., Olden, J. A., and Patterson, R. O. California encephalitis virus prevalence in Yukon mosquitoes during 1973. *Can. J. Public Health* 65:23–28, 1974.

McLean, D. M., Best, J. M., Mahalingam, S., Chernesky, M. A., and Wilson, W. E. Powassan virus: Summer infection cycle, 1964. *Can. Med. Assoc. J.* 91:1360–1362, 1964a.

McLean, D. M., Clarke, A. M., Goddard, E. J., Manes, A. S., Montalbetti, C. A., and Pearson, R. E. California encephalitis virus endemicity in the Yukon Territory, 1972. *J. Hyg.* 71:391–402, 1973.

McLean, D. M., Cobb, C., Gooderham, S., Smart, C., Wilson, A. G., and Wilson, W. E. Powassan virus: Persistance of viral activity during 1966. *Can. Med. Assoc. J.* 96:660–664, 1967.

McLean, D. M., Crawford, M. A., Ladyman, S. R.,

Peers, R. R., and Purvin-Good, K. W. California encephalitis and Powassan virus activity in British Columbia, 1969. *Am. J. Epidemiol.* 92:266–272, 1970.

McLean, D. M., deVos, A., and Quantz, E. J. Powassan virus: Field investigations during the summer of 1963. *Am. J. Trop. Med. Hyg.* 13:747–753, 1964b.

McLean, D. M., and Donohue, W. L. Powassan virus: Isolation of virus from a fatal case of encephalitis. *Can. Med. Assoc. J.* 80:708–711, 1959.

McLean, D. M., Grass, P. N., and Judd, B. D. California encephalitis virus transmission by Arctic and domestic mosquitoes. *Arch. Virol.* 55:39–45, 1977a.

McLean, D. M., Grass, P. N., Judd, B. D., Cmiralova, D., and Stuart, K. M. Natural foci of California encephalitis virus activity in the Yukon Territory. *Can. J. Public Health* 68:69–73, 1977b.

McLean, D. M., Grass, P. N., Judd, B. D., Ligate, L. V., and Peter, K. K. Bunyavirus isolations from mosquitoes in the western Canadian Arctic. *J. Hyg.* 79:61–72, 1977c.

McLean, D. M., Ladyman, S. R., and Purvin-Good, K. W. Westward extension of Powassan virus prevalence. *Can. Med. Assoc. J.* 98:946–949, 1968.

McLean, D. M., and Larke, R. P. B. Powassan and Silverwater viruses: Ecology of two Ontario arboviruses. *Can. Med. Assoc. J.* 88:182–185, 1963.

McLean, D. M., Smith, P. A., Livingstone, S. E., Wilson, W. E., and Wilson, A. G. Powassan virus: Vernal spread during 1965. *Can. Med. Assoc. J.* 94:532–536, 1966.

McLean, R. G., and Bowen, G. S. Vertebrate hosts. In T. P. Monath, ed., *Saint Louis encephalitis*, pp. 381–450. Washington: Am. Public Health Assoc., 1980.

McLintock, J., Curry, P. S., Wagner, R. J., Leung, M. K., and Iversen, J. O. Isolation of snowshoe hare virus from *Aedes implicatus* larvae in Saskatchewan. *Mosq. News* 36:233–237, 1976.

Marenko, V. F., Dunaev, N. B., Egorova, L. S., and Fedorova, T. N. [Experimental mixed infection in muskrats (Omsk hemorrhagic fever and tularemia).] *Vopr. Virusol.* 5:545–550, 1974.

Meyer, K. F., Haring, C. M., and Howitt, B. The etiology of epizootic encephalomyelitis in horses in the San Joaquin Valley, 1930. *Science* 74:227–228, 1931.

Mitchell, C. J., Francy, D. B., and Monath, T. P. Arthropod vectors. In T. P. Monath, ed., *St. Louis encephalitis*, pp. 313–379. Washington: Am. Public Health Assoc., 1980.

Moulton, D. W., and Thompson, W. H. California group virus infections in small, forest-dwelling mammals of Wisconsin. *Am. J. Trop. Med. Hyg.* 20:474–482, 1971.

Muckenfuss, R. S., Armstrong, C., and McCordock, H. A. Encephalitis: Studies on experimental transmission. *Public Health Rep.* 48:1341–1343, 1933.

Murphy, F. A. Evolution of rhabdovirus tropisms. In E. Kurstak and K. Maramorosch, eds., *Viruses, evolution and cancer*, p. 699. New York: Academic Press, 1973.

Nelson, R. L., Tempelis, C. H., Reeves, W. C., and Milby, M. M. Relation of mosquito density to bird: mammal feeding ratios of *Culex tarsalis* in stable traps. *Am. J. Trop. Med. Hyg.* 25:644–654, 1976.

Newhouse, V. F., Burgdorfer, W., and Corwin, D. Field and laboratory studies on the hosts and vectors of the snowshoe hare strain of California virus. *Mosq. News* 31:401–408, 1967.

Newhouse, V. F., Burgdorfer, W., McKiel, J. A., and Gregson, J. D. California encephalitis virus: Serologic survey of small wild mammals in northern United States and southern Canada, and isolation of additional strains. *Am. J. Hyg.* 78:123–129, 1963.

Osterieth, P. M., and Deleplanque-Liegeois, P. Presence d'anticorps vis-a-vis des virus transmis par arthropodes chey le chimpanze (*Pan troglodites*). Comparaison de leur etat immunitaire a celui de l'homme. *Ann. Soc. Belge Med. Trop.* 40:205–214, 1961.

Patterson, W. C., Jenny, E. W., and Holbrook, A. A. Experimental infections with vesicular stomatitis in swine: I. Transmission by direct contact and feeding infected meat scraps. *Proc. U.S. Livestock Sanit. Assoc.* 59:368–378, 1955.

Pavri, K. M., and Singh, K. R. P. Demonstration of antibodies against the virus of Kyasanur Forest disease (KFD) in the frugivorous bat *Rousettus leschenaulti*, near Poona, India. *Indian J. Med. Res.* 53:956–961, 1965.

———. Kyasanur Forest disease infection in the frugivorous bat, *Cynopterus sphinx*. *Indian J. Med. Res.* 56:1202–1204, 1968.

Pinger, R. R., Rowley, W. A., Wong, Y. W., and Dorsey, D. C. Trivittatus virus infection in wild mammals and sentinel rabbits in central Iowa. *Am. J. Trop. Med. Hyg.* 24:1006–1009, 1975.

Pool, W. A., Brownlee, A., and Wilson, D. R. The etiology of louping-ill. *J. Comp. Pathol.* 43:253–290, 1930.

Proctor, S. J., and Sherman, K. C. Ultrastructural changes in bovine lingual epithelium infected with vesicular stomatitis virus. *Vet. Pathol.* 12:362–377, 1975.

Rad'kova, O. A., and Vorob'eva, N. N. [Isolation of OHF viruses from coldblooded animals in a natural focus.] *Izv. Sib. Otd. Akad. Nauk SSSR, Ser. Biol. Med. Nauk* 2:180–182, 1971.

Rajagopalan, P. K., Paul, S. D., and Sreenivasan, M. A. Involvement of *Rattus blanfordi* (Rodentia: Muridae) in the natural cycle of Kyasanur Forest disease virus. *Indian J. Med. Res.* 57:999–1002, 1969a.

———. Isolation of Kyasanur Forest disease virus from the insectivorous bat *Rhinolophus rouxi* and from *Ornithodoros* ticks. *Indian J. Med. Res.* 57:805–808, 1969b.

Ravdonikas, O. V., Chumakov, M. P., Solovey, E. A., Ivanov, D. I., and Korsh, P. V. [Importance of the marsh-burrow inhabiting *Ixodes apronophorus*

P. Sch. tick in Omsk hemorrhagic fever virus circulation in a natural focus. In M. P. Chumakov, ed. *Viral hemorrhagic fevers: Crimean hemorrhagic fever, Omsk hemorrhagic fever, hemorrhagic fever with renal syndrome.*] *Trudy Inst. Polio. Virus. Entsef. Akad. Med. Nauk SSSR*, 19:485–491, 1971.

Ravdonikas, O. V., Korsh, P. V., and Ivanov, D. I. [Landscape characteristics of the distribution area of Omsk hemorrhagic fever.] *Trudy Inst. Polio. Virus. Entsef. Akad. Med. Nauk SSSR* 12:441–448, 1968.

Reid, H. W., Barlow, R. M., Boyce, J. B., and Inglis, D. M. Isolation of louping-ill virus from a roe deer (*Capreolus capreolus*). *Vet. Rec.* 98:116, 1976.

Ribelin, W. E. The cytopathogenesis of vesicular stomatitis virus infection in cattle. *Am. J. Vet. Res.* 29:66–73, 1958.

Ritter, D. G., and Feltz, E. T. On the natural occurrence of California encephalitis virus and other arboviruses in Alaska. *Can. J. Microbiol.* 20:1359–1366, 1974.

Rosenthal, L. J., and Shechmeister, I. L. Comparison of microtiter procedures with the plaque technique for assay of vesicular stomatitis virus. *Appl. Microbiol.* 21:400–404, 1971.

Sanmartin, C., Mackenzie, R. B., Trapido, H., Barreto, P., Mullenax, C. H., Gutierrez, E., and Lesmes, C. Encefalitis equina venezolana en Colombia, 1967. *Bol. Ofic. Sanit. Panam.* 74:108–137, 1973.

Scherer, W. F., Dickerman, R. W., Ordonez, J. V., Seymour, C., III, Kramer, L. D., Jahrling, P. B., and Powers, C. D. Ecologic studies of Venezuelan encephalitis virus and isolations of Nepuyo and Patois viruses during 1968–1973 at a marsh habitat near the epicenter of 1969 outbreak in Guatemala. *Am. J. Trop. Med. Hyg.* 25:161–162, 1976.

Scherer, W. F., Ordonez, J. V., Jahrling, P. B., Pancake, B. A., and Dickerman, R. W. Observations of equines, humans and domestic and wild vertebrates during the 1969 equine epizootic and epidemic of Venezuelan encephalitis in Guatemala. *Am. J. Epidemiol.* 95:255–266, 1972.

Schliessmann, D. J., and Calheiros, L. B. A review of the status of yellow fever and *Aedes aegypti* eradication programs in the Americas. *Mosq. News* 34:1–9, 1974.

Seibold, H. R., and Sharp, J. B., Jr. A revised concept of the pathologic changes of the tongue in cattle with vesicular stomatitis. *Am. J. Vet. Res.* 21:35–51, 1960.

Seymour, C., and Dickerman, R. W. Venezuelan encephalitis virus infection in neotropical bats: III. Experimental studies on virus excretion and nonarthropod transmission. *Am. J. Trop. Med. Hyg.* 27:307–312, 1978.

Seymour, C., Dickerman, R. W., and Martin, M. S. Venezuelan encephalitis virus infection in neotropical bats: I. Natural infection in a Guatemalan enzootic focus. *Am. J. Trop. Med. Hyg.* 27:290–296, 1978a.

_____. Venezuelan encephalitis virus infection in neotropical bats: II. Experimental infections. *Am. J. Trop. Med. Hyg.* 27:297–306, 1978b.

Shah, K. V. Experimental infection of lactating monkeys with Kyasanur Forest disease virus. *Acta Virol.* 9:71–75, 1965.

Shah, K. V., Aniker, S. P., Murthy, D. P. N., Rodrigues, F. M., Jayadeviah, M. S., and Prasanna, H. A. Evaluation of the field experience with formalin-inactivated mouse brain vaccine of Russian spring-summer encephalitis against Kyasanur Forest disease. *Indian J. Med. Res.* 50:162–174, 1962.

Shinner, J. J. St. Louis virus encephalomyelitis. *Arch. Pathol.* 75:309–322, 1963.

Shope, R. E., and Woodall, J. P. Ecological interaction of wildlife, man and a virus of the Venezuelan equine encephalomyelitis complex in a tropical forest. *J. Wildl. Dis.* 9:198–203, 1973.

Singh, K. R. P., Goverdhan, M. K., and Bhat, H. R. Transovarial transmission of Kyasanur Forest disease virus by *Ixodes petauristae*. *Indian J. Med. Res.* 56:628–632, 1968a.

Singh, K. R. P., Goverdhan, M. K., and Ramachandra Rao, T. Experimental transmission of Kyasanur Forest disease virus to small mammals by *Ixodes petauristae*, *I. ceylonensis*, and *Haemaphysalis spinigera*. *Indian J. Med. Res.* 56:594–609, 1968b.

Sizemova, G. A. [Clinical picture of Omsk hemorrhagic fever (OHF) associated with epizootics among muskrats.] *Trudy Inst. Polio. Virus. Entsef. Akad. Med. Nauk SSSR* 12:449–452, 1968.

Smith, C. E. G., Varma, M. G. R., and McMahon, D. Isolation of louping ill virus from small mammals in Ayrshire, Scotland. *Nature* 203:992–993, 1964.

Srihongse, S. Vesicular stomatitis virus infections in Panamanian primates and other vertebrates. *Am. J. Epidemiol.* 90:69, 1969.

Steelman, C. D., Gassie, J. M., and Crowen, B. R. Laboratory and field studies on mosquito control in waste disposal lagoons in Louisiana. *Mosq. News* 27:57–59, 1967.

Suarez, O. M., and Bergold, G. H. Investigations of an outbreak of Venezuelan equine encephalitis in towns of eastern Venezuela. *Am. J. Trop. Med. Hyg.* 17:875–880, 1968.

Sudia, W. D., Coleman, P. H., and Chamberlain, R. W. Experimental vector-host studies with Tensaw virus, a newly recognized member of the Bunyamwera arbovirus group. *Am. J. Trop. Med. Hyg.* 18:92–97, 1969.

Sudia, W. D., McLean, R. G., Newhouse, V. F., Johnston, J. G., Jr., Miller, D. L., Trevino, H., Bowen, G. S., and Sather, G. Epidemic Venezuelan equine encephalitis in North America in 1971: Vertebrate field studies. *Am. J. Epidemiol.* 101:36–50, 1975.

Sudia, W. D., and Newhouse, V. F. Epidemic Venezuelan equine encephalitis in North America: A summary of virus-vector-host relationships. *Am. J. Epidemiol.* 101:1–13, 1975.

Sudia, W. D., Newhouse, V. F., and Chappell, W. A. Venezuelan equine encephalitis virus vector studies following a human case in Dade County, Florida, 1968. *Mosq. News* 29:596–600, 1969.

Sulkin, S. E., Allen, R., and Sims, R. Studies of arthropod-borne virus infections in Chiroptera: I. Susceptibility of insectivorous species to experimental infection with Japanese B and St. Louis encephalitis viruses. *Am. J. Trop. Med. Hyg.* 12:800–814, 1963.

Tarasevich, L. N., Tagil'tsev, A. A., Bogdanov, I. I., and Shmel'kov, Yu. A. [Survival of Omsk hemorrhagic fever in gamasid mites in bird nests of southern Omsk oblast.] *Sborn. Trud. Ekol. Virus* 2:140–144, 1974.

Tarasevich, L. N., Tagil'tsev, A. A., and Mal'kov, G. B. [Data on the virological examination of ixodid ticks and fleas in the south of Omsk oblast.] *Med. Parazit.* 38:705–707, 1969.

Tatarintsev, N. M. [Remote sequelae of Omsk hemorrhagic fever.] *Sov. Med.* 31:97–100, 1968.

Taufflieb, R., Robin, Y. and Cornet, M. 1971. [Yellow fever virus in African wildlife.] *Cah. ORSTOM, ser. Ent. Med. Parisitol.* 9:351–371, 1971.

Tempelis, C. H., and Washino, R. K. Host-feeding patterns of *Culex tarsalis* in the Sacramento Valley, California, with notes on other species. *J. Med. Ent.* 4:315–318, 1967.

Tesh, R. B., Chaniotis, B. N., and Johnson, K. M. Vesicular stomatitis virus, Indiana serotype: Multiplication and transmission by experimentally infected phlebotomine sandflies (*Lutzomyia trapidoi*). *Am. J. Epidemiol.* 93:491, 1971.

_____. Vesicular stomatitis virus (Indiana serotype): Transovarial transmission by phlebotomine sandflies. *Science* 175:1477, 1972.

Tesh, R. B., Peralta, P. H., and Johnson, K. M. Ecologic studies of vesicular stomatitis virus: I. Prevalence of infection among animals and humans living in an area of endemic VSV activity. *Am. J. Epidemiol.* 90:255, 1969.

Tesh, R., Saidi, S., Javadian, E., Loh, P., and Nadim, A. Isfahan virus, a new vesiculovirus. *Am. J. Trop. Med. Hyg.* 26:299–306, 1977.

Theiler, M., and Downs, W. C. *The arthropod-borne viruses of vertebrates*. London: Yale University Press, 1973.

Thomas, L. A., Kennedy, R. C., and Eklund, C. M. Isolation of virus closely related to Powassan virus from *Dermacentor andersoni* collected along North Cache La Poudre River, Colorado. *Proc. Soc. Exp. Biol. Med.* 104:355–359, 1960.

Timoney, P. Powassan virus infection in the grey squirrel. *Acta Virol.* 15:429, 1971.

Timoney, P. J., Donnelly, W. J. C., Clements, L. O., and Fenlon, M. Encephalitis caused by louping ill virus in a group of horses in Ireland. *Equine Vet. J.* 8:113–117, 1976.

Trainer, D. O., and Hanson, R. P. Serologic evidence of arbovirus infections in wild ruminants. *Am. J. Epidemiol.* 90:354–358, 1969.

Trainer, D. O., and Hoff, G. L. Serologic evidence of arbovirus activity in a moose population in Alberta. *J. Wildl. Dis.* 7:118–119, 1971.

Trapido, H., Goverdhan, M. K., Rajagopalan, P. K., and Rebello, M. J. Ticks ectoparasitic on monkeys in the Kyasanur Forest disease area of Shimoga District, Mysore State, India. *Am. J. Trop. Med. Hyg.* 13:763–772, 1964.

Valle, M. Factors affecting plaque assay of animal viruses with special reference to vesicular stomatitis and vaccinia virus. *Acta Pathol. Microbiol. Scand., Ser. B,* suppl. 219, 69 pp., 1971.

Varma, M. G. R., Pudney, M., Leake, C. J., and Peralta, P. H. Isolation in a mosquito (*Aedes pseudoscutellaris*) cell line (Mos. 61) of yellow fever virus strains from original field material. *Intervirology* 6:50–56, 1976.

Varma, M. G. R., Webb, H. E., and Pavri, K. M. Studies on the transmission of Kyasanur Forest disease virus by *Haemaphysalis spinigera* Neumann. *Trans. R. Soc. Trop. Med. Hyg.* 54:509–516, 1960.

Vorob'eva, A. M., Dokuchaeva, Yu. I., and Vershinina, T. A. [Combined foci of tick-borne encephalitis and Omsk hemorrhagic fever in southern taiga of Irtysh region.] *Mater. 6. Simp. Izuch. Virus. Ekol. Svyazan. Ptits.,* pp. 29-30. Omsk: 1971.

Warren, A. J. Landmarks in the conquest of yellow fever. In G. K. Strode, ed. *Yellow fever,* pp. 1–37. New York: McGraw-Hill, 1951.

Webb, H. E. Kyasanur Forest disease virus in three species of rodents. *Trans. R. Soc. Trop. Med. Hyg.* 59:205–211, 1965.

Webb, H. E., and Burston, J. Clinical and pathological observations with special reference to the nervous system in *Macaca radiata* infected with Kyasanur Forest disease virus. *Trans. R. Soc. Trop. Med. Hyg.* 60:325–331, 1966.

Webb, H. E., and Chatterjea, J. B. Clinico-pathological observations on monkeys infected with Kyasanur Forest disease virus, with special reference to the hemopoietic system. *Br. J. Haematol.* 8:401–413, 1962.

Webb, H. E., and Rao, R. L. Kyasanur Forest disease: A general clinical study in which some cases with neurological complications were observed. *Trans. R. Soc. Trop. Med. Hyg.* 55:284–98, 1961.

Wellings, F. M., Lewis, A. L., and Pierce, L. V. Agents encountered during arboviral ecological studies: Tampa Bay, Florida, 1963 to 1970. *Am. J. Trop. Med. Hyg.* 21:201–213, 1972.

Wenger, F. Venezuelan equine encephalitis. *Teratology* 16:359–362, 1977.

West, G. P., ed. *Encyclopedia of animal care,* 11th ed., pp. 433–434. Baltimore: Williams and Wilkins, 1975.

Whitney, E. Serologic evidence of group A and B arthropod-borne virus activity in New York State. *Am. J. Trop. Med. Hyg.* 12:417–424, 1963.

Whitney, E., and Jamnback, H. The first isolation of Powassan virus in New York State. *Proc. Soc.*

Exp. Biol. Med. 119:432–435, 1965.

Whitney, E., Jamnback, H., Means, R. G., Roz, A. P., and Rayner, G. A. Isolation and characterization of California encephalitis complex from *Aedes cinereus. Am. J. Trop. Med. Hyg.* 18:123–131, 1969.

Williams, H., and Thorburn, H. Serum antibodies to louping-ill virus. *Scottish Med. J.* 7:353–355, 1962.

Williams, H., Thorburn, H., and Ziffo, G. S. Isolation of louping ill virus from the red grouse. *Nature* 200:193–194, 1963.

Woodall, J. P. Discussion of dynamics of VEE virus transmission in the Aura Forest. In *Venezuelan encephalitis.* Pan Am. Health Org. sci. publ. no. 243, pp. 273–275, 1972.

———. Virus research in Amazonia. *Atas do Simposio sobre a biota Amazonica* 6(Patalogia):31–63, 1967.

Work, T. H., Rodriguez, F. R., and Bhatt, P. N. Virological epidemiology of the 1958 epidemic of Kyasanur Forest disease. *Am. J. Public Health* 49:869–874, 1959.

Work, T. H., and Trapido, H. Summary of preliminary report of investigations of the Virus Research Center on epidemic disease affecting forest villages and wild monkeys of Shimoga District, Mysore. *Indian J. Med. Sci.* 11:340–341, 1957.

World Health Organization. Dengue fever. *Wkly. Epidemiol. Rec.* 52:243, 1977.

World Health Organization. Dengue surveillance. *Wkly. Epidemiol. Rec.* 51:373, 1976.

World Health Organization. Technical guide for a system of yellow fever surveillance. *Wkly. Epidemiol. Rec.* 45:493–500, 1971.

Young, N. A., and Johnson, K. M. Antigenic variants of Venezuelan equine encephalitis virus: Their geographic distribution and epidemiologic significance. *Am. J. Epidemiol.* 89:286–307, 1969.

Yuill, T. M. Vesicular stomatitis. In J. H. Steele and G. W. Beran, eds. *Handbook of zoonoses,* sect. B, Viral zoonoses. West Palm Beach: CRC Press, 1980.

Yuill, T. M., and Hanson, R. P. Serologic evidence of California encephalitis virus and western equine encephalitis virus infection in a population of snowshoe hares. *Zoon. Res.* 3:153–163, 1964.

Yuill, T. M., Iversen, J. O., and Hanson, R. P. Evidence for arbovirus infections in a population of snowshoe hares: A possible mortality factor. *Bull. Wildl. Dis. Assoc.* 5:248–253, 1969.

Zarnke, R. L. Occurrence of selected microbial pathogens in Alberta wild mammals. Ph.D. thesis, University of Wisconsin, 1978.

Zarate, M. L., and Scherer, W. F. Contact spread of Venezuelan equine encephalomyelitis virus among cotton rats via urine or feces and the naso- or oropharynx. *Am. J. Trop. Med. Hyg.* 17:894–899, 1968.

6 *Foot-and-Mouth Disease*

R. S. HEDGER

Synonyms: **Aphthous fever, hoof-and-mouth disease.**

Foot-and-mouth disease (FMD) is an acute, febrile, highly contagious viral disease of ruminants and pigs, characterized primarily by the formation of vesicles and subsequently by erosions on the tongue, in the mouth, and on the feet. Numerous wild species including buffalo, deer, antelope, peccaries, and European hedgehogs are susceptible. In domestic animals the disease is a problem of worldwide concern occurring over wide areas of Europe, Asia, Africa, and South America.

HISTORY AND DISTRIBUTION. Although FMD is not mentioned in the works of ancient writers, it has long been recognized as a disease of domestic ruminants and pigs, and it has been known for many years that wild ungulates may also be affected. The majority of early reports of FMD in wild species, whether free living or in zoological gardens, were based on clinical observations during concurrent outbreaks of disease in domestic animals; few were substantiated by virus isolation or the demonstration of specific antibody. In the light of present knowledge, however, there can be little doubt that at least some of these reports represented occurrences of FMD.

In the United States in 1924, during a campaign to eradicate FMD in California, more than 22,000 deer were slaughtered, 10% of which showed lesions typical of FMD (McVicar et al. 1974). Magnusson (1939) reported that a young moose (*Alces alces*) found near an infected farm had typical signs of infection. In Europe the disease has been described in free living fallow deer (*Dama dama*) (Bartels and Classen 1936) during an epizootic in cattle in the same area and in roe deer (*Capreolus capreolus*) and red deer (*Cervus elaphus*) (Cohrs and Weber-Springe 1939). Kvitkin (1959) and Ogryzkov (1963) have described both experimental and naturally occurring FMD in reindeer (*Rangifer tarandus*). In great Britain, McLaughlan and Henderson (1947) found infected hedgehogs (*Erinaceus europaeus*) in the vicinity of outbreaks in cattle. The hedgehogs had lesions on

their feet, tongues, and snouts. It has also been shown that hedgehogs could harbor latent FMD virus infection during hibernation and then transmit the disease on awakening in the spring (Hulse and Edwards 1937).

Several authors have described outbreaks of FMD in zoological gardens. Urbain et al. (1938) gave an account of an outbreak in the Paris zoo in which 32 out of 250 animals believed to be susceptible were reported as affected. Positive cases were recorded in gaur (*Bos gaurus*), Asiatic buffalo (*Bubalus bubalis*), bison (*Bison bison*), deer (*Cervus eldi*), wild boars (*Babirussa bàbirussa*) from the Celebes, bushbuck (*Tragelaphus scriptus*), warthogs (*Phacochoerus aethiopicus*), and tapirs (*Tapirus indicus* and *T. terrestris*).

During an outbreak of FMD in the Zurich zoo in 1949, bison and yak (*Bos grunniens*) were described as clinically affected (Allenspach, 1950), and in South America, Grosso (1957) described an outbreak of disease in the Buenos Aires zoo, mentioning Asiatic buffalo, American bison, Columbian deer (*Odocoileus columbianus*), and grizzly bears (*Ursus arctos*) as being affected. Unfortunately none of these cases of FMD was confirmed by virus isolation.

In Africa, where in many territories FMD is endemic and wild animals of many species share their habitat with domestic animals, there has long been interest in the role played by wild animals in the perpetuation and spread of FMD. Many species have been incriminated. In 1947 Rossiter and Albertyn described lesions indicative of FMD in 6 of 70 game animals shot on farms where cattle were infected with FMD. Lesions were seen in 2 impala (*Aepyceros melampus*), 2 waterbuck (*Kobus ellipsiprymnus*), a kudu (*Tragelaphus strepsiceros*), and a sable antelope (*Hippotragus niger*). Lesions on both tongue and feet were encountered in only one animal, an impala. Scrapings from one impala inoculated into guinea pigs produced lesions typical of FMD. In 1964 Macaulay published a checklist of no less than 29 different species of nondomestic animals reported throughout the world to have been infected with FMD. Of these, 19 were African species, and Macaulay mentioned that 5 East African species had been proved to be susceptible to artificial infection in the laboratory; namely, East African hedgehog (*Atelerix albiventris*), procupine (*Hystrix galeata*), mole rat (*Tachyoryctes splendens*), wild rat (*Arvicanthis abyssinicus nubilans*), and hyrax (*Dendrohyrax* spp.).

A few of the earlier reports of FMD in free living African wildlife were confirmed by virus isolation or transmission experiments. In Southern Rhodesia in 1932, virus isolated from fresh foot lesions of a kudu shot during an outbreak of disease in cattle was inoculated into cattle, which developed typical lesions of FMD (Hooper-Sharpe 1937). Curiously, this virus was subsequently typed in 1948 at the World Reference Laboratory for Foot-and-Mouth Disease as the prototype South African Territories type 1 (SAT 1) virus. Later, Lambrechts et al. (1956) succeeded in transmitting FMD to kudu by intradermolingual inoculation of vesicular fluid from infected cattle. The kudu developed extensive lesions on all four feet but no tongue lesions. In South Africa, Meeser (1962) described the isolation of type SAT 3 virus from clinically infected impala in the Kruger National Park.

ETIOLOGY. FMD is caused by a picornavirus approximately 24 nm in diameter and containing an RNA core. There are seven distinct immunological types of virus: O, A, C, SAT 1, SAT 2, SAT 3, and Asia 1. Infection with one type of virus does not confer immunity to challenge with another type. Within each immunological type are a number of antigenically different strains or subtypes. Differences among strains within a type may be such that vaccination with one strain may not necessarily protect an animal from infection with a widely different strain.

Types O, A, and C virus occur in Europe, South and Central America, Asia, and Africa. Types SAT 1, 2, and 3 are normally limited to Africa. Type SAT 1, however, caused an extensive epizootic in the Middle East in 1962–1963 but has since not been recorded outside Africa. Type Asia 1 occurs in Asia. Australasia, Central and North America, and Japan have been free of FMD for many years.

FMD virus is highly resistant to external influences, including the common disinfectants, and may survive outside the host for considerable periods in body fluids, animal products, and contaminated materials such as bedding, fodder, and clothes, particularly in conditions of high relative humidity and low temperatures. It is, however, susceptible to pH changes and is readily inactivated by sodium carbonate (4%), sodium hydroxide (1%), formalin, and citric acid (0.2%).

HOST RANGE. Reports of naturally occurring FMD incriminate many wild species mainly in the order Artiodactyla. In some free living populations, infection has been confirmed by virus isolation; in others, it has been indicated by the demonstration of specific antibody. Many species other than artiodactyls have been infected experimentally, and it is possible, particularly where contact infection has been demonstrated, that some may be potential or actual natural hosts.

Table 6.1 lists nondomestic species that have been shown to be, or reported as, susceptible to FMD virus. Zoological classification is according to Morris (1965), and distinction is drawn between reports of natural infection based on clinical grounds (without notation) and those where infection was confirmed by

TABLE 6.1   Wildlife Hosts of Foot-and-Mouth Disease.

Order and Family	Genus and Species	Common Name	Reference Natural Infection	Experimental
Artiodactyla				
Bovidae	*Tragelaphus scriptus*	bushbuck	Condy et al. 1969[a]	
	Tragelaphus strepsiceros	greater kudu	Hooper-Sharpe 1937[b]	Hedger et al. 1972[c]
	Taurotragus oryx	eland	Condy et al. 1969[a]	
	Boselaphus tragocamelus	nilgai	Mukhopad Hyay et al. 1975[b]	
	Bos gaurus	gaur	Urbain et al. 1938	
	Bos grunniens	yak	Prasad et al. 1978[b]	
	Syncerus caffer	African buffalo	Hedger et al. 1969[ab]	Hedger et al. 1972[cd]
	Bison bison	American bison	Urbain et al. 1938	
	Sylvicapra grimmia	duiker	Condy et al. 1969[a]	

TABLE 6.1 (Continued)

Order and Family	Genus and Species	Common Name	Natural Infection	Reference Experimental
	Kobus			
	ellypsiprymnus	waterbuck	Condy et al. 1969[a]	
	Redunca arundinum	reedbuck	Condy et al. 1969[a]	
	Hippotragus equinus	roan antelope	Condy et al. 1969[a]	
	Hippotragus niger	sable antelope	Anon. 1971[b]	
	Oryx gazella	oryx	Condy et al. 1969[a]	
	Damaliscus lunatus	tsessebe	Condy et al. 1969[a]	
	Damaliscus korrigum	topi	Condy et al. 1969[a]	
	Alcelaphus			
	buselaphus	hartebeest	Macaulay 1964	
	Connochaetes			
	taurinus	wildebeest (gnu)	Macaulay 1964	Anderson et al. 1975[c]
	Raphicerus melanotis	grysbok	Condy et al. 1969[a]	
	Aepyceros melampus	impala	Meeser 1962[b]	Hedger et al. 1972[d]
	Gazella thomsoni	Thomson's gazelle	Hedger 1976 (2)[a]	
	Saiga tatarica	Saiga antelope	Kindyakov et al. 1972[b]	
	Rupicapra rupicapra	chamois	Stroh 1933	Ercegovac et al. 1968[c]
	Capra ibex	ibex	Hediger 1940	
Cervidae	*Muntiacus muntjak*	Indian muntjac		Gibbs et al. 1975[d]
	Dama dama	fallow deer	Bartells and Claasen 1936	Forman and Gibbs 1974[d]
	Cervus nippon	sika deer		Gibbs et al. 1975[i]
	Cervus eldi	eld's deer	Urbain et al. 1938	
	Odocoileus			
	columbianus	Columbian deer	Grosso 1975	
	Odocoileus			
	virginianus	white-tailed deer	McVicar et al. 1974	McVicar et al. 1974[d]
	Mazama simplicornis	catinga deer	Yida et al. 1974[b]	
	Alces alces	moose		Dzuhina and Sviridov, 1965[c]
	Rangifer tarandus	reindeer	Orgryskov 1964	Kvitkin 1959[c]
	Capreolus capreolus	roe deer	Cohrs and Weber-Springe 1939	Forman et al. 1974[d]
Suidae	*Potamochoerus*			
	porcus	bush pig	Condy et al. 1969[a]	Hedger et al. 1972[c]
	Sus scrofa	wild boar	Urbain et al. 1938	Wilder et al. 1964[d]
	Phacochoerus			
	aethiopicus	warthog	Condy et al. 1969[a]	Hedger et al. 1972[d]
	Babirussa babirussa	babirusa	Urbain et al. 1938	Ercegovac et al. 1968[c]
Tayasuidae	*Tayassu tajacu*	collared peccary		Dardiri et al. 1969[d]
Camelidae	*Lama guanico*	guanaco		Mancini 1952
	Lamas pacos	alpaca		Mancini 1952
	Vicugna vicugna	vicuna		Mancini 1952
	Camelus			
	dromedarius	Arabian camel		K. H. Ahmed Ibrahim, personal communication, 1978[c]
Insectivora Erinaceidae	*Erinaceus europaeus*	European hedgehog	McLaughlan and Henderson 1974[b]	Edwards 1931[d]
	Atelerix albiventris	East African hedgehog		Macaulay 1964[d]

TABLE 6.1 *(Continued)*

Order and Family	Genus and Species	Common Name	Reference Natural Infection	Reference Experimental
Talpidae	*Talpa europaea*	common mole		Capel Edwards 1971[c]
Edentata Dasypodidae	*Dasypus novemcinctus*	nine-banded armadillo		Wilder et al. 1974[d]
Lagomorpha Leporidae	*Oryctolagus cuniculus*	European rabbit		Gibbs 1931[c]
Rodentia Sciuridae	*Sciurus carolinensis*	gray squirrel		Capel-Edwards 1971[c]
	Funambulus pennanti	Indian squirrel		Tewari et al. 1976[c]
Cricetidae	*Mesocricetus auratus*	golden hamster		Komarov 1954[c]
	Arvicola terrestris	water vole		Capel-Edwards 1971[c]
Rhizomyidae	*Tachyoryctes* sp.	East African mole rat		Macaulay 1964[c]
Muridae	*Arvicanthis abyssinicus nubilans*	African field rat		Macaulay 1964[c]
	Rattus norvegicus	brown rat		Capel-Edwards 1971[c]
Hystricidae	*Hystrix galeata*	large porcupine		Macaulay 1964[d]
Hydro- choeridae	*Hydrochoerus hydrochoeris*	capybara		Rosenberg and Gomes 1978[c]
Capro- myidae	*Myocastor coypus*	coypu		Capel-Edwards 1971[d]
Dasy- proctidae	*Dasyprocta aguti*	aguti		Federer 1969[d]
Chin- chillidae	*Chinchilla laniger*	chinchilla		Dellers 1963[c]
Proboscidea Elephan- tidae	*Loxodonta africana*	African elephant	Piragina 1970[b]	Howel et al. 1973[c]
	Elephas maximus	Indian elephant	Pyakural et al. 1976[b]	
Hydracoidea Procaviidae	*Dendrohyrax* sp.	hyrax		Macaulay 1964[c]
Carnivora Ursidae	*Ursus arctos*	grizzly bear	Grosso 1957	
	Selenarctos thibetanus	Asiatic black bear	Neugebauer 1976	
Marsupialia and Monotremata	various species	kangaroos, wallabies, wombats, etc.		Snowdon 1968[c]

[a] Virus isolated.
[b] Antibody demonstrated.
[c] By inoculation.
[d] Contact infection.

virus isolation or by the demonstration of antibody. Similar distinction is made between experimental infection by inoculation and contact infection.

TRANSMISSION. Transmission of FMD is primarily from the infected animal itself, especially during the early febrile stage when virus is present in the blood, organs, tissues, and body fluids. Affected animals shed virus in vesicular epithelium, vesicular fluid, saliva, milk, feces, urine, semen, vaginal secretions, and possibly in other body fluids during and immediately after periods of maximum viremia. Virus is excreted not only during the clinical manifestations of disease but also prior to the development of clinical signs (Burrows 1968). In some species, such as the African buffalo (Condy and Hedger 1974; Hedger 1976a), infection may take place and virus may be excreted in the total absence of clinical signs.

Indirect transmission may occur through the dissemination of virus in meat, milk, hides, and other animal products; or through fomites such as vehicles, buildings, utensils, bedding, and fodder. The virus is resistant to external influences, and its survival for many weeks has been reported on various contaminated objects at ambient temperature (Cottral 1969). Virus may also be transmitted mechanically by living vectors, especially man who combines freedom of movement with rapid transportation.

A number of investigations have strongly indicated that in certain circumstances FMD virus can be transmitted by the airborne route. It has been demonstrated that pigs particularly, but also cattle, sheep, goats, and deer, can excrete high levels of virus into the air, probably in their breath, when infected with FMD (A. Donaldson, personal communication; Forman et al. 1974; Hyslop 1965; Sellers and Parker 1969). Infected hedgehogs have also been shown to excrete virus in their breath (Edwards 1934). In conditions of high relative humidity (above 60%), airborne virus is capable of long-term survival and may be transported over considerable distances (Sellers et al. 1973). An aerosol dose containing very little virus is capable of producing disease in cattle (Eskildson 1969), but the dose of virus required to infect by the alimentary route is several-thousand-fold higher (Sellers 1971). There is little information yet available on the amount of virus required for infection of other species by inhalation. In light of these findings, less emphasis is now placed on the importance of birds as vectors of FMD.

Although the carrier state in cattle, sheep, and goats as a normal sequel to infection is well documented, proven incidents of transmission from domestic virus carriers to susceptible animals are rare indeed. Transmission of infection from virus-carrying African buffalo, however, has been observed on at least two occasions (Condy and Hedger 1974; Hedger et al. 1972) and may be a normal method of transmission in this species.

SIGNS. Clinical signs in FMD vary considerably in different species. In domestic cattle, following a short incubation period of from 2 to 8 days, the disease is characterized by an initial period of pyrexia with temperatures ranging from 40°C to 41.1°C, depression, and anorexia. Painful vesicles develop on the dorsal surface of the tongue, dental pad, lips, buccal mucosa, and muzzle. The vesicles vary in size, but in severe cases may involve the greater part of the dorsal surface of the tongue. Rupture usually occurs within 24 hours, releasing vesicular fluid containing as much as 10^8 infective units of virus per milliliter. The vesicular epithelium is shed, salivation is profuse, and strips of ropey saliva may hang from the muzzle.

Subsequent to or concurrent with the mouth lesions, vesicles may appear on one or more feet, especially in the clefts or on the coronary bands, causing severe pain and lameness. Vesicles may also occur on the teats and udder, sometimes resulting in secondary bacterial mastitis.

Sucking calves may die from an acute myocarditis (tiger heart) often in the absence of other signs. In sheep and goats the infection may be subclinical or, if disease is apparent, so mild that it is not recognized. Lesions in the mouth are small and transient, but on the feet they may be severe, leading to exungulation. Lameness is marked and, in goats, agalactia is a feature. In pigs also, the feet are commonly affected, and lameness is characteristic.

Clinical signs in deer vary according to species. In a recent series of experiments (Forman and Gibbs 1974; Gibbs et al. 1975) red, fallow, roe, muntjac, and sika deer were infected with two types of FMD virus both artificially and by contact. All five species were susceptible. The disease was particularly severe in roe and muntjac, several of which died. In both species vesicular lesions occurred in the mouth and commonly on all four feet, particularly on the interdigital coronary band and bulbs of the heels. The appearance and distribution of lesions were similar to those in sheep. Clinical disease, however, was mild or inapparent in red, fallow, and sika deer. Vesicular epithelium from all five species contained large amounts of virus, usually in excess of $10^{8.0}$ TCID$_{50}$ per gram. Following infection most fallow, sika, and some red deer became virus carriers. The duration of the carrier state was not studied in sika or red deer, but virus persisted in fallow for only up to 63 days.

McVicar et al. (1974), who demonstrated experimental contact transmission of FMD from white-tailed deer (*Odocoileus virginianus*) to other deer, from deer to cattle, and from cattle to deer, reported that the clinical syndrome was intermediate in severity between that seen in cattle, sheep, and goats similarly exposed. Lesions occurred in both mouth and feet. One deer remained a virus carrier for 11 weeks after infection.

Khukhorov et al. (1974), describing a type A$_{22}$ outbreak in Russia which spread to Saiga antelope (*Saiga tatarica*), described numerous erosions on the mucous membranes of the lips, tongue, and hard palate. Apthae or erosions were found near the cleft of the hoof and close to the heel in the majority of Saiga examined.

In Africa, Meeser (1962) described the disease in impala as severe. There was no salivation, even though the dental pad was a frequent site of vesicle formation. Lameness was often so severe that a limb was carried. No lesions were seen in the interdigital space, but vesicles commonly formed on the bulb of the heels. Thimbling (exungulation) occurred and the entire hoof was sometimes shed. Mortality was high in young animals. Hedger et al. (1972) noted similar signs after experimental infection. Impala did not become virus carriers. These same workers also reported the experimental infection, both by inoculation and by contact of a number of other species of African wildlife. Disease was severe in kudu, vesicles occurring on the tongue, muzzle, and all four feet and accessory digits, and all the infected kudu became virus carriers. The carrier state persisted for up to 140 days.

In warthogs and the bush pig (*Potamochoerus porcus*) the disease was similar to that in domestic swine. Lesions were mainly confined to the feet but also occurred on the foreleg, kneeling pads, and accessory digits in the warthog. Thimbling occurred in the bush pig. Snout lesions occurred in one bush pig and a single buccal lesion in one warthog. Neither species became virus carriers.

None of four wildebeest succumbed to either natural or artificial infection, and no antibody responses were elicited. Anderson et al. (1975), using a different virus type, also found difficulty infecting wildebeest, although mild lesions and antibody responses were recorded in some animals.

Naturally occurring type 0 has been confirmed in the Indian elephant (*Elephas maximus*) in Nepal (Pyakural et al. 1976) and type A in African elephant (*Loxodonta africana*) in a circus in Italy (Piragino 1970). Lesions, particularly in the mouth, were described as very severe in the Indian elephant.

Howell et al. (1973) also noted very severe lesions in African elephant following intradermolingual inoculation of virus. Although the epidermis of the elephant tongue is very thin and delicate, vesicles were distended and very firm. When punctured, the contents did not readily escape, and vesicles appeared to contain numerous fine septae between which the fluid was trapped. Foot lesions were severe with partial or complete separation and sloughing of the footpad. In spite of the severity of lesions, contact infection to uninoculated control elephants in the same pens did not take place. Nor have there been reports of infections in African elephants in the wild, and 353 elephant sera collected at random from different African countries, often during outbreaks of FMD in both domestic and wild animals, were negative for antibodies.

A number of small mammals have been shown to be susceptible to experimental infection (Capel-Edwards 1971). Contact infection took place from cattle to coypu (*Myocastor coypus molina*), which developed vesicular lesions in all four feet. The agouti (*Dasyprocta aguti*) has also been shown to be highly susceptible to contact infection with FMD (Federer 1969), with lesions occurring on the tongue and in the mouth.

Perhaps most important of all wild species found to be susceptible to FMD virus is the free living African buffalo in which infection normally takes place in the total absence of observable clinical signs (Hedger 1976a). Although infection is normally not apparent, even small herds of buffalo have been shown to be capable of maintaining multiple virus types over an indefinite period and independent of infection in other species.

PATHOGENESIS. There is considerable evidence to suggest that the main route of infection in domestic cattle, and presumably in wild ruminants, is via the pharynx (Burrows 1972). It has been shown also that the lower respiratory tract (Eskildson 1969), the nasal passages (Korn 1957), and the udder (Burrows et al. 1971) may afford alternative portals of entry for the virus. In swine, airborne virus initiated infection in the lower respiratory tract while ingested virus infects the tonsils (Terpstra 1972). Following infection, virus is distributed to predilection sites in the mouth and feet via the lymph and blood. A demonstrable viremia can be detected for about 3 days after the appearance of clinical signs. An important aspect of FMD is the prodromal phase during which virus can be recovered from various secretions and excretions in the absence of clinical signs. This phase may be as long as 9 days in cattle and may be even more prolonged in swine (Burrows 1972). Some aspects of pathogenicity, particularly infectivity in different species, may vary according to the type or strain of virus.

Of particular interest in the pathogenesis of FMD is the part apparently played by the pharynx. The pharynx provides the route of infection, prodromal excretion of virus is from the pharynx, and the pharynx harbors the virus in carrier animals after infection.

PATHOLOGY. The histology of the typical vesicle has been described as "balloon degeneration" and commences with a swelling of the nucleus and cytoplasm of infected cells in the stratum spinosum of the epidermis. Vacuolation, separation, and necrosis of affected cells results in the formation of microvesicles that eventually coalesce to form macroscopic lesions (Burrows 1972). Although small differences may exist, it is not possible to distinguish histologically between the viral vesicular diseases.

In the acute and often fatal form of FMD in young bovines and swine, and possibly in some wild species, the most significant lesions are found in the heart muscles. Macroscopically the areas of degeneration and necrosis of the myocardial fibers appear as whitish stripes, giving the characteristic condition of "tiger heart."

DIAGNOSIS. The diagnosis of FMD is usually based on clinical evidence. When a highly contagious disease showing vesicular lesions on the tongues and feet affects numbers of bovines, swine, sheep, goats, or other susceptible species such as impala at the same time, a provisional diagnosis of FMD can be made.

Diagnosis is confirmed either by direct complement fixation tests using triturated vesicular epithelium or vesicular fluid from fresh cases of disease as antigen against type specific sera, or by virus isolation in tissue cultures or experimental animals. The complement fixation test is rapid and specific. If samples are taken from unruptured or recently ruptured vesicles, results may be achieved within 2–3 hours of the samples arriving in the laboratory.

The similarity of the clinical signs in FMD and other vesicular diseases emphasizes the need for rapid differential diagnosis. FMD must be differentiated from vesicular stomatitis, swine vesicular disease, vesicular exanthema of swine, and other possible nonspecific forms of stomatitis and bluetongue. On the basis of domestic animal susceptibility, FMD affects cattle, sheep, goats, and swine but not horses; vesicular stomatitis affects cattle, pigs, and horses, and swine vesicular disease and vesicular exanthema affect only swine. Complement fixation tests, using vesicular tissues or isolated viruses as antigens against specific antisera, will also differentiate the first three of these diseases. Bluetongue in South Africa, characterized by mouth and foot lesions, may be readily mistaken for FMD (Henning 1949). Bluetongue, however, is usually confined to sheep, cattle only rarely being affected. It can only be transmitted by inoculation and does not spread by contact.

Other diseases of wild ruminants that may be confused with FMD include epizootic hemorrhagic disease of deer, mucosal disease, rinderpest, and malignant catarrhal fever.

Diagnosis of FMD in wildlife is frequently hindered by the age of the lesions in suspect cases and the consequent absence of suitable vesicular material for either complement fixation or virus isolation. In such cases confirmation of disease, in species that become virus carriers after infection, may be obtained by the isolation and characterization of virus from esophageal-pharyngeal samples (Hedger 1976). Such methods have been particularly useful in studies of free living African buffalo in which infection occurs in the absence of clinical signs. Useful additional evidence of the nature of the infection may be provided by serologic tests.

THE ROLE OF WILDLIFE. With such an imposing range of hosts shown to be susceptible to FMD virus, this chapter would not be complete without some comment on their possible role in the spread and maintenance of FMD. Many species have been shown to be susceptible under experimental conditions by inoculation only. In others the conditions under which contact transmission has taken place hardly parallel those of the natural state. Even when natural infection has taken place in captivity in zoological gardens, conditions where animals are fed, housed, and kept in close proximity to other species do not relate to those in the wild, particularly in relation to airborne transmission.

It is, therefore, very probable that under natural conditions many hosts would not represent a danger to domestic stock. For example, on experimental evidence, Capel-Edwards (1971) suggested that brown rats (*Rattus norvegicus*), because of their close association with farm animals and their ability to migrate considerable distances under pressure, could play a significant role in the epidemiology of FMD. However, Hugh-Jones (1970), in an analytical study of the very extensive 1967–1968 epizootic of FMD in England, found no evidence of the involvement of rats in the spread of disease.

Many other hosts, when infected under natural conditions, are probably incidentally infected during concurrent disease in domestic animals and are not themselves responsible for or capable of maintaining virus. Thus Ercegovac and Popovic (1970), searching for the primary source of individual outbreaks of disease in Yugoslavia, were unable to prove in a single case that wild game animals were the cause. Similarly, Cohrs and Weber-Springe (1939) concluded that the danger of spread by deer of FMD under European conditions was not very great. Although several species of deer have been shown to be susceptible to contact infection and even to carry virus for a period after infection, there was no indication of their involvement during the 1967–1968 epizootic in England.

Incidental hosts can, however, on occasion, play an important part in the epizootiology of FMD. In 1967 in Kazakhstan in the USSR, infection spread from cattle into a very large population of Saiga antelope, estimated at over 1 million. Large-scale migration of the Saiga led to widespread dissemination of disease and infection of cattle in distant places (Kindyakov et al. 1972). Whether an incidental host becomes a maintenance host may depend in some degree on population dynamics. If a susceptible wild population is large enough and sufficiently concentrated, virus may be maintained by direct animal-to-animal transmission. It is possible that this may be the situation in the Kruger National Park in South Africa where isolations of virus from impala have been made regularly during the 1960s and 1970s.

In Africa free living buffalo have been shown to maintain the virus of FMD independent of disease in other species, thus providing a reservoir for their possible future infection. Spillover, however, of this very infectious virus into other species is a surprisingly rare occurrence. This may be due in part to the transience of normal contact among animals of different species.

REFERENCES

Allenspach, V. von. Die Maul- und Klauenseuche im Zoologischen Garten Zurich. *Schweiz. Arch. Tierheilkd.* 92:42–47, 1950.

Anderson, E. C., Anderson, J., Doughty, W. J., and Drevmo, S. The pathogenicity of bovine strains of foot-and-mouth disease virus for impala and wildebeest. *J. Wildl. Dis.* 11:248–255, 1975.

Anon. Rep. Dir. Vet. Services, Rhodesia, 1971.

Bartels, and Claassen, P. Zur Frage der Erkrankung des Wildes an Maul- und Klauenseuche und ihre Bedeutung fur die Verschleppung in Klauenviehbestaenden. *Ber. Muench. Tieraerztl. Wochenschr.* 52:(14)230–233, 1936.

Burrows, R. Early stages in virus infection: Studies in vivo and in vitro. In *Microbial pathogenicity in man and animals*, pp. 303–332. Symp. Soc. Gen. Microbiol. No. 220. Cambridge: University Press, 1972.

_____. Excretion of foot-and-mouth disease virus prior to the development of lesions. *Vet. Rec.* 82:287–288, 1968.

Burrows, R., Mann, J. A., Greig, A., Chapman, W. G., and Goodridge, D. The growth and persistence of foot-and-mouth disease virus in the bovine mammary gland. *J. Hyg., Camb.* 69:307–321, 1971.

Capel-Edwards, M. The susceptibility of small mammals to foot-and-mouth disease virus. *Vet. Bull.* 41:815–823, 1971.

Cohrs, P., and Weber-Springe, W. Maul- und Klauenseuche beim Reh und Hirsch. [Foot and mouth disease in roe deer and red deer.] *Dtsch. Tieraerztl. Wochenschr.* 47:97–103, 1939. Abstr. *Vet. Bull.* 9:767, 1939.

Condy, J. B., and Hedger, R. S. The survival of foot-and-mouth disease in wildlife in Rhodesia and other African territories. *J. Comp. Pathol.* 79:27–31, 1969.

_____. The survival of foot-and-mouth disease virus in African buffalo with non-transference of infection to domestic cattle. *Res. Vet. Sci.* 16:182–185, 1974

Cottral, G. E. Persistence of foot-and-mouth disease virus in animals, their products and the environment. *Bull. Off. Int. Epizoot.* 71:549–568, 1969.

Dellers, R. W. Experimental foot-and-mouth disease in chinchillas. *Vet. Rec.* 75:1226, 1963.

Dardiri, A. H., Yedloutschnig, R. J., and Taylor, W. D. Clinical and serological response of white-collared peccaries to African swine fever, foot-and-mouth disease, vesicular stomatitis, vesicular exanthema of swine, hog cholera and rinderpest virus. *Proc. U.S. Anim. Health Assoc.* 73:437–452, 1969.

Dzupina, S. I., and Sviridov, A. A. Foot-and-mouth disease in moose under experimental conditions. *Veterinariya (Moscow)* 42(5):47–48, 1965. Abstr. *Wellcome FMD Bull.* 69/57, 1969.

Edwards, J. T. In Progress report: Foot-and-mouth disease. *Res. Comm.* 4:165–179, 1931.

––––––. Further experiments with hedgehogs. Foot-and-Mouth Disease Research Committee. Unpublished papers 214B and 223B, 1934.

Ercegovac, D., Golosin, R., Parjevic, D., Borojevic, M. and Calic, Z. Potential role of certain wild animals in the epizootiology of foot-and-mouth disease. *Acta Vet.* 18:119–126, 1968. Abstr. *Wellcome FMD Bull.* 70/81, 1970.

Ercegovac, D., and Papovic, S. A. field evaluation of the role of game in the epizootiology of foot-and-mouth disease. *Vet. Glasn.* 24:459–463, 1970. *Abstr. Wellcome FMD Bull.* 71/144, 1971.

Eskildson, M. K. Experimental pulmonary infection of cattle with foot-and-mouth disease virus. *Nord. Vet. Med.* 21:86–91, 1969.

Federer, K. E. Susceptibility of the agouti (*Dasyprocta aguti*) to foot-and-mouth disease virus. *Zentralbl. Vet. Med.* 16(9):847–853, 1969.

Forman, A. J., and Gibbs, E. P. J. Studies with foot-and-mouth disease in British deer (red, fallow and roe): I. Clinical disease. *J. Comp. Pathol.* 84:215–220, 1974.

Forman, A. J., Gibbs, E. P. J., Baber, D. J., Herniman, K. A. J., and Barnett, I. T. Studies with foot-and-mouth disease virus in British deer (red, fallow and roe): II. Recovery of virus and serological response. *J. Comp. Pathol.* 84:221–229, 1974.

Gibbs, Y. M. In Progress report: Foot-and-mouth disease. *Res. Comm.* 4:164–165, 1931.

Gibbs, E. P. J., Herniman, K. A. J., and Lawman, M. J. P. Studies with foot-and-mouth disease virus in British deer (muntjac and sika). *J. Comp. Pathol.* 85:361–366, 1975.

Grosso, A. M. La fiebre aftosa en el Jardin Zoologico de Buenos Aires en los ultimos quince anos. [Foot-and-mouth disease in the Buenos Aires zoo.] *Gac. Vet.* 19:54–55, 1957.

Hedger, R. S. Foot-and-mouth disease in wildlife with particular reference to the African buffalo (*Syncerus caffer*). In L. A. Page, ed., *Wildlife diseases*, pp. 235–244. New York and London: Plenum Press, 1976a.

––––––. The maintenance of foot-and-mouth disease in Africa. Ph.D. thesis, University of London, 1976b.

Hedger, R. S., Condy, J. B., and Falconer, J. The isolation of foot-and-mouth disease virus from African buffalo (*Syncerus caffer*). *Vet. Rec.* 84:526–517, 1969.

Hedger, R. S., Condy, J. B., and Golding, S. M. Infection of some species of African wildlife with foot-and-mouth disease virus. *J. Comp. Pathol.* 82:458–461, 1972.

Hediger, H. Uber Maul- und Klauenseuche bei Zoo-

tieren. *Zool. Gart.* 12:298, 1940.

Henning, M. W. *Animal diseases in South Africa,* 2d ed. South Africa: Central News Agency, 1949.

Hooper-Sharpe, G. C. *Ann. Rep. Chief Vet. Surg.,* Southern Rhodesia, 1937.

Howell, P. G., Young, E., and Hedger, R. S. Foot-and-mouth disease in the African elephant (*Loxodonta africana*). *Onderstepoort J. Vet. Res.* 40:41–52, 1973.

Hugh-Jones, M. E. Epidemiological studies of the 1967/68 foot-and-mouth disease outbreak: The possible spread of infection by farm rats (*Rattus norvegicus*). *Br. Vet. J.* 126:368–371, 1970.

Hulse, E. C., and Edwards, J. T. Foot-and-mouth disease in hibernating hedgehogs. *J. Comp. Pathol. Ther.* 50:421–430, 1937.

Hyslop, N. St. G. Airborne infection with the virus of foot-and-mouth disease. *J. Comp. Pathol.* 75:119–126, 1965

Khukhorov, V. M., Pronina, N. A., Korsun, L. N., Karpenko, I. G., Kruglikov, B. A., Ponomareu, I. A., Koshelev, M. I., and Tsedenov, K. E. Foot and mouth disease in saiga antelopes. *Veterinariya* (Moscow) 5:60–61, 1974.

Kindyakov, V. I., Nagumanov, F. M., and Tasbulatov, E. S. The epizootiological significance of contact between wild and domestic animals in relation to foot-and-mouth disease. *Vopr. Prir. Ochag. Bolezn.* 5:66–63, 1972. Abstr. *Wellcome FMD Bull.* 74/4, 1974.

Komarov, A. The propagation of foot-and-mouth disease virus in the Syrian hamster. *Refuah vet.* 11:198, 1954. *Abstr. Vet. Bull.* 25:477, 1955.

Korn, G. Experimentelle untersuchungen zum virus nachweis im inkubationsstadium der Maul- und Klauenseuche und zu ihrer pathogenese. *Arch. Exp. Vet. Med.* 11:37, 1957.

Kvitkin, V. P. Physiopathology of experimental foot-and-mouth disease in reindeer. *Veterinariya* (Moscow) 36:25–28, 1959. Abstr. *Vet. Bull.* 30:119, 1960.

Lambrechts, M. C., Buhr, W. H. B., and Van der Merwe, J. P. Observations on the transmission of foot-and-mouth disease to game and controlled transmission of the disease from game to cattle and vice versa by means of contact. *J. South Afr. Vet. Med. Assoc.* 27(2):133–137, 1956.

Macaulay, J. W. A check list of nondomestic animals reported to have been infected with foot-and-mouth disease. *Bull. Epizoot. Dis. Afr.* 12:127–128, 1964.

McLaughlan, J. D., and Henderson, W. M. The occurrence of foot-and-mouth disease in the hedgehog under natural conditions. *J. Hyg., Camb.* 45:477–479, 1947.

McVicar, J. W., Sutmoller, P., Ferris, D. H., and Campbell, C. H. Foot-and-mouth disease in white-tailed deer: Clinical signs and transmission in the laboratory. *Proc. 78th Ann. Meet. U.S. Anim. Health Assoc.,* pp. 169–180, 1974.

Magnusson, H. Ein Fall von Maul- und Klauenseuche beim Elch. [A case of foot-and-mouth disease in an elk.] *Dtsch. Tieraerztl. Wochenschr.*

47:509–511, 1939. Abstr. *Vet. Bull.* 10:670, 1940.

Meeser, M. J. N. Foot-and-mouth disease in game animals with special reference to the impala (*Aepyceros melampus*). *J. South Afr. Vet. Med. Assoc.* 33:351–354, 1962.

Morris, D. *The mammals.* London: Hodder & Stoughton in association with the Zoological Society of London, 1965.

Ogryzkov, S. E. The pathology of foot-and-mouth disease in reindeer. Tr. 2. *Vses. Konf. Patol. Anat. Zhivotn., Mosk. Vet. Akad.*, pp. 420–425, 1963. Abstr. *Vet. Bull.* 36:418, 1966.

Piragino, S. Un focalaio di afta epizootica in elefanti da circo. *Zooprofilassi* 25(1–2):17–22, 1970.

Prasad, S., Sharma, V. K., Ramakant, A. K. L., and Singh, B. Isolation of foot-and-mouth disease virus from a yak. *Vet. Rec.* 102:363–364, 1978.

Pyakural, S., Singh, U., and Singh, N. B. An outbreak of foot-and-mouth disease in Indian elephants (*Elephas maximus*). *Vet. Rec.* 99(2):28–29, 1976.

Rosenberg, F. J., and Gomes, I. Susceptibility of capybara (*Hydrochoerus hydrochoeris*) to foot-and-mouth disease. *Bol. Cent. Panam. Fiebre Aftosa* 27–28:43–48, 1977.

Rossiter, L. W., and Albertyn, A. A. L. Foot-and-mouth disease in game. *J. South Afr. Vet. Med. Assoc.* 18:16–19, 1947.

Sellers, R. F. Quantitative aspects of the spread of foot-and-mouth disease. *Vet. Bull.* 41:431–439, 1971.

Sellers, R. F., Barlow, D. F., Donaldson, A. I., Herniman, K. A. J., and Parker, J. Foot-and-mouth disease: A case study of airborne disease. In J. F. P. F. Hers and K. C. Winkler, ed., *Airborne transmission and airborne infection*, pp.

405–412, Utrecht: Oosthoek, 1973.

Sellers, R. F., and Parker, J. Airborne excretion of foot-and-mouth disease virus. *J. Hyg., Camb.* 67:671–677, 1969.

Snowdon, W. A. The susceptibility of some Australian fauna to infection with foot-and-mouth disease virus. *Aust. J. Exp. Biol. Med. Sci.* 46:667–687, 1968.

Stroh, G. Abgeheilte Maul- und Klauenseuche bei Reh und Gemse. *Berl. Muench. Tieraerztl. Wochenschr.* 47:749–750, 1933.

Terpstra, C. Pathogenesis of foot-and-mouth disease in experimentally infected pigs. *Bull. Off. Int. Epizoot.* 77:859–874, 1972.

Urbain, A., Bullier, P. and Nouvel, J. Au sujet d'une petite epizootie de fievre aptheuse ayant sevi sur des animaux sauvage en captivite. *Bull. Acad. Vet. Fr.* 11:59–73, 1938.

Wilder, F. W., Dardiri, A. H., Gay, J. G., Beasley, H. C., Heflin, A. A., and Acree, J. A. Susceptibility of one-toed pigs to certain diseases exotic to the United States. *Proc. 78th Ann. Meet. U.S. Anim. Health Assoc.*, pp. 195–199, 1974a.

Wilder, F. W., Dardiri, A. H., and Yedloutschnig, R. J. Clinical and serological response of the nine-banded armadillo (*Dasypus novemcinctus*) to viruses of African swine fever, hog cholera, rinderpest, vesicular exanthema of swine, vesicular stomatitis and foot-and-mouth disease. *Proc. 78th Ann. Meet. U.S. Anim. Health Assoc.*, pp. 188–194, 1974b.

Yida, O., Pustiglione Netto, L., Suga, O., and Kotait, I. The isolation of foot-and-mouth disease virus from catinga deer. *Biologico (S. Paulo)* 40:216, 1974. Abstr. *Wellcome FMD Bull.* 76/29, 1976.

7 *Feline Panleukopenia*

JAMES L. BITTLE

Synonyms: **Feline infectious enteritis, feline distemper, feline agranulocytosis.**

Feline panleukopenia is an acute viral disease affecting most members of the family Felidae and some animals in closely related families, including Mustelidae, Procyonidae, and Viverridae. The disease is characterized by an enteritis and a depression in hemopoietic centers with a marked decrease in leukocytes from the peripheral circulation.

HISTORY. The disease was first described in 1925 by Kirk and was shown by Verge and Cristoforoni (1928) to be transmitted by filtrates from tissues of infected cats. Hindle and Findlay (1932) in England and Leasure et al. (1934) in the United States confirmed the filtrate transmission.

Lawrence and Syverton (1938) and Lawrence et al. (1940) described the agranulocytosis commonly associated with the disease. Hammon and Enders (1939) characterized the disease more fully, demonstrating the aleukocytosis, the enteric lesions, and the presence of intranuclear inclusion bodies in the intestinal epithelium. Johnson (1964, 1965a, 1966, 1967a) was able to grow the virus in tissue culture and to develop quantitative assay procedures. He also described the chemical and physical properties of the virus.

Kilham et al. (1967) described the congenital transmission of the virus and the resultant cerebellar ataxia occasionally seen in young kittens.

DISTRIBUTION AND HOSTS. Feline panleukopenia disease occurs in widely separated areas of the world, having been reported from England, France, Germany, Sri Lanka, India, Brazil, the United States, Canada, and Australia.

The disease occurs in many members of the Felidae and has been described in the cheetah (*Acinonyx jubatus*), leopard (*Felis pardus*), bobcat (*Lynx rufus*), tiger (*F. tigris*), lynx (*F. lynx*), serval (*F. capensis*), cougar (*F. concolor*), jaguar (*F. onca*), ocelot (*F. pardalis*), margay (*F. tigrina*), lion (*F. leo*), and wildcat (*F. sylvestris*, Europe; *F. ocreata*, Africa). The virus also infects Mustelidae (mink and skunk), Procyonidae (raccoons, lesser panda, kinkajou, coati mundi), and Viverridae (binturong). When inoculated experimentally, the virus will infect ferrets (Kilham et al. 1967). In an epidemiological study in northeastern United States, the disease occurs in a seasonal pattern, mainly during July, August, and September. The birth peaks in April, May, and June, and the resultant addition of large numbers of susceptible kittens to the population causes the development of summertime epidemics (Rief 1976). Goss (1948) compared the susceptibility of different species to the virus from an evolutionary standpoint.

ETIOLOGY. A filterable agent was demonstrated by early investigators to be the cause of feline panleukopenia. Studies by Johnson (1966) have characterized the infectious particle as a DNA virus, which is resistant to ether, low pH, and heat. The virus is classified as a parvovirus containing single-stranded DNA with no envelope; it multiplies intranuclearly and produces inclusion bodies. The virus is very small (20 mμ), and all isolates have been found to be antigenically similar.

A number of investigators have suggested a relationship between feline panleukopenia and mink enteritis virus (Bouillant and Hanson 1965; Burger and Ott 1963; MacPherson 1956; Myers and Fritz 1959; Wills 1952). Johnson (1967b) compared a strain of mink enteritis virus with six strains of panleukopenia virus and found them to have similar chemical and physical properties. The clinical disease in mink closely resembles feline panleukopenia in cats.

TRANSMISSION. Based on observed epizootics, panleukopenia is highly infectious in susceptible cat populations. The most common route of natural infection is by inhalation or ingestion of the virus from infected feces, urine, or saliva, either by direct contact or by fomites on food, hands, clothing, and so on.

The virus is shed in the saliva, feces, and urine of infected cats during the course of the disease and for months after recovery. It has been shown that cats with high levels of serum-neutralizing antibody can shed the virus from their feces for 43 days and from urine for 22 days postinfection (Csiza et al. 1971). The virus also persisted in the lungs of infected cats for 52 weeks and in the kidneys for 57 weeks.

Torres (1941) has shown that fleas may serve as a vector in transmitting the virus to the domestic cat. Bouillant et al. (1965) demonstrated that the housefly may also serve as a vector in transmitting mink enteritis virus to susceptible mink.

The virus is highly resistant to physical changes such as heat and drying and may survive long periods in infected premises. Thus, the persistence of the virus in the infected animal and its extreme stability in the environment establishes a reservoir of infection and ensures its survival.

SIGNS. The signs of panleukopenia in wild animals are very similar to those in the domestic cat. The acute form of the disease is characterized by sudden onset of depression, anorexia, and elevated temperature. The temperature rise may persist for several days and then return to normal with a recurrent elevation after 24–48 hours. In the peracute form, however, the diphasic febrile response may not occur, and the animal may die within 48 hours after onset, showing few of the classic signs.

Gastrointestinal signs, including vomiting and diarrhea, are common and produce severe dehydration. The vomitus is often a bile-stained mixture of mucus and gastric juices, and the feces often contain blood. Abdominal tenderness may also be present.

The virus causes little damage to the intestinal mucosa in the germ-free cat (Rohovsky and Fowler 1971). Thus, the clinical signs observed in this animal are minimal, and the survival rate is very high.

The virus may cross the placental barrier causing reproductive problems such as abortions and fetal resorptions. Kittens infected late in the gestation period or early in postnatal period may develop cerebellar syndrome with signs of incoordination.

PATHOGENISIS. The exact mode of natural infection has not been determined. Experimentally, the virus may infect by inhalation or ingestion. The high concentration of virus in the intestinal epithelium and surrounding lymph nodes suggests the oral or nasal pharyngeal region as the primary site of infection.

Hindle and Findlay (1932) could not produce neurological signs in cats inoculated intracerebrally, although they did develop typical signs of illness. However, Johnson et al. (1967) described an ataxia syndrome in neonatal kittens shown to be caused by panleukopenia virus.

The virus of panleukopenia has an affinity for cells undergoing active stages of mitosis. Therefore, in very young animals, the infection may be widespread and highly lethal. If infection occurs during gestation, the fetus may be aborted or resorbed. In the period prior to birth or shortly after, the virus will infect the cerebellum causing a cortical hypoplasia, and kittens will show signs of incoordination. In older susceptible animals, the hemopoietic tissue and intestinal mucosa are the main sites for viral replication and destruction.

The virus multiplies extensively in the lymphatic system, thus being spread throughout all tissues. The virus also replicates in the epithelial mucosal cells, particularly in the lower ileum region. The low incidence of virus-induced lesions in the intestinal mucosa of germ-free cats implies that other factors may be responsible for the destructive nature of this virus in that area.

PATHOLOGY. At necropsy, the animal appears dehydrated, with evidence of vomiting and diarrhea. The intestine is usually empty of solids but may contain a small amount of bile-stained fluid.

The gross pathology in the small intestine varies considerably, but careful examination will reveal some change throughout its length. The most common lesion is found in the lower portion of the ileum and consists of a hemorrhagic enteritis. The mesenteric lymph nodes are swollen, and the marrow of the long bones appears to be fluid.

Microscopically, the most obvious changes are in the lymph tissue and the bone marrow. Hammon and Enders (1939) described the pathology of the ileocecal lymph nodes as the marked depletion of adult lymphocytes and injury to the cells forming in the germinal centers. The sinusoids are crowded with mononuclear phagocytes containing erythrocytes. The bone marrow is hypoplastic.

The lesions are not consistent throughout the small intestine, but the most obvious changes occur in the epithelial cells lining the crypts and acini of the posterior ileum. These cells degenerate, leaving areas denuded. Sections taken at the proper time will show cells containing intranuclear inclusion bodies. The inclusion will be found in various stages, but in the most pronounced one, the inclusion fills most of the cell and is surrounded by a halo of marginated chromatin. According to Jubb and Kennedy (1962), observation of inclusions depends on the time of necropsy and the use of rapid-acting acid fixations such as Zenker's fluid.

Inclusion bodies may also be found in the lymph tissue, liver, and renal tubules, although they are more difficult to differentiate than in the intestinal epithelium.

In very young kittens, the thymus is reduced in size, and there is a primary immunosuppressive effect on T-cell activity (Schultz et al. 1975). There is cerebellar hypoplasia with a decrease of granular and Purkinje cells.

DIAGNOSIS. The disease is diagnosed by the characteristic clinical signs which include depression, anorexia, elevated temperature, emesis, and diarrhea. The leukocyte count will fall below 4,000/mm^3, with lymphocytes and polymorphonuclear cells gradually disappearing from the circulation.

A comparison of acute and convalescent serum samples will show a rise in serum-neutralizing antibodies 2–3 weeks postinfection.

On necropsy, gross and microscopic lesions primarily affecting the bone marrow and small intestine are seen. Intranuclear inclusion bodies may be found chiefly in the epithelial cells of the small intestine.

There is no marked anemia, and the dehydration may cause a hemoconcentration with a raised packed-cell volume.

PROGNOSIS. The mortality from the acute disease has been estimated to be between 60% and 90%. However, it is likely that the disease occurs in a mild form in many felines, causing a high morbidity but overall lower mortality. The variation in morbidity and mortality with this disease can probably be accounted for by a number of factors, such as the virulence of the strain causing the infection, individual animal susceptibility, and other agents that may act synergistically with feline panleukopenia virus, producing a more severe syndrome (Bittle et al. 1961; Carlson et al. 1977; Rohovsky and Fowler, 1971). In general, the ability of an animal to survive infection probably depends upon the degree to which it can immunologically respond before the virus produces its destructive effect.

Since the destruction of hemopoietic tissue can be measured by the decrease in circulating leukocytes, the prognosis may be based on the ability of the bone marrow to respond. A rapid increase in circulating leukocytes is a good sign

of recovery. The extent of damage to the intestinal mucosa, with resulting dehydration, is also an important factor in the animal's ability to survive.

IMMUNITY. Susceptibility to infection is related to the absence of antibody. Maternal passive antibody will protect young animals for a period after birth. The half-life of serum-neutralizing maternal antibody was shown to be 9.5 days (Scott et al. 1970). Kittens with a titer of 1:30 were protected, and this level can persist for approximately 8 weeks in kittens born to queens that transmitted high antibody levels to their offspring. Active immunity is conferred either by surviving natural infection or by artificial immunization. Animals recovering from natural infection are thought to be immune for the rest of their lives.

TREATMENT. The virus exerts its destructive effect before actual symptoms of the disease can be recognized. Therefore, treatment is primarily of a supportive nature. The regulation of body fluids and electrolyte balance may be accomplished by administering a balanced electrolyte solution. Ott (1964) suggested that intravenous transfusion of whole blood at the rate of 11–22 ml/kg body weight on a daily basis is beneficial. Donor animals must be tested for other pathogens such as feline leukemia virus. The anorexia, emesis, and diarrhea should be treated conservatively. Overhandling and overtreatment may aggravate the symptoms.

After vomiting subsides, usually in 48 hours, small amounts of liquid in the form of milk or meat broths may be given. Kaolin or similar compounds help in the control of diarrhea.

Antibiotic therapy to control secondary bacterial infection is also a good procedure, broad-spectrum antibiotics being preferred. Panleukopenia virus has not been shown to be affected by any of the known antiviral drugs including isoprinosine (Glasgow and Galasso 1972), 6-azauridine, and 5-iododeoxyuridine (Steffenhagen et al. 1976).

CONTROL. Inactivated vaccines have been available for many years and in general have been quite successful in controlling panleukopenia. The early vaccines were prepared from the tissues of infected cats and were difficult to standardize. The newer inactivated vaccines are prepared from infected tissue cultures and are highly antigenic and safe (Bittle et al. 1970).

Modified live virus (MLV) vaccines are also

available and confer very good immunity; however, they should not be used in species where they have not been proved safe or recommended by the manufacturer. Some of the MLV virus vaccines are shed from the vaccinated animals and may infect susceptible animals in contact with them. This is a problem if the virus infects pregnant queens, where abortions or other congenital effects may occur.

Vaccines have also been prepared from mink enteritis virus isolated from mink and will protect mink and cats against panleukopenia just as panleukopenia virus vaccines will cross-protect mink against mink enteritis (Wills and Belcher 1956).

Oral vaccination has not been successful (Schultz and Scott 1973), but exposure of cats in a chamber to aerosolized virus for 1–3 minutes effectively immunized (Scott and Glauberg 1975).

Both inactivated and MLV vaccines confer protection rapidly, usually within 48–72 hours after vaccination.

The question of when to vaccinate is always a problem, because young animals with passive maternal antibody usually do not respond as well as completely susceptible animals. For this reason, at least two doses, one given at 8 weeks and a second at 12 weeks should be administered to ensure long-term protection.

Immune serums may be used prophylactically and do confer protection for a limited time (Hindle and Findlay 1932; Leasure et al. 1934). Their usefulness in treatment may be open to question unless they are considered to be of general supportive value.

The complete decontamination of infected quarters is essential in controlling the spread of this disease. The removal of all organic material is recommended by steam cleaning and washing the area with suitable detergents, followed by the use of an effective viricidal preparation such as sodium hypochlorite. In closed isolation facilities, the quarters that can be sealed off may be decontaminated by gaseous disinfectants such as formaldehyde.

The control of such insect vectors as fleas and flies is necessary. Infected animals should be confined to an isolation area and have no contact with other animals. The excreta from infected animals should be disinfected and great care exercised in its disposal.

Young animals should be held in isolation until properly vaccinated. Cats that have recovered from panleukopenia infection should be allowed contact with vaccinated animals only.

REFERENCES

Bittle, J. L., Emery, J. B., York, C. J., and McMillen, K. Comparative study of feline cytopathogenic viruses and feline panleukopenia virus. *Am. J. Vet. Res.* 22:374, 1961.

Bittle, J. L., Emrich, S. A., and Gauker, F. B. Safety and efficacy of an inactivated tissue culture vaccine for feline panleukopenia. *J. Am. Vet. Med. Assoc.* 157(Dec. 15):2052–2056, 1970.

Bouillant, A., and Hanson, R. P. Epizootiology of mink enteritis. Stability of the virus in feces exposed to natural environmental factors. *Can. J. Comp. Med. Vet. Sci.* 29:125, 1965.

Bouillant, A., Lee, V. H., and Hanson, R. P. Epizootiology of mink enteritis: II. *Mucosa domestica* L. as a possible vector of virus. *Can. J. Comp. Med. Vet. Sci.* 29:148, 1965.

Burger, D., and Ott, R. L. Protection of cats against feline panleukopenia following mink virus enteritis vaccination. *Small Anim. Clin.* 3:611, 1963.

Carlson, J. H., Scott, F. W., and Duncan, J. R. Feline panleukopenia: I. Pathogenesis in germfree and specific pathogen-free cats. *Vet. Pathol.* 14:79–88, 1977.

Csiza, C. K., Scott, F. W., de Lahunta, A., Gillespie J. H. Immune carrier state of feline panleukopenia virus infected cats. *Am. J. Vet. Res.* 32(March):419–426, 1971.

Glasgow, L. A., and Galasso, G. J. Isoprinosine: Lack of antiviral activity in experimental model infections. *J. Infect. Dis.* 126(Aug.):162–169, 1972.

Goss, L. J. Species susceptibility to the viruses of Carre and feline enteritis. *Am. J. Vet. Res.* 9:65, 1948.

Hammon, W. D., and Enders, J. F. A virus disease of cats, principally characterized by aleukocytosis, enteric lesions, and presence of intranuclear inclusion bodies. *J. Exp. Med.* 69:327, 1939.

Hindle, E., and Findlay, G. J. Studies on feline distemper. *J. Comp. Pathol. Ther.* 45:11, 1932.

Johnson, R. H. Isolation of a virus from a condition simulating feline panleukopenia in a leopard. *Vet. Rec.* 76:1,008, 1964.

———. Feline panleukopenia virus: I. Identification of the virus associated with the syndrome. *Res. Vet. Sci.* 6:466, 1965a.

———. Feline panleukopenia virus: II. Some features of the cytopathic effect in feline kidney monolayers. *Res. Vet. Sci.* 6:472, 1965b.

———. Feline panleukopenia virus: III. Some properties compared to a feline herpes virus. *Res. Vet. Sci.* 7:112, 1966.

———. Feline panleukopenia virus: IV. Methods for obtaining reproducible in vitro results. *Res. Vet. Sci.* 8:256, 1967a.

———. Feline panleukopenia virus: In vitro comparison of strains with a mink enteritis virus. *J. Small Anim. Pract.* 8:319, 1967b.

Johnson, R. H., Margolis, G., and Kilham, L. Identity of feline ataxia virus with feline panleukopenia virus. *Nature* 214:175, 1967.

Jubb, K. V. F., and Kennedy, P. C. *Pathology of domestic animals,* vol. 1. New York: Academic Press, 1962.

Kilham, L., and Margolis, G. M. Viral etiology of spontaneous ataxia of cats. *Am. J. Pathol.* 48:991, 1966.

Kilham, L., Margolis, G., Colby, E. D. Cerebellar ataxia and its congenital transmission in cats by feline panleukopenia virus. *J. Am. Vet. Med. Assoc.* 158(March):888–901, 1971.

———. Congenital infections of cats and ferrets by feline panleukopenia virus manifested by cerebellar hypoplasia. *Lab. Invest.* 17:465–480, 1967.

Kirk, H. *The diseases of the cat.* London: Bailliere, Tindall and Cox, 1925.

Lawrence, J. S., and Syverton, J. T. Spontaneous agranulocytosis in a cat. *Proc. Soc. Exp. Biol. Med.* 38:914, 1938.

Lawrence, J. S., Syverton, D. H., Shaw, J. S., and Smith, F. P. Infectious feline agranulocytosis. *Am. J. Pathol.* 16:333, 1940.

Leasure, F. E., Leinhardt, H. F., and Tabernes, F. R. Feline infectious enteritis. *North Am. Vet.* 15:7, 30, 1934.

MacPherson, L. V. Feline enteritis: Its transmission in mink under natural and experimental conditions. *Can. J. Comp. Med. Vet. Sci.* 20:197, 1956.

Myers, V. L., and Fritz, T. E. Histopathologic changes in virus enteritis of mink. *Can. J. Comp. Med. Vet. Sci.* 23:246, 1959.

Ott, R. L. Viral diseases. In E. J. Catcott, *Feline Medicine and Surgery,* 1st ed., p. 72. Wheaton, Ill.: American Veterinary Publications, 1964.

Povey, C. Viral diseases of cats: Current concepts. *Vet. Rec.* (April):293–298, 1976.

Reif, J. S. Seasonality, natality and herd immunity in feline panleukopenia. *Am. J. Epidemiol.* 103:81–87, 1976.

Rohovsky, M. W., and Fowler, E. H. Lesions of experimental feline panleukopenia. *J. Am. Vet. Med. Assoc.* 158(March):872–875, 1971.

Schultz, R. D., Mendel, H., and Scott, F. W. Effect of feline panleukopenia virus infection on development of humoral and cellular immunity. *Cornell Vet.* 66:324–332, 1976.

Schultz, R. D., Mendel, H., and Scott, F. W. Absence of an immune response after oral administration of attenuated feline panleukopenia virus. *Infect. and Immun.* 7(4):547–549, 1973.

Scott, F. W., Csiza, C. K., and Gillespie, J. H. Maternally derived immunity to feline panleukopenia. *J. Am. Vet. Med. Assoc.* 156:439–453, 1970.

Scott, F. W., and Glauberg, A. F. Aerosol vaccination against feline panleukopenia. *J. Am. Vet. Med. Assoc.* 166:147–149, 1975.

Steffenhagen, K. A., Easterday, B. C., and Galasso, C. J. Evaluation of 6-azauridine and 5-iododeoxyuridine in the treatment of experimental viral infections. *J. Infect. Dis.* 133:603–612, 1976.

Torres, E. Infectious feline gastroenteritis in wild cats. *North Am. Vet.* 22:297, 1941.

Verge, J., and Cristoforoni, N. La gastro enterite infectieuse des chats; est-elle due a un virus filtrable? *C. R. Soc. Biol.* 99:312, 1928.

Wills, G. C. Notes on infectious enteritis of mink and its relationship to feline enteritis. *Can. J. Comp. Med. Vet. Sci.* 16:419, 1952.

Wills, G. C., and Belcher, J. The prevention of virus enteritis of mink with commercial feline panleukopenia vaccine. *J. Am. Vet. Med. Assoc.* 128:559, 1956.

8 *Pseudorabies*

DANIEL O. TRAINER

Synonyms: Aujeszky's disease, mad-itch, pseudohydrophobia, peste de cocar (scratching pest), Aoeski disease, *Herpes suis.*

Pseudorabies (Pr) is an infectious, often acute, viral disease that infects the central nervous system of wild mammals, ranch mink, fur farm foxes, and a variety of domestic species including swine, cattle, sheep, dogs, and cats. It is characterized by a marked localized pruritus and fatal termination.

HISTORY AND DISTRIBUTION. At the turn of the century, Aujeszky (1902) initially isolated and identified Pr virus from a naturally infected ox, a dog, and a cat. Subsequent investigations have been summarized by Galloway (1938), Shahan et al. (1947), Hanson (1954), and Baskerville et al. (1973). These and other investigators have reported natural infections of Pr in domesticated and feral swine, sheep, goats, cattle, dogs, and cats.

Until the 1960s the disease in swine was mild with limited mortality among young pigs. In 1962, virulent strains of Pr virus began to appear in swine, and now virulent strains are found throughout the United States. Mortality among adult swine does occur, and Pr often produces abortions and mortality in adult sows.

Naturally infected wildlife species include rats, mice, red fox, mink, arctic fox, roe deer, raccoon, skunks, and field hare. Experimental transmission of Pr virus by inoculation or feeding has been successful in nearly all warmblooded animals in which it has been tried, including a wide variety of wildlife species (Table 8.1). Accounts of human infection are sketchy and of questionable validity.

Since Aujeszky's initial diagnosis of Pr in Hungary, it has been reported to exist in North America, South America, Middle East, Africa, Asia, and most of Europe (Bitsch 1975; Galloway 1938; Shahan et al. 1947). Hanson (1954) summarized the history of Pr in the United States and its widespread geographic occurrence.

ETIOLOGY. Pseudorabies virus is a member of the herpesvirus family now known as the Herpesviridae. It is an enveloped, double-stranded DNA virus with a high guanine-cytosine ratio, 5:3:2 axial symmetry, and icosahedral shape. The capsid is composed of 1,962 hollow capsomeres, 150 of which are hexagonal in shape and 12 of which are pentagonal. The complete virus is about 150 nm, the nucleocapsid 110 nm, and the core 77 nm.

Optimum storage temperatures of the virus are either −30°C or +4°C. The virus survives for several months at refrigerator temperature when stored in 50% glycerol, but freezing in a conventional home freezer (−18°C) can inactivate the virus in less than a month. It is acid, ether, and heat sensitive and may also be destroyed by ultraviolet light, gamma irradiation, boiling, crystal violet, trypsin, 1% sodium hydroxide, 5% phenol, 2% formalin, and lipid solvents such as chloroform and ether.

The virus is relatively stable and has been found to survive on hay and wooden surfaces for 2−7 weeks, depending on temperature, humidity, and whether indoors or outdoors; on rabbit skin pickled in brine for 4 weeks; and in the muscle of animal carcasses for 2−5 weeks, depending on temperature. Survival time is decreased somewhat in the presence of feces (Solomkin and Tutushin 1956; Ustenko 1958).

Pr virus can be propagated and passaged readily in cell cultures derived from many animal species including cattle, swine, rabbits, dog, and monkey, as well as primary chicken embryo cells. Cowdry type A intranuclear inclusions are produced by the virus in a wide variety of mammalian cell cultures. The cytopathic effect of Pr virus in cell cultures is similar to that associated with many other herpesviruses (Gustafson 1975). The cytopathic effect includes vacuolation leading to lysis; foci of cytopathic effect leave the cell sheets pocketed with holes surrounded by infected cells. The virus is easily isolated in cell cultures from animals with acute pseudorabies, but isolation from normal carrier animals is difficult.

TRANSMISSION. Domestic swine are considered to be the principal reservoir of the disease (Gustafson 1975). Infected swine may harbor the virus as symptomless carriers, transmitting it to susceptible individuals of a variety of spe-

TABLE 8.1   Natural and Experimental Pseudorabies Infection in Wildlife.

Common Name	Scientific Name	Reference
Natural Infections		
Arctic fox	*Alopex lagopus*	Ljubashenko et al. 1958
Field hare	*Lepus europaeus*	Grunett and Skoda 1964
Mice	Unknown	Lukashev and Rotov 1939
Mink	*Mustela vison*	Konrad and Blazek 1958; Lapcevic 1964
Norway rat	*Rattus norvegicus*	Shope 1935; Nikitin 1960
Opossum	*Didelphis marsupialis*	Kanitz et al. 1974
Raccoon	*Procyon lotor*	Beran et al. 1977; Kanitz et al. 1974
Red fox	*Vulpes fulva*	Bitsch and Munch 1974
Roe deer	*Capreolus capreolus*	Nikolitsch 1954; Srajber and Kurjakov 1956
Silver and common fox	*Vulpes* spp.	Soldatova 1962; Zwierzchowski 1962
Skunk	*Mephitis mephitis*	Beran et al. 1978
Experimental Infections		
Badger	*Taxidea taxus*	Trainer and Karstad 1963
Brown bat	*Eptesicus fuscus*	Reagan et al. 1953
Buzzard	*Buteo buteo*	Remlinger and Bailly 1934
Cottontail rabbit	*Sylvilagus floridanus*	Trainer and Karstad 1963
Ferret	*Mustela* spp.	Goto et al. 1968; Ohshima et al. 1976
Jackal	*Canis aureus*	Remlinger and Bailly 1934
Mallard duck	*Anas platyrhynchos*	Bemlinger and Bailly 1934
Mink	*Mustela vison*	Goto et al. 1968
Muskrat	*Ondatra zibethica*	Trainer and Karstad 1963
Opossum	*Didelphis marsupialis*	Trainer and Karstad 1963; Kanitz et al. 1974
Porcupine	*Hystrix* spp.	Braga and Faria 1934
Raccoon	*Procyon lotor*	Trainer and Karstad 1963; Kanitz et al. 1974
Red fox	*Vulpes fulva*	Trainer and Karstad 1963
Rhesus monkey	*Macaca mulatta*	Karasszon 1965
Sable	*Martes zibellina*	Tynl'panova and Grabovskii 1964
Skunk	*Mephitis mephitis*	Trainer and Karstad 1963
Sparrow hawk	*Accipiter nisus*	Remlinger and Bailly 1934
White-tailed deer	*Odocoileus virginianus*	Trainer and Karstad 1963
Woodchuck	*Marmota monax*	Trainer and Karstad 1963; Remlinger and Bailly 1934

cies. The virus may be present in the nasal discharge of infected pigs for long periods of time, and transmission to susceptible hosts occurs via contact through abraded skin, inhalation via the intact nasal mucosa, or by ingestion of infected material. Transmission through the sow's milk and by coitus also has been reported.

Although rodents have often been incriminated in the transmission of Pr, recent studies show that rats and mice are quite resistant to infection and are poor shedders of the virus. As a result, they are not considered to be good reservoirs or to play an important role in its spread (Kanitz et al. 1974; McFerran and Dow 1970).

Carnivores such as raccoons, skunks, foxes, opossums, and dogs are readily infected by ingestion of infected carcasses. They in turn can serve as a source of infection for other species,

wild or domestic (Beran et al. 1977; Kirkpatrick et al. 1980).

Fur farm outbreaks of Pr among mink and foxes have been attributed to the feeding of virus-infected pig offal (Bitsch and Munch 1971; Konrad and Blazek 1958; Lapcevic 1964; Ljubashenko et al. 1958; Ugorski 1958). Oyrzanowska and Kita (1966) found it prerequisite to scarify the skin around the buccal cavity of foxes and the oral mucosa of mink before being able to produce infection by feeding infectious rabbit viscera. However, scarification was not needed by Trainer and Karstad (1963) to infect raccoons and foxes by a similar route.

SIGNS. The signs of Pr are variable among individuals and species. Generally, the severity of the signs increases with the length of the incubation period. This was especially noticeable among wildlife species studied by Trainer and Karstad (1963). Pseudorabies, or mad itch, which is almost always fatal, is characterized by various degrees of nervous disorder accompanied by a marked pruritus, usually at the site of infection. Respiratory signs of rhinitis or pneumonia often accompany the infection.

Among naturally infected domestic species, only the pig fails to develop a pruritus. The clinical disease in pigs varies with the age of the pig, strain of virus involved, and past exposure. Mortality rates decrease as the age of infected animals increases. In severe cases, signs may include anorexia, dullness, agalactia, vomiting, opisthotonus, convulsions, spasms of muscle groups, paralysis of certain parts of the body, incoordination, and abortion (Blood and Henderson 1963). A common feature in pregnant sows is abortion. In young pigs, the disease is usually severe, with mortality rates as high as 100%. Paralysis, excessive salivation, respiratory distress, vomiting, and ataxia have been reported in cattle, sheep, dogs, and cats.

Numerous fur farm outbreaks have been reported in the Old World. Signs observed in mink include tonic and clonic spasms, derangements of equilibrium, excitement alternating with depression, and violent itching with self-mutilation (Geurden et al. 1963). Scratching and loss of fur about the head and muzzle was observed by Ljubashenko et al. (1958) in foxes but not in mink. Konrad and Blazek (1958) also failed to observe pruritus among mink.

Observations of experimental Pr in wildlife species concur with those seen on fur farms. For example, a pruritus was produced in infected foxes but not in mink (Oyrzanowska and Kita 1966). Trainer and Karstad (1963) observed pruritus in experimentally infected fox, badger, raccoon, woodchuck, skunk, opossum, and deer, as did Goret and Mariette (1938) in the ferret. Goto et al. (1968) reported the clinical signs in mink and rabbits to be severe, whereas those of ferrets were generally mild. Pruritus was not produced in the sable (Tynl'panova and Grabovskii 1964), big brown bat (Reagan et al. 1953), or the muskrat and cottontail rabbit (Trainer and Karstad 1963).

Anorexia, excessive salivation, clonic spasms, and convulsions were observed in all species studied by Trainer and Karstad (1963), except muskrat and skunk which merely became comatose immediately before death. They also noted tooth grinding in the raccoon and deer as has been reported in the big brown bat (Reagan et al. 1953).

Signs of Pr in the sable include loss of

appetite, depression, dyspnea, frothy salivation, coughing, vomiting, circling, staggering, increased excitability, and finally general weakness and paralysis of the hind limbs, terminating in death (Tynl'panova and Grabovskii 1964).

PATHOGENESIS. Little is known regarding the pathogenesis of Pr in wildlife. In domestic species the natural route of exposure is considered to be through nasal infection. Primary viral multiplication occurs in the cells of the nasopharyngeal mucosa, and the virus gains entry into the central nervous system via the peripheral nerves, passing along them centripetally and causing nerve cell damage resulting in local pruritus and encephalomyelitis (Hurst 1934).

The disease is reported to be strictly neurotropic in domestic ruminants. Experimental studies with cattle have shown that lesions occur in the central nervous system in areas directly associated with the sites of inoculation by peripheral afferent and efferent nerves. Spread of the virus along these peripheral nerve routes has been suggested (Dow and McFerran 1966; Ohshima et al. 1976). Fluorescent antibody studies in rabbits and weaned pigs have shown a predilection of the virus for the ependymal lining and periventricular nervous tissues (Albrecht et al. 1963).

Taga et al. (1957) reported experimental Pr infection in pigs spread from the site of infection by way of the lymphatic system and further viral multiplication in lymph nodes. Ohshima et al. (1976), studying pathologic changes in ferrets, reported findings that support the view that lymphohematogenous spread of virus occurs.

The pathogenesis of the pruritus itself is thought to involve the central nervous system (cerebral cortex) rather than the peripheral nervous system adjacent to the inoculation site (Saiko 1960).

The virus has been recovered from a variety of tissues of experimentally infected wild mammals, with the brain, lungs, adrenals, turbinates, and tonsils being the most consistent sources. The findings were somewhat different in a white-tailed deer, where virus was isolated from the urine, kidney, spleen, sciatic nerve, lumbar and thoracic regions of the spinal cord, and a number of lymph nodes (Trainer and Karstad 1963; Kirkpatrick et al. 1980).

PATHOLOGY. There are no pathognomonic lesions for Pr. Both gross pathology and histopathology vary with the species affected and the route of infection. Natural infection or experimental infection via subcutaneous, intradermal, or intramuscular routes usually results in characteristic skin lesions in most domestic animals and some wild ones. An intense cutaneous irritation develops at the point of inoculation or at the terminal distribution of an infected nerve trunk. This does not take place until the virus reaches the related segment of nerve cord (Jubb and Kennedy 1970). The area becomes denuded of hair, and accompanying lacerations of the skin and underlying tissues result from the animal's licking, rubbing, biting, and scratching because of the pruritus. The subcutaneous tissue of the region is often very edematous, and a bloody exudate may cover the entire area. Although the lesions described are quite spectacular, they do not occur among all species, nor regularly in all cases in a given species.

In severely infected swine, a common finding is congestion and hyperemia of the nasal mucosa and pharynx (Gustafson 1975). Pulmonary congestion, edema, and hemorrhage are frequently observed during the postmortem of infected animals. Petechial hemorrhages in the pericardial sac and thymus, and moderate injection of the meningeal vessels also may occur. Marked meningitis is usually restricted to acute fatal cases.

Major histologic changes occur in the central nervous system. Principal changes consist of a diffuse, nonsuppurative meningoencephalomyelitis and ganglioneuritis. Perivascular cuffing and diffuse and focal gliosis are associated with extensive neuronal and glial necrosis (Olander et al. 1966). Jubb and Kennedy (1970) noted that in naturally acquired infections among domestic animals, inflammatory changes within the brain are nonsuppurative. After intracerebral inoculation the reaction is more severe and is characterized by meningitis and encephalitis in which neutrophils and eosinophils may be abundant. They reported severe ganglioneuritis in paravertebral ganglia and acidophilic intranuclear inclusion bodies in neurons and astroglia. These inclusion bodies occur in all species, including pigs in which they were not found originally.

Information regarding the pathology of Pr among wild species is sparse. Trainer and Karstad (1963) reported that gross pathology and histopathology differ with the species, route of infection, and age of the animal.

Moderate enlargement of the spleen with infarction; pulmonary congestion of the turbinates, adrenals, kidneys, spleen, and liver; along with petechiation of the heart and moderate engorgement of the meningeal vessels were seen in a raccoon, an opossum, and a fox which had died from experimental infection (Trainer and Karstad 1963). Gross pathologic changes were not detected in a deer which had died from experimental Pr. Hyperemia and petechiation of many organs and marked injection of the blood vessels of the brain were the major lesions resulting from experimental infection of sable (Tynl'panova and Grabovskii 1964); pulmonary edema was the most typical finding during an epizootic among mink, arctic fox, and silver fox at a Leningrad fur farm (Ljubashenko et al. 1958).

DIAGNOSIS. Clinical diagnosis of Pr is usually based on the severe pruritus and short course of the disease. However, absence of such specific signs may confuse the diagnosis. A presumptive diagnosis can be made from gross and histopathologic findings, especially when they parallel an appropriate case history.

Isolation of the virus is required for laboratory confirmation of Pr. This is routinely done by inoculation of susceptible laboratory animals, tissue culture, or fluorescent antibody procedures (Kanitz et al. 1974). Samples from suspected cases may include spinal cord from the area of pruritus, local nerve trunks, edematous fluid from the infected area, lymph nodes, tonsils, or brain tissue.

Rabbits are the laboratory animals of choice. When infected with Pr virus, they usually develop frenzied itching with characteristic local inflammation of the skin and die in respiratory failure. Death of inoculated rabbits without an accompanying pruritus has been observed after infection with modified Pr strains (Zuffa and Grigelova 1966). Mice 2–4 weeks old are also very susceptible and can be used as an aid in diagnosis.

Isolation of Pr virus in tissue culture has been shown to be more sensitive and accurate and considerably faster than animal inoculation (Masic and Petrovic 1964). A wide range of tissue culture systems can be used (Kaplan 1969).

The fluorescent antibody test is very useful in the diagnosis of Pr in tissues and in tissue culture (Sabo and Rajcani 1970; Stewart et al. 1967; Kirkpatrick et al. 1980). A number of serologic tests are available, and the most commonly used is the serum neutralization test. Cutaneous allergic tests are available and may be useful in epizootiologic studies (Smith and Mengeling 1977).

IMMUNITY. Information on immunity in wild animals is not available. Antibody levels detected among pigs and horses indicate that natural immunity against Pr exists to some degree within these and possibly other species. In swine, high antibody levels persist for as long as 54 months following outbreaks, and maternal immunity is transferred passively to piglets through colostrum after natural infection. Killed and modified live vaccines have been used successfully in Europe and are available for use in swine in the United States.

TREATMENT AND CONTROL. Treatment and control of Pr in wildlife has not been considered necessary or feasible. Hyperimmune serum produced in horses or swine and concentrated gamma globulin have been used successfully to treat domestic animals in Europe (Popescu 1965).

Control procedures, including proper sanitation, are useful for preventing losses from Pr for captive wildlife and on fur farms. The isolation of infected animals is a primary control step becuase the disease can spread by direct contact (Ljubashenko et al. 1960; Trainer and Karstad 1963). All offal being fed should be thoroughly cooked. Control of rats and small rodents, of practical value in captive animal outbreaks, is of little value for free-ranging wildlife.

REFERENCES

Albrecht, P., Blaskovic, D., Jakubik, J., and Lesso, J. Demonstration of pseudorabies virus in chick embryo cultures and infected animals by the fluorescent antibody technique. *Acta Virol.* 7:289–396, 1963.

Aujeszky, A. Ueber eine neue Infektionskrankheit bei Haustieren. *Zentralbla. Bakteriol. [Orig A].* 32:353–373, 1902.

Baskerville, A., McFerran, J. B., and Dow, C. Aujeszky's disease in pigs. *Vet. Bull.* 43:465–480, 1973.

Beran, G. W., Kunesk, J., and Howard, H. *Epidemiological studies of pseudorabies in Iowa*, p. 30. Pseudorabies Fact Finding Conference. Ames: Iowa State University Press, 1977.

Bitsch, V. A study of outbreaks of Aujeszky's disease in cattle. *Acta Vet. Scand.* 16:420–455, 1975.

Bitsch, V., and Munch, B. On pseudorabies in carnivores in Denmark: I. The red fox. *Acta Vet. Scand.* 12:274–284, 1971.

Blood, C. D., and Henderson, J. A. *Veterinary medicine*. Baltimore: Williams and Wilkins, 1963.

Braga, A., and Faria A. *Rev. Dept. Nacl. Prod. Animal, Rio de Janeiro* 1:53, 1934.

Dow, C., and McFerran, J. B. Experimental studies on Aujeszky's disease in cattle. *J. Comp. Pathol. Ther.* 76:379–386, 1966.

Galloway, I. A. Aujeszky's disease. *Vet. Rec.* 50:745–762, 1938.

Geurden, L. M. G., Devos, A., Viaene, N., and Staelens, M. Aujeszky's disease in mink. *Vlaams Diergeneesk. Tijdschr.* 32:36–47, 1963.

Goret, P., and Mariette, C. Receptivite due furet (*Putorius furo* L.) au virus de la maladie d'Aujeszky inocule par differentes voies. *C. R. Soc. Biol.* 128:871–873, 1938.

Goto, H., Gorham, J. R., and Hagen, K. W. Clinical observation of experimental pseudorabies in mink and ferrets. *Jpn. J. Vet. Sci.* 30:257–263, 1968.

Grunett, Z., and Skoda, R. Epidemiology of the Aujeszky's disease in Czechoslovakia: I. History and geographical distribution. *Vet. Med.* 9:351–360, 1964.

Gustafson, D. P. Pseudorabies. A. D. Leman, et al. *Diseases of swine*, 5th ed., Ames: Iowa State University Press, pp. 209–223, 1981.

Hanson, R. P. The history of pseudorabies in the United States. *J. Am. Vet. Med. Assoc.* 124:259–261, 1954.

Hurst, E. W. Studies on pseudorabies (infectious bulbar paralysis, mad itch): II. Routes of infection in the rabbit with remarks on the relation of the virus to other viruses affecting the nervous system. *J. Exp. Med.* 59:729–749, 1934.

Jubb, K. V. F., and Kennedy, P. C. *Pathology of domestic animals*, 2d ed. New York: Academic Press, 1970.

Kanitz, C. L., Hand, R. B., and McCrocklin, S. M. Pseudorabies in Indiana: Current status, laboratory confirmation and epizootiologic considerations. *Proc. U.S. Anim. Health Assoc.* 78:346–358, 1974.

Kaplan, A. S. Herpes simplex and pseudorabies viruses. *Virol. Monogr.* 5:26–27, 1969.

Karasszon, D. Pathohistological studies on the central nervous system of monkeys inoculated with a modified strain of Aujeszky's virus. *Acta Vet.* 15:405–411, 1965.

Kirkpatrick, C. M., Kanitz, C. L., and McCrocklin, S. M. Possible role of wild mammals in transmission of pseudorabies to swine. *J. Wildl. Dis.* 16(4):601–614, 1980.

Konrad, J., and Blazek, K. Aujeszky's disease in mink. *Sb. Cesk. Akad. Zemedel. Ved.* 3:803–816, 1958.

Lapcevic, E. Aujeszky's disease in mink. *DTW.* 71:273–275, 1964.

Ljubashenko, S. Y., Tynl'panova, A. F., and Grishin, V. M. Aujeszky's disease in mink, arctic fox and silver fox. *Veterinariya* 35:37–41, 1958.

———. Aujeszky's disease in fur animals: Immunization, treatment and epidemiology. *Veterinariya* 37:46–51, 1960.

Lukashev, I. I., and Rotov, V. I. Materialy k epizootologii bolezni aveshki. *Sov. Vet.* 7:51–54, 1939.

McFerran, J. B., and Dow, C. Experimental Aujeszky's disease (pseudorabies) in rats. *BR. Vet. J.* 126:173–178, 1970.

Masic, M., and Petrovic, M. Early diagnosis of Aujeszky's disease by means of a tissue culture technique. *Vet. Glasn.* 18:167–178, 1964.

Nikitin, M. Isolation of Aujeszky's disease virus from wild *Rattus norvegicus. Zool. Zh.* 39:282–287, 1960.

Nikolitsch, M. Aujeszky's disease in roe deer in Yugoslavia. *Wien. Tieraerztl. Monatsschr.* 41:603–605, 1954.

Ohshima, K., Gorham, J. R., and Henson, J. B. Pathologic changes in ferrets exposed to pseudorabies virus. *Am. J. Vet. Res.* 37:591–596, 1976.

Olander, H. J., Saunders, J. R., Gustafson, D. P., and Jones, R. K. Pathologic findings in swine affected with a virulent strain of Aujeszky's virus. *Pathol. Vet.* 3:64–72, 1966.

Oyrzanowska, J., and Kita, J. The source of Aujeszky's disease virus for fur animals. *Med. Weterynar.* 22:579–581, 1966.

Popescu, A. Aujeszky's disease virus: I. Culture in trypsinized cells. II. Preparation of hyperimmune serum by using culture virus. *Lucrarile Inst. Cercetari Vet. Bioprep. Pasteur* 2:143–167, 1965.

Reagan, R. L., Day, W., Marley, R., and Brueckner, A. L. Effect of pseudorabies virus in the large brown bat (*Eptesicus fuscus*). *Am. J. Vet. Res.* 14:331–332, 1953.

Remlinger, P., and Bailly, J. Contribution a l'etude due virus de la "maladie d'Aujeszky." *Ann. Inst. Pasteur* 52:361, 1934.

Sabo, A., and Rajcani, J. Rapid diagnosis of Aujeszky's disease by the fluorescent antibody technique. *Acta Virol. Prague* 14:476–484, 1970.

Saiko, A. A. Pathogenesis of the itching associated with Aujeszky's disease: I. Role of the histidine decarboxylase and the histamine-histaminase systems. II. Role of the acetylcholine-cholinesterase system in the skin. *Sb. Tr. Kharkov Vet. Inst.* 24:186–202, 1960.

Shahan, M. S., Knudson, R. L., Seibold, H. R., and Dale, C. N. Aujeszky's disease (pseudorabies): A review, with notes on two strains of the virus. *North Am. Vet.* 28:440–449, 1947.

Shope, R. E. Experiments on the epidemiology of pseudorabies: II. Prevalence of the disease among middle western swine and the possible role of rats in herd-to-herd infections. *J. Exp. Med.* 62:101–117, 1935.

Smith, P. C., and Mengeling, W. L. A skin test for pseudorabies virus infection in swine. *Can. J. Comp. Med.* 41:364–368, 1977.

Soldatova, R. Aujeszky's disease in silver-gray foxes. *Krolikovod. Zverovod.* (2):23, 1962.

Solomkin, P. S., and Tutushin, M. I. Viability of the virus of Aujeszky's disease in fodder and on products of animal origin. *Veterinariya* 33:49–50, 1956.

Srajber, L., and Kurjakov, B. Incidence of Aujeszky's disease in the Vojvodina Province. *Vet. Glasn.* 10:496–500, 1956.

Stewart, W. C., Carbrey, E. A., and Kresse, J. I. Detection of pseudorabies virus by immunofluorescence. *J. Am. Med. Assoc.* 151:747–751, 1967.

Taga, M., Berbinschi, C., Cristet, I., and Coman, I. Distribution of Aujeszky's disease virus in pigs experimentally infected by various routes. *Anu. Inst. Patol. Igiena. Anim.* 7:221–228, 1957.

Trainer, D., and Karstad, L. Experimental psuedorabies in some wild North American mammals. *Zoon. Res.* 2:135–151, 1963.

Tynl'panova, A., and Grabovskii, A. Susceptibility of sable to the virus of Aujeszky's disease. *Krolikovod. Zverovod.* 7:26–27, 1964.

Ugorski, L. Aujeszky's disease in silver foxes. *Med. Vet.* 14:449–450, 1958.

Ustenko, V. S. Survival of the virus of Aujeszky's disease in the external environment. *Tr. Vses. Inst. Vet. Sanit. Ektoparasitol.* 13:49–59, 1958.

Zuffa, A., and Grigelova, K. Immunization against Aujeszky's disease: II. Cytopathic action and plaque morphology of various virus strains in relation to their virulence for pigs. *Arch. Exp. Veterinaermed.* 20:127–140, 1966.

Zwierzchowski, J. Aujeszky's disease in foxes and mink. *Veterinariya,* pp. 133–140, 1962.

9 Virus B Infection

FRANCES M. LOVE   WILLIAM G. STONE

Synonyms: **Herpesvirus simiae, herpetic stomatitis of monkeys.**

Virus B herpetic infection in animals is a communicable disease usually occurring naturally in monkeys as a mild, inapparent, self-limited form characterized by vesicular or ulcerative lesions of the labial skin and oral or pharyngeal mucous membranes, but occasionally involving the central nervous system or the viscera. The lesions are strikingly similar to the lesions of herpes simplex in man (*Herpesvirus hominis* fever blisters, cold sores, and so on). The lesions usually heal spontaneously in 7–14 days. Central nervous system lesions may be found during necropsy examination even when there is no history of clinical disease.

HISTORY. This variety of herpesvirus infection was first recognized during the investigation of a human fatality. Sabin and Wright (1934) isolated a virus from the central nervous tissue taken from a laboratory worker who died 17 days after being bitten by an apparently normal rhesus monkey. They called it virus B. Gay and Holden (1933) isolated the same agent from the same material and named it virus W. The term used by Sabin and Wright has become universally accepted. Sabin and his co-workers studied the properties of the virus extensively, and even though there have been some additions to their contributions, their work remains definitive. Sabin (1949) reported a second fatal infection which occurred in another laboratory worker under circumstances similar to the first. In all, 20 infections have been reported in man. Additional incidence has been suspected but not reported because the diagnosis was not confirmed. Others have probably occurred but have not been recognized. All but 3 of the infections confirmed in man have been fatal, and the survivors have had central nervous system damage.

Bryan et al. (1975) reported the case of the third survivor of infection, confirmed by isolation of the virus from skin lesions and by serologic testing. This case is unique in that the disease developed 10 years after the last exposure and was presented first with ophthalmic symptoms with a dendritic zoster type ulcer of the cornea, followed by a zoster type skin rash along the distribution of the trigeminal nerve and then by encephalomyelitis. This case was also reviewed by Fierer et al. (1973) and by Roth and Purcell (1977). All known human infections have occurred in persons handling monkeys or monkey tissues.

Epidemiologically, only humans and monkeys are known to have developed the disease by natural transmission. An epidemic of herpetic stomatitis in a monkey colony was observed by Keeble et al. (1958). They isolated a virus from lesions of the oral mucous membranes and identified it as virus B. These authors and other observers have substantiated the observation that the naturally occurring infection becomes even more prevalent under colony conditions. Although the disease does not present a major health problem in infected lower primates, its importance lies in the increasing possibility of infection of personnel in zoos, hospitals, and laboratories in pharmaceutical production and research involving monkeys or monkey tissues. It may even pose a threat to owners of primate pets.

DISTRIBUTION. Virus B is a natural pathogen of certain primates. Its course is apparently similar to other herpeslike viruses which occur as natural parasites of humans, pigs, horses, chickens, and cows.

The incidence of virus B is higher in rhesus (*Macaca mulatta*) and cynomolgous (*M. philippinensis*) monkeys than in other monkey species. Keeble (1960) reported an incidence of 2.3% in his series of 1,400 rhesus monkeys. Orcutt et al. (1976) found that 73% of adult macaques, 36.6% of young adults, and 12.4% of juvenile rhesus monkeys captured in the wild were seropositive for virus B antibodies. Because the incidence has been shown to increase under colony conditions, it is likely that when monkeys are confined in close proximity for any considerable period of time almost 100% infection is achieved. However, Orcutt et al. (1976) found only one seroconversion upon retesting after the second test with serial samples taken at 2-week intervals for five times. Di Giacomo and Shah (1972) have shown that colony-reared rhesus monkeys may be kept free of virus B.

Vervet monkeys (*Cercopithecus pygerythrus*) are known to harbor the virus under unusual circumstances, but most African and South American monkeys have not been shown to be naturally infected under the conditions of their native habitats. Nevertheless, there is good reason to assume that most primates are susceptible when exposed and are potentially capable of transmitting the virus to other susceptible species. Also important is the ability of virus B to persist in a latent form in monkeys (Vizoso 1975).

Although the incidence of virus B infection in man is small, the seriousness of the disease and the increasing number of contacts between man and monkeys justifies the concern with the possibility of human infection. Monkey kidney cell cultures and monkey nerve tissues from apparently normal animals have both yielded virus B (Melnick and Banker 1954; Wood and Shimada 1954) and should be considered a source of infection, just as should direct contact with infected animals. Serum-neutralizing antibodies can be detected in an unexpectedly high percentage of monkeys that have no clinical symptoms. An incidence of 100% of neutralizing antibodies has been reported in some colonies (Hartley 1966). It has been shown that in India there is a natural increase in the clinical disease in monkeys during the monsoon and postmonsoon seasons (Hartley 1964; Keeble 1960).

ETIOLOGY. The nature of virus B is of great interest biologically. It easily passes bacterial filters, indicating an average particle size of 125 mμ. The virus consists of a central core with icosahedral symmetry, 162 capsomeres, and a capsule with a limiting membrane. Green (1965) classified it with DNA viruses. The herpesvirus group includes a number of agents that are probably closely related immunologically. The best known of these are the agents of human herpes, simian herpes, marmoset herpes, pseudorabies of swine, and human varicella. Rhinopneumonitis of horses and infectious laryngotracheitis of chickens are also classified in this group. Recently a common antigen in human herpes simplex, bovine herpetic mammilitis, and virus B has been identified (Norrild et al. 1978). Herpesvirus of marmosets has been isolated too recently to know much about its biological relationships.

All these may have originated with the same virus and later adapted to specific hosts. The theory has been advanced that virus B is the more "complete" of this group antigenically and may be closer to the common ancestor than the herpesvirus of man or the others in this class (Burnet 1955). In each instance the naturally occurring virus has become so adapted that it causes little damage when infecting its specific host. In exceptional instances, usually in the young of the species, the first infection with the host-specific virus may be serious or even fatal. Cross-specific infection of simian virus in man is almost always fatal.

TRANSMISSION. The naturally occurring infection in monkeys appears to follow closely the patterns of herpetic infection in man. Under colony conditions the virus probably spreads by way of salivary contamination of the food or water, bites or scratches of the skin, and possibly through aerosols. The virus has been isolated from saliva (Chappell 1960); it has never been isolated from the feces or urine. Animal attendants and laboratory workers are infected through bites or other breaks in the skin contaminated with monkey saliva, monkey kidney cell cultures, or during necropsy examination of infected tissues. Other sites of primary entry suggested by studying the course of infections in man are the pharynx, nose, and eye. There is no known instance of natural passage from a monkey to any other species of animal other than man, and there is no known transmission from one human being to another.

In the laboratory, using inoculum from infected persons or primates, the rabbit is the only common animal easily infected by a number of routes. Guinea pigs and young mice are resistant but can be infected by direct intracerebral inoculation. Results are usually unpredictable. Infection in these species is achieved more uniformly by injections of material that has been serially passed through susceptible species or monkey tissue cultures. The virus has been propagated on the chorioallantoic membrane of the embryonated chicken egg, using a serially passed virus inoculum (Burnet et al. 1939).

SIGNS. An epidemic of clinical stomatitis under colony conditions was described by Keeble (1960). He was able to reproduce the clinical disease by reinoculation of monkeys. He described lesions on the tongue, buccal mucous membrane, and mucocutaneous junction of the lips grossly similar to lesions observed in human infections with *H. hominis*. These lesions are circumscribed, vesicular eruptions which rapidly become shallow ulcerations and then pass through stages of crusting and scale formation followed by desiccation and healing, usually without scars. The process takes about 7–14 days. He isolated virus B from these mouth lesions. The animals observed were without generalized symptoms and continued to behave and eat normally. A mucopurulent nasal discharge occurred in some instances, and occasionally there was slight conjunctivitis. Keeble also described thick scabs at the sites of bites and scratches on the body. These did not yield virus, but herpeslike type A inclusion bodies were seen when the tissue was examined microscopically.

Signs of infections produced in the laboratory vary somewhat according to the site of inoculation. Injections into the skin of rabbits produce vesiculation, crusting, and scabbing. The infection is spread systemically either along the nerve tracts or by viremia. Both result finally in encephalomyelitis. Injections into the eye produce vesicular conjunctivitis followed by a similar chain of events. In other animals direct intracerebral inoculation causes diffuse encephalitis. The disease may produce various symptoms in humans, but a notably consistent feature is viral encephalomyelitis. The detailed clinical signs in humans have been reviewed in the literature (Davidson and Hummeler 1960; Love and Jungherr 1962; Ruch 1959; Scott and Tokumaru 1965).

PATHOGENESIS. Although the exact pathogenesis of the disease is uncertain, several possibilities are suggested. Lesions of both man and monkey have occurred in skin, mucous membrane, nerve tissue, and viscera, indicating the pantropic nature of the virus. Latency, which is characteristic of *H. hominis* infection in humans, has only recently been demonstrated with virus B in monkeys (Vizoso 1975). The virus has been isolated from blood (Chappell 1960) and sera (Keeble 1960) under experimental conditions, and the occurrence of viremia in natural infections is almost certain.

Once the virus gains access to the body, it propagates in the cells of the invaded tissue at the point of entry. From studies of tissue cultures, it is thought to spread by the fusion of infected cells with contiguous cells. After intracellular multiplication of the virus and destruction of the cells, released virus may invade other cells at the site or become disseminated by the blood. If the invaded cell is a neuron and the tissue is a nerve trunk, the virus can pass directly along the nerve pathway to the brain and spinal cord. The specific neurological findings probably correlate with the point of entry. In the monkey, oral entry is correlated with central nervous system lesions located in the roots and brainstem nuclei of cranial nerves. Because the course of the disease is usually mild in monkeys, such correlations are more strikingly demonstrated by examples from human infections. In humans, bites on the extremities are usually followed by ascending myelitis that terminates in diffuse encephalitis. The widespread and remarkable visceral pathology in human infections indicates the development of viremia. The pathologic changes are remarkably similar in all species of animals susceptible to infection, the differences being mainly in the degree of severity. For example, infected monkeys characteristically have little change in the adrenal glands, whereas these are markedly altered in humans and rabbits.

PATHOLOGY. Grossly, the characteristic mucous membrane lesion is found on the lingual or buccal mucosa and is first vesicular, then ulcerative (Hartley 1966; Keeble 1960). In the fully developed lesion, there is a thin, whitish membrane over a central necrotic area which is surrounded by a sharp line of erythema. Healing occurs by granulation and a gradual replacement of epithelium. There is usually no scarring. Microscopically, there is an initial swelling and degeneration of the epithelial cells, an intermediate stage during which eosinophilic inclusion bodies are seen, and finally the destruction of cells and the development of necrosis. The necrotic membrane is underlain by an area of leukocytic infiltration. Syncytial masses, the herpetic giant cells, are sometimes found in the advancing periphery of the lesion.

Epidermal lesions develop a fine reddish brown scab following vesiculation. Histologically, they are similar to the mucous membrane lesions. In monkeys, the pathologic changes occur in liver, spleen, and central nervous system. Because of the usual benignity of the disease in these species, findings have been made incidentally during postmortem examination or through experimental infection. Tracts of the cranial nerves, sensory nuclei, reticular substance, anterior horn cells, and brainstem nuclei show inflammatory changes. Except for the eosinophilic inclusions occasionally found in the neuron cell nucleus, the changes are those of nonspecific microglial proliferation and perivascular cuffing with lymphocytes.

DIAGNOSIS. The clinical disease occurring naturally in monkeys may be described as a benign and usually insignificant herpetic stomatitis or dermatitis (Hartley 1966; Keeble

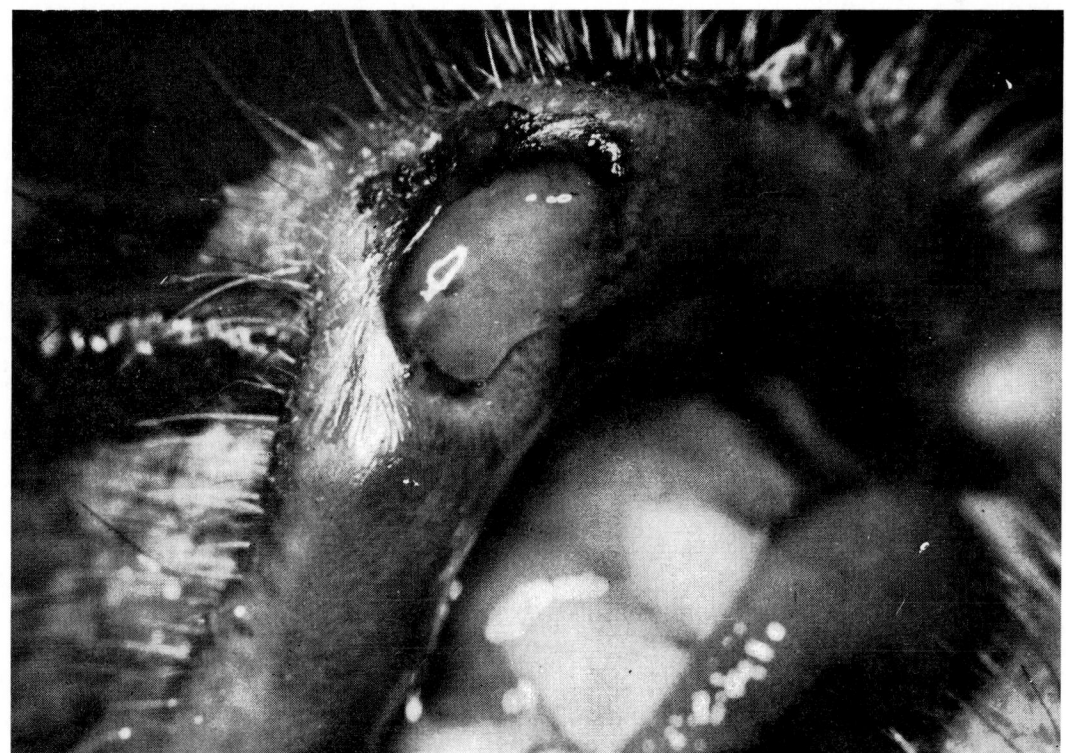

FIG. 9.1 Characteristic virus B ulceration on labial mucous membrane. (Courtesy of E. V. Hartley.)

1960). To diagnose the disease in these species, the animal is examined for herpeslike vesicles or ulcers near the mouth or on oral, lingual, or pharyngeal mucous membranes. Figure 9.1 shows the characteristic ulceration on the labial mucous membrane. Laboratory confirmation can be sought by histologic examination of the tissues, isolation of the virus, or demonstration of rising titers of neutralizing antibodies against a known virus B strain. Diagnosis in humans must depend on a history of exposure to monkeys or monkey tissues in cases exhibiting signs of a myelitis or encephalitis. Isolation and identification of the virus of simian herpes is accomplished by culturing material from localized lesions or tissue from the central nervous system or viscera. Monkey kidney cell cultures, rabbit kidney cell cultures, and the chorioallantoic membrane of the chick embryo have all been used successfully. Intracerebral inoculation of rabbits, monkeys, and suckling mice may also be used to isolate the virus.

When a viral agent has been isolated, it is best identified by antibody neutralization titrations against known antiserum and virus B strains inoculated intracerebrally into suckling mice. Such isolation and identification requires special equipment and highly trained personnel because of the seriousness of accidental infection; hence, the procedure will not ordinarily be available, and without it the diagnosis can only be tentative.

PROGNOSIS. In monkeys the disease is almost asymptomatic and is usually detected only by careful, deliberate observation. Rhesus monkeys are probably the true natural host; therefore, the disease is most frequently diagnosed in this species. Cynomolgous monkeys are thought to be more seriously affected and may suffer occasional fatalities (Burnet et al. 1939). Insufficient evidence prevents a valid estimate of the seriousness of the disease in other primates; when clinical symptoms appear in man, the infection is almost always fatal. Natural infection is not known to occur in species other than primates, suggesting a high degree of immunity to cross-infection. Under laboratory conditions virus B is almost always fatal for rabbits; and the prognosis varies in monkeys, mice, and guinea pigs according to the virulence of the virus, previously attained immunity, or natural resistance of the test animal.

IMMUNITY. Various studies indicate that naturally occurring antibodies can be demonstrated in up to 73% of rhesus and cynomolgous monkeys arriving in a compound (Burnet 1955; Krech and Lewis 1954; Orcutt et al. 1976; Pierce et al. 1958). When the animals are housed together under colony conditions, the percentage rises and may even approach 100%. Naturally occurring antibodies have not been reported in African or South American monkeys. The recurrence of clinical symptoms has not been reported in monkeys once infected.

The antigenic compositions of *H. simiae* and *H. hominis* are very similar, and a recognized relation exists between the serologic reactions of the two viruses. Antisera against *H. hominis* or *H. simiae* will neutralize the human virus, but virus B, except in very low titers, is not neutralized by antisera against *H. hominis* (Burnet et al. 1939). This observation led to the hypothesis that there is a group activity, with virus B being the older in evolution and closer to some common ancestral virus. From this it is postulated that virus B is a more complete antigen—a thesis not yet established in fact. A comprehensive review of the conflicting evidence in the literature and some work completed by Cabasso et al. (1967) indicate that a large percentage of individuals having serologic activity against herpes simplex virus will also show neutralizing action against virus B, but in very much lower titers. Of related interest is the finding that some human placental gamma globulin preparations show high titers against virus B. No useful biological product for active immunization has yet been developed. Efforts to produce a safe, effective killed vaccine for virus B have been unsuccessful (Hull 1971).

TREATMENT. Because the infection in the monkey causes no special discomfort or disability, no treatment is required. Other than supportive measures, there is no definitive treatment for the infection in humans. Large doses of gamma globulin, given after the appearance of the clinical signs, have not been effective. The first two patients who recovered were given corticosteroids, but the effectiveness of this treatment is difficult to assess. Survival of the third infected person followed intensive treatment with prednisone, gamma globulin, and cytosine arabinosine, but again the role of these agents is unclear. Major emphasis must be placed on prevention.

All minor wounds, such as cuts, scratches, and abrasions, should be protected before monkeys or monkey tissues are handled. Wounds acquired during work with animals or tissues, particularly bites, should receive immediate treatment. The virus is susceptible to oxidizing agents, soap and water, and certain antiseptics. It is advisable to flood the wound immediately with fresh 3% hydrogen peroxide USP, then to wash it with soap and water. To prevent nonviral infections, the treatment should include an application of iodine antiseptic. It has been customary in many locations to administer 15 or 20 ml of human gamma globulin prophylactically, but the efficacy of this practice has not been definitely established. Klenerman et al. (1975) have reviewed methods used in the hospital in treatment of wounds from animals potentially infected with neurotropic viruses.

CONTROL. Monkeys and monkey tissues must always be considered potentially contaminated with virus B. Although it is possible that African and South American monkeys are not as frequently infected, rhesus and cynomolgous monkeys are always suspect. Any susceptible species that has been in close contact with monkeys should also be considered as a possible source of infection. Wherever monkeys or monkey tissues are used, the potential infection should be recognized. Comprehensive programs should be instituted to prevent the dissemination of virus within colonies of monkeys and to protect the personnel engaged in handling the animals from the possibility of being infected. Muchmore (1973) has reviewed the clinical care of nonhuman primates.

The protection of personnel begins with a comprehensive training program for all who handle monkeys or monkey tissues. Mandatory refresher courses should be given periodically by well-trained personnel. Standard operating procedures and safety checklists should be supplied to personnel for study.

Protective clothing should be provided, and such clothing should be carefully selected and correlated with the task being performed. Suitable sterile containers for tissues and cell cultures should be provided, and strict procedures for the disposal of discarded materials, tissues, and dead animals should be established (Stone 1962). Installations housing monkeys are likely to be using them for different purposes, and no single universally applicable system exists. Therefore, these general principles must be adapted to each specific application.

REFERENCES

Bryan, B. L., Espana, C. D., Emmons, R. W., Vijayan, N., Hoeprich, P. D., Recovery from encephalomyelitis caused by *Herpesvirus simiae.* Report of a case. *Arch. Int. Med.* 135(6):868–870, 1975.

Burnet, F. M. *Principles of animal virology.* New York: Academic Press, 1955.

Burnet, F. M., Lush, D., and Jackson, A. V. Propagation of herpes B., and pseudorabies viruses on the chorio-allantois. *Aust. J. Exp. Biol. Med. Sci.* 17:35, 1939.

Cabasso, V. J., Chappell, W. A., Avampato, J. E., and Bittle, J. Correlation of B virus (BV) and herpes simplex virus (HSV): Antibodies in human sera. *J. Lab. Clin. Med.* 70:172–178, 1967.

Chappell, W. A. Animal infectivity of aerosols of monkey B virus. *Ann. N. Y. Acad. Sci.* 85:931–934, 1960.

Davidson, W. L., and Hummeler, K. B virus infection in man. *Ann. N. Y. Acad. Sci.* 85:970–979, 1960.

Di Giacomo, R. F., and Shah, K. V. Virtual absence of infection with *Herpesvirus simiae* in colony-reared rhesus monkeys (*Macaca mulatta*) with a literature review on antibody prevalence in natural and laboratory rhesus populations. *Lab. Anim. Sci.* 22(1):61–67, 1972.

Espana, C. Viral epizootics in captive nonhuman primates. *Lab. Anim. Sci.* 24(1):167–176, 1974.

Fierer, J., Bazely, P., and Braude, A. I. Herpes B presenting as ophthalmic zoster: A possible latent infection reactivated. *Ann. Intern. Med.* 79(2):225–228, 1973.

Gay, F., and Holden, M. The herpes encephalitis problem. *J. Infect. Dis.* 53:287–303, 1933.

Green, M., Major groups of animal viruses. In F. L., Horsfall, and I. Tamm, eds., *Viral and rickettsial infections of man.* Philadelphia: Lippincott, 1965.

Hartley, E. G., Naturally occuring B virus in cynomolgous monkeys. *Vet. Rec.* 76:555, 1964.

———. B virus disease in monkey and man. *Brt. Vet. J.* 122:46–50, 1966.

Hull, R. N. B virus vaccine. *Lab. Anim. Sci.* 21(6):1068–1071, 1971.

Keeble, S. A. B virus infection in monkeys. *Ann. N. Y. Acad. Sci.* 85:960–969, 1960.

Keeble, S. A., Christofinis, G. J., and Wood, W. Natural virus B infection in rhesus monkeys. *J. Pathol. Bacteriol.* 78:189–199, 1958.

Klenerman, L., Coid, C. R., and Aoki, F. Y. Treatment

of wounds from animals suspected of carrying neurotropic viruses. *Brt. Med. J.* 3:740–741, 1975.

Krech, U., and Lewis, L. J. Propagation of B virus in tissue cultures. *Proc. Soc. Exp. Biol. Med.* 87:174–178, 1954.

Love, F. M., and Jungherr, E. Occupational infection with virus B of monkeys. *J. Am. Med. Assoc.* 179:804–806, 1962.

Melnick, J. L., and Banker, D. D. Isolation of B virus (herpes group) from the central nervous system of a rhesus monkey. *J. Exp. Med.* 100:181–194, 1954.

Muchmore, E. Clinical care of nonhuman primates. Synopsis and evaluation of a workshop held at the National Institutes of Health, Bethesda, Maryland, March 1973. *J. Med. Primatol.* 2:341–352, 1973.

Norrild, B., Ludwig, H., and Rott, R. Identification of a common antigen of herpes simplex virus, bovine herpes mammilitis, and B virus. *J. Virol.* 25:712–717, 1978.

Orcutt, R. P., Pucak, G. J., Foster, H. L., Kilcourse, J. T., and Ferrell, T. Multiple testing for the detection of B virus antibody in specially handled rhesus monkeys after capture from virgin trapping grounds. *Lab. Anim. Sci.* 26:70–74, 1976.

Pierce, E. C., Pierce, J. D., and Hull, R. N. B-virus: Its current significance. Description and diagnosis of a fatal human infection. *Am. J. Hyg.* 68:242–250, 1958.

Roth, A. M., and Purcell, T. W. Ocular findings associated with encephalomyelitis caused by *Herpesvirus simiae.* *Am. J. Ophthalmol.* 84:345–348, 1977.

Ruch, T. C. *Diseases of laboratory primates,* pp. 410–417, Philadelphia: Saunders, 1959.

Sabin, A. B. Fatal B virus infection in a physician working with monkeys, *J. Clin. Invest.* 28:808, 1949.

Sabin, A. B., and Wright, A. M. Acute ascending myelitis following a monkey bite with isolation of a virus capable of reproducing the disease. *J. Exp. Med.* 59:115–136, 1934.

Scott, T. F. N., and Tokumaru, T. The herpesvirus group. In F. L. Horsfall and I. Tamm, eds., *Viral and rickettsial infections of man,* pp. 892–914. Philadelphia: Lippincott, 1965.

Stone, W. G. Management practices in a normal monkey colony, *Proc. Anim. Care Panel* 12:99–106, 1962.

Vizoso, A. D. Recovery of herpes simiae (B virus) from both primary and latent infections in rhesus monkeys. *Br. J. Exp. Pathol.* 56:485–488, 1975.

Wood, W., and Shimada, F. T. Isolation of strains of virus B from tissue cultures of cynomolgous and rhesus kidney. *Can. J. Public Health* 45:509–518, 1954.

10 Simian Herpesviruses, Excluding B Virus

NORVAL W. KING, JR.

Herpesvirus Hominis

Synonyms: **Herpesvirus simplex.**

HISTORY. Infection with *Herpesvirus hominis,* more commonly known as *H. simplex* (HVS), is one of the oldest viral infections known to humans. In fact, the word *herpes,* derived from the Greek verb *herpein* (to creep), has been used in medicine since the time of Hippocrates (fifth century B.C.) for various spreading, ulcerative lesions of the skin. The first published clinical description of HVS infection as we know it today in humans (herpes febrilis, or cold sores) dates back to the seventeenth century (Morton 1694). Since that time the clinical spectrum of human HVS infections has been greatly expanded to include genital infections (herpes genitalis), gingivostomatitis, encephalitis, keratitis, Kaposi's varicelliform eruption, and generalized neonatal disease. In addition to humans, a wide variety of laboratory animals including several species of nonhuman primates are also susceptible to experimental and natural infection by this virus.

DISTRIBUTION AND HOSTS. Humans are the only known natural reservoir host for HVS. Primary infection occurs principally in young children as an acute gingivostomatitis, which usually heals with no adverse effects. Serologic surveys indicate that up to 90% of the human population has been infected by the time of adolescence or early adulthood. Furthermore, a significant percentage of infected persons suffer recurrent episodes of secondary *H. hominis* infection in the form of cold sores, fever blisters, or genital lesions despite the presence of neutralizing antibodies in their serum. Recurrent lesions are presumed to result from activation of a latent infection that persists for life, possibly in certain sensory ganglia of infected individuals. The virus can also be isolated sporadically from oral secretions of a significant portion of the human population in the absence of visible lesions. These latter two categories of people serve as the source of infection for children as well as various susceptible animal spe-

cies. Rabbits, guinea pigs, mice, rats, hamsters, and Cebus monkeys have been experimentally infected with HVS. There are several species of nonhuman primates that are reportedly susceptible to spontaneous as well as experimental infection with this virus. These include gibbons (*Hylobates lar*) (Emmons and Lennette 1970; Smith et al. 1969); owl monkeys (*Aotus trivirgatus*) (McClure and Keeling 1971; Melendez et al. 1969); marmosets (*Saguinus* spp.) (Hull 1973), and tree shrews (*Tupaia glis*) (McClure et al. 1972).

ETIOLOGY. Two recognized variants of HVS have been isolated from human patients. These are designated types 1 (HVS-1) and 2 (HVS-2) and differ in a number of biological properties including the general pattern of disease that they produce. These differences have been extensively reviewed by Nahmias and Roizman (1973). In general, HVS-1 causes lesions in nongenital sites and HVS-2 causes genital lesions and generalized infection of neonates as the result of delivery through an infected birth canal. Spontaneous infection in nonhuman primates is principally with HVS-1 although certain species (*Cebus* spp.) have been experimentally infected with HVS-2 (Nahmias et al. 1971).

HVS is antigenically related to at least two other herpesviruses that affect nonhuman primates, *Herpesvirus simiae* and SA-8. Using the serum neutralization test, there is a one-way cross between HVS and *H. simiae*. Antiserum to *H. simiae* neutralizes HVS to relatively high titers, whereas antiserum to HVS has very little neutralizing effect on *H. simiae*. In contrast, a two-way cross exists between HVS and SA-8, and the degree of cross-neutralization between these two agents can be markedly enhanced by the addition of complement to the system (Hampar et al. 1969). One has to be aware of these antigenic relationships when attempting to identify the causative agent of a herpesvirus infection of nonhuman primates using serologic methods alone.

TRANSMISSION. Direct or indirect contact of susceptible individuals with clinically or latently infected humans who are excreting the virus is the most frequent route of transmission of HVS-1; venereal transmission is the most common mode for HVS-2. Newborn infants may acquire localized or generalized infection with HVS-2 during delivery through an infected birth canal.

SIGNS AND PATHOLOGY. HVS may cause several different patterns of clinical disease, depending on the strain of the virus involved and the age, species, and status of the immune system of the affected host. Human infections with HVS have been extensively reviewed by Nahmias and Roizman (1973).

Several species of nonhuman primates are susceptible to natural and experimental infection with HVS. The character of the disease produced is also variable depending on the species. In owl monkeys (*Aotus trivirgatus*) HVS produces an epizootic disease with high morbidity and mortality. Following an incubation period of approximately 7 days, affected animals develop oral, labial, and cutaneous ulcers, conjunctivitis, anorexia, pruritis, weakness, and incoordination. Death invariably occurs within 2–3 days after the onset of clinical signs. Lesions are widely disseminated and both grossly and microscopically identical to those produced in this species by *H. tamarinus*. Encephalitis occurs somewhat more frequently with HVS infection than with *H. tamarinus*, but this is variable (Tate et al. 1971). The encephalitis in owl monkeys is similar to that produced by HVS in humans, the lesions being most extensive in the temporal lobes of the cerebral cortex but also extending into the frontal, parietal, and occipital lobes. Lesions may be found in the thalamus and basal ganglia as well. The brain lesions are characterized by widespread necrosis of neurons with the presence of intranuclear inclusion bodies in many of the affected nerve cells. Gliosis and perivascular cuffing are variable. In addition to the brain lesions, there are widely disseminated foci of necrosis in most organs and tissues of the body. These are especially common in the skin, oral mucosa, liver, spleen, lymph nodes, and adrenal glands. Intranuclear inclusion bodies occur commonly in these lesions.

Spontaneous HVS infection in tree shrews (*Tupaia glis*) is remarkably similar to that in owl monkeys. In gibbons (*Hylobates lar*) spontaneous HVS infection may occur as a fatal encephalitis or as a localized vesicular dermatitis from which the animal recovers.

Marmosets (*Saguinus* spp.) and Cebus monkeys (*Cebus* spp.) are susceptible to experimental infection with HVS. The resultant disease in marmosets is clinically and pathologically identical to spontaneous *H. tamarinus* infection in marmosets and owl monkeys and spontaneous HVS infection in owl monkeys.

Cebus monkeys are susceptible to experimental infection with HVS, and the lesions produced are similar to those that occur naturally in humans. When inoculated into the conjunctiva, skin, or female genital tract, the virus produces localized vesicular or necrotic lesions that heal in 7–10 days. This genus has been used as an animal model for human genital infection with HVS-2 (Nahmias et al. 1971).

DIAGNOSIS. Because of the marked similarity of HVS infection in nonhuman primates to *H. tamarinus* infection in the same species, it is not possible to make a definitive diagnosis of HVS infection based on histopathology alone. Similarly, the close antigenic relationship of HVS to *H. simiae* and SA-8 makes diagnosis of HVS infection by serologic methods alone somewhat difficult. Isolation and identification of the virus from affected tissues is the most definitive means of establishing the diagnosis of HVS infection in nonhuman primate species.

PROGNOSIS. Spontaneous HVS infection in most species of nonhuman primates is a highly fatal disease. The exception is the gibbon (*Hylobates lar*) in which the infection may occur only as a localized vesicular disease from which the animal recovers. Experimental HVS-2 infection in Cebus monkeys is also characterized by self-limiting localized vesicular or ulcerative lesions which resolve; however, the virus may persist as a latent infection in the regional sensory ganglia (Reeves et al. 1976).

IMMUNITY. Although it is known that immunosuppression and immunodeficiency in human patients predisposes them to infection by several herpesviruses including HVS, *H. varicella-zoster*, and cytomegalovirus, the precise role of the immune system in the control of such infections in immunocompetent patients is poorly understood. A large percentage of the human population is latently infected with HVS as a consequence of primary infection during childhood and remains so for life, despite the presence of circulating neutralizing antibodies to the virus. Some of these patients unfortunately suffer recurrent lesions at regular or erratic intervals for many years. The role of the immune system in the control or expression of localized HVS infection including its putative oncogenicity has been the subject of considerable investigation and recent hypotheses (Lehner et al. 1975). It does appear clear, however, that although the immune system is ineffective in excluding HVS from the infected host, it is probably exceedingly important in preventing the development of fulminating systemic infections that occur when the system is severely compromised. It has been possible to effectively immunize marmosets and owl monkeys against HVS using an experimental attenuated live vaccine derived by plaqueing techniques (Daniel et al. 1978). The three commercially available HVS vaccines approved for human use are reportedly of equivocal value in preventing recurrent lesions in human patients (Nahmias and Roizman 1973).

TREATMENT AND CONTROL. There is no effective treatment for widely disseminated, systemic HVS infection in nonhuman primates. In those species in which spontaneous or experimental infection is characterized by localized lesions, specific therapy is generally not required, for the lesions heal naturally in 7–10 days.

The principal method of control of HVS infection in nonhuman primates is to minimize their contact with humans who are the reservoir hosts for this virus. This is not always practical and, therefore, the experimental vaccine developed by Daniel et al. (1978) has been used by several laboratories that maintain large colonies of marmosets and owl monkeys.

Herpesvirus Tamarinus

Synonyms: **Herpesvirus T, Herpesvirus platyrrhinae, and marmoset herpesvirus.**

HISTORY. *Herpesvirus tamarinus* was originally isolated independently by Holmes et al. (1964) and Melnick et al. (1964) in 1963 from tissues of white-tipped tamarins (*Saguinus nigricollis*) and cotton-topped marmosets (*S. oedipus*), respectively, dying of a generalized herpetic disease. It is also quite possible that this same virus was the unidentified herpesvirus responsible for an "inclusion body hepatitis" of red-mantled marmosets described by Sauer and Bishop the same year. In 1966 Hunt and Melendez described in detail the epidemiologic, clinicopathologic, and virologic features of a

spontaneous outbreak of *H. tamarinus* infection in a colony of owl monkeys (*Aotus trivirgatus*) and suggested that squirrel monkeys (*Saimiri sciureus*), with which the affected owl monkeys had been housed, may have been the source of the virus. The subsequent isolation of *H. tamarinus* from throat and anal swabs of two clinically healthy squirrel monkeys, one of which was from the above-described group and the other from a closed colony at another institution, clearly demonstrated that the squirrel monkey may become latently infected with *H. tamarinus* and serve as its reservoir host (Melendez et al. 1966). The serologic data of Holmes et al. were in agreement with this finding and further suggested that the cinnamon ringtail (*Cebus albifrons*) and spider (*Ateles* spp.) monkeys might also serve as reservoir hosts for this virus.

To date, however, *H. tamarinus* has not been isolated from natural infections of these latter two species. In 1967 King et al. provided the first description of the clinicopathologic features of spontaneously occurring *H. tamarinus* infection in squirrel monkeys, and Daniel et al. (1967) reported the isolation of the virus from the lesions of the same animals. The disease in this species is characterized by ulcerative cheilitis, glossitis, and stomatitis from which the animals recover but remain latently infected. These studies further substantiated the assertion that the squirrel monkey is the principal reservoir host for *H. tamarinus*.

DISTRIBUTION AND HOSTS. As already indicated, a high percentage of squirrel, cinnamon ringtail, and spider monkeys naturally have significant neutralizing antibodies to *H. tamarinus*, indicating prior infection and recovery. Although all three species could presumably serve as reservoir hosts for this virus and, as such, periodically excrete it, this has only been demonstrated in the squirrel monkey. Accordingly, this species is generally regarded as the principal source of the virus. In marmosets (*Saguinas* spp.) and owl monkeys, *H. tamarinus* produces an epizootic disease of high morbidity and mortality.

ETIOLOGY. *Herpesvirus tamarinus* has all of the physicochemical properties of the Herpetoviridae family of viruses (Fenner 1976). It will replicate in a wide range of cell cultures; these have been enumerated by Daniel et al. (1972). Infected cells become rounded, swollen, and refractile, and eventually detach from the monolayer. Polykaryocytes are also a prominent feature of its cytopathogenic effect. Typical herpes type intranuclear inclusion bodies are present in infected cells. When grown in cell cultures beneath an agar overlay, the wild type strain of *H. tamarinus* forms a heterogeneous population of well-defined plaques of various sizes. With cloning procedures, the wild type strain can be separated into two variants, one that uniformly produces large plaques and another that consistently produces small plaques (Daniel and Melendez 1968c). These variants have been shown to differ in their production of in vitro markers (Daniel and Melendez 1968a), their immunological properties (Daniel and Melendez 1968b), and in their infectivity for certain laboratory animals (Daniel and Melendez 1970). More importantly the small-plaque variant of *H. tamarinus* was subsequently shown to be immunogenic but nonpathogenic for marmosets and owl monkeys. This property has led to its use as an effective vaccine against infection by the wild type strain of *H. tamarinus* in these species (Daniel et al. 1976, 1978). The large-plaque variant retained its pathogenicity for these species.

TRANSMISSION. In most outbreaks of fatal *H. tamarinus* infection in marmosets and owl monkeys, the original source of the infection can usually be traced back to direct or indirect contact of the affected species with latently infected squirrel monkeys. The latter species periodically excrete the virus in their oral secretions and feces while manifesting no evidence of clinical disease. In addition to direct contact, aerosols and contaminated fomites may also be important in the transmission of the disease.

SIGNS AND PATHOLOGY. Primary infection in the reservoir host, the squirrel monkey, is characterized by a necrotizing cheilitis, glossitis, and stomatitis that generally heals in 7–10 days. Owl monkeys and marmosets also develop necrotic lesions of their labial and oral mucosae but almost invariably die within a few days of the occurrence of such lesions. These tissues contain focal areas of necrosis of the mucosa with the presence of typical herpesvirus intranuclear inclusion bodies in swollen epithelial cells. Multinucleate epithelial giant cells with or without inclusion bodies may also be present in the lesions. Fatally affected owl monkeys and marmosets have widely disseminated focal or diffuse areas of necrosis of virtually all visceral organs and tissues. Intranuclear inclusion bodies are commonly found in the parenchymal cells of affected tissues and organs. Multinucleate giant cells may or may not be present in such lesions.

DIAGNOSIS. Definitive diagnosis can only be made by virus isolation and identification. The clinicopathologic features of natural *H. hominis* infection in marmosets and owl monkeys are virtually identical to those of *H. tamarinus* infection; hence, these two infections cannot be differentiated on the basis of histopathologic examination alone. In squirrel monkeys a rise in antibody titers to *H. tamarinus* in convalescent serum samples is indicative of infection with this virus.

PROGNOSIS. The prognosis for *H. tamarinus* infection in squirrel monkeys is good, for these animals usually survive the infection and become asymptomatic carriers of the virus. The prognosis for owl monkeys and marmosets infected with *H. tamarinus* is poor, for the mortality rate is exceptionally high in these species. There is serologic and virologic evidence that a small percentage of marmosets may survive the primary infection and become carriers of the virus (Holmes et al. 1966; Murphy et al. 1971).

IMMUNITY. Reference has already been made to the immunogenic properties of the small plaque variant of *H. tamarinus*. This strain effectively immunizes owl monkeys and marmosets against the pathogenic wild type and large-plaque strains and has been employed as a vaccine by several institutions using these species (Daniel et al. 1976, 1978).

TREATMENT AND CONTROL. There is no effective treatment for generalized *H. tamarinus* infection in owl monkeys and marmosets. General supportive therapy is all that is required to promote recovery of squirrel monkeys with oral lesions.

The most effective means of controlling the infection in owl monkeys and marmosets is to prevent them from coming in contact with the reservoir hosts for the virus, particularly the squirrel monkey. Vaccination may also be used on an experimental basis as an effective means of control.

Spider Monkey Herpesvirus

Synonyms: **None.**

HISTORY. Spider monkey herpesvirus (SMV) was originally isolated in 1964 from the brain of a 5.5-month-old female black-handed spider monkey (*Ateles geoffroyi*) that had been born and reared at the Roeding Park Zoo, Fresno, California (Hull et al. 1972). The animal died following a brief illness characterized by listlessness and the presence of ulcerative lesions on the lips, nares, tongue, palate, and gums. No other isolates of SMV have been reported to date.

DISTRIBUTION AND HOSTS. Serologic studies revealed a high incidence and high titer of antibody to SMV in adult spider monkeys (*A. geoffroyi* and *A. fusiceps*), and in occasional capuchin monkeys (*Cebus apella, C. albifrons,* and *C. capucinus*). Sera from juvenile spider monkeys had a much lower incidence. Squirrel monkeys (*Saimiri sciureus*), marmosets (*Saguinus* spp.), and wooly monkeys (*Lagothrix lagotrichi*) were rarely antibody positive. From this data it was concluded that the spider monkey is the most likely natural host for SMV, but on rare occasions it can be fatal for this host.

Experimentally, SMV occasionally produces a focal hepatitis and an encephalitis in rabbits and a disseminated herpetic disease in marmosets resembling infection with *Herpesvirus tamarinus*. SMV produces localized skin lesions in guinea pigs and is fatal when inoculated intracerebrally into suckling and weanling mice. Rhesus and African green monkeys are not affected by experimental infection with SMV.

ETIOLOGY. SMV is antigenically related to *H. tamarinus* such that SMV antiserum neutralizes *H. tamarinus* at titers fourfold to eightfold lower than those of the homologous virus, but only high-titered *H. tamarinus* antiserum contains SMV-neutralizing antibodies. Thus SMV appears to be more broadly antigenic than *H. tamarinus*. The growth properties of SMV in certain cell cultures is also similar to *H. tamarinus*. This virus is different from *H. ateles*, a latent herpesvirus of spider monkeys that produces malignant lymphoma when experimentally inoculated into marmosets and rabbits.

TRANSMISSION. Natural transmission of SMV would appear to be via the horizontal route, based on the low incidence of antibody to SMV in juvenile spider monkeys and the high incidence in adult members of these species. Oropharyngeal secretions may be the most likely source of the virus from latently infected individuals.

SIGNS AND PATHOLOGY. Grossly, the one fatally affected *A. geoffroyi* from which SMV was isolated had ulcerations of the lips, nares, and oral mucosae, inflamed lungs, congestion of the meninges, and ulcers on the skin of the back and axilla. The tissues from this animal apparently were not examined histopathologically.

Experimentally infected marmosets die of a disseminated herpetic disease indistinguishable grossly or microscopically from spontaneous *H. tamarinus* or *H. hominus* infection of this species. They have numerous focal areas of necrosis in the liver, spleen, kidneys, and adrenals with eosinophilic, intranuclear inclusion bodies in affected parenchymal cells.

DIAGNOSIS AND PROGNOSIS. Diagnosis of SMV infection in a fatally infected animal can only be made with certainty by virus isolation. One can detect latently or previously infected animals by serologic methods.

The high incidence of antibodies to SMV in adult spider monkeys appears to indicate that most infected animals recover from their primary infection with this virus.

TREATMENT AND CONTROL. There is no effective treatment for SMV infection. The simplest control measure to prevent the occurrence of this infection is to avoid exposure of uninfected juvenile animals with known infected animals.

Simian Varicellalike Herpesviruses

Synonyms: **None.**

HISTORY. Seven simian herpesviruses have been isolated from spontaneous diseases of nonhuman primates that resemble varicella-zoster of man. Liverpool vervet monkey virus (LVV) was originally isolated from vervet monkeys (*Cercopithecus aethiops*) dying of a fatal exanthematous disease while housed at the Liverpool School of Tropical Medicine in 1966 (Clarkson et al. 1967). Similarly, patas monkey herpesvirus (PHV) was first isolated in 1967 from the lesions of patas monkeys (*Erythrocebus patas*) also dying of a generalized exanthematous disease at another laboratory in England (McCarthy et al. 1968). In 1968 and again in 1973 in the United States a virus antigenically related to LVV and PHV but referred to as Delta herpesvirus (DHV) was isolated from patas monkeys dying of a fatal exanthematous disease at the Delta Regional Primate Research Center in Covington, Louisiana (Migaki et al. 1971; Riopelle et al. 1971; Wolf et al. 1974). Medical Lake macaque virus (MLMV) was originally isolated from pig-tailed macaques (*Macaca nemestrina*), Japanese macaques (*M. fuscata*), and cynomolgous or crab-eating macaques (*M. fascicularis*) involved in three outbreaks of a relatively mild varicellalike disease while housed at the Medical Lake Field Station of the Washington Regional Primate Research Center (Blakely et al. 1973; Lourie et al. 1971). *Herpesvirus cyclopis* (HVC) was isolated in 1975 from six Formosan macaques (*M cyclopis*) that developed a generalized vesicular disease at the New England Regional Primate Research Center (Jackman et al. 1977). In 1971 chimpanzee herpesvirus (HC) was isolated from a mild exanthematous disease of chimpanzee (*Pan troglodytes*) (McClure and Keeling 1971). Finally gorilla herpesvirus (HG), which produces a spontaneous, mild, exanthematous disease of gorillas (*Gorilla gorilla*), was isolated in 1972 from an animal housed at the Moscow zoo (Marennikova et al. 1974).

DISTRIBUTION AND HOSTS. The origin of the infection in each of the outbreaks of varicellalike disease described has not been determined. Because of the close antigenic relationship of certain of these agents to human *Herpesvirus varicella-zoster* (HVZ), the question has been raised whether human carriers of HVZ may constitute the source. This question has not been resolved experimentally. The susceptible simian hosts for these agents are enumerated above.

ETIOLOGY. All seven of these herpesviruses have certain features in common. They are all highly cell associated and in this regard resemble HVZ of man. Each has been isolated from one or more nonhuman primate species with a cutaneous vesicular disease resembling human varicella-zoster. There are, however,

differences in the severity of the diseases produced: some are highly fatal; others are relatively mild and are followed by recovery. Several of the agents are very closely related antigenically and may be the same or variants of the same virus, a fact difficult to discern from the available literature. LVV, PHV, and DHV are all closely related antigenically to one another and to HVZ based on serologic tests (Allen et al. 1974; Ayres 1971; Felsenfeld and Schmidt 1975). MLMV also cross-reacts serologically with HVZ, but its relationship to LVV, PHV, and DHV has not been reported (Wenner et al. 1977). Inasmuch as the incidence of titers to these viruses is higher in captive monkeys than in those that are newly captured, it is possible that these four agents may in fact be human HVZ that has been slightly modified by passage through susceptible simian hosts. However, this has not been proved. HVC differs from MLMV serologically but has not been compared with LVV, PHV, DHV, or HVZ viruses.

TRANSMISSION. The mode of transmission of these simian varicellalike viruses is presumed to be by direct contact and aerosols, as has been proposed for HVZ in man. Wenner et al. (1975) demonstrated the presence of MLMV in the urine of experimentally infected *Macaca fascicularis*.

SIGNS AND PATHOLOGY. Infection with any of these seven viruses usually has an abrupt onset. The morbidity is generally high, but mortality varies considerably depending upon the particular virus involved. The incubation period is essentially the same for all these agents and is 10–14 days in length. The first signs of disease consist of the development of a maculopapular rash, which progresses to vesicle formation and eventual crusting. The lesions are generally 1–3 mm in diameter but may become confluent. They can be found anywhere on the body surface but generally spare the palms of the hands and soles of the feet. The abdominal and inguinal areas are commonly affected. Focal ulcerative lesions may also occur on the oral and lingual mucosae. In fatal infections death usually occurs 48–72 hours after the onset of the rash. At necropsy a wide variety of visceral organs contain focal areas of necrosis and hemorrhage. These include the liver, spleen, lymph nodes, gastrointestinal tract, and adrenals. The lungs and heart may contain lesions. The brain is generally not affected.

Microscopically the cutaneous lesions begin as focal areas of ballooning degeneration of cells of the stratum malpighii with intercellular edema. This progresses to the formation of fluid-filled vesicles surrounded by necrotic epidermal cells that contain typical herpetic eosinophilic inclusion bodies in their nuclei. Multinucleate giant cells containing intranuclear inclusion bodies are commonly found in and adjacent to the vesicles. Affected visceral organs contain focal and confluent areas of necrosis and hemorrhage. Eosinophilic intranuclear inclusion bodies are present in parenchymal cells adjacent to the areas of necrosis. These visceral lesions are essentially identical to those produced by other widely disseminated, systemic herpesvirus infections discussed in this chapter.

DIAGNOSIS. Definitive diagnosis can only be made by virus isolation and identification, and because of the close antigenic relationship of several of these viruses (LVV, PHV, DHV, HVZ) to one another, even this can be difficult. The most important differential diagnosis that has to be made is to distinguish these viral infections from the one caused by *Herpesvirus simiae*. This should be possible by serologic methods and by the fact that *H. simiae* is not a cell-associated herpesvirus.

PROGNOSIS. The prognosis varies with each of the seven viral infections. In general, infections with LVV, PHV, and DHV are characterized by a high morbidity and moderate to high mortality. Infection with MLMV has a relatively low morbidity and mortality rate. The number of animals affected in the reported outbreak of HC infection is too few to draw conclusions regarding its morbidity (6/11) and mortality (2/6) rate. Gorillas and chimpanzees acquiring infections with HG and HC apparently suffer only a mild exanthematous disease from which they recover with no adverse consequences.

IMMUNITY. Animals that have recovered from one of these infections are generally immune to reinfection by the same virus. The extent to which they are immune to other closely related viruses has not been thoroughly studied.

TREATMENT AND CONTROL. There is no effective treatment for the widely disseminated, fatal forms of these infections. Those animals that are less severely affected will usually recover on their own with only minimal supportive therapy.

Inasmuch as the source of these viruses has not been determined in the reported outbreaks, it is difficult to adopt control measures that

might be effective in preventing their occurrence. The fact that several of these agents are similar to HVZ would make it imperative that individuals with active varicella-zoster infection and others exposed to such persons not be allowed contact with nonhuman primate species. It simply would not be practical or even possible to identify personnel with latent HVZ for purposes of excluding them from contact with susceptible nonhuman primate species.

Simian Cytomegaloviruses

Synonyms: **Salivary gland virus.**

HISTORY. The first reported examples of cytomegalovirus (CMV) infections in nonhuman primates consisted of microscopic descriptions of the rather characteristic inclusion bodies produced by this group of herpesviruses in the salivary glands of 2 *Cebus fatuellus* (*apella*) and in the kidneys of 31 *Macaca mulatta* (Cowdry and Scott 1935a). The lesions were regarded as incidental findings and were not associated with clinical disease. Twenty years later the histopathologic features of a CMV disease of chimpanzees (*Pan troglodytes*) were reported in 8 of 12 animals (Vogel and Pinkerton 1955). Characteristic inclusion bodies were found in the acinar cells of the salivary glands in all 8 and also in the adrenal glands of 3 and the myocardium of 1 of the affected animals.

The first reported isolation of a CMV from a nonhuman primate appears to be an agent referred to as SA-6 (simian agent-6) isolated from spontaneously degenerating kidney cell cultures derived from African green or vervet monkeys (*Cercopithecus aethiops*) (Malherbe and Harwin 1957). This same agent was also subsequently isolated from the salivary glands of the same species in which there was histologic evidence of CMV infection (Malherbe and Harwin 1963). In the same year Black et al. reported the isolation of a CMV from salivary gland tissue and four separate lots of kidney cell cultures derived from African green monkeys. These authors stated that their isolate did not resemble any of the seven African green monkey agents described in the original report of Malherbe and Harwin (1957) and that, based upon complement-fixing antibody studies, infection with their isolate was common in African green monkeys held in captivity. This was further substantiated in a subsequent report documenting the occurrence of cytomegaloviruses as common adventitious contaminants of primary African green monkey kidney cell cultures obtained from several commercial sources (Smith et al. 1969). Salivary gland inclusion disease was reported as an incidental finding in 6 Philippine tarsius (*Tarsius syrichta*) which died or were sacrificed at intervals varying from 3 days to 18 months after being received at the Oregon Regional Primate Research Center (Smith and McNulty 1969). The lesions were confined to the salivary glands and were not the cause of death in these animals.

Almost 35 years after the original description of CMV inclusion bodies in the kidneys of rhesus monkeys, a virus of this description was isolated from the urine of clinically healthy rhesus monkeys (Asher et al. 1969). The virus was subsequently characterized in detail, and it was found that the rhesus CMV and African green monkey are similar in biological behavior and antigenically related to each other and to human CMV (Asher et al. 1974). The viruses are not, however, identical. There is also a single pathologic report of a generalized CMV infection in a gorilla (*Gorilla gorilla*), but virus isolation was not attempted (Tsuchiya et al. 1969). In 1972 a CMV was isolated from oral and anal swabs from 1 of 6 adult owl monkeys (*Aotus trivirgatus*) from which samples were taken (Ablashi et al. 1972). A survey of sera of 21 owl monkeys revealed that 15 (71%) had antibodies to the owl monkey CMV isolate. This virus was characterized further by Chopra et al. (1972).

DISTRIBUTION AND HOSTS. Cytomegaloviruses are relatively host specific and are known to occur naturally only in those species from which they have been isolated. The few serologic surveys that have been done with selected simian CMVs indicate that they occur commonly in their respective hosts as latent infections. Dissemination and clinical disease associated with these agents is exceedingly rare in nonhuman primates.

ETIOLOGY. The CMV group of herpesviruses is relatively host specific. In contrast to the lymphotropic herpesviruses, they replicate in vitro in monolayers of cells derived from their natural host and only rarely in cells of other species. They are strongly cell associated, replicate slowly, are cytolytic both in vitro and in vivo, and produce marked hypertrophy of the nuclear and cytoplasmic portions of the affected cells with the presence of intranuclear and cytoplasmic inclusion bodies. This latter cytopathic effect is generally regarded as sufficiently

characteristic to permit the diagnosis of CMV infection on the basis of histopathologic findings alone.

Both rhesus and African green monkey CMVs grow well in human and in heterologous monkey fibroblasts as well as in fibroblasts of the natural host, but human CMV grows only in human cells. Owl monkey CMV grows well in monolayers of owl monkey kidney cells.

African green monkey sera with complement-fixing antibody to African green monkey CMV also fixes complement with at least one strain (Ad 169) of human CMV, but human sera with antibody to human CMV fails to react with African green monkey CMV (Asher et al. 1974). African green monkey CMV and rhesus CMV differ antigenically, but both viruses and human CMV appear to share some antigenic determinants. Serum-neutralization tests indicate that owl monkey CMV is not neutralized by antiserum to rhesus CMV.

As mentioned, all CMVs are strongly cell associated. After replicating in the nucleus of infected cells, the infectious particles accumulate in large lysosomelike structures in the cytoplasm, thus accounting for the presence of the small cytoplasmic as well as the large intranuclear inclusion bodies characteristically seen in cells infected with CMVs.

TRANSMISSION. Rhesus monkeys infected with CMV persistently shed infectious virus in their urine for as long as 4 years with no evidence of clinical disease. Virus excretion in the saliva from active lesions in the salivary glands is also a potential source of the virus. Transmission therefore probably results from exposure to these infected excretions. It has been reported that offspring of chronically infected rhesus monkeys become infected early in life, possibly even in utero although this has not been proved (Asher et al. 1974).

SIGNS AND PATHOLOGY. Most simian species infected with CMV exhibit no clinical evidence of disease. In many cases infection has merely been recognized incidentally during the routine histopathologic examination of tissues from animals dying or sacrificed for other reasons. Microscopically the salivary glands, kidneys, and adrenals have been the most common sites affected. The lesions are characterized by marked hypertrophy (cytomegaly) of affected parenchymal cells with the presence of prominent large, usually amphophilic, inclusion bodies in their enlarged nuclei and aggregates of small basophilic inclusions in the expanded cytoplasm. In most instances necrosis is not a prominent feature of the lesion, and consequently, massive inflammatory cellular infiltrates are not commonly found either. The affected organ may contain a modest infiltration of mononuclear inflammatory cells. Only in one of the disseminated cases in a chimpanzee has extensive necrosis and neutrophilic inflammatory cell infiltration been a feature of simian CMV infection. This is quite unlike the devastating CMV of human neonates or immunosuppressed patients where tissue necrosis may be extensive.

DIAGNOSIS AND PROGNOSIS. Diagnosis of CMV infection is established by virus isolation, serologic methods, or by microscopic examination of affected tissues.

CMV infection in simians is almost invariably a subclinical infection, hence the prognosis is good. Animals probably remain infected for life, during which they persistently excrete the virus in their saliva and urine.

TREATMENT AND CONTROL. There is no effective treatment for subclinical CMV infection in nonhuman primates.

Control measures for CMV infections should be directed toward eliminating the possibility of direct or indirect contact of susceptible individuals with known carriers of the virus.

Other Simian Herpesviruses

Other herpesviruses that have been isolated incidentally from cell cultures derived from various nonhuman primate species but for which there is little or no evidence of natural disease are shown in Table 10.1. Several of these agents, however, are pathogenic when experimentally introduced into new nonhuman primate species and are being studied as models for certain human diseases.

Table 10.1.   Other Simian Herpesviruses.

Virus	Species	Reference
AT-46	Spider monkeys (*Ateles geoffroyi*)	Melendez et al. 1972
SA-8	African vervet monkeys (*Cercopithecus aethiops*)	Malherbe and Harwin 1958, 1963
SA-15	African vervet monkeys (*C. aethiops*)	Malherbe and Harwin 1958, 1963
SA-8	baboons (*Papio ursinus*)	Malherbe and Strickland-Cholmley 91969
SA-15	baboons (*P. ursinus*)	Malherbe and Strickland-Cholmley 91969
Herpesvirus aotus type 1	owl monkeys (*Aotus trivirgatus*)	Daniel et al. 1971
H. aotus type 2	owl monkeys (*A. trivirgatus*)	Melendez and Daniel 1971
H. aotus type 3	owl monkeys (*A. trivirgatus*)	Daniel et al. 1973
Cebus herpesvirus	capuchin monkeys (*Cebus albifrons*)	Lewis et al. 1974
Cebus herpesvirus	capuchin monkeys (*C. apella*)	Lewis et al. 1974
Tree shrew herpesvirus	tree shrews (*Tupaia glis*)	Daniel et al. 1972; McCombs et al. 1971
H. saimiri	squirrel monkeys (*Saimiri sciureus*)	Melendez et al. 1968
H. ateles	spider monkeys (*Ateles geoffroyi*)	Melendez et al. 1971, 1972
Rhesus leukocyte-associated herpesvirus	rhesus monkeys (*Macaca mulatta*)	Frank et al. 1973
H. papio	baboons (*Papio hamadryas*) baboons (*P. anubis*) baboons (*P. papio*) baboons (*P. cynocephalus*)	Deinhardt et al. 1976; Falk et al. 1976; Gerber et al. 1977; Lapin et al. 1975; Rabin et al. 1977
H. pongo	orangutan (*Pongo pygmaeus*)	Rasheen et al. 1977

REFERENCES

Herpesvirus Hominus

Daniel, M. D., Barahona, H., Melendez, L. V., Hunt, R. D., Sehgal, P., Marshall, B., Ingalls, J., and Forbes, M. Prevention of fatal herpes infections in owl and marmoset monkeys by vaccination. In D. J. Chivers and E. H. R. Ford, eds. *Recent Advances in Primatology*, vol. 4, pp. 67–69. London: Academic Press, 1978.

Emmons, R. W., and Lennette, E. H. Natural *Herpesvirus hominis* infection of a gibbon (*Hylobates lar*). *Arch. Gesamte Virusforsch.* 31:215–218, 1970.

Hampar, B., Stevens, D. A., Martos, L. M., Ablashi D. V., Burroughs, M. A. K., and Wells, G. A. Correlation between the neutralizing activity of human serum against herpes simplex virus and a simian herpesvirus (SA-8). *J. Immunol.* 102:397–403, 1969.

Lehner, T., Wilton, J. M. A., and Shillitoe, E. J. Immunological basis for latency, recurrences and putative oncogenicity of herpes simplex virus. *Lancet* 2(July):60–62, 1975.

McClure, H. M., and Keeling, M. E. Viral diseases noted in the Yerkes Primate Center colony. *Lab. Anim. Sci.* 21:1002–1010, 1971.

McClure, H. M., Keeling, M. E., Olberding, B., Hunt, R. D., and Melendez, L. V. Natural *Herpesvirus hominus* infection of tree shrews (*Tupaia glis*). *Lab. Anim. Sci.* 22:517–521, 1972.

Melendez, L. V., Espana, C., Hunt, R. D., Daniel, M. D., and Garcia, F. G. Natural herpes simplex infection in the owl monkey (*Aotus trivirgatus*). *Lab. Anim. Sci.* 19:38–45, 1969.

Morton, R. *Pyretologia, pars Altera*, pp. 15–16. London, 1694.

Nahmias, A. J., London, W. T., Catalano, L. W., Jr., Fucillo, D. A., Sever, J. L., and Graham, C. Genital *Herpesvirus hominis* type 2 infection: An experimental model in Cebus monkeys. *Science* 171:297–298, 1971.

Nahmias, A. J., and Roizman, B. Infection with herpes-simplex viruses 1 and 2: A three-part series. *N. Engl. J. Med.* 289:667-674, 719–725, 781–789, 1973.

Reeves, W. C., Di Giacomo, R. F., Alexander, E. R., and Lee, C. K. Latent *Herpesvirus hominis* from trigeminal and sacral dorsal root ganglia of Cebus monkeys. *Proc. Soc. Exp. Biol. Med.* 153:258–261, 1976.

Smith, P. C., Yuill, T. M., Buchanan, R. D., Stanton, J. S., and Chaicumpa, V. The gibbon (*Hylobates lar*): A new primate host for *Herpesvirus hominis*: I. A natural epizootic in a laboratory colony. *J. Infect. Dis.* 120:292–297, 1969.

Herpesvirus Tamarinus

Daniel, M. D., Barahona, H., Melendez, L. V., and Forbes, M. Vaccination of monkeys against fatal herpes infections. *Fed. Proc.* 35:569, 1976.

Daniel, M. D., Barahona, H., Melendez, L. V., Hunt, R. D., Sehgal, P., Marshall, B., Ingalls, J., and Forbes, M. Prevention of fatal herpes infections in owl and marmoset monkeys by vaccination. In D. J. Chivers and E. H. R. Ford, eds. *Recent advances in primatology*, vol. 4, pp. 67–69. London: Academic Press, 1978.

Daniel, M. D., Karpas, A., Melendez, L. V., King, N. W. and Hunt, R. D. Isolation of *Herpes-T* virus from a spontaneous disease in squirrel monkeys (*Saimiri sciureus*). *Arch. Gesamte Virusforsch.* 22:324–331, 1967.

Daniel, M. D., and Melendez, L. V. *In vitro* markers for the characterization of *Herpes-T* variants. *Bact. Proc.* 68:163–164, 1968a.

Daniel, M. D., and Melendez, L. V. Isolation of *Herpes-T* variants and their immunological properties. *Fed. Proc.* 27:734, 1968b.

Daniel, M. D., and Melendez, L. V. Long term maintenance of cell cultures under agar overlay and development of *Herpes-T* plaques. *Proc. Soc. Exp. Biol.* 127:919–925, 1968c.

Daniel, M. D., and Melendez, L. V. Pathogenicity studies in rabbits, hamsters, mice and embryonated eggs with *Herpes-T* variants. *Arch. Gesamte Virusforsch.* 32:45–52, 1970.

Daniel, M. D., Melendez, L. V., Hunt, R. D., and Trum, B. F. The herpesvirus group. In *Pathology of simian primates*, 2, pp. 592–611. Basel: Karger, 1972.

Fenner, F. Classification and nomenclature of viruses, p. 51. *Second Report of the International Committee on Taxonomy of Viruses*. Basel: Karger, 1976.

Holmes, A. W., Caldwell, R. G., Dedmon, R. E., and Deinhardt, F. Isolation and characterization of a new herpes virus. *J. Immunol.* 92:602–610, 1964.

Holmes, A. W., Devine, J. A., Nowakowski, E., and Deinhardt, F. The epidemiology of a herpes virus infection of New World monkeys. *J. Immunol.* 90:668–671, 1966.

Hunt, R. D., and Melendez, L. V. Spontaneous *Herpes-T* infection in the owl monkey (*Aotus trivirgatus*). *Pathol. Vet.* 3:1–26, 1966.

King, N. W., Hunt, R. D., Daniel, M. D., and Melendez, L. V. Overt *Herpes-T* infection in squirrel monkeys (*Saimiri sciureus*). *Lab. Anim. Care* 17:413–423, 1967.

Melendez, L. V., Hunt, R. D., Garcia, F. G., and Trum, B. F. A latent *Herpes-T* infection in *Saimiri sciureus* (squirrel monkey). In R. N. Fiennes, *Some recent developments in comparative medicine*, p. 393. New York: Academic Press, 1966.

Melnick, J. L., Midulla, M., Wimberly, I., Barrera-Oro, J. G., and Levy, B. M. A new member of the herpesvirus group isolated from South American marmosets. *J. Immunol.* 92:596–601, 1964.

Murphy, B. L., Maynard, J. E., Krushak, D. H., and Fields, R. M. Occurrence of a carrier state for *Herpesvirus tamarinus* in marmosets. *Appl. Microbiol.* 21:50–52, 1971.

Sauer, R. M., and Bishop, R. W. Inclusion body hepatitis in marmosets. *Lab. Anim. Care* 13:790–792, 1963.

Tate, C. L., Lewis, J. C., Huxsoll, D. L., and Hilde-brandt, P. K. Herpesvirus T as the cause of encephalitis in an owl monkey (*Aotus trivirgatus*). *Lab. Anim. Sci.* 21:743–745, 1971.

Spider Monkey Herpesvirus

Hull, R. N., Dwyer, A. C., Holmes, A. W., Nowakowski, E., Deinhardt, F., Lennette, E. H., and Emmons, R. W. Recovery and characterization of a new simian herpesvirus from a fatally infected spider monkey. *J. Natl. Cancer Inst.* 49:225–231, 1972.

Simian Varicellalike Herpesviruses

Allen, W. P., Felsenfeld, A. D., Wolf, R. H., and Smetana, H. F. Recent studies on the isolation and characterization of Delta herpesvirus. *Lab Anim. Sci.* 24:222–228, 1974.

Ayres, J. P. Studies of the Delta herpesvirus isolated from the patas monkey (*Erythrocebus patas*). *Lab Anim. Sci.* 21:685–695, 1971.

Blakely, G. A., Lourie, B., Morton, W. G., Evans, H. H., and Kaufmann, A. F. A varicella-like disease in macaque monkeys. *J. Infect. Dis.* 127:617–625, 1973.

Clarkson, M. J., Thorpe, E., and McCarthy, K. A virus disease of captive vervet monkeys (*Cercopithecus aethiops*) caused by a new herpesvirus. *Arch. Gesamte Virusforsch.* 22:219–234, 1967.

Felsenfeld, A. D., and Schmidt, N. J. Immunological relationship between Delta herpesvirus of patas monkeys and varicella-zoster virus of humans. *Infect. Immun.* 12:261–266, 1975.

Jackman, D. A., King, N. W., Daniel, M. D., Sehgal, P. K., and Fraser, C. E. O. *Herpesvirus cyclopis*, a new herpesvirus isolated from *Macaca cyclopis*. *Abstracts of the 77th Annual Meeting of the American Society for Microbiology*, New Orleans, La., p. 348, 1977.

Lourie, B., Morton, W. G., Blakely, G. A., and Kaufmann, A. F., Epizootic vesicular disease in macaque monkeys. *Lab Anim. Sci.* 21:1079–1080, 1971.

McCarthy, K., Thorpe, E., Laursen, A. C., Heymann, C. S., and Beale, A. J. Exanthematous disease in patas monkeys caused by a herpes virus. *Lancet* 2:856–857, 1968.

McClure, H. M., and Keeling, M. E. Viral diseases noted in the Yerkes Primate Center colony. *Lab. Anim. Sci.* 21:1002–1010, 1971.

Marrenikova, S. S., Maltseva, N. N., Shelukhina, E. M., Shenkman, L. S., and Korneeva, V. J. A generalized herpetic infection simulating small-pox in a gorilla. *Intervirology* 2:280–287, 1974.

Migaki, G., Seibold, H. R., Wolf, R. H., and Garner, F. M. Pathologic conditions in patas monkeys. *J. Am. Vet. Med. Assoc.* 159:549–556, 1971.

Riopelle, A. J., Ayres, J. P., Seibold, H. R., and Wolf, R. H. Studies of primate diseases at the Delta Center, Medical Primatology, 1970. *Proceedings of the 2nd Conference on Experimental Medical Surgery on Primates*, New York, 1969, pp. 826–838. Basel: Karger, 1971.

Wenner, H. A., Abel, D., Barrick, S., and Seshumurty, P. Clinical and pathogenetic studies of Medical Lake Macaque virus infections in cynomolgous monkeys (simian varicella). *J. Infect. Dis.* 135:611–622, 1977.

Wenner, H. A., Barrick, S., Abel, D., and Seshumurty, P. The pathogenesis of simian varicella virus in cynomolgous monkeys. *Proc. Soc. Exp. Biol. Med.* 150:318–323, 1975.

Wolf, R. H., Smetana, H. F., Allen, W. P., and Felsenfeld, A. D. Pathology and clinical history of Delta herpesvirus infection in Patas monkeys. *Lab. Anim. Sci.* (pt. 2)24:86, 1974.

Simian Cytomegaloviruses

Ablashi, D. V., Chopra, H. C., and Armstrong, G. R. A cytomegalovirus isolated from an owl monkey. *Lab. Anim. Sci.* 22:190–195, 1972.

Asher, D. M., Gibbs, C. J., and Lang, D. J. Rhesus monkey cytomegalovirus: Persistent asymptomatic viruria. *Bacteriol, Proc. Abstr.* V269, 1969.

Asher, D. M., Gibbs, C. J., Jr., Lang, D. J., and Gajdusek, D. C. Persistent shedding of cytomegalovirus in the urine of healthy rhesus monkeys. *Proc. Soc. Exp. Biol. Med.* 145:794–801, 1974.

Black, P. H., Hartley, J. W., and Rowe, W. P. Isolation of a cytomegalovirus from African green monkey. *Proc. Soc. Exp. Biol. Med.* 112:601–605, 1963.

Chopra, H. C., Lloyd, B. J., Jr., Ablashi, D. V., and Armstrong, G. R. Morphologic studies of a cytomegalovirus isolated from an owl monkey. *J. Natl. Cancer Inst.* 48:1333–1337, 1972.

Cowdry, E. V., and Scott, G. H. Nuclear inclusions suggestive of virus action in the salivary glands of the monkey, *Cebus fatuellus. Am. J. Pathol.* 11:647–658, 1935a.

———. Nuclear inclusions in the kidneys of *Macacus rhesus* monkeys. *Am. J. Pathol.* 11:659–668, 1935b.

Malherbe, H., and Harwin, R. Seven viruses isolated from the vervet monkey. *Br. J. Exp. Pathol.* 38:539–541, 1957.

———. The cytopathic effects of vervet monkey viruses. *S. Afr. Med. J.* 37:407–411, 1963.

Smith, A. A., and McNulty, W. P., Jr. Salivary gland inclusion disease in the tarsier. *Lab. Anim. Care* 19:479–481, 1969.

Smith, K. O., Thiel, J. F., Newman, J. R., Harvey, E., Trousdale, M. D., Gehle, W. D., and Clark, G. Cytomegaloviruses as common adventitious contaminants in primary African green monkey kidney cell cultures. *J. Natl. Cancer Inst.* 42:489–497, 1969.

Tsuchiya, Y., Isshiki, O., and Yamada, H. Generalized cytomegalovirus infection in a gorilla. *Jp. J. Med. Sci. Biol.* 23:71–73, 1970.

Vogel, F. S., and Pinkerton, H. Spontaneous salivary gland virus disease in chimpanzees. *Arch. Pathol.* 60:281–285, 1955.

Other Simian Herpesviruses

Daniel, M. D., Melendez, L. V., Hunt, R. D., and Trum, B. F. The herpesvirus group. In *Pathology of Simian Primates*, p. 2, pp. 592–611. New York: Karger, 1972.

Daniel, M. D., Melendez, L. V., King, N. W., Barahona, H. H., Fraser, C. E. O., Garcia, F. G., and Silva, D. Isolation and characterization of a new virus from owl monkeys: *Herpesvirus aotus* type 3. *Am. J. Phys. Anthropol.* 38:497–500, 1973.

Daniel, M. D., Melendez, L. V., King, N. W., Fraser, C. E. O., Barahona, H. H., Hunt, R. D., and Garcia, F. G. *Herpesvirus aotus:* A latent herpesvirus from owl monkeys (*Aotus trivirgatus*). Isolation and characterization. *Proc. Soc. Exp. Biol. Med.* 138:835–845, 1971.

Deinhardt, F., Falk, L. A., Nonoyama, M., Wolfe, L., Bergholz, C., Lapin, B., Yakovleva, L., Agrba, V., Henle, G., and Henle, W. Baboon lymphotropic herpesvirus related to Epstein-Barr virus (EBV). Abstracts of the Third Herpesvirus Workshop. Cold Spring Harbor *Symp. Quant. Biol.* 64:1976.

Falk, L. A., Deinhardt, F., Nonoyama, M., Wolfe, L. G., Bergholz, C., Lapin, B., Yakovleva, L., Agrba, V., Henle, G., and Henle, W. Properties of a baboon lymphotropic herpesvirus related to Epstein-Barr virus. *Int. J. Cancer* 18:798–807, 1976.

Frank, A. L., Bissell, J. A., Rowe, D. S., Dunnick, N. R., Mayner, R. E., Hopps, H. E., Parkman, P. D., and Myers, H. M., Jr. Rhesus leukocyte-associated herpesvirus: I. Isolation and characterization of a new herpesvirus recovered from rhesus monkey leukocytes. *J. Infect. Dis.* 128:618–629, 1973.

Gerber, P., Kalter, S. S., Schidlovsky, G. Peterson, W. D., Jr. and Daniel, M. D. Biologic and antigenic characteristics of Epstein-Barr virus related herpesviruses of chimpanzees and baboons. *Int. J. Cancer* 20:448–459, 1977.

Lapin, B. A., Agrba, V. Z., Yakovleva, L. A., Sangulia, I. A., Timanovskaja, V. V., Chuvirov, G. N., and Kokosha, L. V. The establishment of lymphoblastoid suspension cell lines, containing herpes-like virus, from hemopoietic organs of hamadryas baboons with malignant lymphoma.

Rep. USSR Acad. Med. Sci. 222:244–246, 1975. (In Russian.)

Lewis, M. A., Frye, L. D., Gibbs, C. J., Jr., Chou, S. M., Cutchins, E. C., and Gajdusek, D. C. Isolation and characterization of two new unrelated herpesviruses from capuchin monkeys. *Microbiol. Proc. Abstr.* V336:256, 1974.

McCombs, R. M., Brunskwig, J. P., Mirkovic, R., and Benyesh-Melnick, M. Electron microscopic characterization of a herpes-like virus isolated from tree shrews. *Virology* 45:816–820, 1971.

Malherbe, H., and Harwin, R. Neurotropic virus in African monkeys. *Lancet* 2:530, 1958.

———. The cytopathic effects of vervet monkey viruses. *S. Afr. Med. J.* 37:407–411, 1963.

Malherbe, H., and Strickland-Cholmley, M. Simian herpesvirus SA-8 from a baboon. *Lancet* 2:1427, 1969.

Melendez, L. V., Castellanos, H., Barahona, H. H., Daniel, M. D., Hunt, R. D., Fraser, C. E. O., Garcia, F. G., and King, N. W. Two new herpesviruses from spider monkeys (*Ateles geoffroyi*) *J. Natl. Cancer Inst.* 49:233–238, 1972.

Melendez, L. V., Castellanos, H., Hunt, R. D., Barahona, H. H., Daniel, M. D., Fraser, C. E. O., and Garcia, F. G. Spider monkey herpesviruses and malignant lymphomas. *Proceedings of the 19th Meeting of the Advisory Committee of Medical Research*. Washington, D.C.: Pan American Health Organization, 1971.

Melendez, L. V., and Daniel, M. D. Herpesviruses from South American monkeys. In *Medical primatology*, pp. 686–693. Proc. 2nd Conf. Exp. Med. Surg. Primates, Basel: Karger, 1971.

Melendez, L. V., Daniel, M. D., Hunt, R. D., and Garcia, F. G. An apparently new herpesvirus from primary kidney cultures of squirrel monkeys (*Saimiri sciureus*) *Lab. Anim. Care* 18:374–381, 1968.

Rabin, H., Newbauer, R. H., Hopkins, R. F., Dzhikidze, E. K., Shevtsova, Z. V., and Lapin, B. A. Transforming activity and antigenicity of an Epstein-Barr-like virus from lymphoblastoid cell lines of baboons with lymphoid disease. *Intervirology* 8:240–249, 1977.

Rasheen, S. Rongey, R. W., Nelson-Rees, W. A., Rabin, H., Newbauer, R. H., Bruszuresky, E. G., and Gardner, M. B. Establishment of a cell line with associated Epstein-Barr-like virus from a leukemic orangutan. *Science* 198:407–409, 1977.

11

Herpesviruses of Wild Ungulates, Including Malignant Catarrhal Fever Virus

W. PLOWRIGHT

Although there has been very little systematic investigation of herpesvirus infections of wild ungulates, a few exceptions are provided by herpesviruses that have an economic significance as pathogens of domesticated species and their usual wild reservoir hosts, which are seldom or never clinically affected. Among these are the agents of malignant catarrhal fever and pseudo-lumpy skin disease (herpes mammillitis) of cattle. The primary stimulus for the study of these infections came from their effects on cattle; in other cases (for example, infectious bovine rhinotracheitis) the involvement of wild hosts was discovered incidentally or as a result of serologic surveys. There is little doubt that wild ungulates will be shown to harbor many as yet unknown herpesviruses when the necessary effort is devoted to their detection.

The nomenclature and classification of herpesviruses is still in dispute. However, if the subfamily of the usual natural host is used in designating virus species, then infectious bovine rhinotracheitis virus becomes bovine herpesvirus 1; the agent of pseudo-lumpy skin disease is bovine herpesvirus 2; orphan herpesviruses are designated bovine herpesvirus 3; and malignant catarrhal fever virus (in its usual African form) becomes alcelaphine herpesvirus 1, after the subfamilies Bovinae and Alcelaphinae, respectively.

Malignant Catarrhal Fever

Synonyms: **Malignant head catarrh, snot- siekte, bosartige katarrhalfieber, coryza gangreneux.**

Malignant catarrhal fever (MCF) is an acute generalized disease of cattle and domestic buffalo, characterized clinically by high fever, severe inflammatory and degenerative changes in the mucosae of the upper respiratory and alimentary tracts, ophthalmia, generalized lymphadenopathy, and signs of meningoencephalomyelitis. The disease has an extremely high mortality rate, but the morbidity rate is irregular and usually low. There is no good evidence for transmission by contact among cattle, and the vast majority of cases can be associated with close contact between cattle and sheep or wildebeest, which are presumed reservoir hosts. The virus from sheep has not yet been isolated and characterized, whereas that from wildebeest was demonstrated by Mettham (1923) in South Africa and first isolated in East Africa in 1959 (Plowright et al. 1960).

HISTORY. In Europe, MCF has probably been recognized as a distinct entity since the end of the eighteenth century, and its differentiation from rinderpest has been documented for some time. Attempts to transmit infection to cattle by feeding or inoculation of fomites and diseased tissues almost invariably failed, and environmental or host factors were often stressed in its etiology. Since 1929 when Gotze and Liess first used large quantities of blood from sheep-associated bovine cases to transmit MCF successfully to cattle, there have been many further demonstrations of its infectious nature (Plowright 1964, 1968). Selman et al. (1974, 1978), Snowden (1972), and Pierson et al. (1974) have reported successful transmissions to cattle, but numerous attempts to demonstrate or isolate the putative virus have failed.

In Africa, snotsiekte was apparently well known to the pioneers and hunters who journeyed into the interior of the southern part of the continent in the early nineteenth century. Cumming (1950) remarked that infection was acquired when cattle grazed over areas previously frequented by wildebeest. Mettam (1923), who first reported on the transmission of snotsiekte, considered that this disease differed

126

from European MCF in its easy experimental transfer to cattle; the absence of skin, horn, and hoof involvement; and the marked, constant enlargement of lymph nodes. Following the work of Gotze and Liess (1929) and their own studies of snotsiekte in East Africa, Daubney and Hudson (1936) concluded that snotsiekte must become a synonym of malignant catarrh, a viewpoint supported by Du Toit and Alexander (1938) and Wyssman (1938).

No evidence has yet been brought forward that MCF, as derived from sheep or other potential reservoir hosts, differs clinicopathologically in a significant way from snotsiekte acquired by close contact with wildebeest in Africa (Selman et al. 1974, 1978; Storz et al. 1976).

DISTRIBUTION AND HOST RANGE. Malignant catarrhal fever, as a clinicopathologic entity, has been reported from all continents and most countries. Confirmation of diagnosis has commonly been based on histopathologic evidence that is probably conclusive for members of the Bovidae. Sometimes, however, the clinical features alone have been used; these can be misleading, especially in species that do not belong to the proven host range.

Among domesticated species, the disease is limited to cattle (*Bos taurus, B. indicus*) and buffalo (*Bubalis bubalis*), but the host range of the causal agent almost certainly includes sheep in Africa as well as other continents (De Koch and Neitz 1950; Piercy 1954; Plowright 1964). There is one report of MCF in a domestic goat that eventually recovered (Altmann et al. 1973).

The range of free-living and captive wild species in which MCF has been reported is continually widening; a summary of available information is given in Tables 11.1 and 11.2. In addition to the captive species mentioned, typical lethal infection was established experimentally in an eland (*Taurotragus oryx*) by inoculation of virulent cattle blood infected with a wildebeest isolate (Plowright 1964). Surprisingly, three African buffalo (*Syncerus caffer*) failed to react when given a similar inoculation, and virus was never recovered from their blood, which was usually sampled once a week. Since the buffalo belongs to the subfamily Bovinae, one would expect a susceptibility similar to that of cattle and many antelopes. Camels were not susceptible to inoculation with virulent cattle blood and failed to develop antibody to wildebeest virus.

Among other species found to be unaffected

TABLE 11.1 Free-living Species in which Malignant Catarrhal Fever Has Been Reported.

Family[a]	Subfamily[a]	Genus and Species	Common Name	Method of Diagnosis	Reference
Antilocapridae	Antilocaprinae	*Antilocapra*	pronghorn antelope	clinical	Skinner 1922
Bovidae	Bovinae	*Bison bison*	American bison	clinicopathologic	Pierson et al. 1974; Ruth et al. 1977
	Rupicaprinae	*Rupicapra rupicapra*	chamois	clinicopathologic	Hofer, quoted by Otte 1928
Cervidae	Odocoileinae	*Capreolus capreolus*	roe deer	clinicopathologic	Otte 1928
	Cervinae	*Axis axis*	axis deer	clinicopathologic	Clark et al. 1970, 1972
	Odocoileinae	*Odocoileus virginianus*	white-tailed deer	clinicopathologic	Clark et al. 1970, 1972
		O. hemionus	mule deer	clinicopathologic	Pierson et al. 1974

[a] The classification used is that of Simpson (1945), as followed by Morris (1965).

TABLE 11.2 Captive Species in which Malignant Catarrhal Fever Has Been Reported.

Family[a]	Subfamily[a]	Genus and Species	Common Name	Method of Diagnosis	Reference
Bovidae	Bovinae	*Bos gaurus*	gaur	clinicopathologic	Hanichen and Ernst 1969
		B. banteng	banteng	clinicopathologic	Roken and Bjorklund 1974
		Boselaphus tragocamelus	nilgai	clinicopathologic	Roken and Bjorklund 1974
		Tragelaphus spekei	sitatunga	clinicopathologic	Roken and Bjorklund 1974
		Bison bonasus	European bison	clinicopathologic	Balsai 1973; Altmann et al. 1973
		T. strepsiceros	greater kudu	clinicopathologic	Boever and Kurka 1974
Cervidae	Cervinae	*Elaphurus davidianus*	Pere David's deer	clinicopathologic	Huck et al. 1962; Tong et al. 1961
		Cervus nippon	sika deer	clinicopathologic	Sanford et al. 1977
		C. elaphus	red deer	clinicopathologic	Reid et al. 1975
	Odocoileinae	*Alces alces*	elk (American moose)	clinicopathologic	Andersson 1953; Altmann et al. 1973
		Odocoileus virginianus	white-tailed deer	clinicopathologic	Wobeser et al. 1973; Wyand et al. 1971
		Rangifer tarandus	reindeer	clinicopathologic	Altmann et al. 1973
Giraffidae	Giraffinae	*Giraffa camelopardalis*	giraffe	clinical	Dieckerhoff 1903

[a] The classification used is that of Simpson (1945), as followed by Morris (1965).

following experimental infection with wildebeest virus are horses, sheep, dogs, and chickens. Cats, goats, ducks, pigeons, and doves have also been found to be nonsusceptible; the blood of these animals also remained nonvirulent for cattle (Mettam 1923). Rabbits are susceptible to sheep-associated (Daubney 1959; De Koch and Neitz 1950; Mansjoer 1955) and wildebeest-derived strains (Daubney and Hudson 1936; Piercy 1955; Plowright 1964) as well as one from deer (Huck et al. 1961). Guinea pigs, mice, and rats develop clinical disease after inoculation of tissues of affected cattle, but Kalunda (1975) recently reported on production of the typical disease syndrome in both guinea pigs and golden hamsters. Embryonated eggs could not be infected successfully (Blood et al 1961; Huck et al. 1961; Piercy 1955), but wildebeest virus grew in 8–day embryonated eggs inoculated into the yolk sac (Danskin 1955).

TRANSMISSION. There is no good evidence for contact transmission of MCF from cattle to cattle; this applies to the sheep-associated disease (Blood et al. 1961; Gotze and Liess 1929, 1930; Rinjard 1935); and the wildebeest-derived form (Kalunda 1975; Mettam 1923; Piercy 1952; Plowright 1968). Rabbit-to-rabbit transmission by contact has also not been reported in spite of extensive use of these animals for experimental purposes.

There are also many records of the failure to transmit MCF to cattle by the feeding or inoculation of excretions of sick animals or of tissues and excretions of carrier sheep. Where success has been claimed, there is considerable doubt about the nature of the disease transmitted (Stenius 1952; Zanzucchi 1934). Some failures to transmit wildebeest-derived virus to other species are summarized in Table 11.3. Hence, it is clear that cattle, like many wild mammals, constitute dead-end hosts for both types of virus.

Natural transmission among wildebeest, as probably in other alcelaphine hosts, is apparently by a combination of vertical and horizontal routes. Transplacental infection has been proved by the recovery of virus from fetuses or the blood of wildebeest calves estimated to be 1 week of age or less (Plowright 1965a,b). Horizontal transmission among the rest of the annual calf crop, which is dropped within a period of a few weeks, probably accounts for an increasing prevalence of viremia during early life, reaching 40% on a single sampling during the 2nd month (Plowright 1965a). Evidence of contact transmission from a congenitally in-

TABLE 11.3 Species to which Malignant Catarrhal Fever Was Not Transmissible.

Family[a]	Subfamily[a]	Genus and Species	Common Name	Method of Diagnosis	Reference
Bovidae	Bovinae	Syncerus caffer	African buffalo	clinical, virus recovery	Plowright 1964
	Caprinae	Ovis aries	sheep (East African and merino)	clinical, virus recovery	Plowright 1964
Camelidae	Camelinae	Camelus dromedarius	dromedary (camel)	clinical, virus recovery, antibody development	Plowright, unpublished

[a] The classification used is that of Simpson (1945), as followed by Morris (1965).

fected animal was also presented in a group of captive wildebeest calves (Plowright 1965b). The presence of material antibody of high titer in the serum of calves up to 5 months old did not prevent infection, and the retention of serum antibody by all free-living wildebeest over 12 months old showed that they invariably acquired an active immunity and were not rendered immunologically tolerant by in utero infection (Plowright 1967).

Congenital infection of the bovine fetus can occur, as shown by the production of infected calves in at least four successive pregnancies of one cow; three of these calves were clinically normal at birth. The dam had originally undergone inapparent experimental infection and must have retained MCFV in her tissues for at least 80 months (Plowright et al. 1972).

Virus excretion by wildebeest is probably by the nasal route (Rweyemamu et al. 1974), with the seasonal distribution of the disease in cattle probably attributable to the greater frequency and quantity of virus in the nasal secretions of calves undergoing initial infection in the first 3–5 months of life. Experimentally, incubation periods in bovine calves varied from 30 to 81 days. Close contact between cattle, demonstrably between viremic wildebeest over 4–5 months old, seldom leads to cases of MCF; one such instance did occur when an adult wildebeest was subjected to experimental severe dehydration stress.

Although hartebeest and topi are known to harbor viruses that have a cattle pathogenicity similar to the wildebeest strains, no cases of MCF in cattle have been attributed to grazing contact with these other species.

Where cases of MCF have occurred in zoos, little information on the source of virus is available. However, in some instances, evidence for close contact with wildebeest on the ranch or in paddocks or housing was obtained (Balsai 1973; Boever and Kurka 1974; Sanford et al. 1977); in others contact with sheep is mentioned (Altman et al. 1973; Pierson et al. 1974; Ruth et al. 1977; Sanford et al. 1977). Sometimes the probable reservoir host could not be determined (Huck et al. 1961; Wobeser et al. 1973).

The incubation period in cattle following contact with presumably infected sheep usually varies between 3 and 6 months (Gotze 1930, 1932) but can be as short as 59 days (Rinjard 1935); these figures are close to the 60–144 days calculated by Pierson et al. (1973).

According to Jubb and Kennedy (1970), the disease in Canada occurs mainly in cattle housed with lambing ewes.

ETIOLOGY. Although there is general agreement that the clinicopathologic features of MCF are essentially the same wherever they occur, nothing is yet known about the etiological agent presumed to be derived from sheep and other reservoir hosts. In countries outside Africa no proof exists that the disease is due to a filterable virus, since all successful transmissions have been accomplished using whole blood or tissue suspensions. There is one report that particles resembling togaviruses were present in the cytoplasm of endothelial and epithelial cells of deer (white-tailed and axis) infected naturally or experimentally with MCF (Clark and Adams 1976), but confirmation of this claim is needed.

The African forms derived from wildebeest are caused by a herpesvirus that can be readily isolated by inoculation of monolayer cell cultures, particularly of primary or secondary bovine thyroid cells (Plowright et al. 1960) (Fig. 11.1), and serially cultivated strains of bovine testis cells at low passage levels. It is necessary to use viable cell suspensions from infected animals as inocula, since no cell-free infectivity has been demonstrated in the tissues of infected cattle (Plowright 1963, 1964) or other species, including wildebeest, which are the natural hosts (Plowright 1965b).

Another method for isolation of virus is to prepare monolayer cultures from the thyroid and adrenal glands of infected cattle and examine them for the typical cytopathic effects; these usually appear after 6–8 days and comprise the development of multinucleate syncytia, with varying degrees of cytoplasmic vacuolation and intranuclear inclusion bodies, which become progressively more basophilic and Fuelgen-positive as they mature (Plowright et al. 1965). Sometimes granular intracytoplasmic inclusions, which are also Feulgen-positive and often paranuclear, may be seen; larger homogeneous cytoplasmic inclusions occasionally occur in the cytoplasm (Plowright 1968).

The methods used for isolation of MCFV from cattle and wildebeest have also been employed successfully for the recovery of similar herpesviruses from the hartebeest (*Alcelaphus buselaphus cokei*) (Reid and Rowe 1973) and the topi (*Damaliscus korrigum*). These techniques have so far failed to demonstrate the etiological agent of sheep-associated MCF (Plowright 1964; Selman et al. 1974, 1978; Snowden 1972; Storz et al. 1976).

Rweyemamu et al. (1974) isolated MCFV from the nasal secretions of 6 of 23 captive wildebeest, including 2 of 3 calves, and sug-

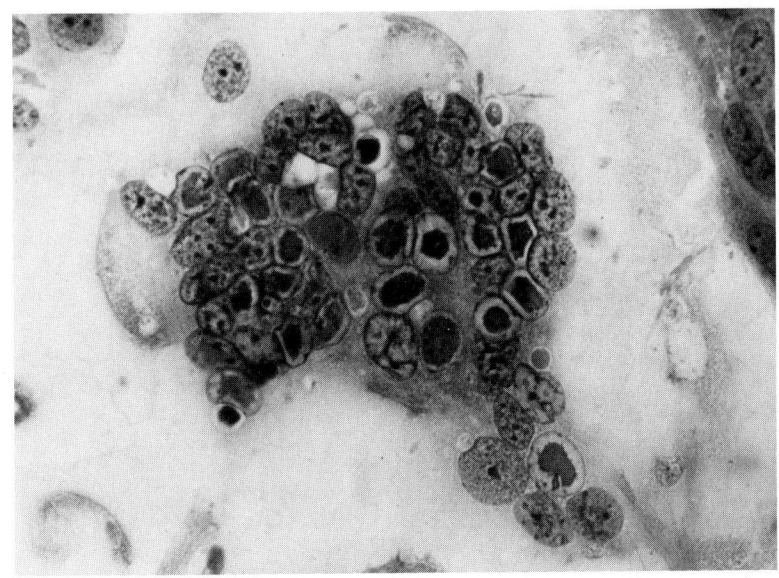

FIG. 11.1 Cytopathic effect of a wildebeest-derived strain of virus in bovine thyroid monolayer, showing syncytium formation with large dense intranuclear inclusion bodies surrounded by clear halos. (Photo by Dr. B. Schieman, 1969.)

gested that this material was a better source of virus than blood, since it was possibly derived from the tonsillar and pharyngeal tissues. In 1 calf only nasal secretions contained cell-free virus, and this was not deposited during clarification by low-speed centrifugation. The same authors found that betamethasone treatment of adult wildebeest (46 mg daily for 7 days) infrequently induced irregular nasal excretion of MCFV, whereas all of 8 wildebeest cows in one experiment developed pustular vulvovaginitis lesions, from which infectious bovine rhinotracheitis virus was isolated.

Reid et al. (1975) suggested that the agents derived from wildebeest and hartebeest should provisionally be designated "alcelaphine" herpesviruses after the subfamily Alcelaphinae, to which some systematists consider they belong. If Simpson's (1945) classification of Bovidae were to be adopted, the appropriate grouping would be "hippotragine," after the Hippotraginae. Whatever the eventual designation, the viruses are typical herpesviruses and strictly cell associated both in the intact hosts and in early culture passages. In the former they are associated with lymphoreticular tissues (lymph nodes, spleen, circulating leukocytes, and bone marrow) and procedures such as freezing and thawing or ultrasonic disruption lead to a complete loss of infectivity; small amounts of cell-free virus may be present in tissue suspensions from experimentally infected rabbits (Plowright, 1964) and nasal secretions of some wildebeest (Rweyemamu et al. 1974).

After passage in cell cultures, wildebeest and hartebeest viruses produce varying quantities of cell-free infectivity; Plowright et al. (1960) reported that this took place after 7–30 passages in a serially cultivated strain of calf kidney cells. The titer of cell-free virus reached $10^{3.3}$ TCD_{50}/ml. After further passages one strain of virus (WC11) attained free-virus titers of $10^{3.8}$–$10^{5.8}$ TCD_{50}/ml in calf thyroid monolayers. This isolate has been used extensively for virus characterization (Plowright et al. 1965) and neutralization tests (Plowright 1967). It was later found that wildebeest viruses recently isolated in calf thyroid monolayers could be propagated readily in secondary calf kidney cultures where they would produce cell-free infectivity up to about $10^{3.5}$ TCD_{50}/ml of medium (Plowright et al. 1975). Even better were monolayers of serially cultivated calf testis cells, which were often highly sensitive for primary isolation of virus from animal tissues. Within 3–5 passages these cells spontaneously released cell-free virus with titers between 10^3 and 10^5 TCD_{50}ml. Comparable amounts of infectious intracellular virus could be released by a single cycle of freezing and thawing (−70 and 37°C.).

Little is known about the stability characteristics of alcelaphine herpesviruses; as expected, their cell-free infectivity is completely inactivated by lipid solvents such as ether and chloroform (Plowright et al. 1965). The WC11 strain of high-passage, cell-free virus was moderately stable in culture maintenance medium containing 5% ox serum; the half-life of two virus stocks at 4°C was 11–14 days. Over periods of 58–70 days at 37°C one stock had a half-life of 9.3 hours; all infectivity was lost within 9–15 minutes at 56°C. At −70°C, or in liquid nitrogen, virus stocks with 2 or 5% bovine serum maintain their titer for periods of many months. The half-life of the infectivity in cattle blood at 4°C, with EDTA or heparin as anticoagulants, was 0.83 and 0.67 days, respectively (Plowright 1964).

Cell suspensions prepared from spleen or lymph node tissues of infected cattle and rabbits, with the addition of 10–20% bovine serum and 10% (v/v) of glycerol or dimethylsulfoxide, maintain their infectivity titer for periods of at least 8–12 months at −70°C or in liquid nitrogen (Plowright 1963, 1964). Similarly, suspensions of cells from infected monolayers can be preserved for periods of many months at −70°C or below. Cell-free infectious virus can be lyophilized with a suitable additive (for example, 0.25% lactalbumin hydrolysate and 5% sucrose) and will then retain its infectivity at −20°C for many years.

Evidence that the wildebeest (or other alcelaphine) herpesviruses are in fact the cause of the majority of African cases of MCF has been obtained by the regular reproduction of the disease in cattle or rabbits, by parenteral inoculation of infected cultured cells (Plowright 1964, 1965a; Rweyemamu et al. 1974), or less consistently, by the intranasal instillation of infected tissue or cultured cell suspensions or of cell-free virus propagated in cell cultures (Plowright 1964). The viruses are in turn recoverable from experimental animals that develop antibody—demonstrable in indirect immunofluorescence (IIF) or virus neutralization (VN) tests—during the incubation or clinical phases (Rossiter et al. 1977). This proof is important because no histopathologic or ultrastructural lesions indicative of herpesvirus infection have yet been found in cattle, rabbits, or any of the wild reservoir hosts.

All the alcelaphine herpesviruses show cross-reactions in neutralization tests. One hartebeest virus (K30 of Reid and Rowe 1973) could be differentiated by significantly higher homologous (hartebeest) titers than were present in wildebeest. The neutralizing antibody detected in topi and oryx (*Oryx beisa*) was always of low titer, again suggesting that antigenic differences exist between the wildebeest virus and the putative indigenous viruses of these species. It should now be possible to ascertain if all have common antigens reacting

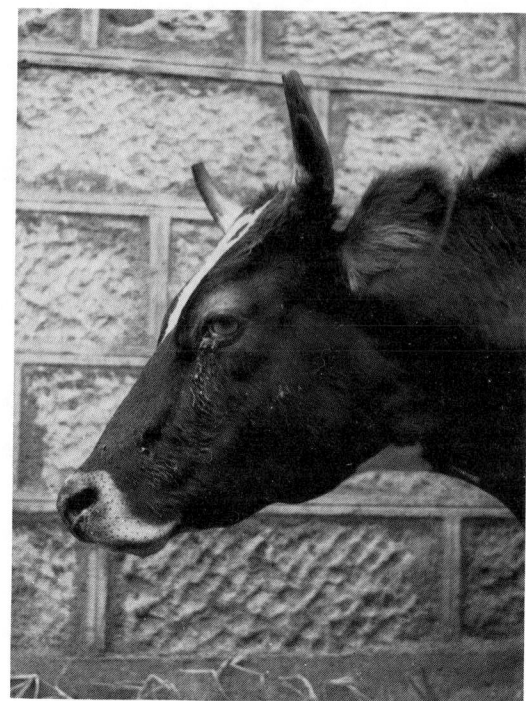

FIG. 11.2   A steer showing ocular and nasal lesions on the 5th day of the malignant catarrhal fever. There is profuse mucopurulent ocular discharge and a wide peripheral zone of corneal opacity. A mucopurulent discharge is also present at the nares. (Photo by Dr. B. Schieman, 1969.)

in IIF (Ferris et al. 1976; Rossiter et al. 1977; Wibberly 1976) and immunodiffusion tests and, incidentally, to investigate any relationship that exists between the sheep-associated and alcelaphine herpesviruses. Attempts to do this have been frustrated by widespread cross-reacting antibodies present in nearly all sheep and many cattle sera.

SIGNS. Although Gotze (1930) described four clinical forms of MCF—peracute, alimentary, head and eye, and mild—most cases fall into the head-and-eye category. Several groups of authors have reported a peracute form in deer, characterized by sudden death (Sanford et al. 1977; Wobeser et al. 1973; Wyand et al. 1971). The mild form, is extremely difficult to diagnose clinically unless virus can be recovered; the mortality in true MCF is more than 90%. The incubation period following experimental inoculation with the non-African agent usually

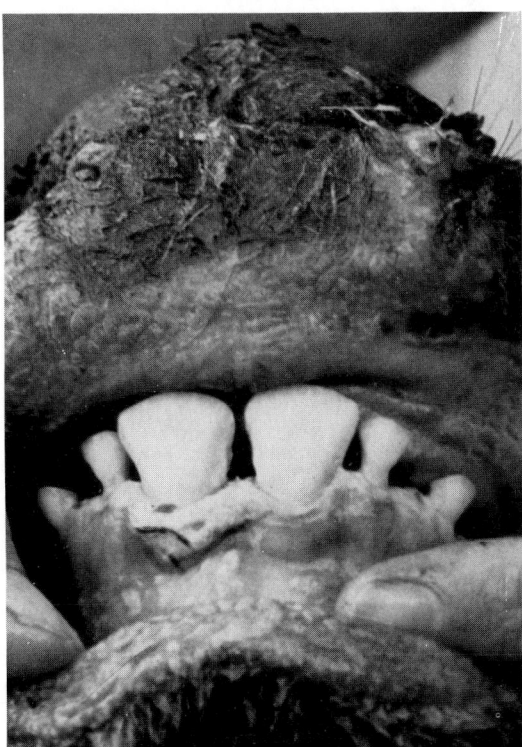

FIG. 11.3 The muzzle of an animal on the 8th day of disease, showing exudate forming adherent scab, with included food material. The gums show necrotic deposits, especially around the alveoli of incisor teeth. (Photo by Dr. B. Schieman, 1969.)

varies between 2 and 8 weeks in cattle (Plowright 1968; Pierson et al. 1974; Selman et al. 1978) and 18 to 48 days in deer (Huck et al. 1961).

The head-and-eye form is usually characterized by sudden onset with unrest, usually high fever, and anorexia. Ocular and nasal discharges at first may be serous or seromucoid but later tend to become more profuse, mucopurulent, and sticky; they leave a trail of matted hair on the cheeks or hang from the nostrils, sometimes in long strings. (See Fig. 11.2.)

The conjunctiva and scleral vessels are usually intensely congested, and examination of the limbus reveals a line of bilateral, corneal opacity that usually appears by the 3rd day of the disease and extends centripetally so that the whole cornea may be involved, resulting in blindness. Cloudiness or whorls of puslike material may be seen in the anterior chamber, and staphyloma may develop terminally in the worst cases. The eye lesions are accompanied by resistance to handling of the head and severe photophobia.

The muzzle rapidly becomes dry and cracked and a serofibrinous exudate appears, which coagulates to form tightly adherent scab, which may become diffuse and, by occluding the rim of the nostrils, exacerbate the dyspnea that develops later (Fig. 11.3). Removal of the deposits leaves ulcerated areas. The visible nasal mucosa is intensely congested with areas of epithelial necrosis and erosion and sometimes with blood-stained discharges, which in the later stages are foul smelling. Noisy breathing and severe dyspnea with the head extended or even extrusion of the tongue point to severe blockage of the upper respiratory pathways.

Excessive salivation with swelling of the lips and frothing is sometimes seen. The oral mucosae are sensitive to handling, showing severe, diffuse congestion from the onset of the disease. This is readily seen on the buccal papillae, the tips of which frequently show necrosis and erosion. Similar lesions also develop around the gums, lower lip, dental pad, and ridges of the palate and on the underside of the free part of the tongue. Excessive thirst or frequent dipping of the muzzle in water has been observed (Tong et al. 1961).

The majority of cattle do not develop diarrhea or dysentery, though these signs have probably been recorded more frequently in wild species, including deer (Clark et al. 1972), bison (Ruth et al. 1977), sitatunga (Roken and Bjorklund 1974), and reindeer (Altmann et al. 1973). The peracute form in cattle may also be accompanied by profuse diarrhea (James et al. 1975) or dysentery (Pierson et al. 1973).

A common but by no means invariable finding is an enlargement of the superficial lymph nodes of the head and neck region and of the body generally. Sometimes swelling of the prescapular and prefemoral nodes can be seen without palpation. The lymphodenopathy may be detectable during the incubation period (Selman et al. 1978) but tends to increase in severity during the clinical phase. Hemolymph nodes show palpable or visible enlargement.

Skin lesions have been frequently reported in wild species as well as cattle. Huck et al. (1961) and Tong et al. (1961) recorded cracking and necrosis of the skin between the toes and hoofs and reddening with ulceration was seen on the perianal skin and vulva. An exudative dermatitis is sometimes seen in cattle, and laminitis is occasionally reported. Cystitis and vaginitis presumably contribute to the frequent dribbling of urine reported by some authors.

Nervous signs, which occur in some cases, may include fine muscular tremors, incoordination, twitching of the ears, and even torticollis.

No clinical signs or lesions referable to MCFV have been observed at any time in free-living wildebeest, hartebeest, or topi populations that have been under continuous observation (Plowright 1964, 1965a; Reid et al. 1975), but in the laboratory a mild pyrexia was observed in two wildebeest calves at the height of the MCF viremia (Plowright 1965b).

PATHOLOGY. The pathology of MCF is variable, depending on the form and duration of the disease, but in the head-and-eye form the necropsy findings are normally characteristic and supplement the clinical findings. In hyperacute or alimentary cases, hemorrhages may be more prominent, and in the more protracted cases the typical epithelial changes of the head-and-eye form become obscured.

Alimentary Tract. The base of the tongue, pharynx, and soft palate show severe congestion, with superficial necrosis and erosion; the tonsils are usually enlarged and congested with the crypts often filled by viscid mucopus. Elongated, brownish erosions are found, especially along the ridges of the esophageal mucosa, and extensive necrosis, occasionally hemorrhagic, is frequently found in the reticulum and, less often, on the pillars of the rumen. Abomasal lesions include diffuse congestion of the fundic and pyloric zones, sometimes with foci of superficial necrosis and erosion, which may be blackened and hemorrhagic.

The small intestine usually shows nothing remarkable, but Peyer's patches are sometimes prominent. Most MCF cases do, however, show congestion with petechiation and blackening of the mucosal folds in the cecum, colon (especially the upper part), and rectum. Fresh or blackened blood, excess mucus, or a blood-stained liquid content are seen in the intestinal form. Necrosis, diphtheresis, and erosion are unusual.

In the liver grayish foci or streaks are sometimes visible on the cut surface or through the capsule; they represent cellular infiltrations. The liver substance may be swollen and friable.

Respiratory Tract. Congestion with more or less extensive necrosis, diphtheresis, erosion, and capillary hemorrhage is almost invariable in the mucosae covering the turbinates and nasal septum. The larynx is congested and often shows hemorrhages or areas of necrosis, especially on the vocal cords. The tracheal mucosa shows similar changes in some animals, hemorrhage being more frequent than in the larynx. Pulmonary changes include a terminal edema, often predominantly interlobular and accompanied by fluid or froth in the bronchial tree. Scattered pneumonic foci may be present, especially in the anterior lobes, but extensive consolidation and pleuritis are unusual.

Urogenital Tract. The kidney cortex may show pale wedge-shaped or irregular areas of cellular infiltration, sometimes with a hemorrhagic periphery resembling anemic infarcts. Occasionally true infarction occurs. The mucosa of the urinary bladder is usually congested and frequently shows hemorrhages or foci of roughening. In females the vaginal mucosa may be congested with areas of necrosis or erosion.

Cardiovascular System. Epicardial petechiae along the coronary grooves are commonly observed as well as a slight to moderate excess of pericardial (also of pleural or peritoneal) fluid, sometimes with fibrin clots.

Lymphopoietic System. The nodes that show the most severe enlargement are those of the head and neck. Visceral nodes generally show less marked involvement. Affected nodes are firm and fleshy with a dense, often pale, cortex and congested medulla; pharyngeal and visceral nodes may be diffusely congested. A gelatinous edema that clots on exposure is frequently seen extending through the capsule into the perinodal connective tissue. The spleen is slightly to moderately enlarged and firm on incision, often with prominent malpighian corpuscles. Hemolymph nodes may be greatly enlarged and darkly congested.

Adrenal Glands. Grayish or hemorrhagic foci often obscure the normal appearance of the transected gland in cattle.

Histopathology and Pathogenesis. The histopathology of MCF has been described by many workers for both the sheep-associated and wildebeest-derived forms (see Jubb and Kennedy 1970). For many decades the characteristic features were regarded as the widespread mononuclear cell (lymphocyte) infiltrations (particularly in perivascular situations) in tissues such as the brain, liver, kidney, lung, and adrenal glands. There is also degeneration and necrosis of epithelia associated with subepithelial cellular infiltrations.

The perivascular infiltrative changes are accompanied by lesions of the blood vessel walls, in which smooth muscle, connective tissue, and endothelial elements undergo degeneration. Similar changes also affect the smooth muscle of hollow viscera and the connective tissues of the capsule and trabeculae of lymph nodes and spleen; these vascular changes resembled those of infectious mononucleosis in humans (Plowright 1953b). The angiitis, with fibrinoid degeneration and necrosis of the media and adventitia, is pathognomonic of MCF

in ruminants and experimental rabbits (Jubb and Kennedy 1970). If the intima is affected, there is a proliferation (often with radial orientation) of endothelial cells (Figs. 11.4 and 11.5); sometimes thrombosis follows, but this is by no means invariable (Fig. 11.6). The vascular lesions are circumscribed and often segmental and occur most frequently in the kidney, brain, and meninges; the capsule and surrounding tissue of the adrenal glands and lymph nodes; and the lung and liver tissue.

Changes in the lymphoid tissues are characterized by a depletion of small lymphocytes and lymphoid follicles through necrosis and phagocytosis, in addition to edema and hemorrhage. Proliferation of larger lymphoblasts, or

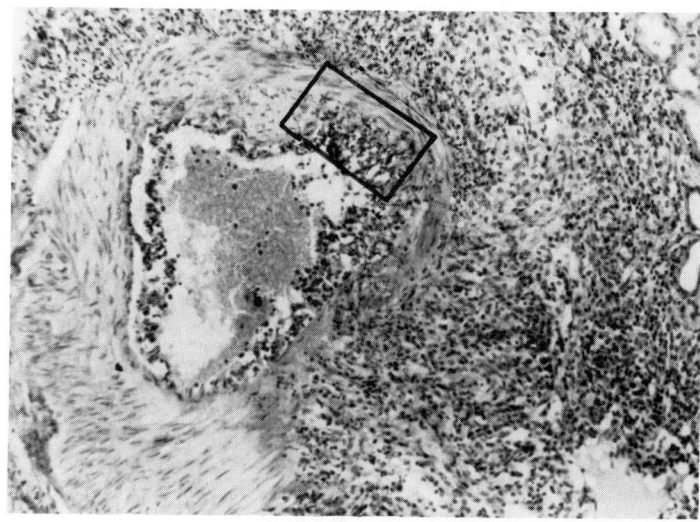

FIG. 11.4 Section of an arcuate artery in the kidney of a heifer with sheep-associated MCF. There is perivascular infiltration and a segmental angiitis. The endothelium is hyperplastic and detaching (×125). (Photo by Dr. B. Schieman, 1969.)

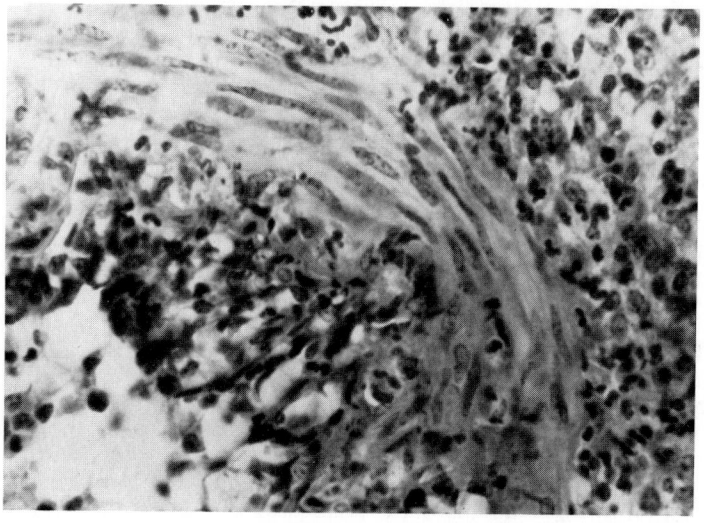

FIG. 11.5 Insert from Figure 11.4 enlarged to show proliferation and radial orientation of endothelial elements. Note polymorphs among perivascular cells (×500). (Photo by Dr. B. Schieman, 1969.)

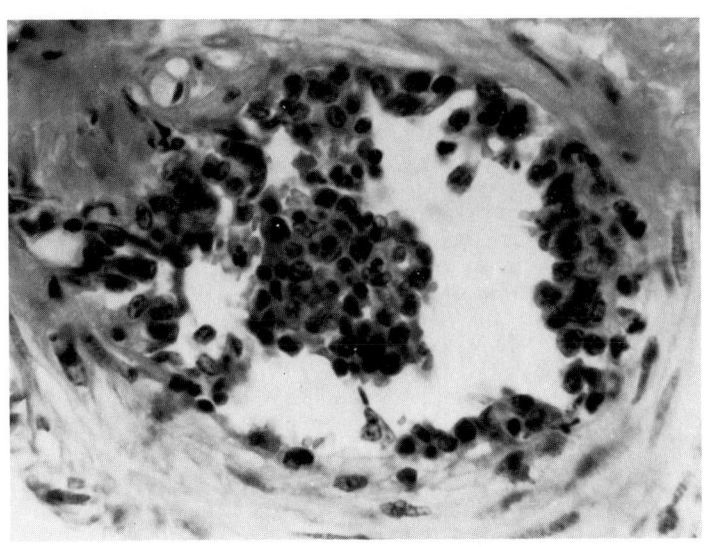

FIG. 11.6 Blood vessel in the mucosa covering the turbinate of an experimental ox. Proliferating endothelial cells block much of the lumen (×500). (Photo by Dr. B. Schieman, 1969.)

abnormal primitive mononuclear cells is observed; these are very difficult to classify. There is simultaneously a considerable increase in the number of macrophages and activated reticulum cells (Plowright 1953b; Jubb and Kennedy 1970). Increases in plasma cells and a broad and active paracortical (thymus-dependent) zone have been reported in cattle (Selman et al. 1974). Areas of semidiffuse, cortical necrosis occur occasionally in lymph nodes or hemolymph nodes, and fibrinoid degeneration of capsular and trabecular connective tissues or of blood vessel walls is not uncommon.

The meningoencephalomyelitis, which is a constant feature of MCF and useful in differential diagnosis, primarily affects the meninges and blood vessel elements; but degenerative changes do occur in neurons, and mononuclear cell infiltration of the choroid plexuses is frequent. The cytoplasmic inclusion bodies described by some authors in neurons of the medulla (Stenius 1952) are not specific for MCF. A remarkable feature of the wildebeest-derived disease is the absence of intranuclear inclusions or other cytological indications, such as syncytium formation, of a herpesvirus infection. It was suggested that the lesions were partially dependent on immunopathologic reactions, possibly associated with the long incubation period and prepatent viremia (Plowright 1968), since the vascular and lymphoreticular responses were manifestations of type III and IV responses of Gell and Coombes (1968; Rweyemamu et al. 1976; Selman et al. 1974). No evidence of antibody-containing complexes was demonstrated in the tissues of reacting rabbits.

The epithelial lesions of MCF are associated primarily with subepithelial edema, lymphoreticular cell infiltration, and degeneration of collagen as well as with the vascular changes. In the skin and other stratified squamous epithelia in particular, these lead to degeneration, microvesicle formation, erosion, and ulceration, usually with little polymorphonuclear reaction.

Cattle with MCF develop a progressive leukopenia from the time of appearance of the lymphadenopathy. All cell types are affected, but there is a relative mononucleosis with the appearance of large and atypical lymphoblasts; a complete eosinopenia and neutrophil shift to the left is usual. Rabbits sometimes show a massive terminal leukocytosis, primarily from large mononuclears (Plowright 1953a).

DIAGNOSIS. The clinical and pathologic findings in the head-and-eye form of MCF are readily recognizable. The combination of mucosal lesions with a bilateral centripetal keratitis, generalized lymphadenopathy, dermatitis, and frequent signs of involvement of the central nervous system should allow a rapid differentiation from mucosal disease and rinderpest. The almost invariable fatal outcome permits a confirmation of the diagnosis by the pathognomonic histopathologic lesions, especially the angiitis, lymphadenopathy, encephalomyelitis, and widespread accumulations of lymphoreticular cells in relation to blood vessels in mucosae and parenchymatous organs. In addition, the sporadic nature of the disease, usually with a history of association with sheep or wildebeest during the previous 2–6 months, and the failure of lateral spread in indicator species all strengthen the diagnosis.

Although the peracute and intestinal forms of the disease may not offer such an easy clinical diagnosis, the histopathology is always pathognomonic if a sufficient range of well-fixed tissues is available, the angiitis being a particularly characteristic feature.

Confirmation by virus recovery or demonstration of neutralizing or other antibodies is as yet only possible for wildebeest-derived cases. Infectivity is demonstrable only in very fresh tissues, especially in suspensions of blood leukocytes or lymph node or spleen cells that are produced in such a manner as to conserve maximum cell viability. Such suspensions may be stored with 10–20% glycerol or dimethyl sulfoxide for periods of months at −70°C or below. They should be injected into permissive cell cultures such as monolayers of calf thyroid or serially passaged calf testis cells; typical cytopathic effects (syncytium formation with Feulgen-positive, intranuclear inclusions) usually develop within 18–21 days (but often within 4–7 days). Moderate amounts of cell-free virus are demonstrable within a few passages, especially in calf testis cells, and can be neutralized by specific antiserum; the specificity of cytopathic effects can also be proved by immunofluorescence tests (Ferris et al. 1976; Wibberley 1976).

Antibody to the wildebeest virus can be detected in reservoir or indicator hosts by IIF tests as well as by VN (Plowright 1967; Reid et al. 1975). The former gives positive results in rabbits and cattle during the incubation period and before the onset of clinical signs. Neutralizing antibody appears later, being frequently absent at the time of death in cattle (Plowright 1968); it is invaluable for a survey of infection in wild reservoir hosts (Plowright 1967; Reid et al. 1975).

IMMUNITY. In wildebeest and other alcelaphine hosts, the calf normally receives passive neutralizing antibody from the dam, and the mean level in serum declines slowly to 4 months of age and then increases steadily from a mean titer of about $10^{-1.2}$ to $10^{-2.3}$ at 13–18 months (Plowright 1967). Thus active infection takes place in the presence of maternal antibody, which does not interfere significantly with the establishment of active immunity. Transfer of maternal antibody may fail for unknown reasons in calves of free-living wildebeest populations, but this does not appear to be associated with disease production in calves that acquire viremia. There is no evidence for the establishment of immunologic tolerance, even in wildebeest calves infected congenitally (Plowright 1967).

Significant clinical disease does not occur in natural reservoir hosts such as wildebeest (and presumably sheep), but persistent infection is frequent, as shown by the recovery of virus from adult animals and the undoubted occurrence of congenital infection of the fetus in older females. Cattle can remain infected at least 80 months after initial inapparent infection (Plowright et al. 1972), those that are affected clinically but recover remain viremic for some months and are solidly immune to parenteral challenge with cell-associated virus for at least 12 months in the absence of further stimulation. On repeated challenge, resistance lasts at least 11 years, and all wildebeest isolates appear to be immunologically homogeneous (Plowright 1968).

Attempts to immunize cattle against MCF have been made using both live attenuated virus and killed virus preparations. One strain of wildebeest virus (WC11) was still capable of causing lethal disease in cattle after 53–59 passages in calf kidney cells. After additional passages (21–30) in calf thyroid monolayers, the same virus, in a dose of $10^{3.8}$–$10^{6.0}$ TCD$_{50}$, was injected by various routes into 16 cattle. Only one showed a delayed, atypical reaction with perforating enteritis, but 11 succumbed to challenge at 56–70 days with virulent blood; the other 4 animals survived, 3 after some clinical reaction. As many as 75 serial rabbit passages failed to attenuate the virus for cattle (Plowright 1968). Reid and Rowe (1973) showed loss of virulence to cattle of a hartebeest isolate following 30 passages in bovine thyroid cells and showed protection against homologous virulent virus but not against wildebeest MCFV.

Formalin-inactivated or live virus, combined with Freund's incomplete adjuvant, produced a good neutralizing antibody response in cattle inoculated parenterally, but there was no significant protection against parenteral challenge with either cell-associated or cell-free virulent virus. It was concluded that neutralizing antibody was not an important component of the resistance mechanism in MCFV infections. More recent work, however, suggests that it may be possible to protect rabbits against parenteral challenge by repeated inoculations of inactivated virulent virus propagated in cell cultures and combined with Freund's complete adjuvant.

TREATMENT AND CONTROL. Intensive symptomatic, supportive, and antibacterial treatments have been widely applied to valuable zoo animals (Altmann et al. 1973), but cattle with typical MCF are seldom regarded as suitable subjects for therapy and may even be sent early for slaughter following confirmation of diagnosis.

Rapid and effective control of MCF can be obtained by preventing contact with reservoir hosts (wildebeest, other alcelaphine antelopes, or sheep and susceptible indicator species). Transfer of infection takes place in housed animals as well as those on pastures. In some instances indirect transfer through contaminated food or water may be implicated, but in cattle this is unusual.

Isolation of sick animals is desirable for treatment and esthetic reasons, but there are no firm indications of contact transmission among indicator hosts.

Infectious Bovine Rhinotracheitis

Synonyms: **None.**

Bovine herpesvirus 1 (BHV-1) is the cause of an infectious disease of the upper respiratory and genital tracts of cattle; it may also be associated with keratoconjunctivitis and encephalomyelitis in this species. It has been isolated from cases of respiratory disease in goats and cases of balanitis, vaginitis, and abortion in swine (Gibbs and Rweyemamu 1977).

DISTRIBUTION AND HOST RANGE. The virus of infectious bovine rhinotracheitis (IBR) and infectious pustular vulvovaginitis (IPV) in cattle is worldwide in distribution but variable in prevalence, as shown by antibody surveys.

In East Africa 24–82% of cattle more than 2 years old had neutralizing antibody for BHV-1, an observation that might explain the high prevalence in game animals (Jessett and Rampton 1975; Rweyemamu 1974).

Surveys in Africa for neutralizing antibody to IBRV have shown that infection with this or a serologically related virus is present in at least 14 free-living wild animal species (Table 11.4). The first reports were those of Kaminjola and Paulsen (1970) and Rweyemamu (1970, 1974). Infection was frequent in buffalo, eland, wildebeest, waterbuck, reedbuck, kob, and hippopotamus but absent in such species as giraffe and Grant's gazelle.

The only signs of disease attributed to the virus in wild species are those of a pustular vulvovaginitis that occurred in 12 of 12 adult female wildebeest treated with betamethasone

(Karstad et al. 1973; Mushi et al. 1978; Rweyemamu et al. 1974). Eight of these were captured and held in temporary pens in the Kajiado District of Kenya. The virus was isolated in these cases and identified by its neutralization with specific antiserum. The appearance of genital lesions presumably resulted from a recrudescence of active infection, such as can be regularly induced in cattle by the administration of corticosteroids. The rate of reactivation pointed to the almost universal presence of BHV-1 in adult female wildebeest from the Kajiado area of Kenya, where at least 56% of cattle more than 2 years old have serologic evidence of infection.

The absence of reported lesions in any wild species is probably a result of the usual need for the presence of extensive and severe disease before it can be observed. Mare (1971) was unable to produce disease in eland by inoculation of virus.

In North America, Hoff et al. (1973) reported the isolation of BHV-1 from pronghorn antelope; in Australia the virus was recovered from the prepuce of 3 of 18 buffalo (*Bubalis bubalis*) (St. George and Philpott 1972) in a population that had serologic evidence of widespread infection. Neutralizing antibody has also been found in the sera of 18 of 50 mule deer in Colorado (Chow and Davis 1964) and in whitetailed deer in New York State (Friend and Halterman 1967). In Canada sera from pronghorn antelope in Alberta and Saskatchewan were positive for neutralizing antibody (Barrett and Chalmers 1975) as were sera from red deer (*Cervus elaphus*) in Scotland (M. Lawman, personal communication, 1976).

Bovine Herpesvirus 2

Synonyms: **Bovine herpes mammillitis virus, Allerton virus.**

Bovine herpesvirus 2 (BHV-2) was first isolated in South Africa (Alexander et al. 1957), and is the cause of a generalized skin eruption of cattle known as pseudo-lumpy skin disease in Africa. It usually produces local vesicular and ulcerative lesions of the skin of the udder, teats, and occasionally the perineum (Gibbs and Rweyemamu 1977) or vulvovaginal mucosae (Povey and James 1973). It is also the cause of similar lesions of the stratified squamous epithelia of the muzzle, nares, mouth cavity,

TABLE 11.4   The Occurrence of Neutralizing Antibody to BHV-1 in Free-living African Game Animals.

Part of Continent[a]	Common Name	Genus and Species	No. Tested	% Positive	Titer Range[b]
E	buffalo	*Syncerus caffer*	140	64	0.48–1.68
S			1334	76	4–256
E	eland	*Taurotragus oryx*	80	43	0.48–1.74
S			31	32	8–22
E	wildebeest	*Connochaetes taurinus*	727	31	0.36–1.80
S			110	20	4–22
E	topi	*Damaliscus korrigum*	63	11	ND[c]
S			23	13	4–6
S	harbebeest	*Alcelaphus buselaphus*	11	45	6–22
S	sable antelope	*Hippotragus niger*	28	61	4–22
S	roan antelope	*H. equinus*	15	40	4–11
E	impala	*Aepyceros melampus*	268	3	0.60–1.56
S			272	0.4	6
E	kob	*Adenota kob*	22	23	ND
S			3	67	8
S	lechwe	*A. lechwe*	95	57	4–90
E	waterbuck	*Kobus ellipsiprymnus*	15	40	3.96–4.20
S			28	96	4–708
E	reedbuck	*Redunca redunca*	10	40	2.76–3.69
S		*R. arundinum*	10	80	32–708
E	Thomson's gazelle	*Gazella thomsonii*	242	20	0.48–1.20
E	hippopotomus	*Hippopotamus amphibius*	188	96	0.72–1.68
S			70	91	6–90

    [a] Figures for East Africa (E) are those provided by Rampton and Jessett (1976); those for South Africa (S) ("mainly"), by Hedger and Hamblin (1978).
    [b] For East Africa these are $\log_{10}$ SN_{50} titers in tube cultures; for South Africa, reciprocals of arithmetic 50% titers in microtiter trays.
    [c] No data.

and forestomachs of cattle. There is one record of naturally occurring, generalized lethal disease in wild buffalo (*Syncerus caffer*) with which this virus was associated in Tanzania, East Africa (Schiemann et al. 1971).

DISTRIBUTION AND HOST RANGE. Although originally regarded as having a restricted distribution, this virus has now been isolated from cattle in South, East, and Central Africa (Cilli and Castrucci 1976; Gibbs and Rweyemamu 1977; Hedger and Hamblin 1977); North America; Europe; and Australia. In the United Kingdom it has been encountered primarily as a cause of ulcerative or gangrenous lesions of the

skin of the udder and teats (Martin et al. 1974). Experimentally, pigs and perhaps sheep and goats develop mild skin lesions following inoculation; neonatal mice, rats, and hamsters develop severe infection, with skin lesions and a high mortality (Gibbs and Rweyemamu 1977). Rabbits and guinea pigs develop mild local lesions following intradermal inoculation.

Serologic surveys indicate that the virus is more widespread in cattle populations than would be expected from the morbidity figures. Tests for neutralizing antibody have shown that 19.5% of 400 bovine sera in western England were positive (Rweyemamu et al. 1969); in Italy, rates varied from 0 to 41.6%; in Bulgaria

23% of farms were affected but the sera from 1,000 cattle and sheep sera from West Germany were negative (Cilli and Castrucci 1976). In Tanzania nearly 84% of all bovine sera from two provinces were positive; the rate in animals less than 1 year old was greater than 70%, rising to 98% in adult cattle 4 years or older. In another province, however, the overall rate was only 20% (Plowright and Jessett 1971). The same authors also found rapid shifts in the proportion of young animals that were seropositive, suggesting the movement of a wave of infection through a large area, which was coincident with an epizootic in the neighboring Serengeti buffalo population. It was remarkable, however, that no disease attributable to BHV-2 had ever been reported in northern Tanzania; the same situation appears to hold in Zambia and Somalia where bovine infection rates varied from 65% to 95% (Cilli and Castrucci 1976; Hedger et al. 1977).

Based on serologic evidence there is virtually universal infection of buffalo (*Syncerus caffer*) populations in East Africa (Table 11.5), which corresponds to the infection rate in many of the local cattle populations. Only a few yearlings and two-year-old animals were devoid of antibody, it was clear that the infection had existed at least since 1967, whereas clinical disease was not present until 1969 in Tanzania and had never occurred in Uganda (Plowright and Jessett 1971).

Surveys for antibody in other game animal populations in East Africa that are in contact with heavily infected buffalo or cattle showed that infection with BHV-2 or a closely related virus probably occurs somewhat infrequently in the giraffe, waterbuck, and hippopotamus. In these species there was no obvious correlation of serologic positivity with age, and antibody titers tended to be low. Occasional positives were also found in eland, oryx, impala, bushbuck, and wildebeest (Table 11.6) but were absent in hartebeest, reedbuck, gazelle, kob, and warthog. Since it is now well established that BHV-2 shares common antigens with *Herpesvirus hominis* (herpes simplex) types 1 and 2, it is possible that different viruses that are serologically related to BHV-2 occur in these species.

TRANSMISSION. There is strong circumstantial evidence that BHV-2 is transmitted to cattle by biting insects and mechanical means such as milking machines. Thus persistence of virus in and transmission by *Byomyia fasciata* has been reported, and Gibbs and Rweyemamu (1977) summarized the evidence for insect transmission in Britain, especially by *Stomoxys calcitrans*. Vector involvement is favored by the reported failure of the infection to spread by contact in cattle; heavy infestations with ticks and lice were also observed on sick buffalo calves (Schiemann et al. 1971). Reactivation of latent infection may also be another means of introduction of the virus to new areas.

ETIOLOGY. The virus causing pseudo-lumpy skin disease and bovine herpes mammillitis is a typical fast-growing herpesvirus that produces large multinucleated syncytia, with Cowdry type A inclusions in many nuclei and a variable degree of cytoplasmic vacuolation. BHV-2 is released readily from infected cells, attaining titers on the order of 10^6 TCD_{50}/ml. A wide variety of cell cultures is susceptible; monolayers of primary bovine kidney or testis cells are perhaps the most suitable for isolation and propagation.

Reciprocal cross-neutralization and kinetic neutralization studies with isolates of different origin indicate that all strains are serologically very similar if not identical, although it is possible that the buffalo (BA) isolate of Schiemann et al. (1971) differs slightly from the others in kinetic neutralization and in cross-immuniza-

TABLE 11.5 Neutralizing Antibody to BHV-2 in East African Buffaloes.

	Country of Origin		
Age Group	Tanzania (Serengeti)	S. Kenya	W. Uganda
6 months	4/4	1/2	1/1
7–18 months	9/9	0/1	1/3
≥2 years	31/33	3/4	56/60

Source: Plowright and Jessett (1971).

TABLE 11.6   Neutralizing Antibody to BHV-2 in East African Game Animals.

Common Name	Genus and Species	No. Positive/ No. Tested	% Positive
Wildebeest	*Connochaetes taurinus*	2/162	1.2
Oryx	*Oryx beisa*	2/3	66
Bushbuck	*Tragelaphus scriptus*	1/8	12
Waterbuck	*Kobus ellipsiprymnus* *K. defassa*	4/14	29
Impala	*Aepyceros melampus*	2/67	3
Giraffe	*Giraffa camelopardalis*	5/33	15
Eland	*Taurotragus oryx*	1/19	5
Hippopotamus	*Hippopotamus amphibius*	20/199	10

Source: Plowright and Jessett (1971).

tion tests (Cilli and Castrucci 1976).

PATHOGENESIS AND CLINICAL SIGNS. The BHV-2 virus replicates and produces its effects primarily in stratified squamous epithelia of the skin and in upper alimentary and respiratory mucosae. It is possible that lesions of the lower genital tract occur occasionally. The propensity to produce a generalized skin eruption, as in pseudo-lumpy skin disease, appears to be unusual except for cattle and, rarely, buffalo in Africa.

In the single natural outbreak of disease recorded in buffalo in Tanzania, clinical signs were observed in several large herds in which young animals (6–12 months old) fell behind the rest and hid in scrub. A considerable mortality was thought to have occurred over a period of about 3 months (Schiemann et al. 1971).

Apart from general cachexia with signs of anemia—probably from helminthic, exoparasitic, and blood protozoal infections—the most striking lesions were well-defined ulcerations on the tongue, palate, and buccal mucosae, with raised edges and a diameter up to 4 cm (Fig. 11.7). Similar lesions were found in the esophagus and rumen (Fig. 11.8). Earlier lesions in one animal showed typical syncytial formations with intranuclear inclusions in the stratum germinativum and stratum spinosum, and tissues from this yielded BHV-2 (strain BA) on inoculation into cell cultures. No generalized skin lesions were observed, but these may have been obscured by reaction to ectoparasites (Schiemann et al. 1971).

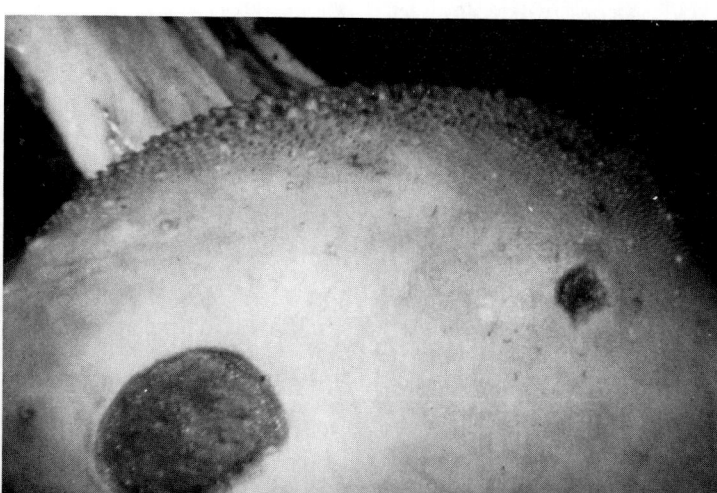

FIG. 11.7   Lateral aspect of the tongue of a Tanzanian buffalo (*Syncerus caffer*) with ulcerated areas showing early regrowth of epithelium. (Photo by Dr. B. Schieman, 1969.)

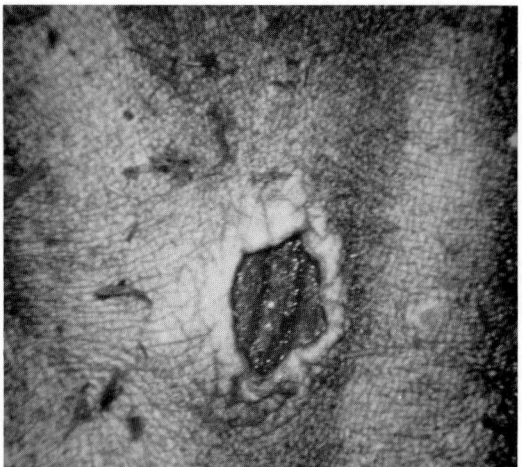

FIG. 11.8 Pillar of rumenal mucosa from another buffalo with a large ulcerated area and raised, well-defined edge. (Photo by Dr. B. Schieman, 1969.)

The BA strain of virus was inoculated intradermally and intravenously into a young, serologically negative buffalo, which exhibited a nearly lethal febrile reaction accompanied by nodules and ulceration of the skin and oral and nasal mucosae and, surprisingly, a keratoconjunctivitis. The skin eruption was generalized, and the lesions developed into areas of deep necrosis. Ticks (*Rhipicephalus appendiculatus*) placed on the buffalo 1 day after infection contained virus up to removal on the 13th day; a virus was present in skin lesions and oral and nasal swabs between days 3 and 10 (Schiemann et al. 1972).

Bovine Herpesvirus 3

Synonyms: **None.**

Although it is generally agreed that the herpesviruses included in this group are not significantly involved in any disease syndrome of cattle, they are isolated often enough from cattle skin lesions, blood, lymphoid tissues, and especially nasal swabs to cause confusion in diagnosis. They have no pathogenicity when inoculated into experimental cattle, sheep, and goats or laboratory hosts such as rabbits, guinea pigs, hamsters, rats, mice, and chickens. They grow readily if somewhat slowly in a wide variety of cell cultures, including bovine, ovine, caprine, and rabbit kidney cells, producing cy-

topathic effects that include formation of intranuclear inclusions of Cowdry type A, but syncytia are seldom if ever observed. Antibody is difficult to detect, but cross-reactions with the prototype strain (Movar 33/63) have been reported with use of neutralization or IIF techniques (Gibbs and Rweyemamu 1977).

Schieman et al. (1971) reported isolation of similar bovine herpesviruses from the lymphoid tissues of three buffaloes in an epidemic of lethal disease involving BHV-2. A similar virus was injected into a serologically negative buffalo, which became viremic but failed to show any clinical or serologic reaction.

Elephant (Loxodontal) Herpesvirus Infection

Synonyms: **None.**

During a cropping operation in the Kruger National Park, South Africa, it was found that 74% of 50 elephants (*Loxodonta africana*) had nodules in the lungs which consisted predominantly of solid masses of lymphoid cells that were sometimes spongy; they also had cavities surrounded by epithelial cells that frequently contained intranuclear inclusions of Cowdry type A and formed syncytial masses. These changes were typical of herpesviruses, and the identification was later proved by electron microscopic examination of the lesions and isolation of the virus.

L. Karstad (personal communication, 1978) reported that elephant lung tissue collected in Tanzania in 1967–1968 by J. G. Debbie contained similar lymphoid nodules with cytomegalic cells containing large intranuclear inclusion bodies.

ETIOLOGY. The herpesvirus associated with the lesions was isolated in monolayers of fetal horse and rabbit kidney cells and found to have the morphologic stability and growth characteristics of a herpesvirus (Erasmus et al. 1971).

PATHOLOGY. The nodules occurred in the lung substance, occasionally beneath bronchial mucosae; some were enveloped by fibrous tissue but were usually easily enucleated. Their diameter varied from 3 to 30 mm, and one to six nodules were found in each animal. Solid lymphoid nodules were most frequent in young animals; a spongy texture from cavities filled with air, fluid, or semifluid material was more common in old animals. The associated lymph nodes were sometimes hyperplastic, and several animals were later found to have foci in the pancreas (Basson et al. 1971).

Histologically the lymphoid nodules contained follicles, with germinal centers and epithelium-lined spaces, sometimes forming confluent cavities. The epithelial cells were apparently derived by metaplasia and hyperplasia of alveolar lining cells that became cuboidal or columnar, some with cytoplasmic vacuolation. Many contained increasingly dense intranuclear inclusions surrounded by a wide, clear halo. Proliferation of epithelial cells sometimes obliterated the cavities and gave rise to solid cords. Syncytium formation was common and eosinophilic bodies appeared in the cytoplasm of these masses.

The association of a herpesvirus with lymphoproliferative lesions and epithelialization of alveolar cells is particularly interesting in view of the possible relationship of pulmonary adenomatosis in sheep to another herpesvirus (Mackay 1969). In this instance (and in malignant catarrhal fever) no cytologic evidence of a herpesvirus infection has been observed.

DIAGNOSIS. No clinical signs are thought to be caused by the herpesvirus unless lesions are complicated by a possible secondary infection in young elephant calves.

The character of the lesions at necropsy can be readily recognized by the syncytia and intranuclear inclusions in epithelial cells. In favorable circumstances the virus can be isolated.

REFERENCES

Malignant Catarrhal Fever

Altmann, D., Kronberger, H., and Schuppel, K. F. Bosartiges Katarrhalfieber (*Coryza gangraenosa*) bei zwei Elchen, zwei Rentieren und eine Hausziege im Thuringer Zoopark Effurt. In *Proceedings of the 15th International Symposium on Diseases of Zoo Animals*, Kolmarden, pp. 41–49. Berlin: Akademie-Verlag, 1973.

Andersson, P. Bovine malignant catarrh in an elk. *Nord. Vet. Med.* 5:847–854, 1953. (Abstr. *Vet. Bull.* 24:305, 1954.

Balsai, A. Bosartiges Katarrhalfieber beim Wisent (*Bison bonasus*). In *Proceedings of the 15th International Symposium on Diseases of Zoo Animals*, Kolmarden, pp. 52–54. Berlin: Akademie-Verlag, 1973.

Berry, D. M., and Wibberley, G. Malignant catarrhal fever antiserum: A proposed international refer-

ence. *Vet. Rec.* 101:170–171, 1977.

Blood, D. C., Rowsell, H. C., and Savan, M. An outbreak of bovine malignant catarrh in a dairy herd: II. Transmission experiments. *Can. Vet. J.* 2:319–325, 1961.

Boever, W. J., and Kurka, B. Malignant catarrhal fever in greater kudus. *J. Am. Vet. Med. Assoc.* 165:817–819, 1974.

Clark, K. A., and Adams, L. G. Viral particles associated with malignant catarrhal fever in deer. *Am. J. Vet. Res.* 37:837–840, 1976.

Clark, K. A., Robinson, R. M., Marburger, R. G., Jones, L. P., and Orchard, J. H. Malignant catarrhal fever in Texas cervids. *J. Wildl. Dis.* 6:373–383, 1970.

Clark, K. A., Robinson, R. M., Weishuhn, L. L., and McConnell, A. Further observations on malignant catarrhal fever in Texas deer. *J. Wildl. Dis.* 8:72–74, 1972.

Cumming, R. G. *Five years of a hunter's life in the interior of South Africa*, vol. 2, p. 373. London: John Murray, 1950.

Danskin, D. Elementary bodies in bovine malignant catarrh. *Nature* 176:518, 1955.

Daubney, R. Suspected bovine malignant catarrh. *Vet. Rec.* 71:493, 1959.

Daubney, R., and Hudson, J. R. Transmission experiments with bovine malignant catarrh. *J. Comp. Pathol.* 49:63–89, 1936.

De Koch, G., and Neitz, W. O. Sheep as a reservoir host of snotsiekte (or bovine malignant catarrh of cattle) in South Africa. *S. Afr. J. Sci.* 46:176–180, 1950.

Dieckerhoff, W. Lehrbuch des Speziellen Pathologie und Therapie fur Tierarzt, 2d ed., vol. 2., pp. 97–112. Berlin: August Hirschwald, 1903.

Du Toit, P. J., and Alexander, R. A. Malignant catarrhal fever and similar diseases. *Proceedings of the 13th International Veterinary Congress*, Zurich. I:553–559, 1938.

Ferris, D. H., Hamdy, F. M., and Dardiri, A. H. Detection of African malignant catarrhal fever virus antigens in cell cultures by immunofluorescence. *Vet. Microbiol.* 1:437–448, 1976.

Gell, P. G. H., and Coombes, R. R. A. *Clinical aspects of immunology*. Oxford: Blackwell Scientific Publications, 1968.

Gotze, R. Untersuchungen uber das bosartige Katarrhalfieber des Rindes: III. *Dtsch. Tieraertzl. Wochenschr.* 38:487–491, 1930.

―――. Bosartige Katarrhalfieber: IV. Mitteilung. *Berl. Muench. Tieraertzl. Wochenschr.* 53: 848–855, 1932.

Gotze, R., and Liess, J. Erfolgreiche Ubertragungsversuche des bosartigen Katarrhalfieber von Rind zu Rind. Identitat mit dem sudafrikanischen Snotsiekte. *Dtsch. Tieraertzl. Wochenschr.* 37:433–437, 1929.

―――. Untersuchungen uber das bosartigen Katarrhalfieber des Rindes: II. Schafe als Ubertrager. *Dtsch. Tieraertzl. Wochenschr.* 38:194–200, 1930.

Hanichen, R., and Ernst, K. Bosartiges Katarrhalfieber bei Gaur und Bantengrindern. *Proceed-*

ings of the 11th International Symposium on Diseases of Zoo Animals, Zagreb, pp. 163–165, 1969.

Huck, R. A., Shand, A., Allsop, P. J., and Paterson, A. B. Malignant catarrh of deer. Vet. Rec. 73:457–465, 1961.

James, M. P., Neilson, F. J. A., and Stewart, W. J. An epizootic of malignant catarrhal fever: I. Clinical and pathological observations. New Zealand Vet. J. 23:9–12, 1975.

Jubb, K. V. F., and Kennedy, P. C. Pathology of domestic animals, 2d. ed., pp. 27–34. New York: Academic Press, 1970.

Kalunda, M. African malignant catarrhal fever; its biologic properties and the response of American cattle. Ph.D. thesis, Cornell University, 1975.

Mansjoer, M. Contribution to the knowledge of penjakit ingusan on cattle and buffaloes in Indonesia, especially the island of Lombok. Indonesian J. Anim. Sci. vol. 62, 1955. (Abstr. Vet. Bull. 25:621, 1955.)

Mettam, R. W. M. Snotsiekte in cattle. 9th and 10th Reports of the Director of Veterinary Education Research, Union of South Africa, pp. 395–432, 1923.

Morris, D. The mammals: A guide to the living species. London: Hodder and Stoughton, 1965.

Otte, W. Weitere Beitrage zur Aetiologie des bosartigen Katarrhalfiebers. Berl. Muench. Tieraertzl. Wochenschr. 44:875–877, 1928.

Piercy, S. E. Studies in bovine malignant catarrh: I. Experimental infection in cattle. Br. Vet. J. 108:35–47, 1952.

———. Studies on bovine malignant catarrh: V. The role of sheep in the transmission of the disease. Br. Vet. J. 110:508–516, 1954.

———. Studies in bovine malignant catarrh: VI. Adaptation to rabbits. Br. Vet. J. 111:484–491, 1955.

Pierson, R. E., Storz, J., McChesney, A. E., and Thake, D. Experimental transmission of malignant catarrhal fever. Am. J. Vet. Res. 35:523–525, 1974.

Pierson, E. E., Thake, D., McChesney, A. E., and Storz, J. An epizootic of malignant catarrhal fever in feedlot cattle. J. Am. Vet. Med. Assoc. 163:349–350, 1973.

Plowright, W. The blood leucocytes in infectious malignant catarrh of the ox and rabbit. J. Comp. Pathol. 63:318–334, 1953a.

———. The pathology of infectious bovine malignant catarrh in cattle and rabbits. Proceedings of the 15th International Veterinary Congress, Stockholm. 1:323–328, 1953b.

———. Studies on the virus of malignant catarrhal fever in Africa. Proceedings of the 17th Wildlife Veterinary Congress, Hannover, 1963, vol. 2, pp. 519–523, 1963.

———. Studies on malignant catarrhal fever of cattle. D.V.Sc. thesis, University of Pretoria, South Africa, 1964.

———. Malignant catarrhal fever in East Africa: I. Behaviour of the virus in freeliving populations of blue wildebeest (Gorgon taurinus, taurinus Burchell). Res. Vet. Sci. 6:56–68, 1965a.

———. Malignant catarrhal fever in East Africa: II. Observations on wildebeest calves at the laboratory and contact transmission of the infection to cattle. Res. Vet. Sci. 6:69–83, 1965b.

———. Malignant catarrhal fever in East Africa: III. Neutralising antibody in freeliving wildebeest. Res. Vet. Sci. 8:129–136, 1967.

———. Malignant catarrhal fever. J. Am. Vet. Med. Assoc. 152:795–804, 1968.

Plowright, W., Ferris, R. D., and Scott, G. R. Blue wildebeest and the aetiological agent of malignant catarrhal fever. Nature 188:1167–1169, 1960.

Plowright, W., Herniman, K. A. J., Jessett, D. M., Kalunda, M., and Rampton, C. S. Immunization of cattle against the herpes-virus of malignant catarrhal fever: Failure of inactivated culture vaccines with adjuvant. Res. Vet. Sci. 19: 159–166, 1975.

Plowright, W., Kalunda, M., Jessett, D. M., and Herniman, K. A. J. Congenital infection of cattle with the herpesvirus causing malignant catarrhal fever. Res. Vet. Sci. 13:37–45, 1972.

Plowright, W., Macadam, R. F., and Armstrong, J. A. Growth and characterization of the virus of bovine malignant catarrhal fever in East Africa. J. Gen. Microbiol. 39:253–266, 1965.

Reid, H. W., Plowright, W., and Rowe, L. W. Neutralising antibody to herpesviruses derived from wildebeest and hartebeest in wild animals in East Africa. Res. Vet. Sci. 18:269–273, 1975.

Reid, H. W., and Rowe, L. W. The attenuation of a herpes virus (malignant catarrhal fever virus) isolated from hartebeest (Alcelaphus buselaphus Cokei Gunther). Res. Vet. Sci. 15:144–146, 1973.

Rinjard, P. Contribution a l 'etude de l 'etiologie du coryza gangreneux: Conditions de conservation du virus. Rec. Med. Vet. 111:391–406, 1935.

Roken, B. O., and Bjorklund, N-E. Elakartad katarrhalfeber i en djurpark. Proceedings of the 12th Nordic Veterinary Congress, Reykjavik, pp. 197–198. Copenhagen: Carl Mortsen, 1974.

Rossiter, P., Mushi, E. Z., and Plowright, W. The development of antibodies in rabbits and cattle infected experimentally with an African strain of malignant catarrhal fever virus. Vet. Microbiol. 2:57–66, 1977.

Ruth, G. R., Reed, D. E., Daley, C. A., Vorkies, M. W., Wohlgemuth, K., and Shave, H. Malignant catarrhal fever in bison. J. Am. Vet. Med. Assoc. 171:913–917, 1977.

Rweyemamu, M. M., Karstad, L., Mushi, E. Z., Otema, J. C., Jessett, D. M., Rowe, L., Drevemo, S., and Grootenhuis, J. G. Malignant catarrhal fever virus in nasal secretions of wildebeest: A probable mechanism for virus transmission. J. Wildl. Dis. 10:478–487, 1974.

Rweyemamu, M. M., Mushi, E. Z., Rowe, L. W., and Karstad, L. Persistent infection of cattle with the herpesvirus of malignant catarrhal fever and observations on the pathogenesis of the disease.

Br. Vet. J. 132:392–400, 1976.

Sanford, S. E., Little, P. B., and Rapley, W. A. The gross and histopathological lesions of malignant catarrhal fever in three captive Sika deer (*Cervus nippon*) in Southern Ontario. *J. Wildl. Dis.* 13:29–32, 1977.

Selman, I. E., Wiseman, A., Murray, M., and Wright, N. G. A clinico-pathological study of bovine malignant catarrhal fever in Great Britain. *Vet. Rec.* 94:483–490, 1974.

Selman, I. E., Wiseman, A., Wright, N. G., and Murray, M. Transmission studies with bovine malignant catarrhal fever. *Vet. Rec.* 102:252–257, 1978.

Simpson, G. G. The principles of classification and a classification of mammals. *Bull. Am. Mus. Nat. Hist.* 85:1–350, 1945.

Skinner, M. F. The prong-horn. *J. Mammal.* 3:82–105, 1922.

Snowden, W. A. Bovine malignant catarrh, p. 16. *Annual Report, Anim. Health CSIRO,* Australia, 1972.

Stenius, P. I. *Bovine malignant catarrh: A statistical, histopathological and experimental study.* Helsinki: Institute of Pathology, Veterinary College, 1952.

Storz, J., Okuna, N., NcChesney, A. E., and Pierson, R. E. Virologic studies on cattle with naturally occurring and experimentally induced malignant catarrhal fever. *Am. J. Vet. Res.* 37:875–878, 1976.

Tong, E. H., Senior, M., and Halnan, C. R. E. An outbreak of malignant catarrh among the Pere David deer. *Proc. Zool. Soc. (Lond.)* 136:477–483, 1961.

Wibberley, G. Observations on two strains of bovine malignant catarrhal fever virus in tissue culture. *Res. Vet. Sci.* 21:105–107, 1976.

Wobeser, G., Majka, J. A., and Milla, J. H. L. A disease resembling malignant catarrhal fever in captive white-tailed deer in Saskatchewan. *Can. Vet. J.* 14:106–109, 1973.

Wyand, D. S., Helmboldt, C. F., and Nielson, S. W. Malignant catarrhal fever in white-tailed deer. *J. Am. Vet. Med. Assoc.* 159:605–610, 1971.

Wyssman, E. Bosartiges Katarrhalfieber und ahnliche Krankheiten. *Proceedings of the 13th International Veterinary Congress,* Zurich, 1938. I:560–569, 1938.

Zanzucchi, A. Ricerche epidemiologiche, etiopathogenetiche cliniche ed anatomopathologiche sulla febre catarrhale maligna. *Clin. Vet. Milano* 57:689–721, 1934.

Infectious Bovine Rhinotracheitis

Barrett, M. W., and Chalmers, G. A. A serologic survey of pronghorns in Alberta and Saskatchewan, 1970–1972. *J. Wildl. Dis.* 11:157–163, 1975.

Chow, T. L., and Davis, R. W. The susceptibility of mule deer to infectious bovine rhinotracheitis. *Am. J. Vet. Res.* 25:518–519, 1964.

Friend, M., and Halterman, L. G. Serologic survey of two deer herds in New York State. *Bull. Wildl. Dis. Assoc.* 3:32–34, 1967.

Gibbs, E. P. J., and Rweyemamu, M. M. Bovine herpesviruses: I. Bovine herpesvirus 1. *Vet. Bull.* 47:317–343, 1977.

Hedger, R. S., and Hamblin, C. Neutralizing antibodies to bovid herpesvirus 1 in African wildlife with special reference to the Cape buffalo (*Syncerus caffer*). *J. Comp. Pathol.* 88:211–218, 1978.

Hoff, G. L., Richards, S. H., and Trainer, D. O. Epizootic of haemorrhagic disease in N. Dakota deer. *J. Wildl. Manag.* 37:331–335, 1973.

Jessett, D. M., and Rampton, C. S. The incidence of antibody to infectious bovine rhinotracheitis virus in Kenyan cattle. *Res. Vet. Sci.* 18:225–226, 1975.

Kaminjolo, J. S., and Paulsen, J. The occurrence of virus-neutralizing antibodies to infectious bovine rhinotracheitis virus in sera from hippotomi and buffaloes. *Zentralbla. Veterinaermed. [B]* 17:864–868, 1970.

Karstad, A., Drevemo, S., Otema, J. C., and Jessett, D. M. Vulvovaginitis in wildebeest caused by the virus of infectious bovine rhinotracheitis. *J. Wildl. Dis.* 10:392–396, 1973.

Mare, C. J. Susceptibility of the common eland to infectious bovine rhinotracheitis virus. *J. Am. Vet. Med. Assoc.* 159:614–616, 1971.

Mushi, E. Z., Karstad, L., Jessett, D. M., and Rossiter, P. B. Observations on the epidemioloy of the herpesvirus of infectious bovine rhinotracheitis/infectious pustular vulvovaginitis in wildebeest. Submitted for publication. *J. Wildl. Dis.*

Rampton, C. S., and Jessett, D. M. The prevalence of antibody to infectious bovine rhinotracheitis virus in some game animals of East Africa. *J. Wildl. Dis.* 12:2–6, 1976.

Rweyemamu, M. M. Probable occurrence of infectious bovine rhinotracheitis virus in Tanzanian wildlife and cattle. *Nature* 225:738, 1970.

———The incidence of infectious bovine rhinotracheitis antibody in Tanzanian game animals and cattle. *Bull. Epizoot. Dis. Afr.* 22:19–22, 1974.

Rweyemamu, M. M., Karstad, L., Mushi, E. Z., Otema, J. C., Jesset, D. M., Rowe, L., Drevemo, S., and Grootenhuis, J. G. Malignant catarrhal fever virus in nasal secretions of wildebeest: A probable mechanism for virus transmission. *J. Wildl. Dis.* 10:478–487, 1974.

St. George, T. D., and Philpott, M. Isolation of infectious bovine rhinotracheitis virus from the prepuce of water buffalo bulls in Australia. *Aust. Vet. J.* 48:126, 1972.

Bovine Herpesviruses 2 and 3

Alexander, R. A., Plowright, W., and Haig, D. A. Cytopathogenic agents associated with lumpy-skin disease of cattle. *Bull. Epizoot. Dis. Afr.* 5:489–492, 1957.

Cilli, V., and Castrucci, G. Infection of cattle with bovine herpesvirus 2. *Folia Vet. Lat.* 6:1–44, 1976.

Gibbs, E. P. J., and Rweyemamu, M. M. Bovine herpesviruses: II. Bovine herpesviruses 2 and 3. *Vet. Bull.* 47:411–425, 1977.

Hedger, R. S., Hamblin, C., and Akefekwa, G. I. The isolation of bovid herpesvirus 2 from cattle in Zambia. *Vet. Rec.* 101:525–526, 1977.

Martin, W. B., Martin, B., and Lauder, I. M. Ulceration of cows' teats caused by a virus. *Vet. Rec.* 76:15–16, 1974.

Plowright, W., and Jessett, D. M. Investigations of Allerton-type herpes virus infection in East African game animals and cattle. *J. Hyg.* 69:209–222, 1971.

Povey, R. C., and James, Z. H. Bovine herpes mammillitis virus and vulvovaginitis. *Vet. Rec.* 92:232–233, 1973.

Rweyemamu, M. M., Johnson, R. H., and Laurillard, R. E. Serologic findings on bovine herpes mammillitis. *Br. Vet. J.* 125:317, 1969.

Schiemann, B., Plowright, W., and Jessett, D. M. Allerton-type herpesvirus as a cause of lesions of the alimentary tract in a severe disease of Tanzanian buffaloes (*Syncerus caffer*). *Vet. Rec.* 89:17–22, 1971.

Schiemann, B., Gwamaka, B., and Kalunda, M. Pathogenicity for a buffalo (*Syncerus caffer*) of Allerton-type herpesvirus isolated from a Tanzanian buffalo. *J. Wildl. Dis.* 8:141–145, 1972.

Elephant (Loxodontal) Herpesvirus Infection

Basson, P. A., McCully, R. M., De Vos, V., Young, E., and Kruger, S. P. Some parasitic and other natural diseases of the African elephant in the Kruger National Park. *Onderstepoort J. Vet. Res.* 38:239–254, 1971.

McCully, R. M., Basson, P. A., Pienaar, J. G., Erasmus, B. J., and Young, E. Herpes nodules in the lung of the African elephant (*Loxodonta africana;* Blumenbach, 1797). *Onderstepoort J. Vet. Res.* 38:225–236, 1971.

Mackay, J. M. K. Tissue culture studies of sheep pulmonary adenomatosis (jaagsiekte). *J. Comp. Pathol.* 79:141–146, 147–154, 1969.

12 Other Poxvirus Infections

THOMAS M. YUILL

A number of poxviruses have been described in free-ranging and captive wild mammals. This chapter discusses some of those pox viral infections, other than the fibromas-myxoma viruses, for which there is some evidence (either virus isolation or antibodies) for infection in the wild.

Monkeypox

Synonyms: **None.**

HISTORY AND DISTRIBUTION. Outbreaks of severe poxlike disease have been reported in free-living monkeys in India, Brazil, Panama, and Trinidad. However, the etiology of these epizootics was not established (Arita and Henderson 1968). The first confirmed outbreak of monkeypox occurred in cynomolgous monkeys (*Macaca iris*) in the Copenhagen zoo in 1958 (von Magnus et al. 1959). Subsequently, there were nine outbreaks in captive nonhuman primates through 1968, in the Netherlands, France, and the United States (McConnell et al. 1962; Prier and Sauer 1960; Arita et al. 1972). The virus was isolated from the tissues of apparently normal West and central African wild primates, suggesting that the virus is enzootic there (Ladnyj et al. 1972; Marennikova et al. 1972b; Shelukhina et al. 1975). In these same areas in Africa, there have been 35 human monkeypox cases with six deaths (Breman et al. 1977b; Center for Disease Control 1979).

ETIOLOGY. The virus is morphologically typical of poxviruses, measuring 200 by 250 nm (von Magnus et al. 1959). The biological characteristics (growth and lesions in embryonated chicken eggs, RK-13 rabbit continuous cell cultures, and the skin of live rabbits) of the monkeypox virus strains studied are identical (Rondle and Sayeed 1972), with the exception of a "white pox" virus strain recovered from cell cultures from normal cynomolgous monkeys (Gispen and Brand-Saathof 1972). Monkeypox virus is similar to variola and vaccinia viruses, but it is unique in its ability to produce hemorrhagic lesions in the skin of rabbits (Gispen et al. 1967). There is some antigenic similarity between these three viruses; cross-reaction occurs in hemagglutination inhibition (HI) and neutralization tests.

HOSTS AND TRANSMISSION. The 1959 outbreak in the Rotterdam zoo illustrates the broad host range of monkeypox virus. The index cases were two giant anteaters (*Myrmecophaga tridactyla*). The virus later spread throughout the monkey house, involving orangutans (*Pongo pygmaeus*), chimpanzees (*Pan troglodytes*), a white-handed gibbon (*Hylobates lar*), gorillas (*Gorilla gorilla*), vervet monkeys (*Cercopithecus hamlyni*), squirrel monkeys (*Saimiri sciurus*), and a marmoset (*Callithrix jacchus*) (Peters 1966). Four of 10 outbreaks in primate colonies occurred in cynomolgous monkeys, and the virus has been isolated from cell cultures from this species, but there is no evidence to suggest that these monkeys are infected in the wild (Arita et al. 1972; McConnell et al. 1962). An outbreak also occurred in a colony of Indian langurs, with deaths of infected *Presbytis entellus* and *P. cristatus* (Espana, 1971b). Antibodies have been found in apparently healthy zoo primates, including talapoins (*Cercopithecus talapoin*), cotton-top marmosets (*Saguinus oedipus*), and greater bushbabies (*Galago crassicaudatus*), indicating that asymptomatic infection (Kalter et al. 1974) or mild undetected disease occurs. Baboons (*Papio cynocephalus*) developed clinical disease following experimental inoculation with the virus, and the infection spread to other baboons housed in the same room, presumably via aerosols (Heberling and Kalter 1971). Rhesus (*Macaca mulatta*) and cynomolgous monkeys have been infected experimentally also, as have rabbits, suckling mice and rats; guinea pigs and hamsters developed antibody but no lesions following inoculation with monkeypox virus (Gispen et al. 1967; Lourie et al. 1972; Marennikova and Seluhina 1976).

The epizootiology of monkeypox virus is not well understood. In parts of central and West Africa, neutralizing and hemagglutination-inhibiting antibody has been found in wild subhuman primates, including chimpanzees, *Cercopithecus aethiops, Cer. mona, Cer. petaurista, Cer. diana, Cer. nictitans, Colobus badius,* and *Col. polykromos* (Gipsen et al. 1976; Breman et al. 1977a,b). Human infection has occurred in rural areas of West and central Africa. The source of these infections presumably was wild primates or other infected wildlife. Human-to-human transmission is not common; only two possible such cases have been reported (Arita and Henderson 1976; Center for Disease Control 1979). Antibodies have been found in wild mammals in the areas where human cases occurred. Neutralizing and HI antibodies were detected in sera from pangolins (*Phataginus tricuspis*), African giant squirrels (*Protexerus strangeri*), a field mouse (*Crocidura* spp.), the multimammate mouse (*Mastomys* spp.), a rusty-bellied rat (*Lophuromys sikapusi*), blue duiker (*Cephalophus monticola*), and two bird species, in addition to *Cercopithecus* monkeys (Breman et al. 1977b). However, these latter results should be interpreted with some caution because of the possibility of serologic cross-reactions with other members of the orthopox virus group. Isolation of monkeypox virus from chimpanzees and monkeys in Africa provides further evidence of the healthy carrier state in nature (Foster et al. 1972) and helps to provide a logical explanation for the sudden appearance of outbreaks in captive animals.

PATHOLOGY. Both naturally and experimentally infected captive primates have similar gross lesions, but the severity may vary with the species, the given individual, and the occurrence of secondary bacterial infection (Gispen et al. 1967; Wenner et al. 1968, 1969a,b). Mortality may be low; in a large rhesus colony in Pennsylvania, morbidity was approximately 10%, while mortality was less than 5% (Sauer et al. 1960). Papules appear on the face, in the mouth and on the tongue, arms, soles of the feet, palms of the hands, and sometimes on the trunk. In severe cases, internal organs are affected, and lesions may resemble those of smallpox in humans. In the liver, fat accumulates in parenchymal cells, there may be focal to scattered necrosis of hepatocytes, and proliferation or pycnosis of sinusoid epithelium with lymphatic infiltration. Large mononuclear cells may be present, some of which may have a rim of basophilic cytoplasm similar to that found in Councilman cells. Characteristic interstitial nephritis with mononuclear infiltrates is seen in the kidneys. Subcortical edema and hyperemia of the vasa recta, with lymphocytes and some eosinophils, are present. Either mitosis or necrosis may occur in renal tubules. In the spleen, there may be swelling and proliferation or pycnosis of the endothelium of the red pulp. In the lung, there may be focal intra-alveolar edema and swelling, with epithelial desquamation. Polymorphonuclear infiltrates are observed in the alveolar walls.

DIAGNOSIS. The appearance of characteristic pox lesions in several primate species point to monkeypox. Rapid tentative diagnosis can be made by silver staining of vesicular fluids from poxlike lesions to demonstrate elementary bodies (Gispen et al. 1967). Definitive diagnosis requires isolation and characterization of the virus (Prier et al. 1960). Variolalike pocks with microscopic acidophilic poxlike inclusions are produced following inoculation of virus-containing material onto the chorioallantoic membrane of embryonated chicken eggs. Cytopathic effect (CPE) occurs in inoculated monkey, pig, or rabbit kidney cell cultures. Monkeypox virus can be differentiated from variola or cowpox viruses on the basis of ceiling temperatures, characteristic hemorrhagic monkeypox lesions in rabbit skin following intradermal inoculation, serial propagation of the virus in rabbit skin or rabbit cell cultures, and the production of CPE in pig embryo kidney cells (von Magnus et al, 1959; Marennikova et al. 1972a). Agar gel has been used to identify isolates, although partial cross-reactions may occur with other viruses of the group (Gispin 1972). Serologic diagnosis may also be established on the basis of a significant rise in complement-fixing or neutralizing antibodies (Hall et al. 1973; Heberling and Kalter 1971).

TREATMENT AND CONTROL. Control of monkeypox virus infection in wild primates or other wildlife is not practical. However, captive primates can be protected from monkeypox infection by vaccination with vaccinia virus (Gispen et al. 1967; McConnell et al. 1964). Noninfectious subunit antigen prepared from a soluble fraction of disrupted virions also provided protection from live virus challenge (Olsen et al. 1977). Antibiotics may be useful in cases of secondary bacterial infection.

Yaba

Synonyms: **None.**

HISTORY AND DISTRIBUTION. Yaba virus infection was first recognized in a rhesus monkey colony in Yaba, Nigeria, where it caused an outbreak of subcutaneous tumors (Andrewes et al. 1959). The only other reported outbreak was in another rhesus monkey colony but may have been of laboratory origin, rather than the result of transmission from carrier animals (Ambrus et al. 1969). Serologic evidence indicates that Yaba virus occurs naturally in wild African and Southeast Asian primates, but Yabalike tumors have not been reported in free-ranging animals (Downie 1974; Tsuchiya and Tagaya 1971).

ETIOLOGY. Yaba virus has characteristic poxvirus morphology (de Harven and Yohn 1966). Although both Yaba and Tanapox viruses cause tumors in monkeys, cross-react serologically (Espana 1971a; Nicholas 1970), and provide partial reciprocal protection to challenge (Downie and Espana 1973), they have been shown to be clearly different viruses (Downie and Espana 1972, 1973). There is some serologic cross-reaction with vaccinia virus, also (Olsen and Yohn 1970; Olsen et al. 1971). However, vaccinia- or monkeypox-immune primates are susceptible to experimental Yaba virus infection (Nicholas and McNulty 1968; von Magnus et al. 1959).

HOSTS AND TRANSMISSION. The epidemiology of Yaba virus in nature has not been established. The first outbreak occurred in rhesus monkeys, an Asian species, housed in an outdoor colony in Africa (Bearcroft and Jamieson 1958). The source of the virus was not determined. Colony outbreaks have occurred mainly in rhesus monkeys and in *Macaca nemestrina*, as well as baboons (*Papio nigerae*) and a young *P. papio* (Ambrus et al. 1963; Andrewes et al. 1959; Niven et al. 1961). No direct transmission among cage mates occurred; biting arthropods were suspected virus vectors. One person exposed to the virus in the laboratory was infected, and humans have been shown to be susceptible to experimental infection (Grace and Mirand 1963). Other experimentally infected primate species include *M. fasicularis* and *Cercopithecus aethiops* (Ambrus et al. 1963; Wolfe et al. 1968b). New World monkeys and laboratory mice and rabbits did not develop lesions following inoculation with the virus (Bearcroft and Jamieson 1958; Espana 1971b; Niven et al. 1961; Yohn et al. 1964).

Yaba virus-neutralizing antibody was found in *C. aethiops, Erythrocebus patas, P. anubis, Colobus* spp., the chimpanzee from Africa, and in cynomolgous monkeys from Malaysia, but not in Indian rhesus monkeys or in several South American primates (Downie 1974; Tsuchiya and Tagaya 1971).

The virus replicates in *Cercopithecus* spp. kidney and fetal human kidney primary cell cultures, and in LLC-MK$_2$ and BSC-1 monkey cell lines (Downie and Espana, 1973; Levinthal and Schein 1964; Noyes 1965).

PATHOLOGY. Rhesus monkeys in the outdoor colony in Nigeria developed subcutaneous tumors 25–45 mm in diameter and 25 mm high. The tumors often became ulcerated. The tumors were associated with the lymphatics of the nose, hands, feet, and limbs, and involved the mesodermal tissues mainly, without affecting the overlying epithelium (Downie and Espana 1972). The tumor mass was made up of pleomorphic cells, some with eosinophilic cytoplasmic inclusions (Bearcroft and Jamieson 1958; Behbehani et al. 1968). General cellular degeneration, rather than necrotic foci, was characteristic of the regression phase (Sproul et al. 1963). Inoculation of monkeys with tumor tissue suspensions resulted in the formation of histiocytomas in the skin, subcutaneous spaces, and the visceral organs. Infection with aerosolized virus produced pulmonary, nasal, and subcutaneous tumors that were invasive to bronchioles, lymphatics, and blood vessels (Wolfe et al. 1968b). The tumors regressed within 1–2 months.

DIAGNOSIS. The virus can be isolated from tumor tissue by inoculation of BSC-1 cells. Infected cells have characteristic focal proliferation (Downie and Espana 1973). Viral antigens in tumor tissue can be demonstrated by immunodiffusion (Olsen and Yohn 1970). Yaba virus infection can be diagnosed by a significant rise in complement-fixing and neutralizing antibody (Hall et al. 1973; Wolfe et al. 1968a). However, complement-fixing antibody response is not correlated with development or regression of the tumors (Behbehani et al. 1968; Metzgar et al. 1962).

TREATMENT AND CONTROL. The rarity of Yaba virus outbreaks have not prompted any special control measures. Ambrus et al. (1969)

suggested thorough cleaning and disinfection of animal quarters and arthropod control. Secondary bacterial infection may be treated with antibiotics.

Tanapox

Synonyms: **None.**

HISTORY AND DISTRIBUTION. Tanapox virus infection (benign epidermal monkeypox) was first recognized in 1957 and was seen again in 1963 among people living along the Tana River in Kenya (Downie et al. 1971). Later, several outbreaks of Tanapox occurred in the United States among captive primates, with spread to humans (Casey et al. 1967; Crandell et al. 1969; Espana 1971b; Hall and McNulty 1967; Nicholas and McNulty 1967).

ETIOLOGY. Virus recovered from human and primate colony cases was shown to be a poxvirus (Downie et al. 1971; Espana et al. 1971), differentiable from Yaba virus or other poxviruses of man (Downie and Espana 1972). The original African human strain is serologically identical to the strains from outbreaks in captive primates in California and Oregon (Downie and Espana 1972).

HOSTS AND TRANSMISSION. The source of human Tanapox in Africa is unknown but is presumed to have been wild primates. The outbreaks followed periods of flooding when people and animals were crowded on islands along the river. *Mansonia* spp. mosquitoes were suspected vectors (Downie et al. 1971). Outbreaks have occurred in nonhuman primates in captivity but have not been detected in the wild. Disease has occurred most frequently in rhesus monkeys, and also in *Macaca speciosa, M. nemistrina, M. radiata, M. iris, Presbytis entellus,* and *Cyanopithecus niger,* and in humans, primarily animal caretakers (Crandell et al. 1969; Espana 1971b; Hall and McNulty 1967; McNulty et al. 1968). Several other primate species and laboratory mammals did not develop lesions following inoculation (Espana, 1971b; Hall and McNulty, 1967), although curiously, nodules did occur in the German checker rabbit (Crandell et al. 1969).

Neutralizing antibody has been found in *Cercopithecus aethiops, Erythrocebus patas, Papio anubis, Colobus* spp., and chimpanzees

from Africa, and in *Macaca iris* from Malaysia, but not in *M. mulatta* from India or in various primates from South America (Downie 1974).

The virus has been grown in several cell cultures, including human thyroid, BSC-1, vervet monkey kidney (Downie and Espana 1972), embryonic rhesus monkey kidney, and African green monkey kidney (Espana et al. 1971).

PATHOLOGY. In primates, the growths occurred on the face and limbs, and the animals did not behave as though ill (Espana, 1971b). The epidermal acanthosis is similar in both naturally infected primates and humans (Casey et al. 1967; Crandell 1969). The tumors are flat, approximately 10 mm in diameter, and up to 3 mm high. The epidermis is hyperplastic. Epidermal and hair follicle cells balloon, cytoplasm and nucleus are vacuolated, and granular pleomorphic eosinophilic cytoplasmic inclusion bodies occur (Wolfe et al. 1968b). There are few infiltrates into the dermis (Downie et al. 1971; McNulty et al. 1968). Later, lesions may become secondarily infected by bacteria, and a fibrinonecrotic exudate may be seen, with an intense inflammatory reaction in the underlying dermis (Kupper et al. 1970). In cell cultures, ultrastructurally, two types of intracytoplasmic virus "factories" may be seen. Tanapox virus, unlike Yaba virus, develops myelin figures and cylindrical tubules within the cell (Espana et al. 1971).

DIAGNOSIS. Diagnosis can be established by isolation of the virus in cell cultures. In BSC-1 cells, Tanapox virus produces a granular response, with nuclear vacuoles, followed by cell degeneration (Downie and Espana 1973). Serologic diagnosis can be established by a significant rise in neutralizing and complement-fixing antibodies to the virus (Downie and Espana 1972; Hall et al. 1973; Nicholas 1970).

TREATMENT AND CONTROL. No satisfactory methods for treatment or prevention have been developed. Antibiotics may be used for treatment of secondary bacterial infection.

Gerbilpoxes

Synonyms: **None.**

A poxvirus was isolated from an apparently healthy wild gerbil (*Tatera kempii*) from Nigeria (Lourie et al. 1975). The virus is of typical orthopox morphology, but differs from ectromelia, rabbitpox, vaccinia, monkeypox, and cowpox based on pocks on the chorioallantois of chicken eggs, ceiling temperatures, and susceptibility of mice, rabbits, and cell cultures to infection. However, by agar gel precipitation there is some antigenic relationship of gerbilpox virus with monkeypox, vaccinia, and variola. The extent and significance of infection in wild gerbil populations and its mode of transmission are unknown.

Poxvirus was also isolated from apparently healthy big gerbils (*Rhombomys opimus*) and yellow susliks (*Citellus fulvus*) captured in Turkmenistan, USSR. This virus is similar to one isolated from felids and giant anteaters in the Moscow zoo and white rats, to "whitepox" from primates, and to the African gerbilpox virus. Experimental inoculation of big gerbils and yellow susliks produced disseminated disease (Marennikova 1979).

Raccoonpox

Synonyms: **None.**

Raccoonpox virus was isolated from upper respiratory tissue from two raccoons (*Procyon lotor*) in a field survey (Alexander et al. 1972). These animals were captured in a mixed forest-grassland area near Aberdeen, Maryland. No disease was reported in these raccoons. Hemagglutination-inhibiting antibody was found in 22 of 92 (24%) raccoons captured in the same area. The virus produced cell rounding and granularity in monkey kidney cell cultures and pocks on the choriollantoic membrane of embryonated chicken eggs. There was some reciprocal serologic cross-reactivity between hemagglutinating antigens and antisera of raccoonpox and vaccinia viruses, but not between raccoonpox and monkeypox viruses. Other characteristics of the virus and its natural history, pathogenesis, and impacts on raccoon populations have not been reported.

Marsupial Pox

Synonyms: **None.**

Epidermal papillomas were described in quokka (*Setonix brachyurus*) on Rottnest Island, off of the coast of Western Australia (Papadimitriou and Ashman 1972). The papillomas were up to 50 mm in size and were usually located on the dorsum of the tail of these marsupials. The lesions were characterized by hyperkeratosis and acanthosis, with thickened rete pegs and parakeratotic cells with inclusion bodies in the stratum corneum. Virus "factories" with mature and immature poxviruses were seen by electron microscopy. Fibrillar nuclear inclusions were present in the nuclei of some infected cells. The virus was not propagated or characterized. The mode of transmission is unknown.

Similar papillamota were observed in captive Australian kangaroos, including a red kangaroo (*Magaleia rufa*) in New South Wales (Bagnall and Wilson 1974) and one in Victoria (P. Presidente, cited in McKenzie et al. 1979), and an eastern (*Macropus giganteus*) and a western (*Mac. fuliginosus*) gray kangaroo (McKenzie et al. 1979). The lesions were grossly and microscopically similar to those of the quokkas and to molluscum contagiosum in humans. There was intense dermal inflammation in the lesions of the eastern gray kangaroo. The viruses in the lesions measured approximately 175–200 nm by 250–300 nm and were of characteristic poxvirus morphology. The source of the infections in the kangaroos and its transmission mechanisms are unknown.

REFERENCES

Alexander, A. D., Flyger, V., Herman, Y. F., McConnell, S. J., Rothstein, N., and Yager, R. H. Survey of wild mammals in a Chesapeake Bay Area for selected zoonoses. *J. Wildl. Dis.* 8:119–125, 1972.

Ambrus, J. L., Felt, E. T., Grace, J. T., and Owens, G. A virus-induced tumor in primates. *Natl. Cancer Inst. Monogr.* 10:447–458, 1963.

Ambrus, J. L., Sandstrom, H. V., and Kawinski, W. "Spontaneous" occurrence of Yaba tumor in a monkey colony. *Experientia* 25:64–65, 1969.

Andrewes, C. H., Allison, A. C., Armstrong, J. A., Bearcroft, G., Niven, J. S. F., and Pereira, H. G. A virus disease of monkeys causing large superficial growths. *Acta Union Int. Contra Cancerum* 15:760–763, 1959.

Arita, I., Gispen, R., Kalter, S. S., Teong Wah, L., Marennikova, S. S., Netter, R., and Tagaya, I. Outbreaks of monkeypox and serological surveys in nonhuman primates. *Bull. WHO* 46:625–631, 1972.

Arita, I., and Henderson, D. A. Smallpox and monkeypox in nonhuman primates. *Bull. WHO* 39:277–283, 1968.

———. Monkeypox and whitepox viruses in West and Central Africa. *Bull. WHO* 53:347–353, 1976.

Bagnall, B. G., and Wilson, G. R. Molluscum contagiosum in a red kangaroo. *Aust. J. Dermatol.*
15:115–120, 1974.

Bearcroft, W. G. C., and Jamieson, M. F. An outbreak
of subcutaneous tumors in rhesus monkeys. *Nature* 182:195–196, 1958.

Behbehani, A. M., Bolano, C. R., Kamitsoka, P. S.,
and Wenner, H. A. Yaba tumor virus: I. Studies
on pathogenesis and immunity. *Proc. Soc. Exp.
Biol. Med.* 129:556–561, 1968.

Breman, J. G., Berena Bernadou, J., and Nakano, J.
H. Poxvirus in West African nonhuman primates: Serological survey. *Bull. WHO*
55:605–612, 1977a.

Breman, J. G., Nakano, J. H., Coffi, E., Godfrey, H.,
and Gautun, J. C. Human poxvirus disease after
smallpox eradication. *Am. J. Trop. Med. Hyg.*
26:273–281, 1977b.

Casey, H. W., Woodruff, J. M., and Butcher, W. I.
Electron microscopy of benign epidermal pox
disease of rhesus monkeys. *Am. J. Pathol.*
51:431–446, 1967.

Center for Disease Control. Monkeypox in humans:
West Africa. *Morbid. Mortal. Wkly. Rep.*
28:135–136, 1979.

Crandell, R. A., Casey, H. W., and Brumlow, W. B.
Studies on a newly recognized poxvirus of monkeys. *J. Infect. Dis.* 119:80–88, 1969.

de Harven, E., and Yohn, D. S. The fine structure of
the Yaba monkey tumor poxvirus. *Cancer Res.*
26:995–1008, 1966.

Downie, A. W. Serological evidence of infection with
Tana and Yaba pox viruses among several species of monkey. *J. Hyg.* 72:245–250, 1974.

Downie, A. W., and Espana, C. Comparison of Tanapox virus and Yaba-like viruses causing epidemic disease in monkeys. *J. Hyg.* 70:23–32, 1972.

———. A comparative study of Yaba and Tanapox
viruses. *J. Gen. Virol.* 19:37–49, 1973.

Downie, A. W., Taylor-Robinson, C. H., Caunt, A. E.,
Nelson, G. S., Manson-Bahr, P. E. C., and
Matthews, T. C. H. Tanapox: A new disease
caused by a poxvirus. *Br. Med. J.*, pp. 363–368,
1971.

Espana, C. A pox disease of monkeys transmissible to
man. *In Medical primatology 1970*, pp. 694–708,
2nd Conf. Exp. Med. Surg. Prim. Basel: Karger,
1971a.

———. Review of some outbreaks of viral disease in
captive nonhuman primates. *Lab. Anim. Sci.*
21:1023–1031, 1971b.

Espana, C., Brayton, M. A., and Ruebner, B. H. Electron microscopy of the Tana poxvirus. *Exp. Mol.
Pathol.* 15:34–42, 1971.

Foster, S. O., Brink, E. W., Hutchins, D. L., Pifer, J.
M., Lourie, B., Moser, C. R., Cummings, E. C.,
Kuteyi, O. E. K., Eke, R. E. A., Titus, J. B.,
Smith, E. A., Hicks, J. W., and Foege, W. H.
Human monkeypox. *Bull. WHO* 46:569–576,
1972.

Gispen, R. Antigenic differentiation of monkeypox.
*Int. Symp. Smallpox Vacc. Symp. Ser. Immu-
nobiol. Stand.* 19:23–26, 1972.

Gispen, R., and Brand-Saathof, B. "White" poxvirus
strains from monkeys. *Bull WHO* 46:585–592,
1972.

Gispen, R., Brand-Saathof, B. B., and Hekker, A. C.
Monkeypox-specific antibodies in human and
simian sera from the Ivory Coast and Nigeria.
Bull. WHO 53:355–360, 1976.

Gispen, R., and Kapsenberg, J. G. *Verslagen en me-
dedelingen betseffende de Volkogezondheid.* The
Hague: Gezondheidsraad, 1968.

Gispen, R., Verlinde, J. D., and Zwart, P. Histopathological and virological studies on monkeypox.
Arch. Gesamte Virusforsch. 21:205–216, 1967.

Grace, J. T., Jr., and Mirand, E. A. Human susceptibility to a simian tumor virus. *Ann. N.Y. Acad.
Sci.* 108:1123–1128, 1963.

Hall, A. S., and McNulty, W. P., Jr. A contagious pox
disease in monkeys. *J. Am. Vet. Med. Assoc.*
151:833–838, 1967.

Hall, R. D., Olsen, R. G., Pakes, S. P., and Yohn, D. S.
Differences in clinical and convalescent-phase
antibodies of rhesus monkeys infected with
monkeypox, Tanapox and Yaba poxviruses. *Infect. Immun.* 7:539–546, 1973.

Heberling, R. L., and Kalter, S. S. Induction, course
and transmissibility of monkeypox in the baboon
(*Papio cynocephalus*). *J. Infect. Dis.* 124:33–38,
1971.

Kalter, S. S., Heberling, R. L., and Cooper, R. W.
Serologic testing of various primate species
maintained in a single outdoor breeding colony.
Lab. Anim. Sci. 24:636–645, 1974.

Kupper, J. L., Casey, H. W., and Johnson, D. K.
Experimental Yaba and benign epidermal monkeypox in rhesus monkeys. *Lab. Anim. Care*
20:979–988, 1970.

Ladnyj, I. D., Ziegler, P., and Kima, E. A human
infection caused by monkeypox virus in Basan-
kusu Territory, Democratic Republic of the
Congo. *Bull. WHO* 46:593–597, 1972.

Levinthal, M. J., and Schein, H. M. Propagation of a
simian tumor agent (Yaba virus) in cultures of
human and simian renal cells as detected by
immunofluorescence. *Virology* 23:268–270,
1964.

Lourie, B., Bingham, P. G., Evans, H. H., Foster, S.
O., Nakano, J. H., and Herrmann, K. L. Human
infection with monkeypox virus: Laboratory investigation of six cases in West Africa. *Bull
WHO* 46:633–639, 1972.

Lourie, B., Kemp, G. E., Nakano, J. H., and Setzer, H.
W. Isolation of poxvirus from an African rodent.
J. Infect. Dis. 132:677–681, 1975.

McConnell, S. J., Herman, Y. F., Mattson, D. E., and
Erickson, L. Monkeypox disease in irradiated
cynomolgus monkeys. *Nature* 195:1128–1129,
1962.

McConnell, S. J., Herman, Y. F., Mattson, D. E.,
Huxsoll, D. L., Lang, C. M., and Yager, R. H.
Protection of rhesus monkeys against monkey-
pox by vaccinia virus immunization. *Am. J. Vet.
Res.* 25:192–195, 1964.

McKenzie, R. A., Fay, F. R., and Prior, H. C. Poxvirus

infection of the skin of an eastern gray kangaroo (*Macropus giganteus*). *Aust. Vet. J.* 55:188–190, 1979.

McNulty, W. P., Jr., Labitz, W. C., Hu, F., Maruffo, C. A., and Hall, A. S. A pox disease in monkeys transmitted to man. *Arch. Dermatol.* 97:286–293, 1968.

Marennikova, S. S. Field and experimental studies of poxvirus infections in rodents. *Bull. WHO* 57: 461–464, 1979.

Marennikova, S. S., and Seluhina, E. M. Susceptibility of some rodent species to monkeypox virus, and course of the infection. *Bull. WHO* 53:13–20, 1976.

Marennikova, S. S., Seluhina, E. M., Mal 'ceva, N. N., Cimiskjan, K. I., and Macevic, G. R. Isolation and properties of the causal agent of a new variola-like disease (monkeypox) in man. *Bull WHO* 46:599–611, 1972a.

Marennikova, S. S., Seluhina, E. M., Mal 'ceva, N. N., and Ladnyj, I. D. Poxviruses isolated from clinically ill and asymptomatically infected monkeys and a chimpanzee. *Bull WHO* 46:613–620, 1972b.

Metzgar, R. S., Grace, J. T., Jr., and Sproul, E. E. Immunologic studies of subcutaneous virus-induced histiocytomas in primates. *Ann. N.Y. Acad. Sci.* 101:192–196, 1972.

Nicholas, A. H. A poxvirus of primates: II. Immunology. *J. Natl. Cancer Inst.* 45:907–914, 1970.

Nicholas, A. H., and McNulty, W. P. In vitro characteristics of a poxvirus isolated from rhesus monkeys. *Nature* 217:745–746, 1968.

Niven, J. S. F., Armstrong, J. A., Andrewes, C. H., Pereira, H. G., and Valentine, R. D. Subcutaneous "growths" in monkeys produced by a poxvirus. *J. Pathol. Bacteriol.* 81:1–14, 1961.

Noyes, W. F. Observations on two poxtumor viruses. *Virology* 25:566–669, 1965.

Olsen, R. G., Blakeslee, J. R., Mathes, L., and Nakano, J. H. Preparation and evaluation of a noninfectious monkeypox virus vaccine. *J. Clin. Microbiol.* 6:50–54, 1977.

Olsen, R. G., Mathes, L. E., and Yohn, D. S. Serologic relationship among simian poxviruses. *Bacteriol. Proc.*, p. 191, 1971.

Olsen, R. G., and Yohn, D. S. Immunodiffusion analysis of Yaba poxvirus structural and associated antigens. *J. Virol.* 5:212–220, 1970.

Papadimitriou, J. M., and Ashman, R. B. A poxvirus in a marsupial papilloma. *J. Gen. Virol.* 16:87–89, 1972.

Peters, J. C. An epizootic of monkeypox at Rotterdam Zoo. *Int. Zoo Yearbook* 6:274–275, 1966.

Rondle, C. J. M., and Sayeed, K. A. R. Studies on the monkeypox virus. *Bull. WHO* 46:577–583, 1972.

Prier, J. E., and Sauer, R. M. A pox disease of monkeys. *Ann. N.Y. Acad. Sci.* 85:951–959, 1960.

Prier, J. E., Sauer, R. M., Malsberger, R. G., and Sillaman, J. M. Studies on a pox disease of monkeys: II. Isolation of the etiological agent. *Am. J. Vet. Res.* 21:381–384, 1960.

Sauer, R. M., Prier, J. E., and Buchanan, R. S. Studies on a pox disease of monkeys: I. Pathology. *Am. J. Vet. Res.* 21:377–380, 1960.

Shelukhina, E. M., Maltseva, N. N., Shenkman, L. S., and Marennikova, S. S. Properties of two isolates (MK-7-73 and MK-10-73) from wild monkeys. *Br. Vet. J.* 131:746–747, 1975.

Sproul, E. E., Metzgar, R. S., and Grace, J. T., Jr. The pathogenesis of Yaba virus-induced histiocytomas in primates. *Cancer Res.* 26:671–675, 1963.

Tsuchiya, Y., and Tagaya, I. Sero-epidemiological survey on Yaba and 1211 virus infections among several species of monkeys. *J. Hyg.* 69:445–451, 1971.

von Magnus, D., Andersen, E. K., Petersen, K. B., and Birch-Andersen, A. A pox-like disease in cynomolgus monkeys. *Acta Pathol. Microbiol. Scand.* 46:156–176, 1959.

Wenner, H. A., Bolano, C. R., Cho, C. T., and Kamitsuka, P. S. Studies on the pathogenesis of monkeypox. III. Histopathological lesions and sites of immunofluorescence. *Arch. Gesamte Virusforsch.* 27:179–197. 1969a.

Wenner, H. A., Cho, C. T., Bolano, C. R., and Kamitsuka, P. S. Studies on the pathogenesis of monkeypox: II. Dose-response and virus dispersion. *Arch. Gestamte Virusforsch.* 27:166–178, 1969b.

Wenner, H. A., Macasaet, F. D., Kamitsuka, P. S., and Kidd, P. Monkeypox: I. Clinical virologic and immunologic studies. *Am. J. Epidemiol.* 87:551–566, 1968.

Wolfe, L. G., Adler, A., and Griesemer, R. A. Immunologic response of monkeys to aerosols of Yaba virus. *J. Natl. Cancer Inst.* 41:1197–1203, 1968a.

Wolfe, L. G., Griesemer, R. A., and Farrell, R. L. Experimental aerosol transmission of Yaba virus in monkeys. *J. Natl. Cancer Inst.* 41:1175–1195, 1958b.

Yohn, D. S., Grace, J. T., Jr., and Haendiges, V. A. A quantitative cell culture assay for Yaba tumor virus. *Nature* 202:881–883, 1964.

13 Myxomatosis and Fibromatosis

THOMAS M. YUILL

Myxomatosis

Synonyms: **None.**

Myxomatosis is an insect-transmitted pox-virus disease of wild and domesticated rabbits. In natural hosts (*Sylvilagus* spp. rabbits) the virus produces small, self-limiting tumors. However, in an exotic host, the European rabbit (domestic or wild *Oryctolagus cuniculus*), the disease is generalized, usually acute, and characterized by proliferative and inflammatory reactions and high mortality.

HISTORY AND DISTRIBUTION. Myxomatosis was first observed by Sanarelli in 1896 in Montevideo, Uruguay, when an outbreak occurred among domestic laboratory rabbits. Unable to demonstrate pathogenic bacteria or a parasite, Sanarelli (1898) perceptively attributed the cause of the disease to a virus, and the filterability of the agent was confirmed in 1911 (Moses 1911). Within 30 years, myxomatosis was reported in Brazil and Argentina (Aragao 1927; Splendore 1909), and subsequently, in Colombia and Panama (Fenner and Ratcliffe 1965). In 1930 the first natural outbreak of myxomatosis outside South America caused losses in commercially raised domestic rabbits in San Diego, California (Kessel et al. 1931). Additional outbreaks have occurred in California, Oregon (Patton and Holmes 1977), and Brazil (Correa et al. 1977).

Aragao (1927) first suggested the use of myxomatosis to control introduced wild *O. cuniculus*, which had become a significant pest species in much of Australia. However, it was not until the late 1930s and early 1940s that interest increased and field testing began. Martin (1936) concluded, on the basis of his experiments at Cambridge, that myxomatosis could suitably control this rabbit in Australia. Unsuccessful attempts at reduction of rabbit populations were made on Skokholm Island, England (Lockley 1955), and on the Vejro and Kattegat islands of Denmark (Bourliere 1956; Fenner and Ratcliffe 1965) from 1936 to 1938. Myxomatosis was successfully introduced into a population of wild rabbits on a Swedish estate in 1938, but the disease disappeared after a period of epizootic spread (Fenner and Ratcliffe 1965). The first attempts to establish myxomatosis in field populations of Australian rabbits were not successful but did suggest the importance of arthropod transmission (Bull and Mules 1944).

During this period, the natural history of myxomatosis in South America became better understood. Aragao (1942, 1943) implicated the wild tapeti (*Sylvilagus brasiliensis*) as the reservoir host and experimentally transmitted the disease by interrupted feeding of *Aedes* spp. mosquitoes. Not until nearly 20 years later was the reservoir species in North America discovered, when the brush rabbit (*S. bachmani*) was found naturally infected in California (Marshall and Regnery 1960).

The great Australian and European epizootics occurred in the 1950s. Myxomatosis was introduced into wild rabbit populations in the Murray River valley, Australia, and soon spread rapidly along the Murray and Darling rivers (Myers 1954). The disease spread to all Australia by 1953 (Fenner and Ratcliffe 1965). News of the Australian epizootics prompted the introduction of myxomatosis into rabbits on a private French estate in 1952, from whence it escaped and spread throughout continental Europe (Bourliere 1956; Giban et al. 1956), the British Isles (Armour and Thompson 1955; Thompson 1956), and finally Scandinavia (Borg and Bakos 1963) and North Africa (Fenner and Ratcliffe 1965).

Another deliberate attempt to control wild European rabbits with myxomatosis was made in Chilean and Argentinian Tierra Del Fuego in 1954. The disease became enzootic there, but its success in reducing rabbit numbers was unevaluated (Fenner and Ratcliffe 1965).

ETIOLOGY. Myxoma viruses are in the *Leporivirus* genus of the Poxviridae family (Fenner 1976, 1979). The two distinct myxoma viruses are designated Aragao's fibroma (Brazilian myxoma), and the Marshall-Regnery fibroma (Californian myxoma) (Fenner and Myers 1978). These viruses differ in the signs they produce and in their soluble antigens. Myxoma virus morphology is typical of poxviruses (Fig. 13.1); the virion measures about 290 nm by 250 nm by 110 nm (Chapple and Westwood 1963; Padgett et al. 1964). Both ovoid and rectangular particles have been seen in a single preparation; the rectangular forms have scalloped margins and no visible internal structure. Envelopes are frequently seen. The surface of the particle comprises irregularly arranged tubular elements and contains an electron-dense central body.

The physical and chemical properties of myxoma virus are similar to those of other poxviruses (Andrewes and Horstmann 1949; Bronson and Parker 1943; Fenner 1953a). Although heat resistant enough to permit effective mechanical transmission by insects, myxoma virus is somewhat more susceptible to heat inactivation than some other poxviruses. The central body of the virus particle is resistant to peptic digestion. Unlike the poxviruses in other subgroups, myxoma virus is ether sensitive.

The antigenic relationship of myxoma virus to the poxvirus group has been established by cross-reactions of internal (group) NP antigens in precipitin and immunofluorescence tests (Takahashi et al. 1959a; Woodroofe and Fenner 1962). The place of myxoma within the *Leporivirus* genus has been similarly established. The close relationship of myxoma and fibroma viruses has been demonstrated by precipitation, complement fixation, cross-neutralization, and vaccination challenge tests and by agglutination of elementary bodies (Berry and Lichty 1936; Fenner 1965; Fenner and Woo-

droofe 1954; Hyde 1939b; Jacotot et al. 1958; Ledingham 1937; Mansi 1957a; Shaffer 1941). The very close relationship of myxoma and fibroma viruses has been further established by experiments demonstrating genetic recombination of these viruses, a phenomenon which occurs only at the genus level (Woodroofe and Fenner 1960).

Antigenic differences in myxoma virus strains from various geographic areas in the Americas have been shown by agar gel precipitation. All Californian strains were identical with the Californian MSW prototype. The Californian strains, however, had fewer antigens than South American strains from Brazil, Uruguay, and Argentina. Strains from Panama and Colombia were more closely related to the North American strains than to the South American ones (Fenner 1965; Fenner and Ratcliffe 1965; Reisner et al. 1963).

TRANSMISSION

Hosts. *Sylvilagus brasiliensis* is the natural host of South American myxomatosis (Aragao 1942, 1943), and *S. bachmani* is the reservoir of Californian myxomatosis (Marshall and Regnery 1960). The susceptibility of other *Sylvilagus* species to infection with Brazilian myxoma virus has been tested (Fenner and Ratcliffe 1965; Marshall and Regnery 1963; Regnery 1971; Regnery and Marshall 1971). Experimentally infected *S. audubonii*, *S. floridanus*, *S. nuttallii*, *S. idahoensis*, and *S. bachmani* developed tumors. Mosquitoes (*Aedes aegypti*) me-

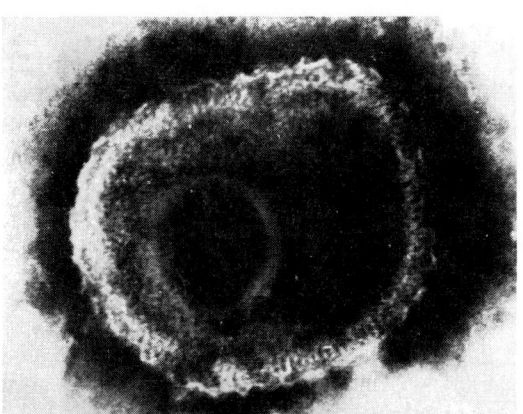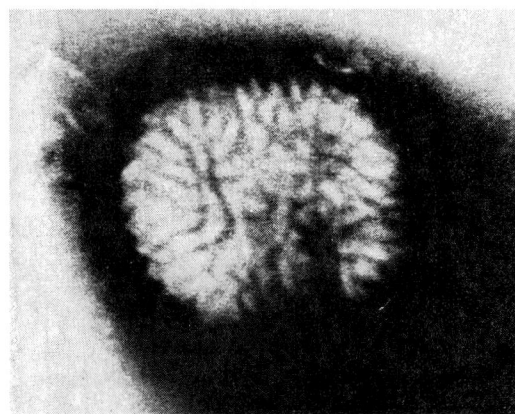

FIG. 13.1 Myxoma virus particles showing irregular tabular arrangement (*left*), and the rectangular type particle (*right*) showing scalloped edges. (Padgett et al. 1964.)

chanically transmitted the virus efficiently enough from the lesions of *S. audubonii* to suggest that this rabbit is a good potential host. Although some mosquito transmission was accomplished from the lesions of *S. floridanus* and *S. nuttallii*, these species were not as good a virus source as was *S. audubonii*. Interestingly, no transmission was accomplished from the lesions of *S. bachmani*, the natural host of the Californian virus. *Sylvilagus nuttallii* was the only species to develop severe disease and die from experimental infection. *Sylvilagus transitionalis* was refractory to infection (Hobbs 1931).

The susceptibility of several New World rabbits to the California myxoma virus was also tested experimentally (Regnery and Marshall 1971). No lesions developed following inoculation of *S. brasiliensis* with this virus. *Sylvilagus audubonii*, *S. idahoensis*, and *S. nuttallii* developed lesions, but the resulting tumors did not contain enough virus to permit mechanical transmission. In contrast, lesions of *S. bachmani* are an excellent source of virus for transmission (Marshall and Regnery 1963), indicating the evolution of a close association of this rabbit with the Californian virus (Fenner and Myers 1978). This association was further illustrated by a natural epizootic among brush rabbits in California (Regnery and Miller 1972). During the spring and summer, 95% of the brush rabbits became infected. However, there was no evidence that myxomatosis affected the rabbit's growth or reproduction.

Myxomatosis vectors have not been extensively studied in the Americas. The South American vector is unknown. In California, myxoma virus has been isolated from wild-caught *Aedes freeborni* (Marshall et al. 1963). This species has successfully transmitted myxomatosis between wild *Sylvilagus* rabbits in the laboratory (Grodhaus et al. 1963).

The European rabbit is extremely susceptible to infection. During the panzootic in European rabbits, natural infections of two species of hares were also found. Generalized infections of the European hare (*Lepus europaeus*) were found in Ireland, England, France, and Italy (Collins 1955; Hudson and Mansi 1955; Jacotot et al. 1954b; Micozzi and Palarchi 1975; Whitty 1955). The brown hare (*L. timidus*) was similarly found infected in Ireland (Anon. 1955). The European hare has been infected experimentally with both European and California strains of myxoma virus (Fenner and Ratcliffe 1965; Jacotot et al. 1955a). On the other hand, two North American hares (*L. californicus* and *L. americanus*) failed to develop lesions following inoculation (Hobbs 1931; Hyde and Gardner 1933; Regnery and Marshall 1971).

Many Australian wild vertebrates were tested and found insusceptible to myxoma virus infection long before the panzootic was started. These included a variety of marsupials and a few other mammals, three species of lizards, and six species of birds (Bull and Dickinson 1937; Fenner and Ratcliffe 1965).

Attempts to infect a variety of domesticated and laboratory animals, as well as man, were unsuccessful. These included guinea pigs, rats, ferrets, pigeons, pigs, chickens, ducks, dogs, horses, cattle, sheep, goats, cats, hamsters, and rhesus monkeys (Bull and Dickinson 1937; Findlay 1929; Hobbs 1928; Sanarelli 1898). Although adult mice develop no lesions when exposed to the virus, intracerebral inoculation of infant mice with myxoma virus does result in some virus multiplication (Andrewes and Harisijades 1955; Claringbold and Sobey 1955). As with many poxviruses, myxoma virus replicates and produces pocks on the chorioallantoic membrane of the embryonated chicken egg (Fenner and McIntyre 1956; Hoffstadt and Pilcher 1938; Lush 1937).

Myxoma virus has been grown in cell cultures, in some cases infecting cells from insusceptible vertebrate species. The virus replicates well in pleural exudate and mononuclear, kidney, heart, testicle, and embryo fibroblast cells from the European rabbit (Chaproniere 1956; Roby et al. 1965; Woodroofe and Fenner 1965). Virus multiplication also took place in chick embryo fibroblasts and human amnion (FL) cells as well as cells from the kidneys of gray squirrels and guinea pigs and rat and hamster embryos (Chaproniere and Andrewes 1957; Takahashi et al. 1959b; Woodroofe and Fenner 1965).

Epizootiology. The basic transmission cycle of myxomatosis in nature is comparatively simple. Transmission is mechanical; the virus is carried on the mouthparts of bloodsucking arthropods from rabbit to rabbit. Unlike viruses of the arthropod-borne virus group, myxoma virus requires no particular vector species and does not multiply in the vector; infected skin, not viremic blood, is the source of the virus carried by the vector (Fenner et al. 1952).

A variety of arthropods have transmitted the virus experimentally, including many mosquito species, fleas, simuliid flies, ticks, rabbit lice, and mites. Primary myxoma lesions or the swollen bases of the ears or the eyelids serve as good sources of virus and are usually accessible to biting arthropods (Fenner and Woodroofe 1953). The distribution of virus in these lesions may be somewhat irregular, however (Day et al. 1956). Mosquitoes feeding on myxoma lesions acquire 10–2,000 rabbit LD_{50} of virus on their mouthparts (Fenner and Ratcliffe 1965). In refeeding, an estimated 12% of the virus is inoculated per probe and the amount of infectious virus declines approximately 20% each day (Day et al. 1956).

Under special circumstances, transmission can occur in the absence of arthropod vectors. Myxoma virus is infectious for European rabbits by the respiratory route, and susceptible rabbits in very close contact with those with advanced disease may become infected (Fenner and Ratcliffe 1965; Sobey and Conolly 1975). Transmission by this means may occur within the warren or outside, when acutely ill individuals blunder into the territory of susceptible rabbits and an encounter ensues (Mykytowycz 1961). There is evidence for mechanical transmission by thistles (*Cirsium vulgarae* and *Arthamus lanatus*) among penned and wild rabbits in certain areas in Australia where these plants were particularly abundant (Dyce 1961).

The myxomatosis panzootics have provided unique insights into the evolution and interaction of populations of vectors, pathogens, and hosts. The Australian epizootic began with a nearly universally fatal infection of an entirely susceptible rabbit host population (Fenner et al. 1953). Within a comparatively short period of time this pattern changed with the selection for attenuated virus and resistant rabbits. There appeared a more nodular type of disease with decreased lethality and a longer course, providing up to a 5 times greater opportunity for mosquito transmission. In Australia selection by the vectors for attenuated virus producing more persistent lesions resulted in a decline in mortality from over 99% to about 90% within 1 year (Fenner 1953b; Fenner et al. 1956; Marshall and Fenner 1960; Mykytowycz 1953). Although virus strains of greatly reduced virulence have appeared from time to time, these strains do not produce sufficient virus content in the skin for efficient arthropod transmission, cause early regression and crusting, and do not persist. Thus, virus virulence declined at first and then stabilized; Douglas and colleagues reported that virus virulence was unchanged for 15 years in Victoria (Dunsmore and Price 1972).

In the face of the sweeping myxomatosis epizootic in Australia, highly susceptible rabbits perished, and a few resistant survivors remained (Fenner 1953b; Marshall and Douglas 1961; Marshall and Fenner 1958; Sobey 1960). Although a resistant rabbit population was selected for, its establishment was slow. Testicular lesions often rendered surviving bucks at least temporarily sterile (Marshall et al. 1955). In one experimental population of 20 bucks convalescent from myxomatosis, 10 were fully fertile. Litters sired by the other 10 contained approximately half the number of progeny sired by unaffected bucks (Sobey and Turnbull 1956). Lowered fertility following infection was also observed among bucks in the field in Australia (Poole 1960) and in myxomatosis convalescent does and bucks in France (Joubert et al. 1972). The removal by predation of sick rabbits which would otherwise have recovered doubtless occurred and, when it did, impeded selection for resistance (Fenner and Ratcliffe 1965; Mykytowycz 1961). Even so, rabbit populations highly resistant to mortality from myxomatosis have emerged in enzootic areas (Douglas 1968). However, this increase in resistance has been associated with a corresponding increase in virulence of field virus strains that produce lesions with sufficient quantities of virus for efficient arthropod transmission (Edmonds et al. 1975).

In Australia the rate and pattern of spread was influenced by mosquitoes, the principal vectors, and was largely confined to wetland areas (Brereton 1953). Outbreaks far distant from the main epizootic appeared and were probably initiated by windblown virus-carrying mosquitoes (Ratcliffe et al. 1952). Two mosquito species (*Culex annulirostris* and *Anopheles annulipes*) are the major Australian vectors (Fenner and Ratcliffe 1965; Myers 1954; Myers et al. 1954), although *C. pipiens australicus* has been implicated in transmission in some areas. Two species of simuliid flies (*Austrosimulium furiosum* and *Siumulium melatum*) have been observed to be abundant in epizootic areas, and both have transmitted myxomatosis to sentinel rabbits in the field (Fenner and Ratcliffe 1965; Mykytowycz 1957). Myxoma virus has been recovered from lice (*Haemodipsus ventricosus*) and mites (*Cheyletiella parasitivorax*) taken from sick wild rabbits, but both of these species were shown to be ineffective vectors (Mykytowycz 1958). The mite *Listrophorus gibbus* was a suspected vector in a winter epizootic among rabbits in New South Wales (Williams 1972). The flea (*Echidnophaga myrmecobu*) transmitted myxomatosis in a population of penned rabbits (Bull and Mules 1944) but was apparently not an efficient vector in the wild (Calaby et al.

1960). In a few areas, myxomatosis epizootics have occurred in winter (Dunsmore et al. 1971) or did not cross fences or enclosures in summer, suggesting that nonflying vectors may have been involved (Fenner and Ratcliffe 1965).

The reappearance of myxomatosis in isolated rabbit populations after several years' absence is difficult to explain. Williams et al. (1972a) suggested that the virus was latent in rabbits. Individual wild rabbits have developed myxomatosis twice, under circumstances that strongly suggest reactivation of a previous infection (Williams and Parer 1972).

The epizootic in Britain followed a different pattern than the Australian one. The disease spread at a much slower rate due to transmission by a sedentary vector, the flea (*Spilopsyllus cuniculi*) (Allan and Shanks, 1955; Armour and Thompson 1955; Lockley 1954). There was no cold-season lull in the epizootic; fleas transmitted the virus during all seasons. The virus was shown to persist on the mouth parts of the fleas for up to 10–12 weeks (Chapple and Lewis 1964; Joubert et al. 1969), suggesting that the virus does not require rapid transmission from host to host to be maintained in the rabbit population. Virus has also been recovered from the soil of warrens several weeks after the death of the rabbits (Joubert et al. 1969), but the significance of the observation is not clear. The virus appears to be continuously maintained in a given locale; but as the rabbit population declines, the area in which the disease is occurring expands (Ross and Tittensor 1980). Following the initial appearance of myxomatosis, epizootics did skip to distant areas. These disjunctions, however, have been credited not to the vector, but to the introduction of diseased animals by persons wishing to eliminate rabbits in particular areas (Ritchie et al. 1954; Thompson 1956). Initially, it appeared that unattenuated virus would be maintained in Britain. In 1955, 2 years after the outbreak of myxomatosis began, the first attenuated strain was found among rabbits in the Sherwood Forest, but the highly virulent strain predominated (Chapple and Bowen 1963; Fenner and Marshall 1955; Hudson and Mansi 1955). The apparent maintenance of highly virulent virus was credited to transmission due to abandonment of dead or dying rabbits by flea vectors. It is now clear that selection for moderately attenuated virus has also taken place in the same way that mosquito-transmitted, milder virus strains have in Australia (Fenner and Chapple 1965; Mead-Briggs and Vaughan 1975; Vaughan and Vaughan 1968). It has been shown that there is considerably more rabbit-to-rabbit movement

by fleas than previously thought and that host abandonment is stimulated by fever, irrespective of survival or death of the rabbit (Mead-Briggs 1964). Also, some evidence suggests that mosquitoes (especially *Ae. detritus* and *Ae. cantans*) may be more important myxomatosis vectors than had been believed previously (Service 1971). Selection for rabbits resistant to myxomatosis occurred in Britain (Ross and Sanders 1977), as it did in Australia.

The influence of the rabbit flea vector on virus virulence was further tested in Australia with the establishment of *S. cuniculi* in the rabbit population and subsequent introduction of highly virulent strains of myxomatosis (Sobey and Conolly 1971; Sobey and Menzies 1969). The attenuated virus strains already present were transmitted more efficiently by the fleas, and predominated over the introduced virulent virus strains (Fullagar 1977; Williams 1971; Williams and Parer 1971). However, the introduction of fleas into Australian rabbit populations has been responsible for changes in the epizootiology of myxomatosis. In some areas of flea infestation, the seasonal occurrence of myxomatosis has shifted from summer to spring, and continuous, low-intensity transmission throughout the year has occurred in other regions (Edmonds et al. 1971).

Myxomatosis vectors have not been described throughout continental Europe, but the situation is probably intermediate between Australia and Britain, with mosquitoes (*Ae. cespius, Ae. detritus, Ae. maculipennis,* and *Culex modestus*) transmitting during warm weather and fleas transmitting throughout the year (Fenner and Ratcliffe 1965; Jacotot et al. 1954a; Joubert et al. 1967, 1972–1973). Although mortality has been very high, attenuated strains were recovered in France 2–3 years after the panzootic began there (Fenner and Marshall 1955; Jacotot et al. 1955b, 1956). Black flies appear to play an occasional secondary role in myxomatosis transmission in France (Joubert and Prave 1973).

SIGNS AND PATHOGENESIS. The pathogenesis of myxoma virus infection has been far more extensively studied in an exotic host, the European rabbit, than in the natural host. This is doubtless due to the greater economic importance and the more spectacular disease associated with infection of the European rabbit, and to the limited availability of natural hosts for experimentation. Virtually all the early descriptions of myxomatosis concerned classic, invariably fatal infections of the European rabbit with South American strains of the virus.

Rabbit Infection. In the European rabbit, infection is initiated by introduction of the virus into the skin, where it multiplies (Fenner and Woodroofe 1953); the skin becomes red and thickened (Hurst 1937a). The virus spreads to the local lymph nodes and by 48–72 hours is found in the cellular constituents of the general circulation and is carried to the organs (Fenner and Woodroofe 1953; Mukai 1960b). The virus may then be found in conjunctival and nasal secretions and in the skin generally. Virus multiplication in the organs increases. By the 6th day, macules about 3 mm in diameter develop away from the site of inoculation, enlarge, and begin to thicken. Bilateral blepharoconjunctivitis and watery to mucopurulent secretions from the nose and eyes may appear (Aragao 1927; Fenner and Woodroofe 1953; Hyde 1936; Moses 1911). The bases of the ears, eyelids, and mucocutaneous junctions become thick and swollen (Fig. 13.2). As the infection progresses over the next few days, the eyelids thicken and may close, and nodular tumors form over the body. Skin lesions may become large, protuberant, and red to blue in color. Blepharitis becomes so marked as to produce the typical leonine head. The testicles may become extremely edematous, causing scrotal rupture. The animal becomes anorexic and then moribund. Dyspnea and stertor, and often opisthotonos, may occur in extremis, with death coming as a terminal convulsion if the animal is disturbed. Survival time is somewhat variable, death in an adult rabbit infected with a virulent

strain usually occurring within 8–12 days (Fenner and Marshall 1957; Fenner and Ratcliffe 1965).

Myxoma virus transmitted to *S. brasiliensis* by mosquito in the laboratory results in a cutaneous tumor which becomes apparent in 1 week and regresses in 2–4 weeks without signs of generalized disease (Aragao 1943). The course of mosquito-transmitted myxomatosis in *S. bachmani* is similar (Grodhaus et al. 1963; Marshall and Regnery 1963).

Strain Variation. Significant variation in clinical disease has been observed following infection of rabbits by various myxoma virus strains or by any given strain (Fenner and Marshall 1957; Fenner and Ratcliffe 1965). For example, the attenuated Australian strain, Uriarra, produces a spectrum of severity in wild rabbits. In mild cases the nodules are numerous but small, and little or no blepharitis or mucocutaneous junction edema results. In moderate cases the nodules are larger, and facial edema and eye and nasal discharges may occur. The eyes do not close, however, and the general condition of the rabbit remains good. In severe cases classic myxomatosis results (Mykytowycz 1956). But even in fatal myxomatosis the manifestations are variable.

In the European rabbit, clinical disease produced by Californian myxomatosis strains is consistently different from that produced by the South American strains. The primary lesion does not become large and nodular but remains small with indistinct edges. Marked blepharoconjunctivitis, with closing of the eyes or

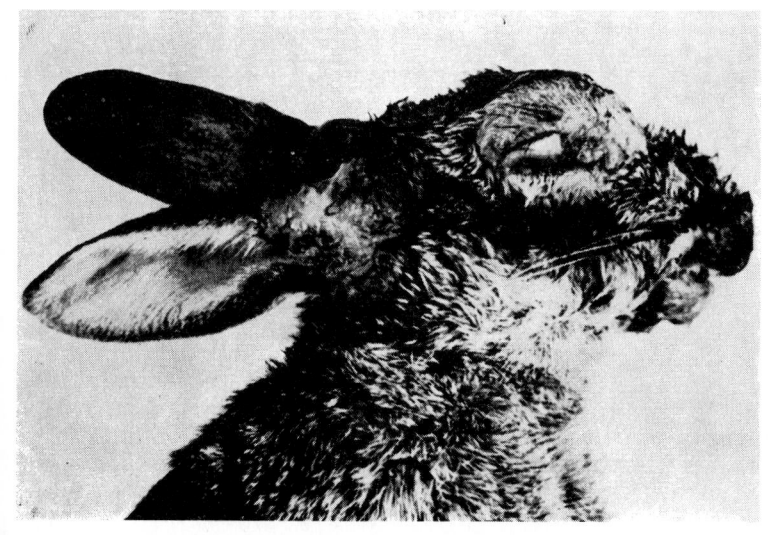

FIG. 13.2 A wild European rabbit (*Oryctolagus cuniculus*) naturally infected with myxomatosis. Note the marked blepharoconjunctivitis and the swelling at the base of the ears. (Borg and Bakos 1963.)

marked edema of the mucocutaneous junctions, is not seen. Secondary skin lesions may not appear. Signs of central nervous system disorder may be seen. Gross hemorrhage into the skin or internal organs is more commonly observed than in infections with the South American strains (Fenner and Ratcliffe 1965).

Host Age. The age of the rabbit partially determines the course of the disease. *Oryctolagus* rabbits infected experimentally at less than 3 weeks of age with fully virulent myxoma virus died faster than adults but with fewer signs of generalized disease (Fenner and Marshall 1954). Even inoculation of a juvenile tapeti (*S. brasiliensis*) resulted in generalized disease with blepharitis, not a small, localized tumor (Aragao 1943). However, other findings indicated that rabbits 10–30 weeks of age inoculated with small doses of myxoma virus survived longer than did adults (Sobey et al. 1970).

Temperature. Ambient temperature has a marked effect on the pathogenesis of myxomatosis in rabbits. Early experimental work demonstrated that high ambient temperatures, with resulting increases in skin and rectal temperatures, modified the disease (Thompson 1938). Later work showed that not only did high temperatures lead to few secondary lesions and early regression but also that the amount of virus in the skin was lower than in animals kept at cooler temperatures (Parker and Thompson 1942). Infection of rabbits in unheated animal quarters with partially attenuated field strains of myxomatosis further documented the relationship of warm temperatures and increased survival, especially in animals with a degree of genetic resistance (Mykytowycz 1956; Sobey et al. 1967). Marshall's (1959) prediction that mortality from the partially attenuated virus strains active in the field would be highest in winter has been supported by subsequent observation. Case fatality of 30% in summer and 86–100% in winter have been reported in a wild rabbit population infected with partially attenuated virus (Dunsmore and Price 1972; Dunsmore et al. 1971; Williams et al. 1972b).

PATHOLOGY

Gross Pathology. Naturally occurring skin lesions of myxomatosis in the brush rabbit are up to 10 mm in diameter. These lesions progress from thickening of the skin to raised, circumscribed areas that become crusted and regress (Regnery and Miller 1972).

The gross and microscopic lesions that occur in European rabbits dying of myxomatosis have been well studied (Ahlstrom 1940; Hurst 1937b; Rivers 1930). At necropsy, involvement of the epidermis, corium, and subcutaneous tissue is seen. The tumors are either gelatinous or fibrous, and hemorrhagic necrosis may be present. The spleen may be normal or enlarged. Malpighian bodies are prominent in the enlarged spleen, and this organ may be dark and soft. The omentum is congested and rolled up, and petechial hemorrhages are present. Hemorrhages may also be seen in the stomach and intestinal walls; in abdominal fascia; under the peritoneum; and in the thymus, coronary vessels, and lungs. Emphysema is occasionally observed. The liver may be mottled or may contain yellow flecks. No gross changes in the kidneys have been noted except for edema in the pelvis in one case. Congestion and discoloration of the adrenals is rare. Both the tunica and the upper poles of the testis may be involved.

Histopathology

SKIN. In myxomatosis, the skin is extensively involved (Hurst 1937a; Hyde 1936; Marcato and Simoni 1977a; Mukai 1960a). In the dermis a mucinous exudate occurs and may extend downward between the bundles of superficial muscles and loose tissue beneath. The margins of the nodular lesions comprise large hyperchromatic stellate or polygonal myxoma cells having oval or swollen nuclei with fragmented chromatin along the nuclear membrane (Fig. 13.3). The cytoplasm of these cells contains inclusions which stain pink to purple with Giemsa stain. The nodular lesion itself is infiltrated by large macrophages and polymorphonuclear cells, many of which are karyorrhectic. Cells in the center of the nodules are few and necrotic and are surrounded by great quantities of mucin. The collagen bundles are swollen.

Changes in the epidermis also occur (Hurst 1937a; Rivers 1926, 1930). The epithelial layer of the epidermis becomes thickened and the cells are swollen. Both proliferation and necrosis are evident (Fig. 13.4). Cells develop vacuolated nuclei and cytoplasmic inclusions. Changes similar to those occurring in variola have been reported (Aragao 1911). In the secondary skin lesions of acute cases, severe epithelial inflammation occurs.

In the dermal vessels one sees vascular changes typical of the disease (Fig. 13.5). Venules and capillaries are most extensively in-

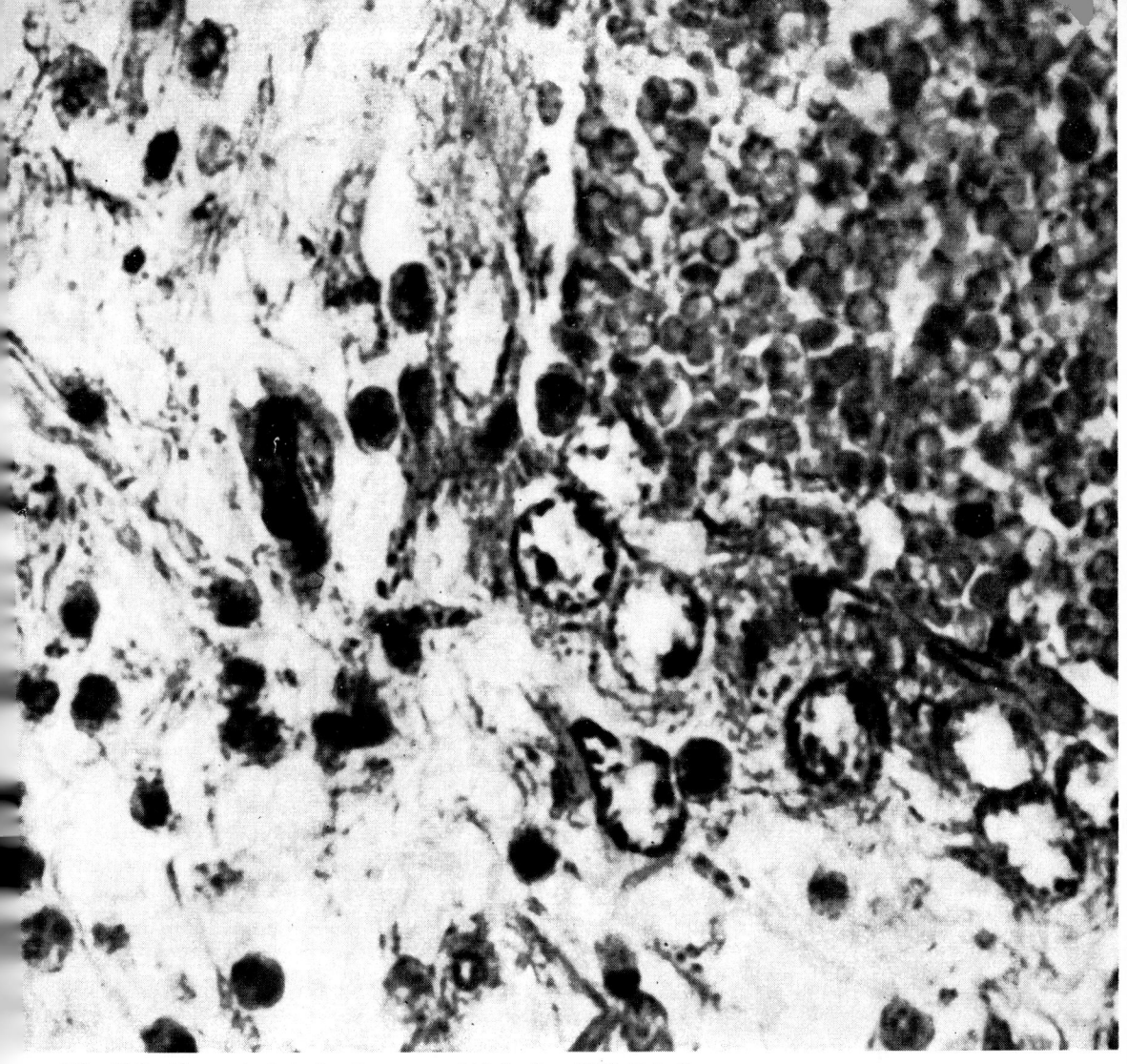

FIG. 13.3 Myxomatosis in the European rabbit (testis ×350). Note the myxoma cells with greatly enlarged nuclei and the fragmented chromatin lying along the nuclear membrane. (Armed Forces Institute of Pathology photograph 59-6364 [615091].)

volved (Hurst 1937a; Hyde 1936), except in North American cases (Patton and Holmes 1977). The vascular endothelium becomes hyperplastic, with numerous mitotic figures. The cells hypertrophy and bulge into the lumen of the vessel. Concentric thickening may occlude the lumen, or the rapidly developing myxoma cells and the infiltrating polymorphonuclear leukocytes may lift the endothelium. The vessel collagen becomes swollen. Extravasated red blood cells are sometimes seen.

LYMPH NODES. The cells of the lymphocytic series degenerate and the reticulum cells proliferate, increasing in size and number (Ahlstrom 1940; Hurst 1937a). Histosyncytial lymphadenitis was commonly seen in naturally occurring cases of myxomatosis in rabbits in Europe (Marcato

and Simoni 1977b). The lymphoid follicles are infected from the periphery inward. Polymorphonuclear leukocytes and occasionally eosinophils, infiltrate into infected areas. Typical blood vessel changes occur, and petechial hemorrhages may result. As the disease progresses, myxoma cells appear in the connective tissue of the hilum and arteries, and neutrophilic infiltration occurs. The end result may be either a necrotic lymph node or one composed of myxoma cells, depending on whether the degenerative or proliferative response predominates.

KIDNEYS. The most common kidney lesion observed is desquamation of the epithelium of the convoluted tubules and ascending loops of Henle (Hurst 1937a). Interstitial hemorrhage, swelling of the endothelial cells of the glo-

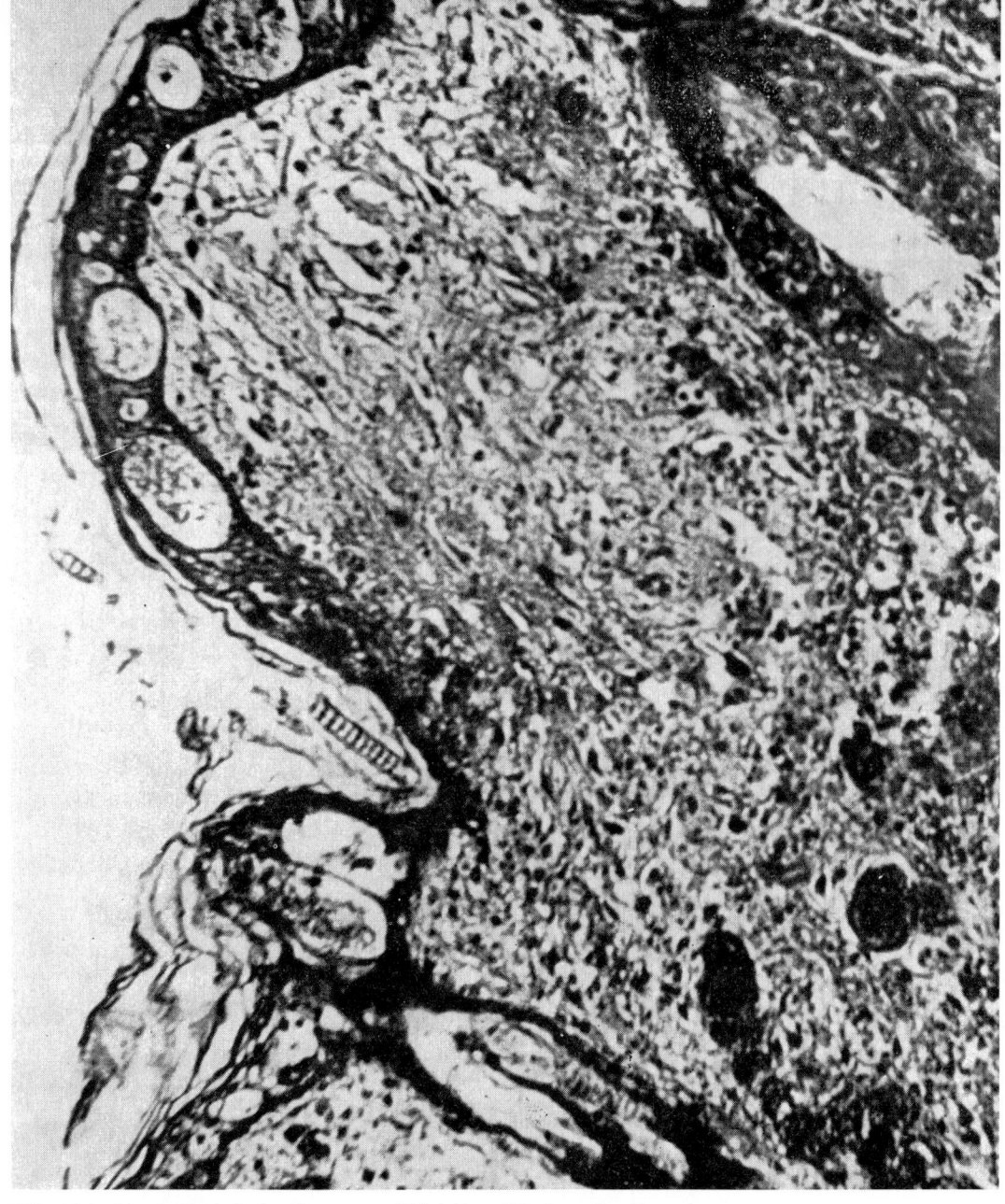

FIG. 13.4 Myxomatosis in the European rabbit (skin ×70). A section through a primary skin lesion. (Armed Forces Institute of Pathology photograph 59-3637 [39095].)

merular tufts, edema of the pelvis, and infarction occur less commonly.

LUNGS. The epithelium of the alveolar sacs proliferates and becomes myxomatous (Ahlstrom 1940; Hurst 1937a). Hemorrhage is seen when the proliferative response has given way to degeneration and necrosis in the alveolar walls. Typical vascular changes are common.

TESTES. Testicular involvement is variable. When lesions occur, they are those of acute inflammation (Hurst 1937a; Rivers 1930). Lesions are most commonly encountered in the rete testis, tunica albugenia, and epididymis. Affected interstitial cells are characterized by swollen, vesicular nuclei, often with chromatin blocks lying along the nuclear membrane. In severe cases the interstitial cells become myx-

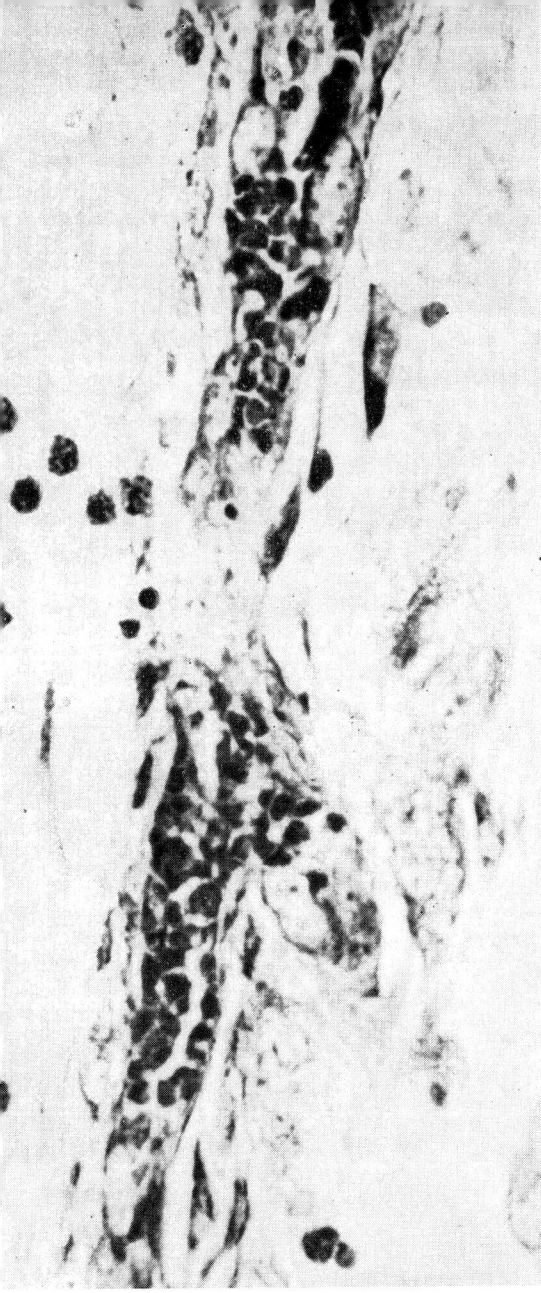

FIG. 13.5 Myxomatosis in the European rabbit (skin ×220). Note the typical vascular changes where myxoma cells bulge into the lumen. (Armed Forces Institute of Pathology photograph 59-6652 [65091].)

lar changes take place. The reticular cells of the splenic pulp do not become stellate but clump together, thickening the walls of the sinuses; fibrin may be present in the sinuses themselves (Hyde and Gardner 1933; Sprunt 1932). Foci of necrotic areas and of stellate cells occur in the malpighian corpuscles.

LIVER. The central lobular veins of the liver are commonly affected. They degenerate, and the nuclei of the endothelial cells do not stain (Ahlstrom 1940; Hurst 1937a; Sprunt 1932). Liver cells in these areas are pyknotic. Karyorrhectic leukocytes may be found in adjacent sinusoids. The sinusoids are greatly dilated, there is a thinning of the cords, and a polymorphonuclear infiltrate is present. Kupffer's cells are greatly enlarged; some are hyperplastic and others degenerate. Myxomatous changes in the bile duct epithelium and portal connective tissue may sometimes be seen (Hyde 1939a).

BONE MARROW. Foci of myxomatous cells have been described in the bone marrow (Ahlstrom 1940; Mukai 1960a). Hyperactivity or degeneration of erythrocytes with accumulation of pigment in the marrow may be seen. Cytotoxic changes in the myelocytic and erythrocytic series has been described. Round, large cells with oval or swollen nuclei containing fragmented chromatin appear at the time of the occurrence of myxomatous cells in other parts of the body and have been considered to be pathognomonic for myxomatosis.

ADRENALS. In most cases the adrenals are normal. In one series of 17 cases, 4 rabbits were observed to have cortical sinusoid congestion. Some cortical cells were degenerative, and hyperchromatic nuclei were seen (Hurst 1937a).

OMENTUM. The omentum is rolled up, thickened, and congested, with polymorphonuclear leukocytic infiltration. Degenerative endothelial and adventitial changes and petechial hemorrhages may occur (Hurst 1937a).

omalike and may be multinucleated. Leukocytes infiltrate the damaged tissue, and a fibrinous exudate is often present. Hemorrhage frequently occurs.

UTERUS AND OVARIES. Scattered myxoma cells may be seen in the muscular layer of the uterus and in the graafian follicles (Sprunt 1932).

SPLEEN. As in the lymph nodes, the lymphocytes in the spleen degenerate and the reticulum cells proliferate and enlarge (Ahlstrom 1940; Hurst 1937a). Leukocytes infiltrate the affected areas and a fibrinous exudate occurs. Typical vascu-

INTRACELLULAR INCLUSIONS. The nature of intra-cytoplasmic inclusions seen in myxomatosis was a point of considerable controversy among early workers. Generally, it has been agreed that these inclusions stained red with Giemsa stain and are of variable size and shape (Hyde 1936; Kato et al. 1963; Rivers 1926). These have been termed type B inclusions (Kamahora et al. 1955; Kato and Cutting, 1959; Kato and Windsor 1958); and have been shown by fluorescent antibody, autoradiography, and Feulgen staining to be sites of virus replication and maturation (Fig. 13.6) (Takahashi et al. 1958).

OTHER HOSTS. During the course of the European epizootics, several investigators reported naturally occurring cases of myxomatosis in the European hare (*Lepus europaeus*). The pathology is very similar to that observed in the European rabbit in nearly all respects (Haag and Haag 1954; Jacotot et al. 1955a; Magallon and Bazin 1953). More hemorrhages have been reported in hares than in rabbits, and comparatively small nodules localized on the forelimb and hind limb have been seen, in one case limiting the movement of humeroradial and femorotibial joints.

Myxoma virus infection of natural hosts (*Sylvilagus* spp.) presents an entirely different picture than in the European rabbit, generalization and death having occurred only in experimental infections of juvenile animals (Fenner and Ratcliffe 1965). Fibromalike, flat, soft skin nodules appear 5–11 days after inoculation by syringe or mosquito bite (Aragao 1942; Grodhaus et al. 1963; Marshall et al. 1963). Young animals tend to have larger, more persistent tumors. The site of inoculation may also influence the persistence of the resulting tumor.

DIAGNOSIS. Diagnosis of myxomatosis in the domesticated European rabbit can be made with reasonable certainty on clinical grounds when a rapid course with blepharoconjunctivites (and the leonine head), terminating in death, occurs. However, various myxoma virus strains may produce disease not typical of this classical picture. In such cases transmissibility of the disease is demonstrable by inoculation of fresh tissue suspensions from diseased animals into susceptible rabbits. Histologic changes associated with myxomatosis should also be seen in either typical or atypical cases.

The differentiation of myxomatosis and fibromatosis of wild *Sylvilagus* rabbits can be made on several points. There is no known

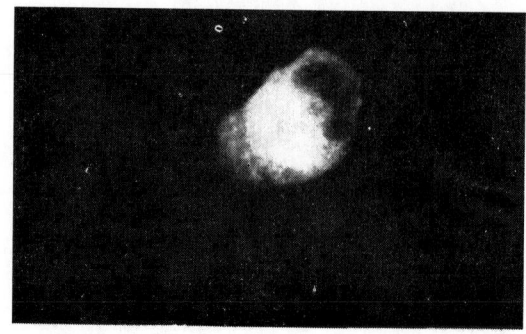

FIG. 13.6 An FL (human amnion) cell infected with myxoma virus showing the B type inclusion demonstrated by immunofluorescence (*above*) and Giemsa stain (*below*). (Takahashi et al. 1959b.)

overlap in the geographic distribution of these two viruses. Fibromatosis is found in central and eastern North America; myxomatosis occurs in California and Oregon and in Central and South America. These two viruses can be easily differentiated on the basis of the disease produced by intradermal inoculation of adult domesticated rabbits with tumor tissue. Infection with myxoma virus produces generalized disease and death, whereas fibroma virus causes only self-limiting skin lesions.

Inoculation of the chorioallantoic membrane of 12-day-old embryonated chicken eggs incubated at 35°C may also be of some differential value. The South America and Panama strains of myxoma virus produce large pocks, the Californian strain of myxoma virus produces minute pocks, and fibroma virus produces lesions too small to count (Fenner and Marshall 1957; Smith 1948).

Antigenic similarities and differences between myxoma and fibroma viruses can be shown by various serologic tests. Although cross-reactive, these two viruses can be distinguished by both complement fixation and precipitation tests when properly controlled (Fenner 1965; Teixeira and Smadel 1941). The plaque technique employing cell cultures is the most convenient precise method for quantifying virus and is useful for virus neutralization tests (Woodroofe and Fenner 1965).

A standard method has been developed for comparing relative strain virulence (Fenner and Marshall 1957). Rabbits of not less than 4 months of age are inoculated intradermally in the flank and held at 21°C. The mean survival time is noted and compared with standard strains. One rabbit passage prior to evaluation is suggested.

A diagnosis of myxomatosis can be established in rabbits surviving acute infection by demonstrating an increase in antibody or the appearance of circulating soluable antigens (Sobey et al. 1966).

IMMUNITY. The protective role of maternal antibody in young, wild *Oryctolagus* rabbits is not well understood. In some instances, offspring of immune does were susceptible to myxoma virus challenge (Hyde and Gardner 1939; Jacotot et al. 1954c; Martin 1936). In cases of passive protection by maternal antibody, the offspring were probably at risk during the following transmission season even though the protection may not have been complete and the young rabbits experienced a mild, localized infection (Fenner and Marshall 1954).

Wild adult European rabbits surviving myxomatosis have been observed to have clinical myxomatosis one or more years after the initial infection (Williams and Parer 1972). Brush rabbits, the natural hosts, are susceptible to reinfection. Eighteen months after primary infection, about half the brush rabbits bitten by virus-carrying mosquitoes in the laboratory developed tumors, some of which in turn served as a source of virus for additional transmission (Fenner and Ratcliffe 1965). Recrudescent infection, or the reversion of immune individuals to the population at risk, must influence the rates of spread and maintenance of the virus in the rabbit population.

TREATMENT. No effective treatment of myxomatosis has been described. Administration of antibiotics is without value (McKercher 1952). Administration of viral suppressive drugs at or shortly after the time of exposure has not been adequately tested. β-Phenylserine has been reported to slightly delay the development of disease and death (Pons and Williams 1961). N-Methylisatin-β-thiosemicarbizone has been

effective in reduction of cases and mortality in smallpox epidemics (Bauer et al. 1962, 1963) and in treating laboratory animals infected with vaccinia virus (Thompson et al. 1953a,b), but its effect against myxomatosis is untested.

CONTROL. The control of myxomatosis among wild European rabbit populations has not usually been desired. Reduction of rabbit populations has lead to desirable ecological changes in Australia, Europe, and Britain (Thomas 1963; Fenner and Myers 1978). Even in continental Europe and in Britain, where hunters feared the loss of the rabbit as a major game species, quarantine, fencing, and extermination practices were not successful in halting the spread of the disease (Armour and Thompson 1955; Ritchie et al. 1954). Protection of commercially reared rabbits in enzootic and epizootic areas has been a problem. Control measures usually proceed along four lines: (1) vaccination, (2) prompt removal of sick and exposed animals, (3) isolation of susceptible animals from arthropod vectors, and (4) exclusion of wild rabbits from the immediate area.

There have been many attempts to make a chemically or physically inactivated myxoma virus vaccine, all of which have been unsuccessful in effectively preventing disease and death (Fisk and Kessel 1931; Jacotot and Vallee 1953; Kessel et al. 1934; McKee 1939). A live, attenuated, and apparently safe vaccine strain of myxoma virus has been derived by multiple passages in rabbit kidney cell cultures (McKercher and Saito 1964). However, this virus strain does revert to virulence when backpassaged in rabbits (Jacotot et al. 1967). Fibroma virus has frequently been used as a living vaccine against myxomatosis because of its close antigenic relationship to myxoma virus and avirulence for adult rabbits (Fenner and Woodroofe 1954; Hyde 1939b; Rowe et al. 1956; Shope 1936a). Results with the fibroma vaccine have been highly variable, however, immunity depending on the strain and the dose employed. Revaccination at 6-month to 1-year intervals is necessary to ensure protection (Durand et al. 1974). Intercutaneous vaccination of domesticated rabbits twice (March and May) with fibroma virus, before the summer myxomatosis transmission season, has been recommended in Europe (Joubert and Brun 1976). Administration of cortisone (50 mg per rabbit) at the time of fibroma virus inoculation and again on postvaccination days 4, 6, and 10 results in larger, more persistent fibromas and longer-lived immunity (Jacotot et al. 1962).

Rabbit Fibromatosis

Synonyms: **None.**

HISTORY AND DISTRIBUTION. Shope's or rabbit fibroma virus was first recovered from a cottontail rabbit in New Jersey in 1932 (Shope 1932a). The transmissibility of the virus and its relationship to myxoma virus was quickly established (Shope 1932b, 1936a,b). During the early 1940s fibroma-infected cottontail rabbits were frequently seen in Michigan and later were reported from Maryland, New York, Missouri, Illinois, Indiana, and Wisconsin and from Ontario (Anon. 1940–1945; Fenner and Ratcliffe, 1965; Haugen 1942; Herman et al. 1956; Karstad, personal communications, 1962–1966; Szczech et al. 1974; Yuill and Hanson 1964). During the 1950s, possible host-vector-virus relationships were investigated in a series of pathogenesis and transmission experiments (Dalmat 1959; Dalmat and Stanton 1959; Kilham and Dalmat 1955; Kilham and Woke 1953). The natural history of the virus has never been described, however.

ETIOLOGY. Classification of Shope's fibroma virus as a poxvirus and its close relationship to myxoma virus is well established. The particle size and morphology of fibroma virus examined by electron microscopy is identical with myxoma virus (Bernhard et al. 1954a,b; Lloyd and Kahler, 1955; Scherrer 1968). The viral nucleic acid is DNA (Roby et al. 1965). Like myxoma virus, fibroma virus is somewhat more heat labile than vaccinia, ectromelia, or fowlpox; is ether sensitive; and produces type B intracytoplasmic inclusions.

The close antigenic relationship of fibroma and myxoma viruses is discussed in the myxomatosis section. Within the myxoma-fibroma pox subgroup, fibroma stands in an intermediate antigenic position between myxoma virus and squirrel and hare fibroma viruses, as demonstrated by agar gel precipitation (Fenner 1965).

TRANSMISSION

Hosts. Although the eastern cottontail rabbit (*Sylvilagus floridanus*) is the natural host of rabbit fibroma virus, attempted transmission to three other *Sylvilagus* species (*S. bachmani, S. nuttallii,* and *S. audubonii*) by inoculation and by mosquito bite has been unsuccessful (Fenner and Ratcliffe 1965). Two species of North American *Lepus* are susceptible. A jackrabbit of undesignated species was successfully infected (Hyde 1936), and two snowshoe hares (*Lepus americanus*) developed flat, transitory lesions of approximately 1 cm in diameter when inoculated intradermally with 300 domestic rabbit ID_{50} of a Wisconsin rabbit fibroma strain (T. M. Yuill, unpublished data). *Lepus europaeus,* however, is refractory to rabbit fibroma infection (Fenner and Ratcliffe 1965). The European rabbit (*Oryctolagus cuniculus*) is susceptible, and a localized tumor is produced at the site of inoculation (Shope 1932a). Natural outbreaks of fibromatosis have occurred in domesticated rabbits in North America (Joiner et al. 1971; Raflo et al. 1973). European rabbits inoculated with fibroma virus at 15 days of age or less usually experience generalized, fatal disease (Duran-Reynals 1940, 1945; Harel and Constantin 1954).

Inoculation of fibroma virus into several species of wild animals from an epizootic area in Maryland failed to produce lesions. These animals included weasels (*Mustela frenata*), opossums (*Didelphis virginianus*), woodchucks (*Marmota monax*), a flying squirrel (*Glaucomys volans*), white-footed mice (*Peromyscus leucopus*), voles (*Microtus pennsylvanicus*), a chipmunk (*Tamias striatus*), a bobwhite quail (*Colinus virginianus*), and eastern box turtles (*Terrapene carolina*) (Herman et al. 1956). Attempts to infect gray squirrels (*Sciurus carolinensis*) were unsuccessful (Kilham et al. 1953). Attempts to infect guinea pigs, laboratory rats and mice, and chickens have also been unsuccessful (Shope 1932a). Rabbit fibroma virus replicates on the chorioallantoic membrane of embryonating hens' eggs but does not produce pocks large enough to count (Shaffer 1941; Smith 1948).

Rabbit fibroma virus has been grown in a variety of cell cultures. Primary rabbit kidney, testicle, spleen, heart, and skin and muscle cells along with continuous cell lines of rabbit kidney and cells from a rabbit papilloma have been used (Constantin and Febvre 1956; Constantin et al. 1956; Roby et al. 1965; Verna 1965; Verna and Eylar 1962). Fibroma virus has also been grown in cell cultures from species which are normally insusceptible to infection, including sheep testicle (Cilli 1958), monkey kidney (Kilham 1958), and cells and tissue from guinea pigs, rats, and man (Chaproniere and Andrewes 1957; Kato et al. 1959).

Epizootiology. The simple rabbit-arthropod-rabbit cycle of transmission for myxomatosis doubtless holds true for fibroma virus as well, but the natural vectors are unknown. Mosquitoes (*Aedes aegypti, Ae. triseriatus, Culex pipiens, C. quinquefasciatus,* and *Anopheles quadrimaculatus*), fleas (*Cediopsylla simplex, Odontopsyllus multispinosus,* and *Hoplopsyllus affinis*), reduviid bugs (*Triatoma infestans, T. phyllosoma pallidipennis,* and *Rhodnius prolixus*), and bedbugs (*Cimex lectularius*) have transmitted the virus between cottontail rabbits in the laboratory (Dalmat 1959; Kilham and Dalmat 1955; Kilham and Woke 1953). An early observation that fibromas invariably occurred on the feet, legs, and noses of infected rabbits led to the speculation that some ground-dwelling vector, perhaps nematode larvae, was responsible (Shope 1951); but tumors were later observed to be just as common at the base of the ears and around the eyes (Dalmat 1959). Although the relationship of the site of development to persistence of arthropod-transmitted fibromas has not been determined, mosquito-transmitted fibromas on the head and nose of one cottontail persisted for only 3 weeks, whereas those on the unshaved feet and legs of another cottontail persisted for 3 months (Kilham and Dalmat 1955).

Naturally occurring fibromas of cottontail rabbits are seen chiefly in the late summer, autumn, and winter (Anon. 1940–1945; Haugen 1942; Herman et al. 1956). These tumors are capable of long persistence and infectivity; the fibroma of one naturally infected cottontail did not regress for 10 months and served as a virus source for mosquitoes during this time (Kilham and Dalmat 1955). Such long-term persistence is probably the main virus overwintering mechanism; however, if flea transmission does occur, the virus may be spread actively during the winter. Although the monthly incidence of disease has not been described, the disease, enigmatically, does not appear in the population during the spring and early summer months.

PATHOLOGY. In the adult natural host, the cottontail rabbit, fibroma virus causes the formation of localized tumors (Fig. 13.7) which, although they may persist for several months, regress and cause little or no apparent damage to the host (Herman et al. 1956; Kilham and Fisher 1954; Shope 1932a). The histologic changes that occur during the course of the infection point to the low virulence and invasive character of the disease. The skin lesions are inflammatory, become granulomatous, and then proliferative (Prose et al. 1971). During the first week of the infection an inflammatory reaction occurs in the corium, accompanied by lymphocytic, neutrophilic, and plasma cell infiltration (Dalmat and Stanton 1959). The vascular changes characteristic of myxomatosis do not occur. Spindle-shaped, fibroblastlike fibroma cells appear during the 2nd week. These cells have abundant cytoplasm, vesicular nuclei, and granular cytoplasmic inclusions (Hyde 1936; Kilham and Fisher 1954; Shope 1932a). During the 3rd week the fibroma cells become round as the inclusions become very large. Rete pegs of epidermis elongate into the tumor mass. Cytoplasmic inclusions may be seen in epidermal cells and become most prominent during the 5th week of infection. At that time, necrotic foci occur, and lymphocytic and neutrophilic infiltrates are seen around the periphery of the fibroma, especially beneath the base. The large pleomorphic fibrocytes in the dermis do not stain well by the alcian blue PAS method (Szczech et al. 1974).

The infection in domesticated (European) rabbits follows a similar but shorter course, with more pronounced epidermal degeneration (Ahlstrom 1938; Fisher 1953; Hurst 1938a). Generalized disease is extremely rare in adults. Tumor regression appears to be associated with cell-mediated immunity (Tompkins et al. 1970).

The inclusion bodies that occur in fibroma virus infections of cottontail or domesticated rabbits or in cell cultures are very similar to those seen in myxoma virus infections (Fisher 1953; Hurst 1938a; Kato and Cutting 1959; Kato et al. 1963).

Poxvirus particles can be seen in the hyperplastic epithelium, the fibroma cells, and occasionally extracellularly in the epidermal prickle cell layer. Tonofibrils are reduced in the hyperplastic epithelium. Desmosomes are usually intact but may be separated occasionally, appearing as hemidesmosomes (Pulley and Shively 1973). Some cells contain long lamellated inclusions in the cytoplasm (Banfield and Kasnic, 1971; Prose et al. 1971).

Age plays an important role in the pathogenesis of fibromatosis. Very young cottontail rabbits develop fibromas which are larger in size and persist longer than those of older cottontails, unless the infection is ameliorated by maternal antibody (Kilham and Dalmat 1955; Yuill and Hanson 1964). Infection of neonatal cottontails produces a generalized fatal disease. The young animals rapidly acquire resistance to generalized infection; although large, persistent tumors may result, the animals survive. It is probable that infection of neonatal cottontails in the wild would be initiated by a virus dose insufficient to produce death. Cottontails 6 days old or less repeatedly bitten by infective *Ae. aegypti* mosquitoes did not die (T. M. Yuill, unpublished data). The course of fibromatosis in neonatal cottontail and European rabbits is different. In young European rabbits generalized disease is more inflammatory than proliferative, and resistance to fatal disease is acquired less rapidly than in cottontails (Duran-Reynals 1940, 1945; Yuill and Hanson 1964). Tumor regression appears to be due to cell-mediated immunity (Tompkins et al. 1970).

DIAGNOSIS. Diagnosis of rabbit fibromatosis in the cottontail can usually be made on the gross appearance of the tumor (Fig. 13.7). The transmissibility of the tumor can be demonstrated by inoculation of cell-free tumor homogenates into adult domesticated rabbits or antibody-free cottontails. The disease should not be fatal. Differentiation of myxomatosis and fibromatosis is discussed in the myxomatosis section. The Shope papilloma of cottontails has occasionally been confused with fibromatosis, but it can be readily differentiated on the basis of gross appearance. The papillomas are hyperkeratinized and very dark in color, often becoming so elongated that they have been described by hunters as "horns." The fibroma is soft and light in color (except when crusted during the regression phase) and is flatter than the papilloma.

Serologic confirmation of fibroma virus infection can be established by demonstrating a significant increase in antibody titer during the course of the disease. Using the domestic rabbit intradermal assay system, Dalmat (1958a) first detected antibody in cottontails 6–8 days after

infection. Maximum titers were reached 51 days postinfection and fell to undetectable levels by days 112–152. It is possible that plaque reduction neutralization tests in cell cultures would be considerably more sensitive and permit detection of convalescent phase antibody for longer periods of time. The addition of leukocytes to the serum-virus mixtures has been reported to enhance neutralization if the donor is immune (Ginder 1955).

TREATMENT AND CONTROL. There is no treatment for rabbit fibromatosis. Development of fibromas in experimentally infected domesticated rabbits has been inhibited by treatment with the interferon inducer synthetic, double-stranded polyinosinic acid–polycytidylic acid (Vilcek et al. 1970). This disease presents little threat to either wild or domesticated rabbits, except for very young individuals. Transmission of fibroma virus from cottontails to domesticated rabbits can be prevented by vector control and screening.

Hare Fibromatosis

Synonyms: **None.**

HISTORY AND DISTRIBUTION. Nodular cutaneous tumors of hares (*Lepus capensis*) were first described in Germany by Dungern and Coca in 1909, and the transmissibility of the tumors to other hares and to domesticated rabbits was demonstrated at that time. Epizootics were subsequently seen in Italy's Po valley (Mello 1929; Leinati et al. 1959) and in Mont-

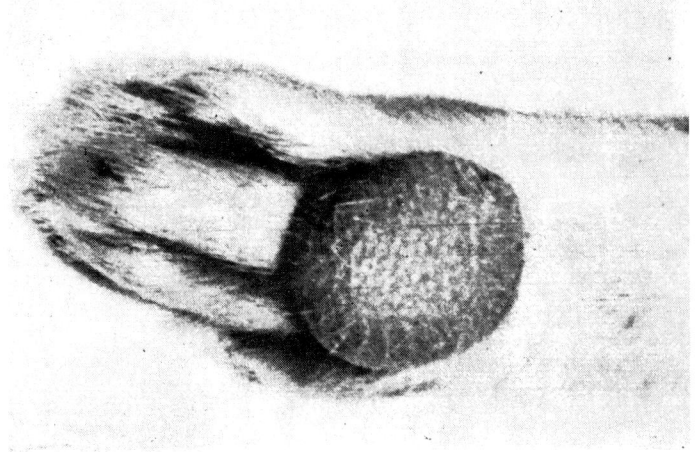

FIG. 13.7 A naturally occurring rabbit fibroma on the forefoot of an eastern cottontail rabbit (*Sylvilagus floridanus*) from Wisconsin. (Yuill and Hanson 1964.)

pellier and Camargne, France (Lafenetre et al. 1960). Similar lesions were seen on *L. capensis* in Kenya (Karstad et al. 1977).

ETIOLOGY. Both European and African hare fibroma viruses appear by electron microscopy to be a typical poxvirus, but other physical and chemical properties have not been determined. European hare fibroma virus is more antigenically akin to rabbit fibroma virus than to myxoma virus by agar gel precipitation tests (Fenner 1965). In vaccination challenge tests, hare fibroma-immune rabbits suffer generalized but not fatal myxomatosis, but myxoma-immune rabbits are refractory to hare fibroma virus challenge (Woodroofe and Fenner 1965). The relationship of the African hare fibroma virus to the European virus, or to other members of the *Leporivirus* genus, has not been studied.

TRANSMISSION

Hosts. In addition to the natural host, the European rabbit is also susceptible to infection by intradermal inoculation of the European virus (Dungern and Coca 1909; Lafenetre et al. 1960; Leinati et al. 1959; Mello 1929). Experimentally infected California jackrabbits (*L. californicus*) developed tumors with sufficient virus content to permit mechanical virus transmission by mosquitoes (Regnery and Marshall 1971). A single unsuccessful attempt was made to infect

a *Sylvilagus* rabbit of undesignated species (Fenner and Ratcliffe 1965). In contrast, the African virus did not produce lesions in domesticated rabbits or on chorioallantoic membranes of chicken eggs or bovine fetal lung, kidney, or muscle cell cultures, or fetal sheep skin cell cultures (Karstad et al. 1977).

Epizootiology. The epizootiology of hare fibromatosis is not understood. The virus is presumably transmitted by arthropod vectors. Of interest is the sharp seasonal incidence of epizootics in Europe, outbreaks having been observed among wild hares exclusively in the late summer and autumn, despite the capture and examination of hares during other seasons, particularly in winter (Lafenetre et al. 1960; Leinati et al. 1959; Mello 1929). The mechanism of interepizootic persistence of the virus is unknown.

PATHOLOGY. The location and size of the tumors on hares is variable (Lafenetre et al. 1960; Leinati et al. 1959). The lesions range in size from 1 cm to 3 cm in diameter and frequently occur at the base of the ear, on the leg and flank, and on the eyelid. The tumors are red gray in color as they develop, becoming whitish and dry and eventually crusting during the regression phase (Fig. 13.8). Lesions on African hares were located on the feet and face (Karstad et al. 1977).

The tumor develops in the dermis. Histologically, the hare fibroma is very similar to the Shope's rabbit fibroma (Karstad et al., 1977; Lafenetre et al. 1960; Leinati et al. 1959). Fibroblastlike cells proliferate rapidly. Large, round cells may arise and become stellate, with large hyperchromatic nuclei and PAS-positive cytoplasmic granules. The epidermis over the rapidly proliferating tumor becomes thin and laminated. Intense infiltration by plasma cells, polymorphonuclear leukocytes, and lymphocytes into and beneath the tumor has been reported.

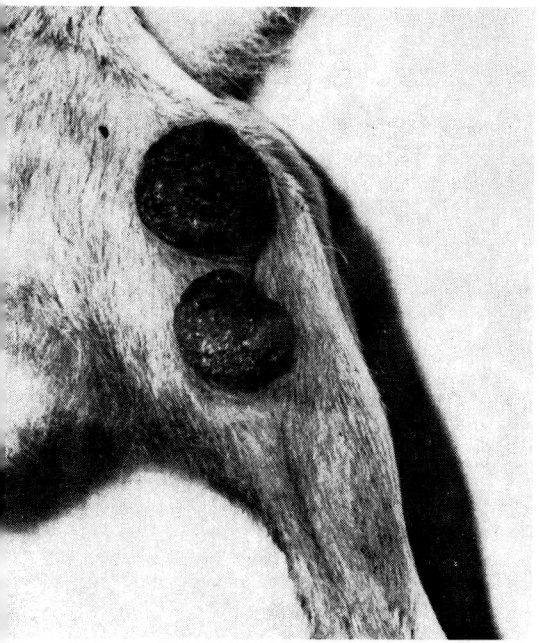

FIG. 13.8 Naturally occurring hare fibromas on the hind leg of a European hare (*Lepus europaeus*) from France. (Courtesy of H. Lafenetre.)

Squirrel Fibromatosis

Synonyms: **None.**

HISTORY AND DISTRIBUTION. The appearance of multiple skin tumors on gray squirrels (*Sciurus carolinensis*) from Maryland was reported in 1953 (Kilham et al. 1953). Unsubstantiated reports of squirrels with skin fibromas have come from New York, Virginia, and North Carolina (Herman and Reilly 1955). Squirrels with skin tumors histologically like viral fibromas have been seen in Ontario (L. H. Karstad, personal communications 1962–1966) and Connecticut (Hirth et al. 1969). Skin lesions were also found on two mature western gray squirrels (*S. griseus griseus*) in California (Regnery 1975).

ETIOLOGY. Squirrel fibroma virus is the least studied of the myxoma-fibroma subgroup. It is morphologically similar by electron microscopy to other poxviruses. A poxvirus group line has been seen in agar gel precipitation studies with this virus, but the soluble antigen and antisera were too weakly reactive to establish relationships with the other members of the myxoma-fibroma subgroup (Fenner 1965). Squirrel fibroma virus has successfully reactivated myxoma virus in cell cultures (Kilham 1958). Rabbit and squirrel fibroma viruses and antisera have been reported to cross-neutralize (Kilham et al. 1953). The California squirrel poxvirus has unusual surface striations and serologically reacts with Californian but not South American myxoma viruses (Regnery 1975).

TRANSMISSION

Hosts. In addition to gray squirrels, woodchucks (*Marmota monax*) are also susceptible to infection with squirrel fibroma virus, and subsequent passage of their tumor suspensions into domesticated rabbits produces small, transitory lesions (Kilham et al. 1953). Inoculation of day-old domesticated rabbits, hamsters, and suckling mice directly with squirrel fibroma suspensions failed to produce lesions (Kirschstein et al. 1958). However, in another trial, domesticated rabbits inoculated with squirrel fibroma virus developed lesions; additional domestic rabbit passage attempts were not successful (Kilham 1955). Squirrel fibroma virus replicated in both rabbit and squirrel kidney cell cultures (Kirschstein et al. 1958).

Epizootiology. The natural history of the squirrel fibroma is not known. Both *Aedes aegypti* and *Anopheles quadrimaculatus* mosquitoes have transmitted the virus from squirrel to squirrel in the laboratory (Kilham 1955). This virus is also presumed to be insect-transmitted in nature.

PATHOLOGY. Although virus-host relationships have been little studied, age appears to play a role in the pathogenesis of fibromatosis in gray squirrels. Naturally infected Maryland squirrels all appeared to be juveniles. The tumors were scattered over the entire body and ranged in size from 2 mm to 25 mm in diameter (Kilham et al. 1953). The results of inoculation of 2- to 4-week-old squirrels was variable; tumors developed only at the site of inoculation in some animals; others developed widely disseminated secondary fibromas. Generalized disease occurred in one squirrel, with multiple lesions developing in the lungs (Kilham 1955). The Connecticut squirrels had single to multiple skin lesions that were hyperkeratotic with papular thickenings (Hirth et al. 1969). Many of these lesions were elevated, flattened, and firm.

The microscopic lesions of squirrel fibroma virus in the gray squirrel are similar to those reported for Shope's rabbit fibroma virus in the cottontail (Kilham et al. 1953). The epidermis is slightly hyperkeratotic, and rete pegs extend down into the tumor mass. Intracytoplasmic inclusions and vacuoles are seen. Foci of fibroblasts are found in the corium and occasionally in the subcutaneous tissue. These areas are infiltrated by plasma cells and lymphocytes. Fibroma cells may also be seen around the vessels, apparently originating from the adventitia. In some lesions from the Connecticut squirrels, the nodules were composed of a mass of fibroblastic cells with an overlying hyperplastic epithelium (Hirth et al. 1969). In the flattened lesions, there was less fibroblastic proliferation and chronic inflammation in the dermis, perhaps as a result of the regression process of these lesions. Unlike the Maryland cases, no lung lesions were observed in the infected squirrels from Connecticut. Although no tests were done to establish serologic relationships of the Connecticut squirrel fibroma with the Maryland (Kilham et al. 1953) virus, poxvirus was observed in the Connecticut cases.

REFERENCES

Ahlstrom, C. G. The histology of the infectious fibroma in rabbits. *J. Pathol. Bacteriol.* 46:461–472, 1938.

———. On the anatomical character of the infectious myxoma of rabbits. *Acta Pathol. Microbiol. Scand.* 17:377–393, 1940.

Allan, R. M., and Shanks, P. L. Rabbit fleas on wild rabbits and the transmission of myxomatosis. *Nature* 175:692, 1955.

Andrewes, C. H., and Harisijades, S. Propagation of myxoma virus in one-day-old mice. *Br. J. Exp. Pathol.* 36:18–21, 1955.

Andrewes, C. H., and Horstmann, D. M. The susceptibility of viruses to ethyl ether. *J. Gen. Microbiol.* 3:290–297, 1959.

Anon. Rose Lake Wildlife Experiment Station Reports 2–7. Michigan Conservation Department, mimeo., 1940–1945.

Anon. Myxomatosis in hares. *Vet. Res.* 67:455, 1955.

Aragao, H de B. Sobre o microbio de myxoma do coelhos. *Brasil-Med.* 25:471, 1911.

———. Myxoma of rabbits. *Mem. Inst. Oswaldo Cruz* 20:225–247, 1927.

———. Sensibilidade do coelho do mato ao virus do myxoma; transmissao pelo *Aedes scapularis* e pelo "stegomyia." *Brasil-Med.* 56:207–209, 1942.

———. O virus do myxoma no coelho do mato (*Sylvilagus minensis*), sua transmissao pelos *Aedes scapularis* e *aegypti*. *Mem. Inst. Oswaldo Cruz* 38:93–99, 1943.

Armour, C. J., and Thompson, H. V. Spread of myxomatosis in the first outbreak in Great Britain. *Ann. Appl. Biol.* 43:511–518, 1955.

Banfield, W. G., and Kasnic, G. Shope fibroma: Electron microscopic structure of associated lamellae. *Ultrastruct. Res.* 37:37–40, 1971.

Bauer, D. J., Dumbell, K. R., Fox-Hulme, P., and Sadler, P. W. The chemotherapy of variola major infection. *Bull. WHO* 26:727–732. 1962.

Bauer, D. J., St. Vincent, L., Kempe, C. H., and Downie, A. W. Prophylactic treatment of smallpox contacts with N-methylisatin-β-thiosemicarbizone. *Lancet* 7306:494, 1963.

Bernhard, W., Bauer, A., Harel, J., and Oberling, C. Les formes intracytoplasmiques du virus fibromateux de Shope. *Bull. Assoc. Frace. Etude Cancer* 41:423–444, 1954a.

Bernhard, W., Harel, J., and Oberling, C. Le virus fibromateux de Shope dans des tumeurs malignes provoquees par lui: Etude au microscope electronique. *C. R. Acad. Sci.* 239:732–734, 1954b.

Berry, G. P., and Lichty, J. A., Jr. Immunological and serological evidence of a close relationship between the viruses of rabbit fibroma (Shope) and infectious myxomatosis (Sanarelli). *J. Bacteriol.* 31:49–50, 1936.

Borg, K., and Bakos, K. Dissemination of myxomatosis by birds. *Nord. Veterinaermed.* 15:159–166, 1963.

Bourliere, F. Biological consequences due to the presence of myxomatosis. *Terre Vie* 103:123–136, 1956.

Brereton, J. le G. Initial spread of myxomatosis in Australia. *Nature* 172:108–110, 1953.

Bronson, L. H., and Parker, R. F. The inactivation of the virus of infectious myxomatosis by heat. *J. Bacteriol.* 45:177, 1943.

Bull, L. B., and Dickinson, C. G. The specificity of the virus of rabbit myxomatosis. *J. Council Sci. Industr. Res. Aust.* 10:291–294, 1937.

Bull, L. B., and Mules, M. W. An investigation of *Myxomatosis cuniculi* with special reference to the possible use of the disease to control rabbit populations in Australia. *J. Council Sci. Industr. Res. Aust.* 17:79–93, 1944.

Calaby, J. H., Gooding, C. D., and Tomlinson, A. R. Myxomatosis in western Australia, *CSIRO Wildl. Res.* 5:89–101, 1960.

Chapple, P. J., and Bowen, E. T. W. A note on two attenuated strains of myxoma virus isolated in Great Britain. *J. Hyg.* 61:161–168, 1963.

Chapple, P. J., and Lewis, N. D. An outbreak of myxomatosis caused by a moderately attenuated strain of myxoma virus. *J. Hyg.* 62:433–441, 1964.

Chapple, P. J., and Westwood, J. C. N. Electron microscopy of myxoma virus. *Nature* 199:199–200, 1963.

Chaproniere, D. M. The effect of myxoma virus on cultures of rabbit tissues. *Virology* 2:599–610, 1956.

Chaproniere, D. M., and Andrewes, C. H. Cultivation of rabbit myxoma and fibroma viruses in tissues of non-susceptible hosts. *Virology* 4:351–365, 1957.

Cilli, V. Aspetti virologici del fibroma di Shope e suoi rapporti con il mixoma di Sanarelli. *G. Mal. Infett. Parassitol.* 10:1017–1040, 1958.

Claringbold, P. J., and Sobey, W. R. The biological assay of myxoma virus. *Br. J. Exp. Pathol.* 36:573–582, 1955.

Collins, J. J. Myxomatosis in the common hare: *Lepus europaeus*. *Irish Vet. J.* 9:268, 1955.

Constantin, T., and Febvre, H. Les corps d'inclusion observes dans les cultures de tissus infectes par le virus de Shope du lapin. *C. R. Soc. Biol.* 150:114–116, 1956.

Constantin, T., Febvre, H., and Harel, J. Cycle de multiplication du virus du fibroma de Shope *in vitro* (souche OA). *C. R. Soc. Biol.* 150:347–348, 1956.

Correa, W. M., Correa, C. N. M., Lavezzo, W., and Lucas, M. W. S. Mixomatose. *Biologico* 43:17–20, 1977.

Dalmat, H. T. Immunity of rabbits to Shope's fibroma virus. *J. Infect. Dis.* 102:179–185, 1958.

———. Arthropod transmission of rabbit fibromatosis (Shope). *J. Hyg.* 57:1–30, 1959.

Dalmat, H. T., and Stanton, M. F. A comparative study of the Shope fibroma in rabbits in relation to transmissibility by mosquitoes. *J. Natl. Cancer Inst.* 22:593–615, 1959.

Day, M. F., Fenner, F., Woodroofe, G. M., and McIntyre, G. A. Further studies on the mechanism of mosquito transmission of myxomatosis in the European rabbit. *J. Hyg.* 54:258–283, 1956.

Douglas, G. W. Observations on the virulence of field strains of myxoma virus and on genetic resistance in wild rabbits in Victoria. *Aust. Verm. Cont. Conf.* p. 86, 1968.

Dungern and Coca. Ueber Hasensarkome, die in Kaninchen wachsen und ueber das Wesen der Geschwulstimmunitaet. *Z. Immunitaetsforsch.* 2:391, 1909.

Dunsmore, J. D., and Price, W. J. A non-winter epizootic of myxomatosis in subalpine south-eastern Australia. *Aust. J. Zool.* 20:405–409, 1972.

Dunsmore, J. D., Williams, R. T., and Price, W. J. A winter epizootic of myxomatosis in subalpine south-eastern Australia. *Aust. J. Zool.* 19:275–286, 1971.

Durand, M., Ravon, D., Guerche, J., and Prunet, P. Etude d'un nouveau vaccin contre la myxomatose. *Rec. Med. Vet.* 150:527–533, 1974.

Duran-Reynals, F. Production of degenerative inflammatory or neoplastic effects in the newborn rabbit by the Shope fibroma virus. *Yale J. Biol. Med.* 13:99–110, 1940.

———. Immunological factors that influence the neoplastic effects of the rabbit fibroma virus. *Cancer Res.* 5:25–39, 1945.

Dyce, A. L. Transmission of myxomatosis on the spines of thistles, *Cirsium vulgare* (Savi) Ten. *CSIRO Wildl. Res.* 6:88–90, 1961.

Edmonds, J. W., Nolan, I. F., Shepherd, R. C. H., and Gocs, A. Myxomatosis: The virulence of field strains of myxoma virus in a population of wild rabbits, *Oryctolagus cuniculus*, with high resistance to myxomatosis. *J. Hyg.* 74:417–418, 1975.

Edmonds, J. W., Shepherd, R. C. H., and Nolan, I. F. Myxomatosis: The occurrence of antibody to a soluble antigen of myxoma virus in wild rabbits, *Oryctolagus cuniculus* (L.), in Victoria, Australia. *J. Hyg.* 81:245–249, 1971.

Fenner, F. Classification of myxoma and fibroma viruses. *Nature* 171:562–563, 1953a.

———. Changes in the mortality rate due to myxomatosis in the Australian wild rabbit. *Nature* 172:228, 1953b.

———. Viruses of the myxoma-fibroma subgroup of the pox viruses: II. Comparison of soluble antigens by gel diffusion tests, and a general discussion of the subgroup. *Aust. J. Exp. Biol. Med. Sci.* 43:143–156, 1965.

———. *Classification and nomenclature of viruses.* New York: Karger, 1976.

———. Portraits of viruses: The poxviruses. *Intervirology.* 11:137–157, 1979.

Fenner, F., and Chapple, P. J. Evolutionary changes in myxoma virus in Britain: An examination of 222 naturally occurring strains obtained from 80 countries during the period October-November 1962. *J. Hyg.* 63:175–185, 1965.

Fenner, F., Day, M. F., and Woodroofe, G. M. The mechanism of the transmission of myxomatosis in the European rabbit (*Oryctolagus cuniculus*) by the mosquito *Aedes aegypti. Aust. J. Exp. Biol. Med. Sci.* 30:139–152, 1952.

———. Epidemiological consequences of the mechanical transmission of myxomatosis by mosquitoes. *J. Hyg.* 54:284–303, 1956.

Fenner, F., and McIntyre, G. A. Infectivity titrations of myxoma virus in the rabbit and the developing chick embryo. *J. Hyg.* 54:246–257, 1956.

Fenner, F., and Marshall, I. D. Passive immunity in myxomatosis of the European rabbit (*Oryctolagus cuniculus*): The protection conferred on kittens born by immune does. *J. Hyg.* 52:321–326, 1954.

———. Occurrence of attenuated strains of myxoma virus in Europe. *Nature* 176:782–783, 1955.

———. A comparison of the virulence for European rabbits (*Oryctolagus cuniculus*) of strains of myxoma virus recovered in the field in Australia, Europe and America. *J. Hyg.* 55:149–191, 1957.

Fenner, F., Marshall, I. D., and Woodroofe, G. M. Studies in the epidemiology of infectious myxomatosis of rabbits: I. Recovery of Australian wild rabbit populations. *J. Hyg.* 51:225–244, 1953.

Fenner, F., and Myers, K. Myxoma virus and myxomatosis in retrospect: The first quarter century of a new disease. In E. Kurstak and K. Maramorosch, eds., *Viruses and environment,* pp. 539–570. New York: Academic Press, 1978.

Fenner, F., and Ratcliffe, F. N. *Myxomatosis.* Cambridge: Cambridge University Press, 1965.

Fenner, F., and Woodroofe, G. M. The pathogenesis of infectious myxomatosis: The mechanism of infection and the immunological response in the European rabbit (*Oryctolagus cuniculus*). *Br. J. Exp. Pathol.* 34:400–411, 1953.

———. Protection of laboratory rabbits against myxomatosis by vaccination with fibroma virus. *Aust. J. Exp. Biol. Med. Sci.* 32:653–668, 1954.

———. Changes in the virulence and antigenic structure of strains of myxoma virus recovered from Australian wild rabbits between 1950 and 1964. *Aust. J. Exp. Biol. Med. Sci.* 43:359–370, 1965.

Findlay, G. M. Notes on infectious myxomatosis of rabbits. *Br. J. Exp. Pathol.* 10:214–219, 1929.

Fisher, E. R. The nature and staining reactions of the fibroma-cell inclusions of the Shope fibroma of the rabbit. *J. Natl. Cancer Inst.* 14:355–364, 1953.

Fisk, R. T., and Kessel, J. F. Immunization studies with the virus of infectious myxomatosis. *Proc. Soc. Exp. Biol. Med.* 29:9–11, 1931.

Fullagar, P. J. Observations on myxomatosis in a rabbit population with immune adults. *Aust. Wildl. Res.* 4:263–280, 1977.

Giban, J., Barthelemy, J., and Aubry, J. L'Epizootie de myxomatose en France chez le lapin de garenne. *Terre Vie* 103:167, 1956.

Ginder, D. R. Resistance to fibroma virus infection. The role of immune leucocytes and immune macrophages. *J. Exp. Med.* 101:43–58, 1955.

Grodhaus, G., Regnery, D. C., and Marshall, I. D.

Studies in the epidemiology of myxomatosis in California: II. The experimental transmission of myxomatosis in brush rabbits (*Sylvilagus bachmani*) by several species of mosquitoes. *Am. J. Hyg.* 77:205–212, 1963.

Haag, E., and Haag, J. Note sur un nouveau cas de myxomatose du lievre en France. *Bull. Acad. Vet. France* 27:479–480, 1954.

Harel, J., and Constantin, T. Sur la malignite des tumeurs provoquees par le virus fibromateux de Shope chez le lapin nouveau-ne et le lapin adulte traite par des doses massives de cortisone. *Bull. Cancer* 41:482–497, 1954.

Haugen, A. O. Life studies of the cottontail rabbit in southwestern Michigan. *Am. Midland Naturalist* 28:204–210, 1942.

Herman, C. M., Kilham, L., and Warbach, O. Incidence of Shope's rabbit fibroma in cottontails at the Patuxent research refuge. *J. Wildl. Manag.* 20:85–90, 1956.

Herman, C. M., and Reilly, J. R. Skin tumors on squirrels. *J. Wildl. Manag.* 20:402, 1955.

Hirth, R. S. Wyand, D. S., Osborne, A. D., and Burke, C. N. Epidermal changes caused by squirrel poxvirus. *J. Am. Vet. Med. Assoc.* 155:1120–1125, 1969.

Hobbs, J. R. Studies on the nature of the infectious myxoma virus of rabbits. *Am. J. Hyg.* 8:800–839, 1928.

———. The occurrence of natural and acquired immunity to infectious myxomatosis of rabbits. *Science* 73:94–95, 1931.

Hoffstadt, R. E., and Pilcher, K. S. The use of the chorioallantoic membrane of the developing chick embryo as a medium in the study of virus myxomatosum. *J. Bacteriol.* 35:353–367, 1938.

Hudson, J. R., and Mansi, W. Attenuated strains of myxoma virus in England. *Vet. Rec.* 67:746–747, 1955.

Hurst, E. W. Myxoma and the Shope fibroma: I. The histology of myxoma. *Br. J. Exp. Pathol.* 18:1–14, 1937a.

———. Myxoma and the Shope fibroma: III. Miscellaneous observations bearing on the relationship between myxoma, neuromyxoma and fibroma viruses. *Br. J. Exp. Pathol.* 18:23–30, 1937b.

———. Myxoma and the Shope fibroma: IV. The histology of fibroma. *Aust. J. Exp. Biol. Med. Sci.* 16:53–64, 1938.

Hyde, K. E. The relationship between the viruses of infectious myxoma and the Shope fibroma of rabbits. *Am. J. Hyg.* 23:278–297, 1936.

Hyde, R. R. The pathogenesis of infectious myxomatosis (Sanarelli) as modified by certain immunizing agents. *Am. J. Hyg.* 30:37–46, 1939a.

———. Infectious myxomatosis of rabbits (Sanarelli) versus the fibroma virus (Shope) with especial reference to the time interval in the establishment of concomitant immunity. *Am. J. Hyg.* 30:47–55, 1939b.

Hyde, R. R., and Gardner, R. E. Infectious myxoma of rabbits. *Am. J. Hyg.* 17:446–465, 1933.

———. Transmission experiments with the fibroma (Shope) and myxoma (Sanarelli) viruses. *Am. J. Hyg.* 30:57–63, 1939.

Jacotot, H., Toumanoff, C., Vallee, A., and Virat, B. Transmission experimentale de la myxomatose au lapin par *Anopheles maculipennis atroparvus* et *A. stephensi*. *Ann. Inst. Pasteur* 87:477–485, 1954a.

Jacotot, H., and Vallee, A. Essasi infructueux de vaccination contre la myxomatose des lapins par anavirus tissulaire. *Ann. Inst. Pasteur* 85:193, 1953.

Jacotot, H., Vallee, A., and Virat, B. Sur un cas de myxomatose chez le lievre. *Ann. Inst. Pasteur* 86:105–107, 1954b.

———. L'Immunite contre la myxomatose des lapins est-elle transmissible de la mere a ses laperaux? *Bull. Acad. Vet. France* 27:465–473, 1954c.

———. Etude sur la transmission experimentale de la myxomatose au lievre. *Ann. Inst. Pasteur* 88:1–10, 1955a.

———. Apparition en France d'un mutant naturellement attenue du virus de Sanarelli. *Ann. Inst. Pasteur* 89:361–364, 1955b.

———. Etude de quelques souches francaises de virus attenue du myxoma infectieux. *Ann. Inst. Pasteur* 90:779–783, 1956.

———. Sur l'immunisation contre le virus du myxome infectieux par inoculation de virus de fibrome de Shope. *Ann. Inst. Pasteur* 94:282–293, 1958.

———. Influence de la cortisone sur l'immunisation du lapin contre la myxomatose par inoculation de virus de Shope fibrome. *Ann. Inst. Pasteur* 103:285–290, 1962.

Jacotot, H., Virat, B., Reculard, P., and Vallee, A. Etude d'une souche attenuee du virus de myxome infectieux obtenue par passages en cultures cellulaires [MacKercher et Saito, 1964]. *Ann. Inst. Pasteur* 113:221–237, 1967.

Joiner, G. N., Jardine, J. H., and Gleiser, C. A. An epizootic of Shope fibromatosis in a commercial rabbitry. *J. Am. Vet. Med. Assoc.* 159:1583–1587, 1971.

Joubert, L., and Brun, A. Prophylaxie medicale a dessein cynegetique de la myxomatose des garennes. *Bull. Soc. Sci. Vet. Med. Comp. Lyon.* 78:101–107, 1976.

Joubert, L., Chippaux, A., Mouchet, J., and Oudar, J. Entretien hivernovernal de virus myxomateux dans les terriers. *Bull. Acad. Vet. France* 42:93–101, 1969.

Joubert, L., Leftheriotis, E., and Mouchet, J. *La myxomatose*. 1. 1972 2. 1973. Paris: L'Expansion Scientifique Francaise, 1972–1973.

Joubert, L., Oudar, J., Mouchet, J., and Hannoun, C. Transmission de la myxomatose par les moustiques en Camargue: Role preeminent de *Aedes caspius* et des *Anopheles* du groupe *maculipennis*. *Bull. Acad. Vet. France* 40:315–322, 1967.

Joubert, L., and Prave, M. Role des simulies (Tetisimulium bezzii Corti, 1914 et Odagmia du groupe ornatum) dans les enzooties hivernales occasionnelles de myxomatose en Haute-Provence. *Lyon Soc. Vet. Med. Comp. Bull.*

74:349–351, 1973.

Joubert, L., Tuaillon, P., Bertrand, M., Girod, J., and Favier, C. Sequelles genitales post-myxomateuses chez la lapine. *Bull. Soc. Sci. Vet. Med. Comp.* 74:27–32, 1972.

Kamahora, J., Kato, S., Baba, E., and Hagiwara, K. Studies on the inclusion bodies of fowl poxvirus. *Med. J. Osaka Univ.* 6:745–754, 1955.

Karstad, L., Thorsen, J., Davies, G., and Kaminjolo, J. S. Poxvirus fibromas on African hares. *J. Wildl. Dis.* 13:245–247, 1977.

Kato, S., and Cutting, W. A study of the inclusion bodies of rabbit myxoma and fibroma virus and a consideration of the relationship between all poxvirus inclusion bodies. *Stanford Med. Bull.* 17:34–45, 1959.

Kato, S., Takahashi, M., Kameyama, S., Morita, K., and Kamahora, J. Studies on the carrier culture of rabbit fibroma and myxoma virus. *Biken's J.* 2:30–34, 1959.

Kato, S., Takahashi, M., Miyamoto, H., and Kamahora, J. Shope fibroma and rabbit myxomia viruses: I. Autoradiographic and cytoimmunological studies on "B" type inclusions. *Biken's J.* 6:127–134, 1963.

Kato, S., and Windsor, C. C. Poxvirus inclusions *in vitro* and *in vivo*. *Fed. Proc.* 17:383, 1958.

Kessel, J. F., Fisk, R. T., and Prouty, C. C. Studies with the California strain of the virus of infectious myxomatosis. *Proc. 5th Pacific Sci. Congr.* 4:2927–2939, 1934.

Kessel, J. F., Prouty, C. C., and Meyer, J. W. Occurrence of infectious myxomatosis in southern California. *Proc. Soc. Exp. Biol. Med.* 28:413–414, 1931.

Kilham, L. Metastasizing viral fibroma of gray squirrels: Pathogenesis and mosquito transmission. *Am. J. Hyg.* 61:55–63, 1955.

——. Fibroma-myxoma virus transformation in different types of tissue culture. *J. Natl. Cancer Inst.* 20:729–738, 1958.

Kilham, L., and Dalmat, H. T. Host-virus-mosquito relations of Shope fibromas in cottontail rabbits. *Am. J. Hyg.* 61:45–54, 1955.

Kilham, L., and Fisher, E. R. Pathogenesis of fibromas in cottontail rabbits. *Am. J. Hyg.* 59:104–112, 1954.

Kilham, L., Herman, G. M., and Fisher, E. R. Naturally occurring fibroma of gray squirrels related to Shope's fibroma. *Proc. Soc. Exp. Biol. Med.* 82:298–301, 1953.

Kilham, L., and Woke, P. A. Laboratory transmission of fibromas (Shope) in cottontail rabbits by means of fleas and mosquitoes. *Proc. Soc. Exp. Biol. Med.* 83:296–301, 1953.

Kirschstein, R. L., Rabson, A. S., and Kilham, L. Pulmonary lesions produced by fibroma viruses in squirrels and rabbits. *Cancer Res.* 18:1340–1344, 1958.

Lafenetre, H., Cortez, A., Rioux, J. A., Pages, A., Vollhardt, Y., and Quatrepates, H. Enzootie de tumeurs cutanees chez la lievre. *Bull. Acad. Vet. France* 33:379–389, 1960.

Ledingham, J. C. G. Studies on the serological interrelationships of the rabbit viruses, myxomatosis (Sanarelli 1898) and fibroma (Shope 1932). *Br. J. Exp. Pathol.* 18:436–449, 1937.

Leinati, L., Mandelli, G., and Carrara, O. Lesioni cutanee nodulari nelle lepri della pianura padana. *Atti. Soc. Ital. Sci. Vet.* 13:429–435, 1959.

Lloyd, B. J., Jr., and Kahler, H. Electron microscopy of the virus of rabbit fibroma. *J. Natl. Cancer Inst.* 15:991, 1955.

Lockley, R. M. The European rabbit-flea, *Spilopsyllus cuniculi*, as a vector of myxomatosis in Britain. *Vet. Rec.* 66:434–435, 1954.

——. Failure of myxomatosis on Skokholm Island. *Nature* 175:906–907, 1955.

Lush, D. The virus of infectious myxomatosis of rabbits on the chorioallantoic membrane of the developing egg. *Aus. J. Exp. Biol. Med. Sci.* 15:131–139, 1937.

McKee, C. M. Immunization against infectious myxomatosis with heat-inactivated virus in conjunction with the type III pneumococcus. *Am. J. Hyg.* 29:165–170, 1939.

McKercher, D. G. Infectious myxomatosis: I. Vaccination. II. Antibiotic therapy. *Am. J. Vet. Res.* 13:425–429, 1952.

McKercher, D. G., and Saito, J. An attenuated live virus vaccine for myxomatosis. *Nature* 202:933–934, 1964.

Magallon, P., and Bazin, J. Myxomatose du lievre. *Bull. Acad. Vet. France* 26:457–463, 1953.

Mansi, W. Serological investigation of myxoma and fibroma viruses: I. Complement-fixation test. *J. Comp. Pathol.* 67:208–216, 1957a.

——. The study of some viruses by the plate gel diffusion precipitin test. *J. Comp. Pathol.* 67:297–303, 1957b.

Marcato, P. S., and Simoni, P. The cutaneous lesions in rabbit myxomatosis: Ultrastructural study. *J. Submicrosc. Cytol.* 9:67–82, 1977a.

——. Ultrastructural researches on rabbit myxomatosis: Lymph nodal lesions. *Vet. Pathol.* 14:361–367, 1977b.

Marshall, I. D. The influence of ambient temperature on the course of myxomatosis in rabbits. *J. Hyg.* 57:484–497, 1959.

Marshall, I. D., and Douglas, G. W. Studies in the epidemiology of infectious myxomatosis of rabbits: VIII. Further observations on changes in the innate resistance of Australian wild rabbits exposed to myxomatosis. *J. Hyg.* 59:117–122, 1961.

Marshall, I. D., Dyce, A. L., Poole, W. E., and Fenner, F. Studies in the epidemiology of infectious myxomatosis of rabbits: IV. Observations of disease behavior in two localities near the northern limit of rabbit infestation in Australia, May 1952-April 1953. *J. Hyg.* 53:12–25, 1955.

Marshall, I.D., and Fenner, F. Studies in the epidemiology of infectious myxomatosis of rabbits: V. Changes in the innate resistance of Australian wild rabbits exposed to myxomatosis. *J. Hyg.* 56:288–302, 1958.

————. Studies in the epidemiology of infectious myxomatosis of rabbits: VII. The virulence of strains of myxoma virus recovered from Australian wild rabbits between 1951 and 1959. *J. Hyg.* 58:485–488, 1960.

Marshall, I. D., and Regnery, D. C. Myxomatosis in a California brush rabbit (*Sylvilagus bachmani*). *Nature* 188:73–74, 1960.

————. Studies in the epidemiology of myxomatosis in California: III. The response of brush rabbits (*Sylvilagus bachmani*) to infection with exotic and enzootic strains of myxoma virus, and the relative infectivity of the tumors for mosquitoes. *Am. J. Hyg.* 77:213–219, 1963.

Marshall, I. D., Regnery, D. C., and Grodhaus, G. Studies in the epidemiology of myxomatosis in California: I. Observations on two outbreaks of myxomatosis in coastal California and the recovery of myxoma virus from a brush rabbit (*Sylvilagus bachmani*). *Am. J. Hyg.* 77:195–204, 1963.

Martin, C. J. Observations of *Myxomatosis cuniculi* (Sanarelli) made with a view to the use of the virus in the control of rabbit plagues. *Bull. Council Sci. Industr. Res. Aust.* vol. 96, 1936.

Mead-Briggs, A. R. Some experiments concerning interchange of the rabbit flea *Spilopsyllus cuniculi* Dale between living rabbit hosts. *J. Anim. Ecol.* 33:13–26, 1964.

Mead-Briggs, A. R., and Vaughan, J. A. The differential transmissibility of myxoma virus strains of differing virulence grades by the rabbit flea *Spilopsyllus cuniculi* (Dale). *J. Hyg.* 75:237–247, 1975.

Mello, U. Di una affezione neoplasica ad andamenio epizootico nelle lepri. *Ann. Staz. Sper. Lotta Mal. Inform. Bestiame Piem. Lig.* 2:47–50, 1929.

Micozzi, G., and Palarchi, M. Mixomatosi spontanea nella lepre. *Vet. Ital.* 26:356–360, 1975.

Moses, A. O virus do mixoma dos coelhos. *Mem. Inst. Oswaldo Cruz* 3:46–53, 1911.

Mukai, S. Experimental studies on the histogenesis of infectious myxoma of rabbits: I. Histopathological study. *Sapporo Med. J.* 17:190, 1960a.

————. Experimental studies on the histogenesis of infectious myxoma of rabbits: II. Generalization of the myxoma virus. *Sapporo Med. J.* 18:263, 1960b.

Myers, K. Studies in the epidemiology of infectious myxomatosis of rabbits: II. Field experiments, August-November 1950, and the first epizootic of myxomatosis in the Riverina Plain of southeastern Australia. *J. Hyg.* 52:47–59, 1954.

Myers, K., Marshall, I. D., and Fenner, F. Studies in the epidemiology of infectious myxomatosis of rabbits: III. Observations on two succeeding epizootics in Australian wild rabbits on the Riverina Plain of southeastern Australia, 1951–1953. *J. Hyg.* 52:337–360, 1954.

Mykytowycz, R. An attenuated strain of the myxomatosis virus recovered from the field. *Nature* 172:448–489, 1953.

————. The effect of season and mode of transmission on the severity of myxomatosis due to an attenuated strain of the virus. *Aust. J. Exp. Biol. Med. Sci.* 34:121–132, 1956.

————. The transmission of myxomatosis by *Simulium melatum* Wharton (Diptera: Simuliidae). *CSIRO Wildl. Res.* 2:1–14, 1957.

————. Contact transmission of infectious myxomatosis of the rabbit, *Oryctolagus cuniculus* (L.). *CSIRO Wildl. Res.* 3:1–6, 1958.

————. Social behavior of an experimental colony of wild rabbits, *Oryctolagus cuniculus* (L.): IV. Conclusion: Outbreak of myxomatosis; third breeding season and starvation. *CSIRO Wildl. Res.* 6:142–155, 1961.

Padgett, B. L., Wright, M. J., Jayne, A., and Walker, D. L. Electron microscopic structure of myxoma virus and some reactivable derivatives. *J. Bacteriol.* 87:454–460, 1964.

Parker, R. F., and Thompson, R. L. The effect of external temperature on the course of infectious myxomatosis of rabbits. *J. Exp. Med.* 75:567–573, 1942.

Patton, N. M., and Holmes, H. T. Myxomatosis in domestic rabbits in Oregon. *J. Am. Vet. Med. Assoc.* 171:560–562, 1977.

Pons, M. W., and Preston, W. S. The *in vivo* inhibition by β-phenylserine of rabies, myxoma and vaccinia viruses. *Virology* 15:164–172, 1961.

Poole, W. E. Breeding of the wild rabbit, *Oryctolagus cuniculus* (L.) in relation to the environment. *CSIRO Wildl. Res.* 5:21–43, 1960.

Prose, P. H., Friedman-Kien, A. E., and Vilcek, J. Morphogenesis of rabbit fibroma virus. *Am. J. Pathol.* 64:467–477, 1971.

Pulley, L. T., and Shively, J. N. Naturally occurring infectious fibroma in the domestic rabbit. *Vet. Pathol.* 10:509–519, 1973.

Raflo, C. P., Olsen, R. G., Pakes, S. P., and Webster, W. S. Characterization of a fibroma virus isolated from naturally-occurring skin tumors in domestic rabbits. *Lab. Anim. Sci.* 23:525–532, 1973.

Ratcliffe, F. N., Myers, K., Fennessey, B. V., and Calaby, J. H. Myxomatosis in Australia: A step towards the biological control of the rabbit. *Nature* 170:7–11, 1952.

Reisner, A. H., Sobey, W. R., and Conolly, D. Differences among the soluble antigens of myxoma viruses originating in Brazil and California. *Virology* 20:539–541, 1963.

Regnery, D. C. The epidemic potential of Brazilian myxoma virus (Lausanne strain) for three species of North American cottontails. *Am. J. Epidemiol.* 94:514–519, 1971.

Regnery, D. C., and Marshall, I. D. Studies in the epidemiology of myxomatosis in California: IV. The susceptibility of six leporid species to Californian myxoma virus and the relative infectivity of their tumors for mosquitoes. *Am. J. Epidemiol.* 94:508–513, 1971.

Regnery, D. C., and Miller, J. H. A myxoma virus epizootic in a brush rabbit population. *J. Wildl. Dis.* 8:327–331, 1972.

Regnery, R. L. Preliminary studies on an unusual poxvirus of the western grey squirrel (*Sciurus griseus griseus*) of North America. *Intervirology* 5:364–366, 1975.

Ritchie, J. N., Hudson, J. R., and Thompson, H. V. Myxomatosis. *Vet. Rec.* 66:796–801, 1954.

Rivers, T. M. Changes observed in epidermal cells covering myxomatous masses induced by virus myxomatosis (Sanarelli). *Proc. Soc. Exp. Biol. Med.* 24:435–437, 1926.

———. Infectious myxomatosis of rabbits: Observations on the pathological changes induced by virus myxomatosum (Sanarelli). *J. Exp. Med.* 51:965–976, 1930.

Roby, R., Tesky, C., and Houlihan, R. B. Inhibition of plaque formation by mxyoma and fibroma viruses with pyrimidine analogues. *Proc. Soc. Exp. Biol. Med.* 120:496–500, 1965.

Ross, J., and Sanders, M. F. Innate resistance to myxomatosis in wild rabbits in England. *J. Hyg.* 79:411–415, 1977.

Ross, J., and Tittensor, A. M. Myxomatosis in selected rabbit populations in Southern England and Wales, 1971–1977. In K. Myers, ed., *Proc. World Lagomorph Congr.*, Guelph, Ont., 12–17 Aug. 1979. IUCN Publ., (in press) 1980.

Rowe, B. Mansi, W., and Hudson, J. R. The use of fibroma virus (Shope) for the protection of rabbits against myxomatosis. *J. Comp. Pathol.* 66:290–298, 1956.

Sanarelli, G. Das myxomatogene Virus. Beitrag zum Studium der Krankheitserreger ausserhalb des Sichtbaren. *Zentralbl. Bakteriol.* 23:865–873, 1898.

Scherrer, P. R. Morphogenese et ultrastructure de virus fibromateux de Shope. *Path. Microbiol.* 31:129–146, 1968.

Service, M. W. A reappraisal of the role of mosquitoes in the transmission of myxomatosis in Britain. *J. Hyg.* 69:105–111, 1971.

Shaffer, J. G. Antigenic relationship of infectious myxoma and fibroma viruses of the rabbit. *Am. J. Hyg.* 34:102–120, 1941.

Shope, R. E. A transmissible tumor-like condition in rabbits. *J. Exp. Med.* 56:793–802, 1932a.

———. A filterable virus causing a tumor-like condition in rabbits and its relationship to virus myxomatosum. *J. Exp. Med.* 56:803–822, 1932b.

———. Infectious fibroma of rabbits: III. The serial transmission of virus myxomatosum in cottontail rabbits, and cross-immunity tests with the fibroma virus. *J. Exp. Med.* 63:33–41, 1936a.

———. Infectious fibroma of rabbits: IV. The infection with virus myxomatosum of rabbits recovered from fibroma. *J. Exp. Med.* 63:43–57, 1936b.

Smith, M. H. D. Propagation of rabbit fibroma virus in the embryonated egg. *Proc. Soc. Exp. Biol. Med.* 69:136–140, 1948.

Sobey, W. R. Myxomatosis: The virulence of the virus and its relation to genetic resistance in the rabbit. *Aust. J. Sci.* 23:53, 1960.

Sobey, W. R., and Conolly, D. Myxomatosis: The introduction of the European rabbit flea *Spilopsyllus cuniculi* (Dale) into wild rabbit populations in Australia. *J. Hyg.* 69:331–346, 1971.

———. Myxomatosis: Passive immunity in the offspring of immune rabbits (*Oryctolagus cuniculus*) infested with fleas (*Spilopsyllus cuniculi* Dale) and exposed to myxoma virus. *J. Hyg.* 74:43–55, 1975.

Sobey, W. R., Conolly, D., and Adams, K. M. Myxomatosis: A simple method of sampling blood and testing for circulating soluable antigens or antibodies to them. *Aust. J. Sci.* 28:354–355, 1966.

Sobey, W. R., Conolly, D., Haycock, P., and J. W. Edmonds. Myxomatosis: The effect of age upon survival of wild and domestic rabbits (*Oryctolagus cuniculus*) with a degree of genetic resistance and unselected domestic rabbits infected with myxoma virus. *J. Hyg.* 68:137–149, 1970.

Sobey, W. R., Menzies, W., Conolly, D., and Adams, K. M. Myxomatosis: The effect of raised ambient temperature on survival time. *Aust. J. Sci.* 30:322–324, 1967.

Sobey, W. R., and Menzies, W. Myxomatosis: The introduction of the European rabbit flea *Spilopsyllus cuniculi* into Australia. *Aust. J. Sci.* 31:404–406, 1969.

Sobey, W. R., and Turnbull, K. Fertility in the rabbits recovering from myxomatosis. *Aust. J. Biol. Sci.* 9:455–461, 1956.

Splendore, A. Uber das Virus myxomatosum der Kaninchen. *Zentralbl. Bakteriol.* 48:300, 1909.

Sprunt, D. H. Infectious myxomatosis (Sanarelli) in pregnant rabbits. *J. Exp. Med.* 56:601–608, 1932.

Szczech, G. M., Carlton, W. W., Hinsman, E. J., and Jacobsen, J. J. Fibroma in Indiana cottontails. *J. Am. Vet. Med. Assoc.* 165:846–849, 1974.

Takahashi, M., Kameyama, S., Kato, S., and Kamahora, J. A study of myxoma virus inclusions by fluorescein-labeled antibody. *Biken's J.* 1:198–200, 1958.

———. Immunological relationship of the poxvirus group. *Biken's J.* 2:27–29, 1959a.

Takahashi, M., Kato, S. Kameyama, S., and Kamahora, J. A study on the multiplication of rabbit myxoma virus with fluorescent antibody technique. *Biken's J.* 2:333–340, 1959b.

Teixeira, J. de Castro, and Smadel, J. E. Further studies on the serological reactions of the soluble antigens of infectious myxomatosis. *J. Bacteriol.* 42:591–603, 1941.

Thomas, A. S. Further changes in vegetation since the advent of myxomatosis. *J. Ecol.* 51:151–186, 1963.

Thompson, H. V. The origin and spread of myxomatosis with particular reference to Great Britain. *Terre Vie* 103:137–152, 1956.

Thompson, R. L. The influence of temperature upon proliferation of infectious fibroma and infectious myxoma viruses in vivo. *J. Infect. Dis.* 62:307–312, 1938.

Thompson, R. L., Davis, J., Russell, P. B., and Hitchings, G. H. Effect of aliphatic oxime and isatin thiosemicarbizone on vaccine infection in the mouse and rabbit. *Proc. Soc. Exp. Biol. Med.* 84:496–499, 1953a.

Thompson, R. L., Minton, S. A., Jr., Officer, J. E., and Hitchings, G. H. Effect of heterocyclic and other thiosemicarbizones on vaccinia infection in the mouse. *J. Immunol.* 70:229–234, 1953b.

Tompkins, W. A. F., Adams, C., and Rawls, W. E. An *in vitro* measure of cellular immunity to fibroma virus. *J. Immunol.* 104:502–510, 1970.

Vaughan, H. E. N., and Vaughan, J. A. Some aspects of the epizootiology of myxomatosis. *Proc. Symp. Zool. Soc. London* 24:289–309, 1968.

Verna, J. E. Cell culture response to fibroma virus. *J. Bacteriol.* 89:524–528, 1965.

Verna, J. E., and Eylar, O. R. Rabbit fibroma virus plaque assay and *in vitro* studies. *Virology* 18:266–273, 1962.

Vilcek, J., Friedman-Kien, A. E., and Prose, P. H. Some biological properties of Poly I-Poly C: Their usefulness in the standardization of interferon inducers. International Symposium on Standardization of Interferon and Interferon Inducers, London, 1969. *Symp. Ser. Immunobiol. Stand.* 14:213–220, 1970.

Whitty, B. T. Myxomatosis in the common hare: *Lepus europaeus. Irish Vet. J.* 9:267–268, 1955.

Williams, R. T. Observations on the behavior of the European rabbit flea, *Spilopsyllus cuniculi* Dale, on a natural population of wild rabbits, *Oryctolagus cuniculus* (L.) in Australia. *Aust. J. Zool.* 19:41–51, 1971.

———. The distribution and abundance of the ectoparasites of the wild rabbit, *Oryctolagus cuni-*culus, in New South Wales, Australia. *Parasitology* 64:321–330, 1972.

Williams, R. T., Dunsmore, J. D., and Parer, I. Evidence for the existence of latent myxoma virus in rabbits (*Oryctolagus cuniculus* (L.)). *Nature* 238:99–101, 1972a.

Williams, R. T., Fullagar, P. J., Davey, C. C., and Kogon, C. Factors affecting the survival time of rabbits in a winter epizootic of myxomatosis at Canberra, Australia. *J. Appl. Ecol.* 9:399–410, 1972b.

Williams, R. T., and Parer, I. Observations on the dispersal of the European rabbit flea, *Spilopsyllus cuniculi* Dale, through a natural population of wild rabbits, *Oryctolagus cuniculus* L. *Aust. J. Zool.* 19:129–140, 1971.

———. The status of myxomatosis at Urana, New South Wales, from 1968 until 1971. *Aust. J. Zool.* 20:391–404, 1972.

Woodroofe, G. M., and Fenner, F. Genetic studies with mammalian poxviruses. IV. Hybridization between several different poxviruses. *Virology* 12:272–282, 1960.

———. Serological relationships within the poxvirus group: An antigen common to all members of the group. *Virology* 16:334–341, 1962.

———. Viruses of the myxoma-fibroma subgroup of the poxviruses: I. Plaque production in cultured cells, plaque-reduction tests, and cross-protection tests in rabbits. *Aust. J. Exp. Biol. Med. Sci.* 43:123–142, 1965.

Yuill, T. M., and Hanson, R. P. Infection of suckling cottontail rabbits with Shope's fibroma virus. *Proc. Soc. Exp. Biol. Med.* 117:376–380, 1964.

14 *African Swine Fever*

W. PLOWRIGHT

Synonyms: **Montgomery's disease, East African swine fever, pestis porcina africana, Afrikanische schweinepest.**

African swine fever virus (ASFV) is the cause of one of the most economically serious and lethal diseases of domestic swine. The ravages of this disease have extended far beyond its cradle of enzootic infection in African wildlife, causing frequent alarms and the initiation of intensive and continuing research programs. However, it apparently produces no overt signs of disease in either the wild Suidae, which were for long regarded as its sole reservoirs, or in the argasid ticks, which in some areas are now known to be highly efficient reservoirs and vectors. The situation could change dramatically if ASFV were to naturally infect other wild vertebrate species such as feral pigs or members of the Tayassuidae and rodents in South America.

Veterinarians in zoological gardens and those conducting wildlife investigations should therefore be familiar with the implications of ASFV infection in species committed to their care, considering the potentially devastating results of a transfer of virus to domestic swine as well as the possible harmful effects in some of their own charges.

Reviews of available information on ASFV are given in Coggins (1974), DeTray (1963), Hess (1971), Neitz (1963), Plowright et al. (1969b), Scott (1965a,b,c) and Walker (1933).

DISTRIBUTION AND HOST RANGE. Until 1957, ASF was limited to the African continent where it had first been described by Montgomery (1921, 1922) in a classical series of studies (1910–1915) to which little was added in the following 45 years. He showed that the epidemiology of the disease in domestic swine in East Africa (Kenya) was consistent with its origin from a virus reservoir in wild swine, particularly warthogs (*Phacochoerus aethiopicus*) but also bush pigs (*Potamochoerus* spp.). He hypothesised that the occurrence of ASF was determined by the carnivorous habits of domestic swine rather than exposure to warthog excretions. It was clearly demonstrated that the two

species of wild Suidae did not react clinically to inoculation with virus, although the agent could be recovered from them for 11–17 days (Montgomery 1921; Walker 1933).

Much later work established that the distribution of ASF in Africa is closely correlated with that of the warthog (Anon. 1962), although some warthog populations in South Africa (Natal, Zululand, Cape Province) are apparently free from infection (Pini and Hurter 1975). The occurrence of the virus in bush pigs is well documented (DeTray 1963; Thomas and Kolbe 1942); but there is only one report of the recovery of ASFV from the much rarer species, the giant forest hog (*Hylochoerus meinertzhageni*) (Heuschele and Coggins 1965a). Reports of virus isolations from the hippopotamus, porcupine, and hyena (Cox 1963) have not been substantiated (Stone and Heuschele 1965). The American white-collared peccary (*Tayassu angulatus*) was not susceptible to inoculation with three strains of ASFV (Salamanca, Tengani, and Dakar) in a dose of 10^5 pig ID_{50} administered intramuscularly or following exposure by contact. Cultures of buffy coat and bone marrow cells from this species did not show hemadsorption (Dardiri et al. 1969).

The virus established itself in domestic swine populations in Africa, particularly in Angola where the infection became enzootic and probably also modified in its virulence for pigs; elsewhere on the continent it was usually self-eliminating or eradicated by slaughter or other veterinary police measures. Outside Africa it was confirmed for the first time in Portugal in 1957 and was thought to have been eliminated by 1958, but it recurred or was reintroduced in 1960 and quickly spread to Spain. It has persisted ever since in the Iberian Peninsula, causing considerable damage; thus, losses in Spain up to 1971 totaled 737,000, with nearly 100,000 pigs slaughtered in control programs during 1971 alone. The disease has since spread on three occasions to France (1964, 1974, and 1976), to Italy (1967–1968), to Cuba (1971), and to Malta, Sardinia, Brazil, and the Dominican Repulic (1978). The only wild vertebrate reported to be affected in these outbreaks was the wild boar in Spain (Botija 1961).

In addition to vertebrates it was also recognized that soft ticks (*Ornithodorus erraticus*) could serve as highly efficient reservoirs and biological vectors of the virus in Spain (Botija 1963). Later it was shown that ASFV was frequently present in collections of *Ornithodorus* from burrows in the Serengeti region of Tanzania (Plowright et al. 1969a,b) and Pini and Hurter (1975) have recently confirmed that ticks infected with ASFV were present in warthog burrows in the western Transvaal of South Africa.

ETIOLOGY. African swine fever virus is a large icosahedral virus, 175–215 mμ in diameter, with a central nucleoid containing double-stranded DNA and a hexagonal, multilayered outer shell, possibly containing at least 812 capsomeres. There are at least five major polypeptides in the virion (Black and Brown 1976) or in virus-infected cells (Dalsgaard et al. 1977). The virus also has an outer envelope derived by budding from the plasma membrane and is sensitive to lipid solvents. The morphology of the virion and its replication in cytoplasmic "factories" are clearly reminiscent of the iridoviruses of insects. The virus is highly resistant to heat, putrefaction, and a wide range of pH values; it persists for months in fresh or processed pig meat products but is inactivated by substituted phenolic disinfectants (Stone and Hess 1973) and is rapidly destroyed by hypochlorite or detergents in the absence of large amounts of protein.

Virus from animal tissues grows readily in glass-adherent cells derived from swine blood leukocytes or bone marrow; the infected cells show hemadsorption of erythrocytes from pigs, warthogs, bush pigs, or giant forest hogs and then undergo cytolysis (Malmquist and Hay 1960). Macrophages from resistant species, such as man, rabbit, guinea pig, hamster, rat, and chicken do not support virus multiplication (Enjuanes et al. 1977). Buffy coat cells from goats are apparently susceptible and show hemadsorption (Dardiri 1966), a finding in line with the reported susceptibility of young goats (Kovalenko et al. 1966). No hemagglutinating activity is demonstrable in virus-infected fluids, but cytoplasmic inclusion bodies containing viral antigens, demonstrable by immunofluorescence, are present in the cell cytoplasm. The virus can be adapted by passage to growth in a number of other primary cultures (for example, pig kidney and chick embryo fibroblasts) or established cell lines, including BHK-21, VERO, and MS.

All strains of ASFV have common antigens

reacting in immunodiffusion, complement fixation, and immunofluorescence tests, and antibodies detectable by these methods are regularly produced in infected survivor animals. However, antibodies neutralizing virus in vitro have not been detected, even in hyperimmunized swine. Pigs surviving infection with one virus isolate usually but not invariably resist challenge by the homologous virus (Montgomery 1921; Walker 1933); but they may succumb to challenge with heterologous strains. This evidence for immunologic variation in ASFV gains support from the fact that antibodies inhibiting hemadsorption to infected cells, which appear in some survivor swine, are specific to the infecting strains and do not cross-react with those induced by other isolates derived from different geographic areas. Some isolates of ASFV lack the capacity to cause hemadsorption (Hess 1971; Vigario et al. 1974) even on isolation from primary outbreaks of disease in Africa (Pini and Wagenaar 1974).

Warthog Populations. Many earlier studies on the occurrence of ASFV in warthog populations in Africa have shown infection to be widespread but have failed to indicate the true prevalence, since antibody tests were seldom performed (DeTray 1963; Heuschele et al. 1965), and attempts to isolate the virus were often made, using mixtures of tissues such as blood or spleen that are now known to be poor sources of the agent (Heuschele et al. 1965). These tissues have also been used in the case of other species such as porcupines and hyenas (Cox 1963) or the hippopotamus (Stone and Heuschele 1965).

More systematic studies on the distribution of ASFV in populations of warthogs in East Africa have shown significant differences between those in northern Tanzania and southern Kenya, on the one hand (the Serengeti region), and those in western Uganda, exemplified by the Queen Elizabeth National Park, on the other. In each of the two areas, over 100 warthogs were shot and samples of individual tissues placed on ice immediately for later detection and titration of virus in pig bone marrow cultures. The samples included blood (with anticoagulant), spleen, lung, liver, kidney, and five lymph nodes, namely, mandibular, parotid, gastrohepatic, superficial inguinal, and bronchial. The results are shown in Figures 14.1 and 14.2 and quantitative data are recorded in Table 14.1.

In the Serengeti region, ASFV was recovered from virtually all animals up to 1 year old, including 6 estimated to be 12 weeks old or less.

Viremia was present in only 2 (7%) of 30 warthogs 1 year old or less, and attempts to demonstrate viremia in an additional 10 animals not more than 7 days old, were successful with 2 of 3 young from one of three litters captured. Undiluted blood was necessary to produce hemadsorption, 1 ml of a 10-fold dilution always failing to do so. These figures coincide with those of Heuschele and Coggins (1969), who found viremia in only 3 of 22 animals in this area but recorded a blood titer of $10^{2.5}$ HAD_{50}/ml in one instance. The rate of virus recovery dropped gradually over succeeding years of life in the Serengeti region, but 21% (4 of 19) of animals aged (4 years or older) still yielded ASFV from one or more tissues (Fig. 14.1).

In western Uganda no virus was present in 6 animals up to 3 months of age, and the infection rate reached a mean maximum of 58% in groups aged 4–12 months. This figure declined to 30% in the 2nd year of life and 8% in all other groups. Hence, infection here was later and became undetectable more rapidly (Fig. 14.1).

The distribution and amount of virus in various tissues from positive warthogs is given in Figure 14.2 and Table 14.1. The tissues most frequently infected in the Serengeti region were the parotid and submaxillary (mandibular) lymph nodes, the former being by far the best source in animals more than 1 year old. Maximal titers of 10^5–10^6 HAD_{50}/g were found in some lymph nodes, but the highest mean figure ($10^{3.8}$ HAD_{50}/g) was always found in the gastrohepatic node. The spleen was not only an infrequent source of virus in both areas examined (6–18% of all positives), but titers were also low, with a mean of $10^{2.0}$ HAD_{50}/g in the Serengeti region. Virus was never recovered from the liver and kidney, and only one isolation was made from lung in a total of 94 positive animals (Fig. 14.2). These negative findings reflect the reliability of the results for virus distribution in other tissues, particularly since highly vascular organs such as lung, liver, and kidney might have been expected to be infected in viremic animals.

In view of the possibility of vertical transmission, ASFV was also sought in the tissues of 52 fetuses derived from 17 warthog sows, 10 of which were infected at the time of death; these fetuses were estimated to be in the 14th–24th weeks of gestation, as judged by weight and crown-rump length. No virus was isolated from lactating mammary tissues from 5 sows, and contrary to hypotheses advanced by Scott (1965a), it was concluded that transplacental and milk transmission did not occur.

TABLE 14.1 The Distribution and Quantity of ASFV in the Tissues of Infected Warthogs in East Africa.

Geographical Area	Age Group	Total No.	PL	ML	IL	BL	GL	Spleen	Blood	Lung
Serengeti (northern Tanzania; southern Kenya)	0–2 months	34	18/31	22/34	16/28	16/31	14/34	6/34	2/30	1/34
		% positive	58	65	57	52	41	18	7	3
		mean titer	3.1	3.1	2.7	3.3	3.6	2.0	(trace)	(2.2)
Do.	>12 months	32	22/31	12/32	10/30	7/30	9/32	2/32	2/29	0/32
		% positive	71	37	33	23	28	6	7	nil
		mean titer	2.7	3.0	2.7	3.1	3.7	2.0	(trace)	...
Queen Elizabeth Park (western Uganda)	all ages	30	15/30	10/29	15/30	17/28	11/30	4/27	0/28	0/28
		% positive	50	35	50	61	37	15	nil	nil
		mean titer	2.8	2.7	3.1	3.6	3.8	2.7	...	...

[a] The abbreviations PL, ML, IL, BL, and GL refer to parotid, mandibular, superficial inguinal, bronchial, and gastrohepatic lymph nodes, respectively.
[b] $\log_{10}$ HAD_{50}/g.

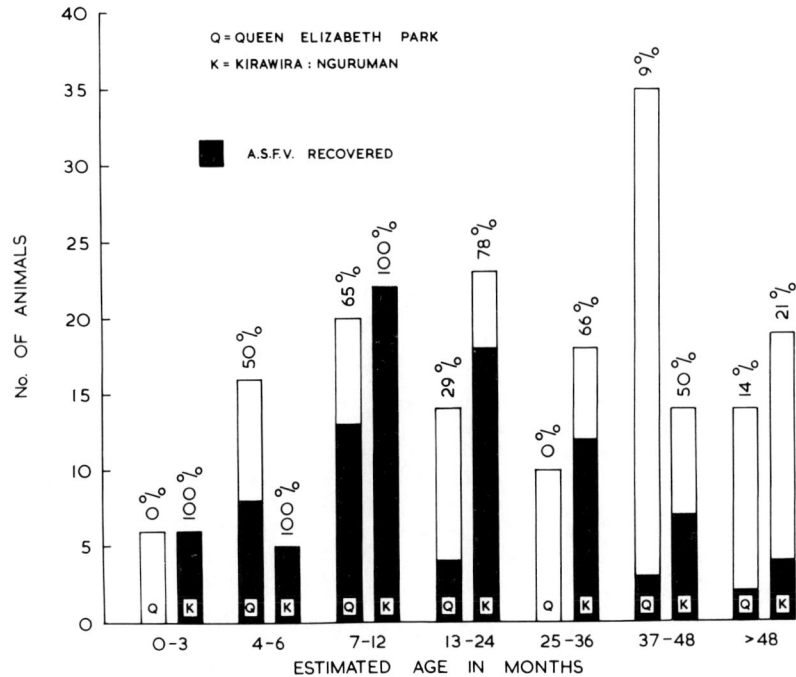

FIG. 14.1 The proportion of warthogs of different age groups with precipitating antibodies to ASFV antigens.

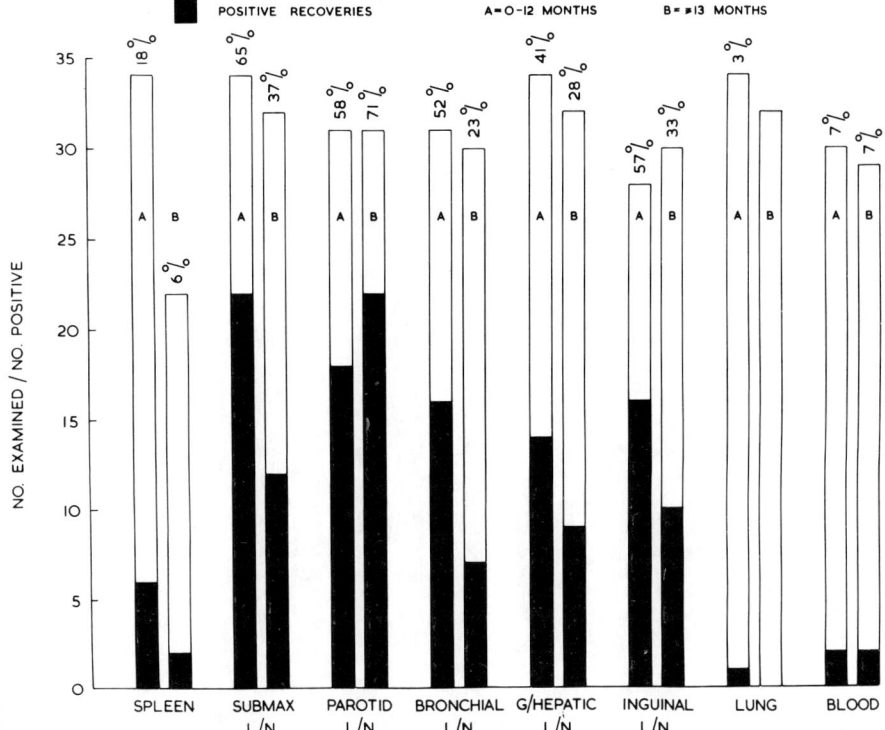

FIG. 14.2 The distribution of virus in Kirawira warthogs shown to be infected with ASFV.

Immunodiffusion tests were performed on the sera of all warthogs, with use of a sonicated extract of infected pig kidney cells as antigen. In the Serengeti region all animals over 4 months of age had antibody, whereas in western Uganda only 50% were positive at 4–6 months, and thereafter 79–93% produced precipitation lines (Fig. 14.3). It was evident that infection was invariable in the former population and probably so in the latter, but a few older animals in Uganda (<10%) may have been serologically negative.

There is a high mortality among warthogs in the first 24 months of life; it may reach 80% and with adverse circumstances be as high as 95% (Child et al. 1968). Jarman (1970, quoted in Pierce 1974) reported that the mean litter size in the western Serengeti dropped from 5.2 for litters farrowed in September to 2.2 by October. There was no suggestion in this population study of failure to thrive or of frank disease caused by ASFV infection. Attempts to experimentally infect warthogs that were assumed not to have been previously exposed have also failed to show pathogenicity of the virus for this species, but Montgomery (1921) did record low-grade fever of about 7–10 days duration. A definitive answer can obviously only be given by virologic and clinicopathologic studies on serologically negative animals infected under close observation.

Bush Pig Populations. Mansveld (1963) stated that the virus was 10 times more frequent in warthogs than in bush pigs. DeTray (1963) recorded the isolation of ASFV from only a few of more than 50 bush pigs in Kenya; the frequency of virus was low.

TRANSMISSION. It is known that there are difficulties in demonstrating transfer of ASFV from warthog to warthog (even ignoring the possibility of previous infection) or from warthog to domestic swine (DeTray 1963; Montgomery 1921; Walker 1933). Virus has not been demonstrated in the excretions of warthogs. Close and prolonged contact between infected warthogs and pigs nearly always failed to result in infection of the latter (DeTray 1963; Heuschele and Coggins 1969; Plowright et al. 1969b). Viremic bush pigs also failed to transfer virus to domestic swine (DeTray 1963).

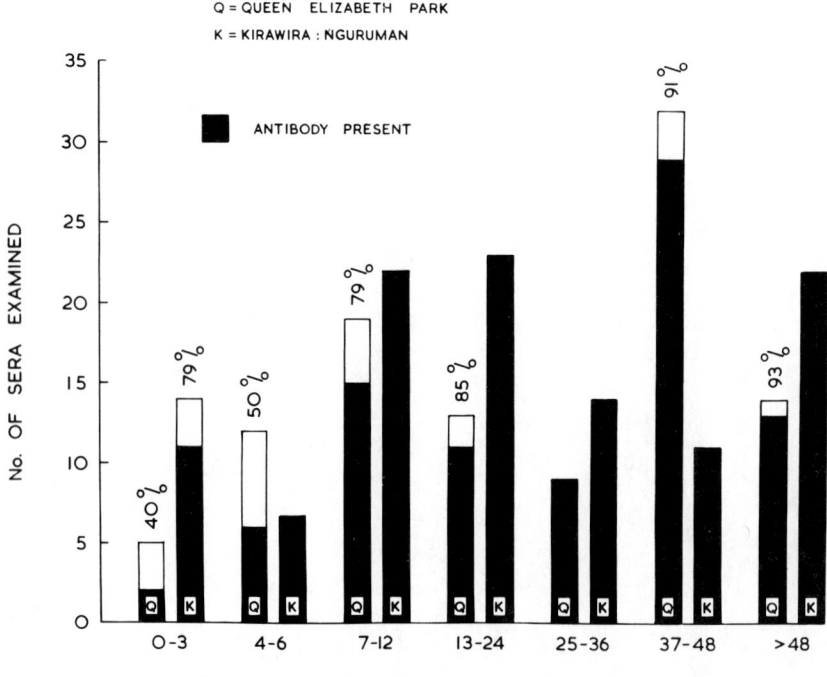

FIG. 14.3 The proportion of warthogs of different age groups from which ASFV was isolated.

The epidemiologic data indicated clearly that the disease usually occurred when warthogs and swine foraged over the same ground, and there was some circumstantial evidence that transfer of virus to domestic swine occurred when warthog carcasses or offal were brought onto farms (DeTray 1963; Heuschele et al. 1965; Montgomery 1921; Pini and Hurter 1975). It was accordingly suggested that ectoparasites such as fleas, lice, argasid or ixodid ticks, and even blood-sucking Diptera might be responsible for virus spread, although no supporting evidence was obtained (DeTray 1963; Montgomery 1921; Walker 1933). Then Botija (1963) reported that the soft tick *Ornithodorus erraticus* in Spain could acquire virus from infected pigs, retain it for long periods, and transmit it to clean swine. Subsequently, Heuschele and Coggins (1965b) showed in East Africa that *O. moubata*, which frequently occurs in large numbers in warthog burrows (Peirce 1974), could acquire virus by feeding on infected swine, and they were able to demonstrate transmission of ASFV by such artificially infected ticks 14 days later. ASFV was not detected, however, in 100 nymphal ticks collected from warthog burrows in southern Kenya, a result recalling that of DeTray (1963).

Later and more extensive investigations in East Africa revealed that *O. moubata* was present in 30–95% of warthog burrows throughout the areas examined, up to an altitude of 1.8 km. The number of ticks in individual burrows varied enormously from less than 10 to more than 30,000 recovered from the roof of one hole in Uganda (Peirce 1974). In the Serengeti region about 30–60% of infested burrows contained ticks infected with ASFV (Table 14.2). The overall rates of infection in tampans varied from 0.28 to 1.35% in this area, but in western Uganda ASFV was extremely infrequent; only 10 isolations were made from about 65,000 ticks, of which 8 came from one small locality on one occasion (Plowright 1977).

Infected tampans contained large amounts of virus, the mean for 216 specimens at various stages of development being $10^{5.6}$ HAD$_{50}$. All developmental and adult forms were infected, including the eggs and unfed first-stage nymphs (Plowright 1977; Plowright et al. 1970b). In addition to this transovarial infection, infected adult males could transmit systemic infection to clean females during copulation, a finding which may explain the 4- to 6-fold increase in infection rates between late nymphal and adult stages (Plowright et al. 1974).

TABLE 14.2 Distribution of *Ornithodorus moubata* and ASFV in Warthog Burrows in East Africa.

Locality	Burrows Infested with Ticks	Burrows with ASFV-infected Ticks	Remarks
Western Uganda (Queen Elizabeth Park)	22/48	2/46 (4%)	Some collections pooled
Northern Tanzania (Kiriwira)	99/112 (88%)	57/96 (59%)	…
Nguruman (southern Kenya)	20/21 (95%)	6/20 (30%)	…
Nairobi National Park	7/19 (37%)	2/5	Some collections pooled
Mara (southern Kenya)	18/60 (30%)	7/18 (39%)	…
Nanyuki (central Kenya)	0/>100	…	…
Maralal (northern Kenya)	11/25 (44%)	2/11	One collection pooled

Source: Plowright 1977.

Clean ticks acquired virus when feeding on infected swine, which have a viremia in the region of 10^6–10^8 HAD$_{50}$/ml, but nothing of this order has ever been recorded in warthogs. Experimental studies showed that as little as 10 or 10^2 HAD$_{50}$ of some strains was sufficient to infect ticks by feeding, but to establish persistent infection in 50% of ticks, 10- to 100-fold more virus was necessary. Other strains required at least 10^5 HAD$_{50}$ to produce any persistent infection. These figures suggest that a viremia in warthogs of at least 10^3–10^4 HAD$_{50}$/ml would be necessary to infect ticks (Plowright et al. 1970b). Attempts to infect porcupines and a striped field mouse (*Arvicanthis* sp.) by parenteral inoculation of ASFV were unsuccessful, but it was not possible to test antbears (*Orycteropus afer*). These species inhabit burrows used by warthogs and might have been regarded as alternative sources of virus for ticks.

The virtual absence of ASFV in Ugandan ticks could not be explained, since the strains of virus circulating there were capable of infecting *Ornithodoros*, even in moderate or low dosage, and Ugandan ticks were susceptible to experimental infection with the usual amounts of virus. Considerable multiplication of virus occurs in the tick, up to 3–4 $\log_{10}$ units (Plowright et al. 1970b). The sites of virus multiplication and persistence have been clearly established (Greig 1972a). Transovarial (Plowright et al. 1970a) and sexual (male-to-female) transmission of ASFV in the tick (Plowright et al. 1974) have been demonstrated in the laboratory and in the field in the former case.

Infected ticks regularly transmit ASFV to pigs during feeding, with incubation periods averaging 5 days, suggesting inoculation of a moderately large dose of virus. Virus is present in tick saliva, in the coxal fluid secreted during engorgement, and in the malpighian excrement and is often voided onto the skin of the vertebrate host. The virus could gain access through the skin if discontinuities were already present or through the bite wounds of other ticks. There is enough virus in infected ticks, which may be crushed and eaten, to infect swine by the nasopharyngeal or oral routes (Plowright 1977).

ASFV shows all the hallmarks of being a virus that is extremely well-adapted to *Ornithodorus* ticks, which depend primarily on warthogs for their blood meals (Plowright 1977). There is much evidence that the virus could be maintained in tick populations for periods of years without viremic vertebrates. The tam-

pans usually feed rapidly, within 30–45 minutes, and then fall off again in the burrow; nevertheless, they are sometimes carried outside (Chorley 1943) and could be deposited on land used for domestic pigs and could transmit ASFV.

In areas where argasid ticks are not present, as in north central Kenya, or where they do not usually function as reservoirs and transmitters, as in western Uganda, the possible vectors of ASFV for warthogs include other ectoparasites such as lice (*Haematopinus phacochoeri* and *Haematomyzus hopkinsi*), fleas (*Echidnophaga*, *Meopsylla*, and *Neotunga* spp.), and the fly (*Auchmeromyia luteola*), the sarcophagous larvae of which are common in warthog burrows (Geigy 1955). Tests on relatively small collections of hard ticks and *Auchmeromyia* in East Africa have always failed to reveal ASFV (Plowright 1977). Previous attempts to show virus maintenance and transmission by the pig louse (*Haematopinus suis*) or fleas gave equivocal results or failed (Botija and Badiola 1966; Heuschele and Coggins 1965b; Kovalenko and Sidorov 1973; Montgomery 1921; Walker 1933). The virus disappears rapidly from the body of engorged lice, and mechanical transfer of virus from contaminated mouth parts does not occur. Even the crushing on the skin of lice carrying virus should occasionally give rise to disease by percutaneous entry through preexisting wounds, since infection through scarified skin can undoubtedly occur (Montgomery 1921). Attempts to produce persistent infection in hard ticks by feeding them on viremic pigs failed in the case of *Rhipicephalus simus* (Plowright 1977), *R. bursa* (Kovalenko and Sidorov, 1973) and *Amblyomma variegatum* (Plowright 1977). Negative results were also obtained with *Anopheles* mosquitoes and a "gadfly" (Kovalenko and Siderov 1973).

The transmission of African swine fever among domestic swine is not difficult to explain since the levels of virus in tissues are very high, about 10^9 HAD$_{50}$/g, and excretion takes place by all the usual routes—pharyngeal, nasal, oral, ocular, and genital secretions, as well as feces and urine (Greig and Plowright 1970). Virus shedding in the early stages of the disease is primarily by the pharyngeal route and reaches a maximum mean of 10^5 HAD$_{50}$/swab by the 2nd and 3rd days of pyrexia; it can begin 24–48 hours prior to the onset of pyrexia in acute cases but is inadequate in amount for regular transmission by contact until 12–24 hours after onset (Montgomery 1921). Subacute and carrier cases excrete less virus at irregular intervals and transmission by contact is accordingly less predictable.

The minimal quantity of virus necessary to infect domestic swine, using a single dose by the nasal and oral routes, was determined to be $10^3 - 10$ HAD_{50} and $10^5 - 10$ or greater HAD_{50}, respectively (Greig 1972; Heuschele 1967; Plowright et al. 1969b). This probably explains the failure to transmit in the prefebrile and early pyrexial stages.

Although Montgomery (1921) concluded from extensive experiments in the open air that aerial transmission did not occur, Wilkinson et al. (1977) found that ASF did spread within 48 hours in loose boxes if pigs were separated by as much as 2.3 m but that aerosol spread was unlikely to be important except in intensive housing systems. It was also found that muzzling of pigs in intimate contact with infected swine or the feeding of virus in baits of sweet potatoes or bananas usually averted the disease (Montgomery 1921). It was concluded by Walker (1933) that the variable outcome of drenching experiments implied entry of virus by discontinuities of the alimentary mucosae.

SIGNS. No clinical effects of ASFV infection have been observed in wild animal reservoirs but this does not mean they do not occur. The fever observed by Montgomery (1921) in two inoculated warthogs (7 months old) may have been caused by ASFV, but it was difficult to observe disease or mortality if the animals remained in their burrows. Sick animals that did emerge would be likely to fall prey to larger predators such as lion or hyena.

The incubation period in swine following contact exposure to acute cases is usually 5–9 days and the time to death thereafter is generally stated to be 4–5 days (DeTray 1963), although strains freshly isolated from warthogs or ticks often require longer to kill pigs than strains from epizootics in swine. Thus for the Tengani (Malawi pig) isolate the mean death time was 2.9 days, whereas for the KWH/12 (Tanzania warthog) strain it was 7 days (Greig and Plowright 1970). The case mortality rate in domestic swine is extremely high for epizootic strains in Africa, exceeding 99% (Montgomery 1921, 1922; Walker 1933), and experimentally such strains allow few survivors (DeTray 1963; Scott 1965a). However, occasional animals, especially perhaps the very young, do survive and remain persistent carriers of virus (De Kock et al. 1940), and rare subclinical infections are encountered experimentally even with fully virulent strains (Montgomery 1921; Walker 1933).

Outbreaks of acute disease in domestic swine are often heralded by a few sudden deaths, followed by a second wave within 7–10 days. The clinical signs are at first those of an acute systemic disease with pyrexia, increasing to around 42°C, listlessness, partial anorexia, huddling together, and unwillingness to stand or move. Some affected pigs show swaying movements of the hindquarters or develop a frank paresis. With progression of the disease many animals show an increasing congestion and cyanosis of the skin of the ears, snout, ventral abdominal wall, and extremities of the limbs.

Seromucoid or mucopurulent discharges are visible at the nares and palpebral rim. The breathing becomes labored and shallow, the pulse rapid. Pregnant females usually abort. Some pigs are constipated, the feces being covered with blood-streaked mucus; others develop watery diarrhea and dysentery, with fresh or altered blood staining the perineum. In the final stages, the temperature falls gradually to subnormal levels, and the animal becomes comatose or develops convulsions and muscular tremors. When lung edema is prominent, a blood-stained watery fluid or froth flows from the nares.

Strains of virus that have prolonged maintenance in swine have begun to lose virulence for this species (as in Angola, Mozambique, Spain, and Portugal) and cause an increasing proportion of subacute, chronic, or even clinically inapparent infections. The first are characterized by clinicopathologic changes that resemble more closely those of acute hog cholera (classical swine fever), but subacute and chronic cases develop a variety of changes not typical of that disease. They include a progressive and necrotizing pneumonia, with serofibrinous pleural and peritoneal effusion and fibrinous pleurisy leading to adhesions. Other animals develop a necrotizing and hemorrhagic dermatitis that affects the skin on pressure points overlying bony protuberances of the limbs (hock, stifle, elbow, shoulder) and leads to deep-seated ulcers. Some cases exhibit a diffuse fibrinous pericarditis with adhesions, which leads to jowl edema, dyspnea on forced exercise, and often sudden death from heart failure. Apart from the skin lesions, painful swellings of limb joints may appear, the periarticular connective tissue being infiltrated by an excess of fibrin-containing fluid.

Subacute and chronic cases probably remain permanent carriers of virus, which they circulate in their blood or excrete periodically in quantities adequate to infect pigs maintained in close contact with them. Carriers became more frequent in Portugal and Spain after culture-attenuated strains of virus had been used for large-scale or field-trial vaccination experiments (Coggins 1974; DeTray 1963; Hess 1971; Scott 1965a).

PATHOGENESIS. In acute experimental infections of pigs, virus usually gains access to the body through the pharyngeal region, either the palatal tonsil (Heuschele 1967) or the dorsal pharyngeal mucosa (Plowright et al. 1968). From these sites it spreads to the local (mandibular and pharyngeal) lymph nodes and then to the blood prior to generalization. Occasionally in young pigs exposed by contact, the bronchial mucosa (Greig 1972b; Wilkinson and Donaldson 1977) or nasal and gastrointestinal mucosae may be involved, followed by the associated lymph nodes.

The primary target cells are macrophages (including monocytes) and reticular cells that undergo necrosis and lysis. The lymphocytes, vascular endothelium, and tunica media of blood vessels appear to be secondarily affected, since viral antigens appear in them (as also in hepatic cells) at later stages of the disease. Injury to the blood vessel walls leads to endothelial degeneration, fibrinoid degeneration of the media, and thrombosis and infarction, which are associated with hemorrhages appearing only a day or so before death. There is a clotting defect that may be partially attributable to virus-induced destruction of megakaryocytes (Colgrove et al. 1969).

The primary and secondary viremias in acute ASF appear as early as 8 hours and 15–24 hours after infection and lead to secondary centers of virus proliferation in a wide range of tissues, particularly the lymph nodes, spleen, liver, and lungs. The viremia is associated largely with the erythrocytes and lymphocytes (Plowright et al. 1968; Wardley and Wilkinson 1977).

In the pneumonic lesions found in some chronic cases, virus replicates in alveolar macrophages, which subsequently degenerate, and viral antigens become associated with immunoglobulins and, in the early stages, with complement and fibrin (Pan et al. 1975). Chronically infected pigs also develop severe hyperplasia of regional lymph nodes on parenteral challenge, suggesting an Arthus type reaction. Coggins (1974) further proposed that the sub-

cutaneous swellings over leg joints, fibrinous pericarditis, pneumonia, and skin ulceration observed in persistently infected swine may have an immunopathologic basis.

Proliferative and necrotic lesions in lymphoreticular tissues such as lymph nodes and spleen have been reported experimentally (Konno et al. 1971) and are increasingly reported in enzootic areas (Henriques et al. 1976).

LESIONS. The lesions in acute cases of ASF resemble those of hyperacute hog cholera. Apart from skin cyanosis, hemorrhages, and discharges, the most striking feature is a hemorrhagic infiltration and enlargement of lymph nodes, particularly the gastrohepatic and renal groups. Sometimes it is cortical but it is often diffuse so that the structures resemble hematomas. Splenic enlargement occurs in infections by some strains in some animals but is often absent; splenic infarcts are less common than in hog cholera. A fleshy enlargement of nodes has been reported in some subacute or chronic cases.

The peritoneal cavity usually contains an excess of fibrin-containing fluid, often with blood clots, and fibrinous exudates are frequent in the other serous cavities. Serosal petechiae or larger hemorrhages and blood streaking are seen on abdominal and thoracic viscera. In subacute or chronic infections, heavy fibrinous deposits, often becoming organized and with adhesions, accompany considerable accumulations of fluid. The heart shows epicardial petechiae or larger blood splashes in acute cases; and endocardium may exhibit massive hemorrhages.

The nasal cavities often contain a blood-stained exudate, and the tonsils are usually hemorrhagic, with crypts filled by mucopus. The tracheal lumen is often filled with watery froth and the mucosa is congested. Similar changes extend into the bronchi and the lung substance, which is swollen and friable; the interlobular septae are often heavily infiltrated by a gelatinous fluid. Petechial or larger hemorrhages are scattered throughout.

The stomach usually exhibits severe fundic congestion and/or hemorrhage, with blood frequently present in the contents; foci of necrotic epithelium or erosions occur, especially in the esophageal zone. The cecum, colon, and rectum often show a blackened or hemorrhagic streaking along mucosal folds, with an excess of mucus and blood streaking in the contents and sometimes a heavy staining by darkened blood. Button ulcers, as in subacute hog cholera, are rare. The liver is often slightly swollen, and the gallbladder wall is thickened by a gelatinous edema that may be hemorrhagic.

The kidneys usually show cortical petechiae varying from a few small points to massive confluent lesions converting the cortex to a hemorrhagic pulp. Perirenal and renal medullary hemorrhage is also frequent, and petechiae are commonly present in the mucosa of the urinary bladder.

Meningeal congestion and cerebral hemorrhages occur, the latter mostly in perivascular locations.

Histologically, the lymphoid lesions are accompanied by extensive destruction of reticular cells, macrophages, and lymphocytes, with a marked tendency to karyorrhexis and pyknosis, leaving granular nuclear debris. There are widespread vascular lesions, including endothelial proliferation, degeneration, and detachment, with hyalinization of the media and accumulation of PAS-positive material. A meningoencephalomyelitis is present with round-cell cuffing of vessels in the brain, neuronal degeneration, and gliosis (De Kock et al. 1940; Maurer et al. 1958).

DIAGNOSIS. In view of the many clinicopathologic similarities between ASF and hog cholera, it is usually necessary to confirm diagnoses reached in field outbreaks by one or more laboratory techniques.

The most commonly employed methods for rapid diagnosis of ASF were, until recent years, the demonstration of infectious virus or virus antigens in mammalian (or acarine) tissues. For the recovery of virus, suspensions of lymph node, spleen, or lung tissue are inoculated into cultures of swine buffy coat or bone marrow cells and examined for hemadsorption (Malmquist and Hay 1960) or for specific immunofluorescence (Botija, 1970). Antigens may also be detected by immunofluorescence in direct impression smears or cryostat sections prepared from these tissues or by complement fixation and immunodiffusion tests against "hyperimmune" pig antiserum, using lymph nodes or liver and kidney tissue as antigen (Boulanger et al. 1967a,b; Coggins and Heuschele 1966; Cowan 1963). These methods often give positive results within 18–24 hours.

Tests for antibodies have become increasingly important as the number of survivor swine has increased. There is a hypergammaglobulinemia in subacute and chronic cases (Pan et al. 1970). ASFV-specific antibodies can be detected by immunofluorescence (Botija et al. 1970); immunodiffusion (Malmquist 1963);

immunoelectroosmophoresis (Pan et al. 1971); and reverse, single radial diffusion (Pan et al. 1974) tests. Antibodies inhibiting hemadsorption (HAdI) of ASFV occur in the serum of some warthogs and swine, but they are not present consistently. Their diagnostic significance is reduced by evidence of strain specificity (Vigario et al. 1974), and some strains do not cause hemadsorption. In western Uganda all virus isolates from warthogs and ticks reacted in HAdI tests with Uganda antiserum, but few with antisera reacted to isolates from other geographical areas. In the Serengeti region only about half the isolates reacted with homologous antiserum.

A definitive proof of the presence of ASFV in animal tissues can be obtained by inoculation of swine, some of which have been immunized against classical swine fever. If all of them react with typical clinicopathologic findings, the agent present is ASFV.

IMMUNITY. Wild swine survive infection without apparently undergoing significant clinical reactions, but they develop antibodies reacting in various serologic tests and often retain virus for prolonged periods, if not for life. Domestic swine undergo more or less severe clinical disease, and the survivors usually resist challenge with homologous and sometimes heterologous strains of virus. They develop antibodies but remain virus carriers and may suffer clinical relapses or death after prolonged periods.

Wild and domestic survivors do develop neutralizing antibodies. Efforts to demonstrate them, whether in serum or tissues, have failed (Hess 1971) as have attempts to transfer resistance passively with antibody. There is apparently no impairment of antibody production in infected animals, since precipitating or complement-fixing antibodies appear as early as 7 days and with 5–6 weeks of infection (Hess and Pan 1977). Cell-mediated immunity, as demonstrated by leukocyte migration inhibition tests is not impaired in ASF (Shimizu et al. 1977) and may contribute to the pathogenesis of chronic lung lesions. Interferon was not produced by ASFV-infected cell cultures, and virus was not inhibited by interferon from pig kidney cells in vitro. An interferon inducer (ds-RNA) did not affect the course of ASF in infected pigs (Wilkinson 1977).

Strains of virus attenuated by prolonged passage in cell cultures have been used in vaccination trials at the laboratory and in field trials in Portugal and Spain. Safe (although producing a transitory febrile response) and effective in many animals in the short term, they often gave rise to persistent infection and severe delayed reactions in the field, especially when animals were subjected to stress. Their use may well have contributed to the widespread circulation in the Iberian Peninsula of strains of reduced virulence for swine, which later infected other countries such as France and Italy; but attenuation for swine had also been observed previously in Angola where vaccine had not been used in the field (see Hess 1971; Scott 1965a). Virus inactivated by a wide variety of agents, including β-propriolactone and acetyl-ethyleneamine, induces antibody production but does not protect against challenge (Coggins 1974).

TREATMENT AND CONTROL. There is no effective treatment for ASF in susceptible swine; the natural reservoir hosts, particularly warthogs, probably do not suffer clinically from infection.

Control of the disease in swine in areas where warthogs are present (that is, in Africa) depends on the prevention of effective contact by double fencing of areas used for pigs and prohibition of entry of warthog carcasses or offal into such units. Montgomery (1922) also advocated that crops fed to pigs should not be accessible to wild swine and that feeding of uncooked meat or meat products should be prohibited.

In areas where the risks of infection from wildlife are high, the prohibition of movement of swine, except internally for slaughter and by permit, may be a necessary adjunct (Mansvelt 1963). In some countries such as Kenya the reduction of warthog populations by payment of a bounty on their snouts has been thought desirable. Such measures are not adequate without a simultaneous effort to disinfest burrows of ectoparasites, especially soft ticks.

If outbreaks of ASF do occur, the only sound course is to destroy and incinerate or bury all the infected herd, paying suitable compensation, and to institute a system of regular veterinary examination of herds in the surrounding area. Restocking should be permitted only after cleansing and disinfection of the premises, disinfestation to deal with any ectoparasites, and a minimum delay of 14 days but preferably 3 months. Small test groups of swine should be introduced when restocking (Scott 1965b).

The problems of control of ASF in Europe, especially Spain and Portugal and probably in new enzootic areas elsewhere, are compounded by the changing clinicopathologic manifestations, with their increasing resemblance to classical swine fever, which is often present concurrently. The much-reduced case mortality rate allows the survival of many more subacute, chronic, or inapparent cases, which disseminate virus directly or indirectly when they are slaughtered and introduced into the food chain. In these circumstances an efficient rapid confirmation of diagnosis is essential, by a laboratory capable of both virus recovery techniques and serologic testing for antibodies. Large-scale serologic surveys are probably essential in these circumstances but have not yet been reported.

Live attenuated vaccines, applied on a significant scale in Portugal, proved highly undesirable because of the tendency to serious delayed reactions under field conditions with dissemination of pathogenic virus by vaccinated swine (Hess 1971). Their use is discouraged, except perhaps where the probability of continuing enzootic infection of swine has been accepted following the failure of eradication measures.

Those responsible for the investigation of wild Suidae in Africa or elsewhere or their international movement to zoological gardens should recognize the potential risks of their infection by ASFV and its transfer to domestic swine. The establishment of known virus-free stocks of warthogs monitored by serologic testing and maintained in strict quarantine is an obvious way of avoiding some of the dangers, but this usually demands the hand-rearing of very young animals from the wild or breeding from virus-free adults in captivity. Some warthog populations in South Africa are fortunately virus free, and these offer the best source of such foundation stock.

REFERENCES

Anon. The geographical distribution of warthog and domestic pigs in Africa. *Bull. Epizoot. Dis. Afr.* 10:91–92, 1962.

Black, D. N., and Brown, F. Purification and physicochemical characteristics of African swine fever virus. *J. Gen. Virol.* 32:509–518, 1976.

Botija, C. S. Comptes-rendues des seances de la conference exceptionelle OIE/FAO sur la peste porcine africaine et la peste equine africaine. *Bull. Off. Int. Epizoot.* 55:378–379, 1961.

———. Reservorios del virus de la peste porcina Africana. *Bull. Off. Int. Epizoot.* 60:895–899, 1963.

———. Diagnosis of African swine fever by immunofluorescence. *Bull. Off. Int. Epizoot.* 73:1037–1044, 1970.

Botija, C. S., and Badiola, C. Presencia del virus de la

peste porcina africana en el *Haematopinus suis*. *Bull. Off. Int. Epizoot.* 66:699–705, 1966.

Botija, C. S., Ordas, A., and Gonzalez, J. G. La inmunofluorescencia indirecta aplicada a la investigacion de anticuerpos de la peste porcina africana. *Bull. Off. Int. Epizoot.* 74:397–417, 1970.

Boulanger, P., Bannister, G. L., Gray, D. P., Ruckerbauer, G. M. and Willis, N. F. African swine fever: II. Detection of the virus in swine tissues by means of the modified direct complement-fixation test. *Can. J. Comp. Med.* 31:7–11, 1967a.

———. African swine fever: III. The use of the agar double-diffusion precipitation test for the detection of the virus in swine tissue. *Can. J. Comp. Med.* 31:12–15, 1967b.

Child, G., Roth, H. H., and Kerr, M. Reproduction and recruitment patterns in warthog (*Phacochoerus aethiopicus*) populations. *Mammalia* 32:5–29, 1968.

Chorley, T. W. An unusual occurrence of *Ornithodoros moubata* (Arachnida). *Proc. R. Entomol. Soc.* 18:27, 1943.

Coggins, L. African swine fever virus: Pathogenesis. *Prog. Med. Virol.* 18:48–63, 1974.

Coggins, L., and Heuschele, W. P. Use of agar diffusion precipitation test in the diagnosis of African swine fever. *Am. J. Vet. Res.* 27:485–488, 1966.

Colgrove, G. S., Haelterman, E. O., and Coggins, L. Pathogenesis of African swine fever in young pigs. *Am. J. Vet. Res.* 30:1343–1359, 1969.

Cowan, K. M. Immunologic studies on African swine fever virus: II. Enhancing effect of normal bovine serum on the complement-fixation reaction. *Am. J. Vet. Res.* 24:756–761, 1963.

Cox, B. F. African swine fever. *Bull. Epizoot. Dis. Afr.* 11:147–148, 1963.

Dalsgaard, K., Overby, E., and Botija, C. S. Crossed immunoelectrophoretic characterization of virus: Specified antigens in cells infected with African swine fever (ASF) virus. *J. Gen. Virol.* 36:203–206, 1977.

Dardiri, A. H. Hemadsorption by African swine fever virus in goat buffy coat culture. *Fed. Proc.* 25:421, 1966.

Dardiri, A. H., Yedloutschnig, R. J., and Taylor, W. D. Clinical and serologic response of American white-collared peccaries to African swine fever, foot-and-mouth disease, vesicular stomatitis, vesicular exanthema of swine, hog cholera and rinderpest viruses. In *Proceedings of the 73rd Annual Meeting of the U.S. Animal Health Association*, pp. 437–452, 1969.

DeKock, G., Robinson, E. M., and Keppel, J. J. G. Swine fever in South Africa. *Onderstepoort J.* 14:31–93, 1940.

DeTray, D. E. The incidence of African swine fever in warthogs in Kenya: A preliminary report. *J. Am. Vet. Med. Assoc.* 138:78–90, 1961.

———. African swine fever. *Adv. Vet. Sci.* 8:299–333, 1963.

Enjuanes, L., Cubero, I., and Vinuela, E. Sensitivity of macrophages from different species to African swine fever (ASF) virus. *J. Gen. Virol.* 34:455–463, 1977.

Geigy, R. Observations sur les phacocheres du Tanganyika. *Rev. Suisse Zool.* 62:139–163, 1955.

Greig, A. The localization of African swine fever virus in the tick *Ornithodoros moubata porcinus*. *Arch. Gesamte Virusforsch.* 29:240–247, 1972a.

———. Pathogenesis of African swine fever in pigs naturally exposed to the disease. *J. Comp. Pathol.* 82:73–79, 1972b.

Greig, A., and Plowright, W. The excretion of two virulent strains of African swine fever virus by domestic pigs. *J. Hyg.* 68:673–682, 1970.

Henriques, R. P., Nunes Petisca, J. L., and Durao, J. Situation actuelle des pestes porcines au Portugal. *Bull. Off. Int. Epizoot.* 85:461–466, 1976.

Hess, W. R. African swine fever virus. *Virol. Monogr.* 9:1–33, 1971.

Hess, W. R., and Pan, I. C. The immune response in African swine fever. Seminar on hog cholera/classical swine fever and African swine fever. Commission of the European Communities, Eur. 5904 En. pp. 602–611.

Heuschele, W. P. Studies on the pathogenesis of African swine fever: I. Quantitative studies on the sequential development of virus in pig tissues. *Arch. Virusforsch.* 21:349–356, 1967.

Heuschele, W. P., and Coggins, L. Isolation of African swine fever virus from a giant forest hog. *Bull. Epizoot. Dis. Afr.* 13:255–256, 1965a.

———. Studies on the transmission of African swine fever by arthropods. *U.S. Livestock Sanit. Assoc. Proc.* 69:94–100, 1965b.

———. Epizootiology of African swine fever in warthogs. *Bull. Epizoot. Dis. Afr.* 17:179–183, 1969.

Heuschele, W. P., Stone, S. S., and Coggins, L. Observations on the epizootiology of African swine fever. *Bull. Epizoot. Dis. Afr.* 13:157–160, 1965.

Konno, S., Taylor, W. D., and Dardiri, A. H. Acute African swine fever: Proliferative phase in lymphoreticular tissue and the reticuloendothelial system. *Cornell Vet.* 61:71–84, 1971.

Kovalenko, Y. R., Burba, L. G., and Siderov, M. A. Symptoms and pathological changes in young goats inoculated with African swine fever virus. *Dokl. Akad. Nauk SSSR* 8:28–31, 1966.

Kovalenko, Y. R., and Sidorov, M. A. Reservoirs and the mechanisms of circulation of African swine fever virus in nature. *S. Biol.* 8:598–606, 1973.

Malmquist, W. A. Serologic and immunologic studies with African swine fever virus. *Am. J. Vet. Res.* 24:450–459, 1963.

Malmquist, W. A., and Hay, D. Haemadsorption and cytopathic effect produced by African swine fever virus in swine bone marrow and buffy coat cultures. *Am. J. Vet. Res.* 21:104–108, 1960.

Mansveld, P. R. The incidence and control of African swine fever virus in the Republic of South Africa. *Bull. Off. Int. Epizoot.* 60:889–894, 1963.

Maurer, F. D., Griesemer, R. A., and Jones, T. C. The pathology of African swine fever: A comparison with hog cholera. *Am. J. Vet. Res.* 19:517–539, 1958.

Montgomery, R. E. On a form of swine fever occurring in British East Africa (Kenya Colony). *J. Comp. Pathol.* 34:159–191, 243–262, 1921.

——. East African swine fever. Bulletin No. 2, Veterinary Department, Colony and Protectorate of Kenya. Nairobi: Government Printer, 1922.

Neitz, W. O. African swine fever. In *Emerging diseases of animals.* FAO agricultural Studies No. 6, pp. 1–70. Rome: FAO, 1963.

Pan, I. C., De Boer, C. J., and Hess, W. R. African swine fever: Application of immunoelectroosmophoresis for the detection of antibody. *Can. J. Comp. Med.* 36:309–316, 1971.

Pan, I. C., De Boer, C. J., and Heuschele, W. P. Hypergammaglobulinaemia in swine infected with African swine fever virus. *Proc. Soc. Exp. Biol.* 134:367–371, 1970.

Pan, I. C., Moulton, J. E., and Hess, W. R. Immunofluorescent studies on chronic pneumonia in swine with experimentally induced African swine fever. *Am. J. Vet. Res.* 36:379–386, 1975.

Pan, I. C., Trautman, R., Hess, W. R., De Boer, C. J., and Tessler, J. African swine fever: Detection of antibody by reverse single radial immunodiffusion. *Am. J. Vet. Res.* 36:351–354, 1974.

Peirce, M. A. Distribution and ecology of *Ornithodoros moubata porcinus* Walton (Acarina) in animal burrows in East Africa. *Bull. Ent. Res.* 64:605–619, 1974.

Pini, A., and Hurter, L. R. African swine fever: An epizootiological review with special reference to the South African situation. *J. S. Afr. Vet. Assoc.* 46:227–232, 1975.

Pini, A., and Wagenaar, G. Isolation of a nonhaemadsorbing strain of African swine fever from a natural outbreak of the disease. *Vet. Rec.* 94:2, 1974.

Plowright, W. Vector transmission of African swine fever virus. Seminar on hog cholera/classical swine fever and African swine fever. Commission of the European Communities. Eur. 5904 En., pp. 575–587, 1977.

Plowright, W., Parker, J. and Peirce, M. A. African swine fever virus in ticks (*Ornithodoros moubata*, Murray) collected from animal burrows in Tanzania. *Nature* 221:1071–1073, 1969a.

——. The epizootiology of African swine fever in Africa. *Vet. Rec.* 85:668–674, 1969b.

Plowright, W., Parker, J., and Staple, R. F. The growth of a virulent strain of African swine fever virus in domestic pigs. *J. Hyg.* 66:117–134, 1968.

Plowright, W., Perry, C. T., and Greig, A. Sexual transmission of African swine fever virus in the tick *Ornithodoros moubata porcinus* Walton. *Res. Vet. Sci.* 17:106–113, 1974.

Plowright, W., Perry, C. T., and Peirce, M. A. Transovarial infection with African swine fever virus in the argasid tick, *Ornithodoros moubata porcinus* Walton. *Res. Vet. Sci.* 11:582–584, 1970a.

Plowright, W., Perry, C. T., Peirce, M. A., and Parker, J. Experimental infection of the argasid tick, *Ornithodoros moubata porcinus*, with African swine fever virus. *Arch. Gesamte Virusforsch.* 31:33–50, 1970b.

Scott, G. R. The virus of African swine fever and its transmission. *Bull. Off. Int. Epizoot.* 63:645–677, 1965a.

——. Prevention, control and eradication of African swine fever. *Bull. Off. Int. Epizoot.* 63:751–764, 1965b.

——. Symposium: The smallest stowaways: I. African swine fever. *Vet. Rec.* 77:1421–1427, 1965c.

Shimizu, M., Pan, I. C., and Hess, W. R. Cellular immunity demonstrated in pigs infected with African swine fever virus. *Am. J. Vet. Res.* 38:27–31, 1977.

Stone, S. S., and Hess, W. R. Effects of some disinfectants on African swine fever virus. *Appl. Microbiol.* 25:115–122, 1973.

Stone, S. S., and Heuschele, W. P. The role of the hippopotamus in the epizootiology of African swine fever. *Bull. Epizoot. Dis. Afr.* 13:23–28, 1965.

Thomas, A. D., and Kolbe, F. F. The wild pigs of South Africa: Their distribution and habits, and their significance as agricultural pests and carriers of disease. *J. S. Afr. Vet. Med. Assoc.* 13:1–11, 1942.

Vigario, J. D., Terrinha, A. M., and Nunes, J. F. Antigenic relationships among strains of African swine fever virus. *Arch. Gesamte Virusforsch.* 45:272–277, 1974.

Walker, J. *East African swine fever.* D.V.M. thesis. Institute of Veterinary Pathology, University of Zurich. London: Bailliere, Tindall and Cox, 1933.

Wardley, R. C., and Wilkinson, P. F. The association of African swine fever virus with blood components of infected pigs. *Arch. Virol.* 55:327–334, 1977.

Wilkinson, P. J. Studies on African swine fever. Seminar on hog cholera/classical swine fever and African swine fever. Commission of the European Communities. Eur. 5904 En., pp. 628–632.

Wilkinson, P. J., and Donaldson, A. I. Transmission studies with African swine fever: The early distribution of virus in pigs infected by airborne virus. *J. Comp. Pathol.* 87:497–501, 1977.

Wilkinson, P. J., Donaldson, A. I., Greig, A., and Bruce, W. Transmission studies with African swine fever virus: Infections of pigs by airborne virus. *J. Comp. Pathol.* 87:487–495, 1977.

15 *Infectious Canine Hepatitis*

VICTOR J. CABASSO

Synonyms: **Hepatitis contagiosa canis, Rubarth's disease, fox encephalitis, encephalitis infectiosa vulpis.**

Infectious canine hepatitis (ICH) virus causes infectious diseases characterized by encephalitis in foxes and by hepatitis in dogs and in skunks. In all species, the virus has an affinity for endothelial cells. ICH virus is reviewed in Cabasso and Wilner (1969).

HISTORY. Although studies of the disease in dogs have been extensive, early knowledge about ICH virus in wildlife came mainly from outbreaks of the disease among ranch foxes. Reports of infection among free-living wild mammals are still few in number.

An epizootic disease in silver foxes, with signs of encephalitis, was reported by Green (1925) and was shown to be caused by a filterable virus (Green et al. 1930) The agent induced focal liver necrosis in dogs infected experimentally, and intranuclear inclusions were demonstrated in various endothelial cells of these animals (Green and Shillinger 1934). The natural occurrence of ICH virus in dogs was first described by Rubarth (1947). It was reported from most parts of the world. The virus was found to be immunologically identical to that responsible for fox encephalitis (FE) by Siedentopf and Carlson (1949). This finding gave rise to some confusion concerning the name of the canine illness, to which some investigators referred for a while as "fox encephalitis in the dog" (Chaddock and Carlson 1950), even though the disease in dogs does not involve the central nervous system. The fox was gradually relegated to second place, and the virus became known primarily as the agent of ICH which could also cause encephalitis in foxes. This virus was eventually identified as a member of the adenovirus group (Rowe and Hartley 1962) and is now termed *Adenovirus canis*.

DISTRIBUTION. ICH virus infection is present in dogs and foxes all over the world. In 1925, Green described an outbreak of fox encephalitis on a ranch in the United States. More recent epizootics of the disease on fox farms were reported from Norway (Kummeneje 1971) and from Poland (Zwierzchowski and Gorski 1974).

Coyotes and timber wolves have also been experimentally infected (Evans et al. 1950; Green et al. 1934). Subsequently, serologic evidence of natural infection of coyotes was reported from western Texas in over 50% of animals tested (Trainer and Knowlton 1968), and ICH antibody was found in 11 of 86 free-living wolves in northern Canada (Choquette and Kuyt 1974). Skunks also were reported as being susceptible to ICH virus infection. Two isolates of the virus were recovered from pooled liver and spleen tissue of two skunks trapped in a Chesapeake Bay area, and sera from 59 of 94 skunks from the same area had neutralizing antibody to these ICH isolates (Alexander et al. 1972). Moreover, two cases of acute, fatal hepatitis occurred in young striped skunks (*Mephitis mephitis*) trapped in southern Ontario, and ICH virus was isolated from their tissues (Karstad et al. 1975).

Bear infection has been described (Chaddock and Carlson 1950) but remains unconfirmed, and an apparent infection may take place in raccoons (Green et al. 1943; Jamison et al. 1973; Parker et al. 1961). Limited susceptibility of the ferret was suggested by frank opacification in the cornea of the eye of animals inoculated with infected dog liver suspension (Cabasso et al. 1954), but Green et al. (1934) and Hudson and Mansi (1953) exposed ferrets to ICH virus with negative results. Mink inoculated with either of two strains of the virus highly pathogenic for dogs developed high levels of neutralizing antibody with no signs of disease except for transient inappetence and depression (Motohashi and Goto 1960). Finally, no ICH antibody could be demonstrated in sera of 25 opossums and 9 woodchucks (Jamison et al. 1973).

Because of this limited knowledge about ICH virus in wildlife species, the information in this chapter is derived mostly from outbreaks of the disease in ranch foxes and, to a much smaller extent, from affected skunks.

ETIOLOGY. *Adenovirus canis* has a diameter of 82 nm (Davies et al. 1961). Electron micrographs of preparations stained with phosphotungstic acid reveal a hexagonal cross section and equilateral triangular faces indicative of icosahedral symmetry, characteristic of all adenoviruses. The complete capsid contains 252 capsomeres.

Adenovirus canis is a DNA virus, is resistant to ether, and is stable under a variety of storage conditions (Chaddock and Carlson 1950; Fastier 1958; Larin 1959). Under specified conditions it agglutinates erythrocytes from several animal species, the hemagglutinin being closely related to the infective particle (Espmark and Salenstedt 1961; Fastier 1957; Shimizu et al. 1960). It produces a soluble complement-fixing antigen separable from the infective particle (Fastier 1957), elicits no interferon in dog kidney tissue culture, and is insensitive to interferon action (Sellers and Fitzpatrick 1963).

ICH virus is related to human adenoviruses. One of the two soluble antigens it produces is ICH specific; the other is common to itself and to human adenoviruses types 5 and 7 (Darbyshire and Pereira 1964; Furminger 1964). Cross complement fixation between ICH virus and human adenovirus antiserum was one-sided (Kapsenberg 1959). There seems to be only one immunologic type of ICH virus.

The first in vitro propagation of ICH virus was in cultures of dog kidney tissue (Cabasso et al. 1954). The characteristic cytopathology was a rounding of the infected cells, followed by their formation into grapelike clusters and subsequent separation from the glass. Assay in tissue culture proved to be a reliable measure of virus infectivity and neutralizing ICH antibody. The virus also grew in cultures of dog testicular tissue (Muller and Thordal-Christensen 1954) and in dog lung, liver, and spleen cultures (Cirstet et al. 1959; Motohashi 1960). ICH also multiplies in cultures of certain other cells: a continuous line of pig kidney and in primary ferret kidney (Fieldsteel and Yoshihara 1957), in pig kidney (Sarkan 1957; Cabasso et al. 1958; Emery and York 1958), and in raccoon kidney (Bolin et al. 1958).

TRANSMISSION. Infection with ICH virus is highly contagious, but it is not airborne. It can be transmitted either by direct contact with affected animals; respiratory tract discharges; saliva, urine or feces; or contact with contaminated utensils, clothing, hands, or syringes (Mark 1952). In ranch foxes under natural conditions the disease has been found to be enzootic in a number of breeding units in which pairs of foxes are grouped with their offspring. When large numbers of animals from such units are brought together on a fur range, the disease reaches epizootic proportions, running a rapid course over a period of about 4 weeks with a mortality of 12–20%. The disease may also take epizootic form in breeding units with small pens placed close together (Green et al. 1930; Zwierzchowski and Gorski 1974). Artificial transmission of FE by infected brain suspension was accomplished in red fox pups less than 1 year of age that were taken from their dens in the wild and raised in isolation (Green et al. 1930). It was equally successful whether carried out by intracranial inoculation, cisternal puncture, or intramuscular inoculation in the hind leg. Whatever the route of infection, the incubation periods, signs of disease, survival rates, and pathologic findings were the same.

In skunks, transmission of an acute fatal hepatitis was readily transmitted from one young animal to another after 15 minutes of contact (Karstad et al. 1975).

SIGNS. The natural disease in foxes appears to have a very sudden onset. Animals may die within a few hours of the first signs of illness, or even before sickness is apparent. A fur ranch epizootic, involving large numbers of foxes, presented the opportunity for close follow-up of signs (Green et al. 1930). The pattern was similar to that seen after experimental inoculation. The incubation period is 2–6 days. In most cases the first sign of illness is loss of appetite. This may be the only evidence of disease or may be followed by other signs in 1 or 2 days. Convulsion, preceded at times by rhinitis, is often the first and major sign and may be followed by death within 10 minutes. Frequently the animal appears hyperexcited and a series of convulsive seizures ensues, which terminate in death. The seizures may be both myotonic and myoclonic. A period of lethargy usually follows the initial convulsion and may give way to agitation, another convulsion, and a return to lethargy. Flaccid and spastic paralyses are common signs in both natural and experimental disease. There may also be muscular twitching, weakness, and finally coma lasting from a few minutes to 24 hours before death. Foxes dying of FE do not generally show any marked loss of weight. Their eyes remain clear with a slight watery discharge. In nonfatal cases an interstitial keratitis involving one or both eyes is occasionally seen. Feces of a sick animal become soft and are mixed with mucus and are sometimes streaked with blood. Occasionally a bloody diarrhea develops, and if there is hemorrhage into the lumen of the bowel, the feces consist of pure blood.

FE can be complicated by other simultaneous infections. Kummeneje (1971) reported a simultaneous infection with toxoplasma in 2 blue fox pups in a ranch with about 400 blue foxes. The signs of disease were minimal, and the rancher did not suspect any infectious disease. Mortality was low. The author has suggested that a better name for FE would be *Hepatitis contagiosa vulpis*.

In striped skunks, *Adenovirus canis* may cause an acute, fatal hepatitis. A report by Karstad et al. (1975) concerned two such cases in young animals trapped in southern Ontario, Canada. The incubation period of the disease occurring in a contact animal was 6 days. The sick animals presented ocular discharge, diarrhea, inappetence, and depression and died 2 days after onset of signs.

PATHOGENESIS. The oropharynx is the most probable route of infection with *Adenovirus canis* in foxes, as it is in dogs. In experiments with the latter, virus has been present in the bloodstream 3–8 hours after intraperitoneal inoculation (Parry et al. 1951). From the blood the virus spreads to the viscera (Larin 1959), including the central nervous system (Green and Shillinger 1934; Rubarth 1947). Virus has been recovered from the blood, spleen, spinal cord, and brain of foxes with FE (Green et al. 1930).

PATHOLOGY. At necropsy examination of foxes dead from natural FE, the only definite gross pathology found is general congestion of many tissues and hemorrhage in various organs, especially the brain. Microscopic examination of tissues mainly reveals injuries of the vascular system, which account for the hemorrhages (Green et al. 1930). This is also the case when the disease is complicated by a simultaneous infection (Kummeneje 1971). Pathognomonic intranuclear inclusions appear in the vascular endothelium, meningeal and hepatic cells, and other tissues (Green et al. 1933).

In natural infection of striped skunks, gross lesions may be limited to the liver, and the kidneys and adrenals may be slightly enlarged (Karstad et al. 1975). Histologic examination will reveal very large, deeply acidophilic or basophilic inclusions in the nuclei of hepatic cells, and at times in cells of the bile duct epithelium and the adrenal cortex. Other lesions found include necrosis of hepatic and renal tubular epithelial cells and infiltrations of mononuclear leukocytes in the periportal tissues, lungs, and meninges.

DIAGNOSIS. The course of natural *Adenovirus canis* infection in foxes or skunks is so rapid and so devoid of significant signs that no reliable diagnosis of the sporadic case is possible on purely clinical grounds. However, extensive range epizootics present fewer problems. Accurate diagnosis of infection can be made after death by the finding of intranuclear inclusions in vascular endothelium and meningeal and hepatic cells (Green et al. 1933; Karstad et al. 1975). They can be revealed in tissue sections or touch preparations stained with hematoxylin and eosin, Giemsa stain, or fluorescein-labeled antibody (Coffin et al. 1953; Davis and Anderson 1950; Rubarth 1947).

PROGNOSIS. Reports on the outcome of *Adenovirus canis* infection in foxes have varied. Green et al. (1930) have indicated that foxes 6 months old or less are very susceptible to FE. Mortality in them from the experimental disease can be as high as 80%. In fur range epizootics the death rate in pups for this age group has been twice that of adults. Young animals carefully reared in quarantine develop a faster resistance with age. In a natural epizootic the overall death rate may be 10–20% of the population.

Equally severe losses were reported by Zwierzchowski and Gorski (1974) during an epizootic on a fox ranch in Poland in 1970 and 1971. However, another outbreak of the disease in blue foxes in Norway caused very few deaths (Kummeneje 1971). In this latter outbreak, toxoplasma occurred as a concomitant infection.

Experience with the natural disease in skunks is very limited, but those cases observed died rapidly after the onset of signs (Karstad et al. 1975). In coyotes, on the other hand, no evidence could be obtained that mortality from *Adenovirus canis* infection was important, despite a seemingly widespread infection (Trainer and Knowlton 1968).

IMMUNITY. Recovery from FE is followed in foxes by a solid and durable immunity. In the wild, several other mammalian species appear to undergo silent infection with *Adenovirus canis*, as indicated by the development of antibody (Choquette and Kuyt 1974; Jamison et al. 1973).

Green et al. (1935) reported some success in preventing FE by the use of a hyperimmune serum. More recently, Zwierzchowski and

Gorski (1974) applied mass vaccination to foxes during the course of a severe outbreak of the disease on a fur ranch in Poland. With a monovalent, commercially available dog vaccine (Canivac H), they reported beneficial results.

REFERENCES

Alexander, A. D., Flyger, V., Herman, Y. F., McConnell, S. J., Rothstein, N., and Yager, R. H. Survey of wild mammals in a Chesapeake Bay area for selected zoonoses. *J. Wildl. Dis.* 8:119–126, 1972.

Bolin, V. S., Jarnevic, N., and Austin, J. A. Infectious canine hepatitis virus studies with special reference to passage of raccoon tissue cultures. *Proc. Soc. Exp. Biol. Med.* 98:414–418, 1958.

Cabasso, V. J., Stebbins, M. R., and Avampato, J. M. A bivalent live virus vaccine against canine distemper (CD) and infectious canine hepatitis (ICH). *Proc. Soc. Exp. Biol. Med.* 99:46–51, 1958.

Cabasso, V. J., Stebbins, M. R., Norton, T. W., and Cox, H. R. Propagation of infectious canine hepatitis virus in tissue culture. *Proc. Soc. Exp. Biol. Med.* 85:239–245, 1954.

Cabasso, V. J., and Wilner, B. I. Adenoviruses of animals other than man. In C. A. Brandley and C. E. Cornelius, eds., *Advances in veterinary science and comparative medicine*, vol. 13. New York: Academic Press, 1969.

Chaddock, T. T., and Carlson, W. E. Fox encephalitis (infectious canine hepatitis) in the dog. *North Am. Vet.* 31:35–41, 1950.

Choquette, L. P. E., and Kuyt, E. Serological indication of canine distemper and of infectious canine hepatitis in wolves (*Canis lupus* L.) in Northern Canada. *J. Wildl. Dis.* 10:321–324, 1974.

Cirstet, I., Coman, I., and Feteanu, A. The culture of the virus of Rubarth's disease *in vitro*. Attempts to adapt the virus to the embryonated chicken egg and to laboratory animals. *Lucrarile Stiint. Inst. Patol. Igiena. Anim.* 9:25–29, 1959.

Coffin, D. L., Coons, A. H., and Cabasso, V. J. A histologic study of infectious canine hepatitis by means of fluorescent antibodies. *J. Exp. Med.* 98:13–20, 1953.

Darbyshire, J. H., and Pereira, H. G. An adenovirus precipitating antibody present in some sera of different animal species and its association with bovine respiratory disease. *Nature* 201:895–897, 1964.

Davies, M. C., Englert, M. E., Stebbins, M. R., and Cabasso, V. J. Electron miscroscopic structure of infectious canine hepatitis (ICH) virus: A canine adenovirus. *Virology* 15:87–88, 1961.

Davis, C. L., and Anderson, W. A. The rapid diagnosis of contagious canine hepatitis by touch preparation of fresh liver tissue. *Vet. Med.* 45:435–437, 1950.

Emery, J. B., and York, C. J. Propagation of infectious canine hepatitis virus in porcine kidney tissue culture. *Science* 127:148, 1958.

Espmark, J. A., and Salenstedt, C. R. Hemagglutina-tion-inhibition test for titration of antibodies against hepatitis *contagiosa canis* (infectious canine hepatitis). *Arch. Gesamte Virusforsch.* 11:64–72, 1961.

Evans, C. A., Dowell, M., and Green, R. G. The effects of viruses on intraocular tissues: I. Infections with the virus of fox encephalitis (Canine hepatitis). *J. Infect. Dis.* 86:1–11, 1950.

Fastier, L. B. Studies on the hemagglutination of infectious canine hepatitis virus. *J. Immunol.* 78:413–418, 1957.

———. The survival of infectious canine hepatitis virus under various experimental conditions. *Vet. Res.* 70:623–626, 1958.

Fieldsteel, A. H., and Yoshihara, G. M. Propagation of infectious canine hepatitis virus in cultures of pig and ferret kidney. *Proc. Soc. Exp. Biol. Med.* 95:683–686, 1957.

Furminger, I. G. S. Relationship between adenoviruses and canine hepatitis virus. *Nature* 202:728–729, 1964.

Green, R. G. Distemper in the silver fox (*Vulpes vulpes*). *Proc. Soc. Exp. Biol. Med.* 22:546–548, 1925.

Green, R. G., Evans, G. A., and Yanamura, H. Y. Susceptibility of the raccoon to fox encephalitis. *Proc. Soc. Exp. Biol. Med.* 53:186–187, 1943.

Green, R. G., Katter, M. S., Shillinger, J. E., and Hanson, K. B. Epizootic fox encephalitis: IV. The intranuclear inclusion. *Am. J. Hyg.* 18:462–481, 1933.

Green, R. G., and Shillinger, J. E. Epizootic fox encephalitis: VI. A description of the experimental infection in dogs. *Am. J. Hyg.* 19:362–391, 1934.

Green, R. G., Ziegler, N. R., Carlson, W. E., Shillinger, J. E., Tyler, S. H., and Dewey, E. T. Epizootic fox encephalitis: V. General and pathogenic properties of the virus. *Am. J. Hyg.* 19:343–361, 1934.

Green, R. G., Ziegler, N. R., Green, B. B., and Dewey, E. T. Epizootic fox encephalitis: I. General description. *Am. J. Hyg.* 12:109–129, 1930.

Green, R. G., Ziegler, N. R., Green, B. B., Shillinger, J. E., Dewey, E. T., and Carlson, W. E. Epizootic fox encephalitis: VII. Nature of the immunity. *Am. J. Hyg.* 21:366–388, 1935.

Hudson, J. R., and Mansi, W. Rubarth's disease (canine virus hepatitis): II. The insusceptibility of ferrets to experimental infusion. *J. Comp. Pathol. Ther.* 63:335–345, 1953.

Jamison, R. K., Lazar, E. C., Binn, L. N., and Alexander, A. D. Survey for antibodies to canine viruses in selected wild mammals. *J. Wildl. Dis.* 9:2–3, 1973.

Kapsenberg, J. G. Relationship of infectious canine hepatitis virus to human adenovirus. *Proc. Soc. Exp. Biol. Med.* 101:611–614, 1959.

Karstad, L., Ramsden, R., Berry, T. J., and Binn, L. N. Hepatitis in skunks caused by the virus of infectious canine hepatitis: *J. Wildl. Dis.* 11:494–496, 1975.

Kummeneje, K. *Encephalitis infectiosa vulpis (Hepatitis contagiosa canis)* in a blue fox farm. *Nord.*

Vet. Med. 23:352–360, 1971.

Larin, N. M. The mechanism of immunity in canine virus hepatitis. *Br. Vet. J.* 115:35–45, 1959.

Mark, J. H. Epizootiology of infectious canine hepatitis. In *Proceedings of the 89th Annual Meeting, American Veterinary Medical Association,* pp. 226–228. Chicago: Am. Vet. Med. Assoc., 1952.

Motohashi, T. Infection and propagation of infectious canine hepatitis virus in various animals and tissue cultures: I. Experiments with dogs. *NIBS Bull. Biol. Res.* 5:25–35, 1960.

Motohashi, T., and Goto, S. An inoculation experiment with dog-passaged strains of infectious canine hepatitis virus in minks. *NIBS Bull. Biol. Res.* 5:49–51, 1960.

Muller, J., and Thordal-Christensen, A. Cultivation of the virus of infectious canine hepatitis (Rubarth) in tissue culture. *Nord. Vet. Med.* 6:767–779, 1954.

Parker, R. L., Cabasso, V. J., Dean, D. J., and Cheatum, E. L. Serologic evidence of certain virus infections in wild animals. *J. Am. Vet. Med. Assoc.* 138:437–440, 1961.

Parry, H. B., Larin, N. M., and Platt, H. Studies on the agent of canine virus hepatitis (Rubarth's disease): II. The pathology and pathogenesis of experimental disease produced by four strains of virus. *J. Hyg.* 49:482–496, 1951.

Rowe, W. P., and Hartley, J. W. A general review of the adenoviruses. *Ann. N.Y. Acad. Sci.* 101:466–474, 1962.

Rubarth, S. An acute virus disease with liver lesions in dogs (*hepatitis contagiosa canis*): A pathologico-anatomical and etiological investigation. *Acta Pathol. Microbiol. Scand.* suppl. 69, 1947.

Sarkan, S. Immunization of dogs with infectious canine hepatitis virus propagated by tissue culture in swine kidney cells. Ph.D. thesis, Cornell University, 1957.

Sellers, R. F., and Fitzpatrick, M. Multiplication, interferon production and interferon sensitivity of viruses in dog kidney tissue culture. *Res. Vet. Sci.* 4:151–159, 1963.

Shimizu, Y., Kunishige, T., and Hirato, K. Immunological studies on the infectious canine hepatitis virus: II. Hemagglutinin. *Jpn. J. Vet. Res.* 8:271–278, 1960.

Siedentopf, H. A., and Carlson, W. E. A comparative study of the fox encephalitis virus and the virus of infectious canine hepatitis. *J. Am. Vet. Med. Assoc.* 115:109–111, 1949.

Trainer, D. O., and Knowlton, F. F. Serologic evidence of diseases in Texas coyotes. *J. Wildl. Manag.* 32:981–983, 1968.

Zwierzchowski, J., and Gorski, J. Attempts at evaluation of effectiveness of vaccination against Rubarth's disease in enzootic focus. *Acta Microbiol. Pol.* 6 (ser. A.):140, 1974.

16 *Aleutian Disease of Mink*

JOHN R. GORHAM   DAVID T. SHEN

Synonyms: **Plasmacytosis.**

Aleutian disease (AD) is a slowly progressive viral disease of mink (*Mustela vison*) characterized by loss of weight, splenomegaly, lymphadenopathy, plasmacytosis, hypergammaglobulinemia, necrotizing arteritis, and proliferative glomerulonephritis. Certain genotypes of mink—Aleutian *aa* or Chediak-Higashi syndrome (C-HS)[1]—are more susceptible to the AD virus and develop a more rapid clinical course of disease than other genotypes (Johnson et al. 1975). C-HS is manifested clinically by partial oculocutaneous albinism, photophobia, increased susceptibility to infection, and a hemorrhagic tendency. AD is currently the most important infectious disease facing the mink industry.

HISTORY. Prior to 1940, only "standard dark" or "wild type" mink were raised. Color phase mutations appeared from time to time but were not raised because their pelts were considered to have little value. One cannot say whether Aleutian disease was present in these first pen-raised mink; at that time problems associated with proper diet and devastating outbreaks of distemper and botulism were the farmers' major worry. If AD was present it was not clinically evident in the more resistant dark herds.

In 1941, an Oregon rancher saved a gunmetal-colored mink for breeding. The color gene that was inherited as an autosomal recessive trait was designated *a* and called the Aleutian gene. By crossing other mutant mink with Aleutian mink (so-called because their pelts resembled those of the Aleutian fox), several substrains were developed and were collectively called blue mink. The pelts of these blue mink were extremely valuable, and a brisk sale of breeding stock followed. Little did these ranchers realize that they were later to provide the industry with millions of sentinel animals for AD.

In the 1940s, Aleutian mink were sold to American and Canadian ranchers, and shortly thereafter, ranchers observed an increased mortality rate in the progeny from these parent strains. The mink were called bleeders because the ragged ulcers on the gingival borders often bled when the mink were handled. These signs are now recognized as being those of AD. Hartsough and Gorham (1956) reported the first gross lesions of AD in blue mink.

Losses from AD increased each year. Before the advent of chicken embryo attenuated distemper vaccines, autogenous tissue vaccines from distemper-infected mink were used in an attempt to control distemper outbreaks. The infectious nature of AD was suggested when outbreaks ensued after the large-scale use of these autogenous products. Helmboldt and Jungherr (1958) recorded that most of the mink on a Connecticut ranch vaccinated with such a vaccine were dead of AD after 6 months. It is now known that the formalin added to the vaccines inactivated the distemper virus component, but the AD virus, which was also present in the vaccine, was remarkably resistant to formalin (Burger et al. 1965; Henson et al. 1962; Karstad et al. 1963).

By 1950, it was obvious that AD was contagious. When mink were brought from farms with AD to clean farms, the disease appeared in the noninfected mink on the new farms. Infected mink established new foci of AD on previously uninfected ranches. Initially, the disease was thought to be confined to the *aa* genotype, because *Aa* and *AA* mink raised on the same farm seemed to be unaffected. But when the uninfected blue mink were sent to ranches where AD was present but unrecognized in the dark mink, the newly purchased blues served as sentinels by rapidly succumbing to AD.

It was believed that mink was the only species susceptible to AD; however, it has now been reported that ferrets inoculated with AD-infective material of mink origin harbor the infective agent for at least 136 days after inoculation (Kenyon et al. 1966, 1967). Histopathologic changes in the liver, spleen, and lymph nodes are similar in infected animals of both species. Lesions and overt signs of AD

---

1. In this chapter the designations Aleutian mink (*aa*), blue mink, and mink with the Chediak-Higashi syndrome (C-HS) are used interchangeably.

develop more slowly in ferrets than in mink; however, in most instances infected ferrets show no signs of disease. In terms of the rapidity with which lesions develop, the ferret appears to be at one extreme of the spectrum, *aa* mink at the opposite extreme, and *Aa* mink intermediate (Ohshima et al. 1978).

Sera from other wild carnivores contained specific antibody to AD by counter immuno-electrophoresis (CIEP). Ingram and Cho (1974) found positive samples in 2 of 100 foxes, 1 of 27 raccoons, and 128 of 196 skunks. The importance of these animals in maintaining the virus in nature is an enigma. Dogs and cats experimentally injected with AD virus have shown a transient positive serologic response with CIEP although they appear normal during a 6-month observation period (Gorham and Shen 1975). The length of persistence of antibody appears to be variable. Until further studies have elucidated the agent's pathogenicity for man, one should be cautious when handling AD virus, particularly highly concentrated laboratory preparations.

ETIOLOGY. Vaccine accidents first suggested that AD was transmissible. Its infectious nature was confirmed independently by several investigators using cell-free filtrates (Henson et al. 1962; Karstad and Pridham 1962; Russell 1962; Trautwein and Helmboldt 1962). Studies have shown that AD virus is a parvovirus (Porter et al. 1977). It is temperature sensitive when propagated in vitro. The size of AD virus ranges from 23 nm to 25 nm (Chesebro et al. 1975; Cho and Ingram 1973; Porter et al. 1977).

Attempts to culture AD virus in vitro were not successful until 1977 (Porter et al. 1977). Investigators found that propagation of AD virus had to be accomplished at 31.8°C and that a highly virulent strain of AD virus, such as the Utah 1 strain, must be used. Although numerous attempts have been made to culture AD virus strains of low virulence, to date all have failed.

AD virus is highly resistant to chemical and enzymatic inactivation. Burger et al. (1965) found that the partly purified AD agent was surprisingly stable to the action of proteolytic enzymes and nucleases but was readily inactivated by boiling or treatment with strong acids, bases, and iodine. Crude tissue preparations showed greater stability toward heat (90–95°C) and 0.4% formalin; however, this can be explained by a possible stabilizing effect of protein impurities on the AD agent. Gray (cited in Karstad 1967), using crude AD-virus-infected

tissue suspensions, reported that the AD agent persisted at 80°C for 30 minutes and at 99.5°C for 3 minutes. A recent evaluation of chemical disinfectants for AD virus showed that 1% formalin, 0.5–1% sodium hydroxide and 3% 0-SYL are effective antiviral agents (Shen and Gorham 1980).

AD virus is easily recovered from the serum, whole blood, feces, urine, saliva, and various tissues of infected mink (Eklund et al. 1968; Gorham et al. 1964; Kenyon et al. 1963). Although the disease is regarded as being slow, the virus replicates rapidly in the mink. The highest viral titers in the spleen, liver, and lymph nodes (10^7 ID_{50}/g) are detected about 10 days after inoculation. Development of antiviral antibody can also be demonstrated about 10 days after inoculation (Porter et al. 1969). Later, the virus titers decline; 2 or more months after infection, spleen titers of 10^5 ID_{50}/g and serum titers of 10^4 ID_{50}/ml can be shown. Using the highly virulent Utah I strain of AD virus, Porter et al. (1969) did not show a difference in the level of viral replication in different mink genotypes. However, Eklund et al. (1968) reported that when the Pullman strain was titered in mink of different genotype, higher virus titers were recorded in *aa* mink than in non-Aleutian mink. The Pullman strain of AD virus is markedly less virulent than the Utah strain (Bloom et al. 1975). By immunofluorescence, Porter et al. (1969) detected viral antigen mainly in the cytoplasm of macrophages in the spleen, lymph nodes, and Kupffer cells.

TRANSMISSION. Both horizontal and vertical transmission of AD virus have been reported (Gorham et al. 1964, 1976; Padgett et al. 1967). When AD-susceptible animals were brought into AD-virus-infected farms, AD was occasionally detected in these mink. Because AD virus was detected in saliva, urine, and feces (Gorham et al. 1964; Kenyon et al. 1963), it is possible that affected mink can transmit the disease to susceptible mink through biting, feces, urine, or handling with contaminated gloves (Larsen 1969). Gorham et al. (1964) reported two possible routes of natural transmission, fecal-oral and saliva-aerosol-respiratory.

Vertical transmission appears to be the most common means of perpetuating AD in mink. The continuing viremia stimulated Haagsma (1969) and Shen et al. (1973) to investigate insect transmission. Haagsma collected fleas from AD-infected animals and prepared a suspension that, when injected into test mink, failed to evoke AD.

Mosquitoes (*Aedes fitchii*) were maintained for as long as 35 days after a blood meal on AD-infected mink. When these mosquitoes were homogenized and injected into C-HS test mink, AD was produced. Even though a vector-pathogen relationship was suggested by this and other studies, the prospect that *A. fitchii* serves as a natural vector remains speculative because experimental transmission of AD virus from mink to mink by this mosquito has not been successful (Shen et al. 1973).

Asymptomatic and even nonpersistent infections by AD virus are common in non-Aleutian and wild mink (An and Ingram 1977, 1978; An et al. 1978; Cho and Greenfield 1978; Larsen and Porter 1975).

Until subjected to experimentation, it can be assumed that C-HS mink are infectious for life. The infectivity of non-C-HS mink is open to question but will probably be related to the outcome of the disease; that is, non-C-HS mink that eventually die from AD probably excrete the virus for life. W. J. Hadlow (personal communication, 1977) found the Pullman virus isolate in the mesenteric lymph nodes of non-C-HS mink 40 months after AD virus injections. The epizootiologic significance of the persistence of AD virus in the mesenteric lymph nodes of non-C-HS mink will eventually have to be resolved.

PATHOLOGY. Gross lesions include emaciation, hepatomegaly with small, pale, pinpoint foci scattered through the liver parenchyma, generalized lymphadenopathy with the spleen and lymph nodes 2−4 times normal size, and nephritis characterized by enlarged kidneys with widespread petechiae early in the course of the disease and by shrunken pale kidneys during the later stages of AD. Histologically, there is marked proliferation and infiltration of plasma cells in practically all organs (Helmboldt and Jungherr 1958; Henson et al. 1966; Obel 1959). The plasmacytosis leads to a marked hypergammaglobulinemia, which may exceed 60% of the total serum proteins. The level of plasma cell proliferation is directly proportional to the serum globulin levels and the severity of vascular changes (Porter and Larsen 1964).

Circulating complexes of infectious virus coupled with antibody are presumed to initiate some of the lesions. The glomeruli in affected kidneys are relatively avascular and contain large amounts of slightly granular, eosinophilic material. The latter represents a proliferation of mesangial matrix as well as deposition of gamma globulin and complement (C3) (Henson

et al. 1968). Deposition of gamma globulin and C3 along the glomerular capillary basement membranes and in the mesangial areas is seen by fluorescent microscopy (Henson et al. 1969). These deposits are seen ultrastructurally as electro-dense granules subendothelially and, less frequently, subepithelially; they most likely represent deposition of antigen-antibody complexes (Henson et al. 1968, 1969). In some animals, viral antigen can also be demonstrated in the glomeruli. Widespread necrotizing arteritis involving the small muscular arteries is also observed. Gamma globulin, complement, and viral antigen are demonstrable in the affected arteries, suggesting that deposition of antigen-antibody complexes initiates arteritis (Porter et al. 1973). Experimentally infected mink immunosuppressed with cyclophosphamide do not develop lesions, but the virus persists in high titer. These findings further incriminate the immune response of the host in the development of the lesions in AD (Cheema et al. 1972).

Lesions occur in all clinically affected mink genotypes, but their development is much more rapid in Aleutian mink than in others. If non-C-HS mink succumb to AD, the lesions are as severe as those in the Aleutian genotype. C-HS is manifested histologically by enlarged cytoplasmic granules in many types of granule-containing cells. Many of the enlarged cytoplasmic granules are lysosomes (Oliver and Essner 1973; White 1966). The impaired degradative activity in C-HS phagocytes appears to be related to delayed delivery of lysosomal enzymes into phagosomes.

Mink with Aleutian disease developed severe anemia within a few months of infection. Evaluation of erythropoiesis and erythrocyte survival demonstrated that the anemia was caused by increased erythrocyte destruction, complicated in some cases by decreased or inadequate erythropoiesis (McGuire et al. 1979).

DIAGNOSIS. AD can be suspected whenever production is poor and mink appear unthrifty despite adequate diet. Affected mink typically are sick for weeks or months and succumb during periods of sudden stress (rapid changes in temperature, environment, diet, or transport). A diagnosis in an individual mink is suggested by chronicity of the course and the signs. Similarly, the gross finding of enlarged kidneys, spleen, lymph nodes, and liver are often sufficiently characteristic for a tentative diagnosis; however, microscopic examination provides the most definitive diagnosis.

Nonspecific Test. Virtually all C-HS mink become hypergammaglobulinemic during the course of the disease. The increased level of gamma globulin can be detected by a simple field test, the iodine agglutination test (IAT) (Gorham et al. 1976). Although IAT detects any increase in gamma globulin levels regardless of the cause, control programs have shown that non-AD-induced increases in gamma globulin are insignificant. A disadvantage of the IAT is the 3-week lag time before gamma globulin reaches a positive level (15% of the total serum proteins); therefore, IAT does not detect AD early enough to prevent transmission. The IAT also detects only 16–65% of the mink with AD antibody as shown by the CIEP tests (Greenfield et al. 1973; Ingram and Cho 1974). Serum protein electrophoresis has also been used to detect and quantify AD antibody (Larsen 1965).

The antibody response in non-C-HS mink is quite different from that in C-HS mink. Depending on whether virus strains are of high or low virulence in an epidemic of AD, the gamma globulin level will (1) never rise, (2) rise and fall and never rise again, or (3) rise and remain high until death. Thus, the nonspecific test has additional disadvantages when dealing with non-C-HS mink.

Specific Tests. Since the report of Porter et al. (1969) of an immunofluorescence technique for the detection of AD virus antigen and antibody, other specific serologic tests have been described (Burger et al. 1978; Cho and Ingram 1972; McGuire et al. 1971). The sensitivity, reproducibility, and specificity of immunofluorescence, complement fixation, and CIEP tests were compared by Crawford et al. (1977). They found all three tests to be reliable and specific for AD virus. The CIEP test is used in eradication programs. Burger et al. (1978) demonstrated the application of an enzyme-linked immunosorbent assay (ELISA) for the detection of AD antibody in mink. The potential of ELISA as a field test is currently under investigation.

IMMUNITY. There is no known immunity to AD virus. All mink, regardless of genotype, are susceptible. No vaccine has been effective in preventing the disease. Until the pathogenetic mechanisms are understood, hope for a vaccine is slight.

No treatment for AD is effective. Antibiotics are ineffective against the AD virus but may help to prevent secondary bacterial infection and prolong life for a short time.

TREATMENT AND CONTROL. AD has been partly controlled by elimination of clinically ill and hypergammaglobulinemic mink. Cho and Greenfield (1978) reported success in eliminating AD from three infected mink ranches by use of the CIEP tests and subsequently pelting all animals that had AD virus antibody. Presently, about 0.5 million mink have been tested by the CIEP in Denmark; as a result, AD has been eradicated on 15 farms in Denmark (M. Henson, personal communication, 1980).

It now appears possible to control and eliminate AD on infected mink ranches by use of the CIEP tests. Rigorous culling of all mink positive for AD virus antibody enables potential AD virus carriers to be eliminated and hence aids in the eradication of AD from infected mink ranches.

REFERENCES

An, S. H., and Ingram, D. G. Detection of inapparent Aleutian disease virus infection in mink. *Am. J. Vet. Res.* 38:1619–1624, 1977.

———. Transmission of Aleutian disease from mink with inapparent infection. *Am. J. Vet. Res.* 39:309–315, 1978.

An, S. H., Depauli, F. J., Wright, P., and Ingram, D. G. Characteristics of inapparent Aleutian disease virus infections in mink. *Am. J. Vet. Res.* 24:200–204, 1978.

Bloom, M. E., Race, R. E., Hadlow, W. J., and Chesebro, B. Aleutian disease of mink: The antibody response of sapphire and pastel mink to Aleutian disease virus. *J. Immunol.* 115:1034–1037, 1975.

Burger, D., Gorham, J. R., and Leader, R. W. Some physical and chemical characteristics of partially purified Aleutian disease virus. In *Slow, latent and temperate virus infections.* National Institute of Neurological Diseases and Blindness monogr. 2, pp. 307–313. Washington, D.C.: U.S. Government Printing Office, 1965.

Burger, D., Srirangnathan, N., and Gorham, J. R. Detection of antibody and antigen in Aleutian disease-virus infected mink with the enzyme-linked immuno-sorbent assay (ELISA). Abstracts of the 78th annual meeting of the American Society for Microbiology, Las Vegas, 1978. Washington, D. C.: American Society for Microbiology.

Cheema, A., Henson, J. B., and Gorham, J. R. Aleutian disease of mink: Prevention of lesions by immunosuppression. *Am. J. Pathol.* 55:543–556, 1972.

Chesebro, B., Bloom, M., Hadlow, W., and Race, R. Purification and ultrastructure of Aleutian disease virus of mink. *Nature* 254:456–457, 1975.

Cho, H. J., and Greenfield, J. Eradication of Aleutian disease mink by eliminating positive counterimmunoelectrophoresis reactors. *J. Clin. Microbiol.* 7:18–22, 1978.

Cho, H. J., and Ingram, D. G. Antigen and antibody in Aleutian disease in mink: I. Precipitation reaction by agar-gel electrophoresis. *J. Immunol.* 108:555–557, 1972.

———. Isolation, purification and structure of Aleutian disease virus by immunological techniques. *Nature N. Biol.* 243:174–176, 1973.

Crawford, T. B., McGuire, T. C., Porter, D. D., and Cho, H. J. A comparative study of detection methods for Aleutian disease viral antibody. *J. Immunol.* 118:1249–1251, 1977.

Eklund, C. M., Hadlow, W. J., Kennedy, R. C., Boyle, C. C., and Jackson, T. A. Aleutian disease of mink: Properties of the etiologic agent and the host responses. *J. Infect. Dis.* 118:510–526, 1968.

Gorham, J. R., Henson, J. B., Crawford, T. B., and Padgett, G. A. The epizootiology of Aleutian disease. In R. H. Kimberlin, ed., *Slow virus diseases of animals and man*, pp. 135–158. Amsterdam: North-Holland Publishing Co., 1976.

Gorham, J. R., Leader, R. W., and Henson, J. B. The experimental transmission of a virus causing hypergammaglobulinemia in mink: Sources and modes of infection. *J. Infect. Dis.* 114:341–345, 1964.

Greenfield, J., Walton, R., and MacDonald, K. R. Detection of Aleutian disease in mink: Serumplate agglutination using iodine compared with precipitation by agar-gel electrophoresis. *Res. Vet. Sci.* 15:382–383, 1973.

Haagsma, J. Epizootiology of Aleutian disease (plasmacytosis) in mink. *Neth. J. Vet. Sci.* 2:19–30, 1969.

Hartsough, G. R., and Gorham, J. R. Aleutian disease in mink. *Nat. Fur News* 28:10–11, 1956.

Helmboldt, C. F., and Jungherr, E. L. The pathology of Aleutian disease in mink. *Am. J. Vet. Res.* 19:212–222, 1958.

Henson, J. B., Gorham, J. R., Leader, R. W., and Wagner, B. M. Experimental hypergammaglobulinemia in mink. *J. Exp. Med.* 116:357–364, 1962.

Henson, J. B., Gorham, J. R., Padgett, G. A., and Davis, W. C. Pathogenesis of the glomerular lesions in Aleutian disease of mink: Immunofluorescent studies. *Arch. Pathol.* 87:21–28, 1969.

Henson, J. B., Gorham, J. R., Tanaka, Y., and Padgett, G. A. Sequential development of ultrastructural lesions in the glomeruli of mink with experimental Aleutian disease. *Lab. Invest.* 19:153–162, 1968.

Henson, J. B., Leader, R. W., Gorham, J. R., and Padgett, G. A. The sequential development of lesions in spontaneous Aleutian disease of mink. *Pathol. Vet.* 3:289–314, 1966.

Ingram, D. G., and Cho, H. J. Aleutian disease in mink: Virology, immunology and pathogenesis. *J. Rheumatol.* 1:74–92, 1974.

Johnson, M. I., Henson, J. B., and Gorham, J. R. The influence of genotype on the development of glomerular lesions in mink with Aleutian disease

virus: A correlated light, fluorescent and electron microscopic study. *Am. J. Pathol.* 81:321–332, 1975.

Karstad, L. Aleutian disease: A slowly progressive viral infection of mink. *Curr. Top. Microbiol. Immunol.* 40:1–21, 1967.

Karstad, L., and Pridham, T. J. Aleutian disease of mink: I. Evidence of its viral etiology. *Can. J. Comp. Med. Vet. Sci.* 26:97–102, 1962.

Karstad, L., Pridham, T. J., and Gray, D. P. Aleutian disease (plasmacytosis) of mink: II. Responses of mink to formalin-treated diseased tissues and to subsequent challenge with virulent inoculum. *Can. J. Comp. Med. Vet. Sci.* 27:124–128, 1963.

Kenyon, A. J., Helmboldt, C. F., and Nielson, S. W. Experimental transmission of Aleutian disease with urine. *Am. J. Vet. Res.* 24:1066–1067, 1963.

Kenyon, A. J., Howard, E., and Buko, L. Hypergammaglobulinemia in ferrets with lymphoproliferative lesions (Aleutian disease). *Am. J. Vet. Res.* 28:1167–1172, 1967.

Kenyon, A. J., Kenyon, B. J., and Hahn, E. C. Protides of the mustelidae: Immunoresponse of mustelids of Aleutian mink disease virus. *Am. J. Vet. Res.* 39:1011–1015, 1978.

Kenyon, A. J., Magnano, T., Helmboldt, C. F., and Buko, L. Aleutian disease in the ferret. *J. Am. Vet. Med. Assoc.* 149:920–923, 1966.

Larsen, A. E., Electrophoresis, IAT and the elusive Aleutian disease. *Nat. Fur News* 37:18–22, 1965.

———. Immunological and viral studies of Aleutian disease in mink. Ph.D. dissertation, University of Utah, 1969.

Larsen, A. E., and Porter, D. D., Pathogenesis of Aleutian disease of mink: Identification of nonpersistent infections. *Infect. Immun.* 11:92–94, 1975.

McGuire, T. C., Crawford, T. B., Henson, J. B., and Gorham, J. R. Aleutian disease of mink: Detection of large quantities of complement-fixing antibody to viral antigen. *J. Immunol.* 107:1481–1482, 1971.

McGuire, T. C., Perryman, L. E., and Gorham, J. R. Mechanisms of anemia in Aleutian disease viral infection of mink. *Vet. Microb.* 4:17–27, 1979.

Obel, A. L. Studies on a disease of mink with systemic proliferation of the plasma cells. *Am. J. Vet. Res.* 20:384–393, 1959.

Ohshima, K., Shen, D. T., Henson, J. B., and Gorham, J. R. Comparison of the lesions of Aleutian disease in mink and hypergammaglobulinemia in ferrets. *Am. J. Vet. Res.* 39:653–655, 1978.

Oliver, C., and Essner, E. Distribution of anomalous lysosomes in the beige mouse: A homologue of Chediak-Higashi syndrome. *J. Histochem. Cytochem.* 21:218–228, 1973.

Padgett, G. A., Gorham, J. R., and Henson, J. B. Epizootiologic studies of Aleutian disease: I. Transplacental transmission of the virus. *J. Infect. Dis.* 117:35–38, 1967.

Porter, D. D., and Larsen, A. E. Statistical survey of

Aleutian disease in ranch mink. *Am. J. Vet. Res.* 25:1226–1229, 1964.

Porter, D. D., Larsen, A. E., Cox, N. A., Porter, H. G., and Suffin, S. C. Isolation of Aleutian disease virus of mink in cell culture. *Intervirology* 8:129–144, 1977.

Porter, D. D., Larsen, A. E., and Porter, H. G. The pathogenesis of Aleutian disease of mink: I. *In vitro* viral replication and the host antibody responses to viral antigen. *J. Exp. Med.* 130:575–593, 1969.

———. The pathogenesis of Aleutian disease of mink: III. Immune complex arteritis. *Am. J. Pathol.* 71:331–338, 1973.

Russell, J. D. Research and control of Aleutian disease. *Nat. Fur News* 34:22–33, 1962.

Shen, D. T., Gorham, J. R., Harwood, R. E., and Padgett, G. A. The persistence of Aleutian disease virus in the mosquito *Aedes fitchii. Arch. Gesamte Virusforsch.* 40:375–381, 1973.

Trautwein, G. W., and Helmboldt, C. F. Aleutian disease of mink: I. Experimental transmission of the disease. *Am. J. Vet. Res.* 23:1280–1288, 1962.

White, J. G. The Chediak-Higashi syndrome: A possible lysosomal disease. *Blood* 28:143–156, 1966.

17 Miscellaneous Viral Infections

L. KARSTAD

Caliciviruses

Synonyms: **None.**

HISTORY. Caliciviruses were first isolated from wild mammals in 1972 when Smith and his coworkers isolated two serotypes from sea lions (*Zalophus californianus*) on San Miguel Island, California, and showed a relationship between the San Miguel sea lion virus (SMSV) and vesicular exanthema swine virus (VESV) (Smith et al. 1973). From 1932 to 1956, vesicular exanthema (VES) was an important disease of swine in the United States (Bankowski 1965). Between 1956 and 1972, VES was not recognized and was thought to be an example of an animal disease eradicated by stringent disease control measures. The isolation of SMSV and recognition of its virtual identity to VESV was therefore viewed with grave concern.

ETIOLOGY. The caliciviruses, SMSV and VESV, which can probably be considered one virus with a multiplicity of antigenic types, together with feline calicivirus, are considered as a possible generic group within the family Picornaviridae. They are small RNA viruses, about 30–40 nm in diameter, resistant to lipid solvents, heat labile, and unstable in acid pH (Fenner 1976).

HOST RANGE AND DISTRIBUTION. SMSV strains have been isolated from sea lions in California and from fur seals (*Callorhinus ursinus*) and elephant seals (*Mirounga augustirostris*) in Alaska (Sawyer et al. 1978; Smith et al. 1973). In addition, serologic evidence of SMSV infection has been found in gray foxes (*Urocyon littoralis*) and in feral swine and donkeys in California (Prato et al. 1977; Smith and Latham 1978). Antibodies to nine VESV serotypes have been found in California sea lions, California gray whales (*Eschrichtius robustus*), sperm whales (*Physeter catodon*), finback whales (*Balaenoptera physalus*), sei whales (*B. borealis*), feral swine, and a feral donkey, all along the California coast (Smith and Latham

1978). These findings led Smith and Latham (1978) to propose that VESV is probably still present and active along the California coast, although it had not been recognized as a cause of disease in swine since it was officially declared eradicated in 1956. Furthermore, their mention of recent calicivirus isolates from *Girella nigricans*, a fish which inhabits tidal pools, illustrated the possibility that such a reservoir may provide a source of infection for both land and marine mammals (Smith and Latham 1978).

Experimentally, SMSV has been transmitted to an African green monkey (*Cercopithecus aethiops*), and antibodies appearing in the sera of research workers and technicians is evidence of exposure and possible human infection (Smith et al. 1978).

PATHOLOGY. VESV causes a vesicular disease of the mouth, lips, and feet of swine that cannot be differentiated on clinical and pathologic grounds from two other important vesicular diseases of swine, vesicular stomatitis and foot-and-mouth disease (Bankowski 1965). Little is known of the pathology of VESV and SMSV in wild animals. The initial isolates of SMSV were made from a population of sea lions that experienced a high rate of abortion and neonatal deaths. Whether SMSV was responsible for the reproductive losses could not be confirmed. SMSV was isolated from vesicles on the flippers of fur seals on St. Paul Island, Alaska (Sawyer et al. 1978), but no histologic description of the lesions was provided.

DIAGNOSIS. Because the pathologic effects of calicivirus infections in wild mammals are not well defined, diagnosis must rely on virus isolation and identification. (Sawyer et al. 1978; Smith and Latham 1978). The virus neutralization test may be used to demonstrate antibodies in the sera of exposed animals, but its value is mainly as an epidemiological tool to provide evidence of past infection.

TREATMENT AND CONTROL. The methods used successfully to eradicate VESV from domestic swine in 1956 were quarantine, slaughter, sanitary disposal of affected swine herds, and cooking of all garbage fed to swine. Control of naturally occurring infections in wild mammals in their marine habitat is impractical. One should be aware, however, of the possible dangers of transporting these viruses by trade in marine mammals for zoos and aquariums and the hazards of interstate commerce in ranch mink foods prepared from the carcasses of slaughtered fur seals (Sawyer et al. 1978; Smith and Latham 1978).

Hog Cholera

Synonyms: **Swine fever.**

Hog cholera is a generalized systemic disease of swine, both wild and domestic. It is a pantropic viral infection characterized by lesions in tissues of the blood vessels, lymph nodes, spleen, and brain. Affected swine become febrile and depressed and may either die acutely or live for variable periods of time with signs of gastrointestinal disease and emaciation.

HISTORY. Hog cholera in wild swine does not differ from its occurrence and appearance in domestic swine (*Sus scrofa*). The student of wildlife disease will find ample information on hog cholera in the standard veterinary textbooks (Leman et al. 1981; Merchant and Packer 1967). A description of the disease in wild swine, particularly in Germany, is given by Wetzel and Rieck (1962).

Hog cholera was first recognized as a new disease of swine in Ohio in 1833. Its possible occurrence earlier is discussed by Hanson (1957). It reached Europe and spread to Germany in the late 1800s. The first report of its occurrence in wild swine describes an outbreak in a fenced park near Munich in 1906 (Wetzel and Rieck 1962). Later, outbreaks occurred also in free-ranging wild swine.

In the Americas, hog cholera in wildlife is limited to the few populations of introduced European wild swine and feral domesticated swine.

DISTRIBUTION. Hog cholera occurs worldwide. A few countries (Canada, for example) have been able to eradicate the disease and, except for occasional chance reintroductions, have

been kept free of hog cholera. Eradication may be difficult in areas where there are large populations of wild or feral swine.

ETIOLOGY. Hog cholera virus is a small, relatively stable virus which is classified, together with the virus of mucosal disease, in the *Pestivirus* genus of the Togaviridae (Fenner 1976).

TRANSMISSION. Transmission occurs naturally by ingestion of contaminated feed and by direct contact with infected swine or virus-contaminated objects. Hog cholera virus is present in the blood and all body organs of infected swine and is shed in all excretions and secretions. The presence of virus in carcasses of dead domestic swine may be a source of exposure for wild swine if carcasses are carelessly disposed of. Hog cholera virus may also be transmitted congenitally from exposed pregnant sows to their offspring. Such newborn pigs may have neurological damage manifested by severe tremors.

SIGNS. Affected wild swine are reported to lose their natural caution. They remain near water, probably because of fever and increased thirst. Weakness, depression, and rapid weight loss occur. There may be staggering, circling, and convulsions. Vomiting and coughing may occur, and diarrhea is common. Depression and profound weakness cause the animals to seek cover and remain quiet in terminal stages of the disease. Few infected swine recover.

PATHOGENESIS. Virus commonly enters the body by invasion and multiplication in cells of the upper digestive tract, tonsils, and lymph nodes. Viremia occurs, usually beginning within 24 hours of exposure. Fever appears about 3 days postexposure, and peak body temperatures are reached 3 or 4 days later (Dunne 1970).

PATHOLOGY. Lesions are variable, depending in part on the age of the animal and the duration of illness. Pigs that die after very short illness may have gross lesions limited to petechial and ecchymotic hemorrhages in the skin and subcutis; on the mucosae of the larynx, trachea, and intestines; and on serosal surfaces of the lungs, heart, and abdominal viscera. Regarded as characteristic are pinhead to pea size hemorrhages in the kidney cortex, marginal hemorrhages in enlarged lymph nodes, and red marginal infarcts in the spleen. Chronically affected pigs may have buttonlike ulcers in the intestines. Pneumonic lung changes are sometimes present.

There are no pathognomonic lesions in hog cholera. Most pigs that die of the disease have nonsuppurative encephalitis, marked by prominent perivascular accumulations of lymphocytes.

DIAGNOSIS AND PROGNOSIS. A presumptive diagnosis of hog cholera may be made upon the recognition of characteristic clinical signs, gross lesions, and histologic findings. Confirmation is made by reproduction of the disease in susceptible swine by inoculation of bacteria-free filtrates of blood or suspensions of tissues (for example, spleen), and protection of other susceptible pigs by simultaneous inoculation of specific antiserum.

The mortality rate is variable, depending on the possibility of previous exposure with virulent or attenuated strains of virus. In unexposed swine it may exceed 90%.

IMMUNITY. Vaccine prophylaxis should be practiced for captive swine in countries where hog cholera commonly occurs. Both inactivated virus and live attenuated virus vaccines are available. These should be used in preference to the older procedure of vaccination with simultaneous injections of virulent virus and antiserum because of the danger of accidental distribution of virulent virus. Immunity to hog cholera virus can be strong and lasting. More durable immunity is obtained from the live vaccines. If inactivated virus vaccine is used, revaccination should be practiced annually.

TREATMENT AND CONTROL. There is no specific treatment. Antibiotic treatment may increase the number of survivors by controlling secondary bacterial infections. Serum from hyperimmunized swine may be used in treatment, but unless given very soon after exposure, it has little beneficial effect.

In isolated outbreaks the best form of control is eradication. All diseased and known exposed swine should be slaughtered and the carcasses burned or otherwise treated to destroy the virus. Contaminated premises must be carefully cleaned and treated with disinfectants. Slaughter of diseased and exposed swine is usually combined with a program of vaccination of swine to create a peripheral buffer zone of immunized animals. It is obvious that these measures may not be practicable in outbreaks of hog cholera in free-ranging animals.

Contagious Ecthyma

Synonyms: **Contagious pustular dermatitis, sore mouth, orf.**

Contagious ecthyma is an infectious disease of sheep and goats characterized by vesicular, pustular, and crusted lesions on the nose and lips. The infective agent is a poxvirus in the Parapoxvirus subgroup (Fenner 1976).

HISTORY. Connell (1954) reported the occurrence of contagious ecthyma in bighorn sheep (*Ovis canadensis*) in Banff National Park, Canada, in the spring and early summer of 1953. Signs of disease were similar to those characteristic for contagious ecthyma in domestic sheep. Diagnosis was confirmed by transmission of infection to a susceptible domestic lamb by inoculation of a suspension of scab material from affected bighorn sheep. A second domestic sheep, previously recovered from contagious ecthyma, was immune to infection with the same inoculum.

TRANSMISSION AND HOSTS. Transmission occurs by contamination of abrasions of mucous membranes or skin, with exudate or scabs. The most susceptible site is the mucocutaneous junction of the lips. Like other pox agents, the virus is very stable in dried scabs.

In addition to its occurrence in domestic sheep and goats (Blood and Henderson 1963) and bighorn sheep (Connell 1954; Samuel et al. 1975), the disease has been reported in chamois (*Rupicapra rupicapra*) and tahr (*Hemitragus jemlaicus*) in New Zealand (Daniel and Christie 1963), in mountain goats (*Oreamnos americanus*) in Canada (Hebert et al. 1977; Samuel et al. 1975), and in muskoxen (*Ovibos moschatus*) in Norway (Kummeneje and Krogsrud 1978).

This disease is a zoonosis. Man becomes infected by contact exposure to infected sheep or goats.

SIGNS. Lesions in sheep and goats develop most commonly on the lips and muzzle, first as vesicles, then as pustules and, finally, scabs. The scabs are firmly attached and persist for several days or weeks, covering raised areas of eroded inflamed skin. Lesions may occur also on the feet and udder, especially in outbreaks in which lip lesions are present in suckling lambs. In bighorn sheep and mountain goats, lesions occurred also in the mouth, particularly on the gingiva and tongue (Fig. 17.1).

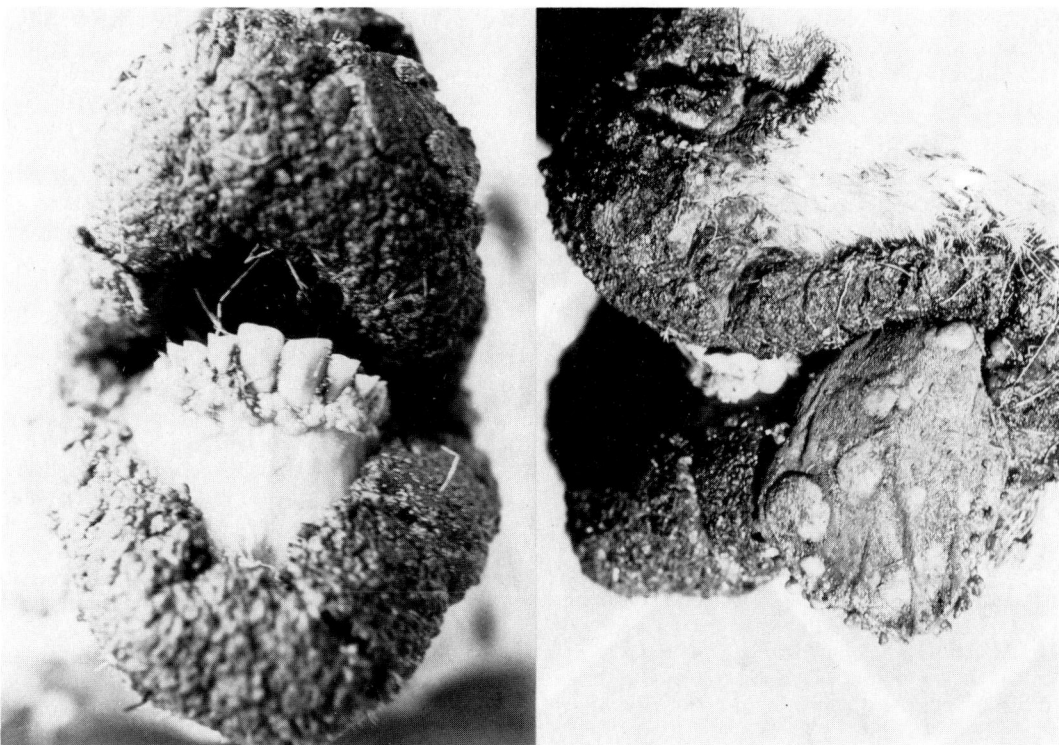

FIG. 17.1   Lesions of contagious ecthyma in a mountain goat (Samuel et al. 1975).

Lesions on the tongue were pale, circumscribed, of varying diameter, and raised slightly above the normal surface. Clusters of pink or reddish brown proliferative papilliform lesions occurred on the gingival mucosa in one case, forming a mass of a size sufficient to interfere with placement of the tongue. In captive muskoxen, the lesions were described as warty or cauliflowerlike and were referred to as papillomas. They occurred around the mouth and nose and also, to a lesser extent, on other parts of the body, for example, the eyelids, neck, chest, and the perineal area.

Secondary bacterial or fungal infections are common, and the ecthyma lesions may become infested with fly maggots. Debilitation, the result of soreness and inability to feed, is a major problem. Deaths have been reported in bighorn sheep, mountain goats, and muskoxen. All five calves born into the captive muskoxen herd in 1975 died as a result of interference with eating and respiration (Kummeneje and Krogsrud 1978).

PATHOGENESIS. Affected cells in the epithelium become swollen and develop intracyto-

plasmic inclusions typical of the poxviruses. Inclusions may be difficult to find after the stage of vesiculation has passed. Infiltration with neutrophils occurs in the affected epithelium, and small pustules develop and coalesce, becoming covered by heavy crusts. Scabs usually persist until healing is well advanced. Lesions in muskoxen were more proliferative and took the form of papillomas.

DIAGNOSIS. Diagnosis is based largely on clinical signs but should be confirmed by histopathology and transmission experiments. Demonstration of poxvirus virions by electron microscopy was used as an adjunct to histopathology by Samuel et al. (1975) and by Kummeneje and Krosgsrud (1978).

TREATMENT AND CONTROL. Treatment is aimed at suppression of secondary bacterial or fungal infections and improvement of the nutritional state of affected animals. In dealing with captive animals, vaccine prophylaxis should be considered. Live ecthyma vaccines, prepared for domestic sheep, should be used with caution on wild species. In one trial, a muskox calf developed a large neoplastic mass after inoculation of contagious ecthyma vaccine into the skin of the thigh, the usual site for vaccination of domestic sheep (Kummeneje and Krosgsrud 1978). Apparently muskoxen are extremely susceptible to infection with the virus of contagious ecthyma and react to infection with greater cell proliferation than is seen in sheep and goats. The papilliform proliferative gum lesions (Samuel et al. 1975) of bighorn sheep and mountain goats may be intermediate in this regard.

Sealpox

Synonyms: **None.**

In 1969, a nodular proliferative skin disease of California sea lions (*Zalaphus californianus*) was shown to be caused by a poxvirus (Wilson et al. 1969). Subsequently the same or a similar virus was shown to be the cause of pox in South American sea lions (*Otaria byronia*) and harbor seals (*Phoca vitulina*) (Wilson and Poglayen-Neuwall 1971; Wilson et al. 1972).

Sealpox has been found in captive and free-living harbor seals on the Atlantic coast in Nova Scotia, in captive sea lions in inland aquariums, and in free-living sea lions in the rookeries of the Pacific coast of California and the coasts of South America. Thus the virus or viruses involved appear to be well adapted to their pinniped hosts. Transmission occurs probably by contamination of skin abrasions. In captivity and in the wild, the social behavior of pinnipeds ensures plenty of opportunity for contacts, both direct bodily contact and indirect contact with heavily used sand and rocks in beach areas where seals and sea lions normally congregate.

The gross appearance of pox in pinnipeds resembled a focal neoplastic skin disease. The firm nodular lesions were round or oval, broadly based, 0.5–3.0 cm in diameter, and raised 0.5–1.5 cm above the normal skin surface (Fig. 17.2). They occurred on any part of the body but were most numerous about the head and flippers; in these areas they often became confluent and frequently fissured and suppurating. Although they were usually covered with hair, they frequently ulcerated and became crateriform.

Histologically the most characteristic change was hypertrophy and hyperplasia of cells of the stratum spinosum. The enlarged spinosum cells had a rarefied or vacuolated cytoplasm, containing acidophilic inclusion bodies. Some cells contained several granular or irregularly shaped cytoplasmic inclusion bodies; others contained only one large inclusion. Poxvirus virions, approximately 200 nm by 300 nm, were easily demonstrated in the inclusion bodies by electron microscopy of ul-

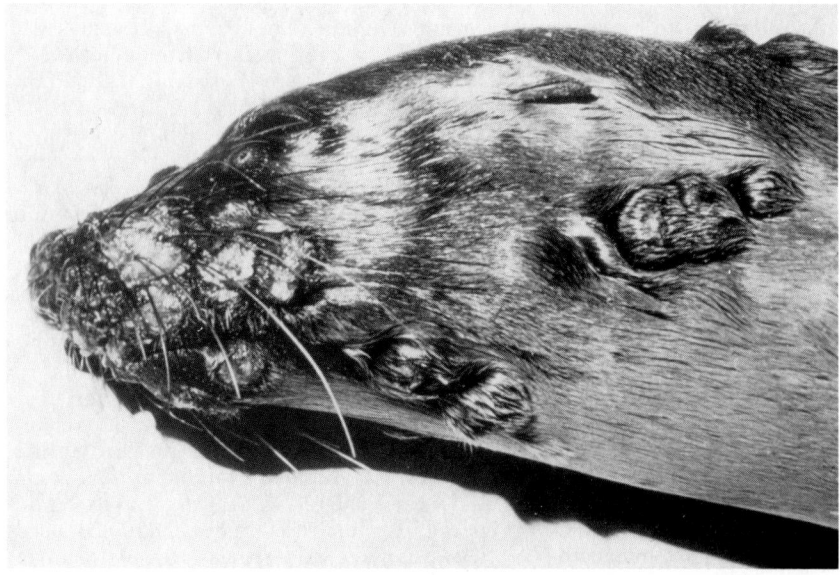

FIG. 17.2 Pox lesions on a California sea lion (Wilson et al. 1969).

trathin sections. Similar virions were demonstrable in ground-up tissues by negative staining. In size and morphology, the sealpox virions were similar to those of ecthyma and bovine papular stomatitis, in the Paravaccinia group of the poxviruses (Wilson and Sweeney 1970).

Other commonly observed changes were moderate hyperkeratosis, parakeratosis, and a variable degree of dermal inflammation, characterized by infiltration with leukocytes and fibrosis.

The incubation period in sealpox was 3–5 weeks. Some of the affected seals and sea lions died, but in these cases death was due, at least in part, to complicating factors such as lungworms and bacterial infections. In animals which survived, the lesions began to regress after about a month but remained visible for 15–18 weeks (Wilson et al. 1972).

Cowpox

Synonyms: Variola, variolavaccinia.

Eruptive and nodular proliferative skin lesions are the characteristic responses to infection with viruses of the Poxvirus family. Several outbreaks of cowpox or cowpoxlike virus infection have occurred in zoo animals, species in which pox is not known to occur in the natural environment.

Cowpox or cowpoxlike virus infections have been reported in okapi (*Okapi johnstoni*), in elephants (*Elephas maximus*), and in a variety of large cats and anteaters (*Myrmecophaga tridactyla*), all in zoos or circuses (Baxby 1977). Only minor differences from classical cowpox virus have been found in the viruses isolated. This, together with the frequently mysterious appearance of cowpox in cattle or humans, has led to speculation about the possible existence of reservoirs other than cattle. This hypothesis has borne fruit in the case of the cowpoxlike virus outbreak in the Moscow zoo. There the probable source of the virus was traced to white rats brought into the zoo as animal food, then to a rat farm outside of the zoo, and finally to free-living rodents (gerbils, *Rhombomys opimus*, and susliks, *Citellus fulvus*) (Marennikova and Ladnyj, cited in Baxby 1977). A number of human infections have occurred in zoo personnel, some characterized by severe and prolonged conjunctivitis.

OKAPI. In 1968, an outbreak of cowpox occurred in five okapi at the Rotterdam zoo (Zwart et al. 1971). Lesions were round, 1–2 cm in diameter, flattened or umbilicated, and covered with brownish scabs. They occurred mainly on the sides of the neck, on the eyelids, and around the nostrils and lips. Soft, pale lesions occurred also in the mouth, particularly on the tongue. The youngest animal, a calf of 2 months, refused to eat and died.

Histopathology of skin lesions revealed ballooning degeneration of prickle cells, vesiculation, and the presence of large eosinophilic intracytoplasmic inclusions. A virus isolated from skin lesions and propagated on the chorioallantoic membranes of hen eggs and in cell cultures was identified as cowpox virus on the basis of the hemorrhagic appearance of the lesions in chicken embryo membranes, temperatures of propagation, and by gel precipitation, using vaccinia antiserum and a 10% suspension of infected membranes. The source of infection was not determined.

ZOO CATS AND ANTEATERS. In 1973 an outbreak of cowpox occurred in Felidae (lions, black panthers, cheetahs, pumas, jaguars, and ocelots) and in giant anteaters (*Myremecophada tridactula*) at the Moscow zoo (Marennikova et al. 1977). The disease occurred in two forms, dermal and pulmonary. All animals with the pulmonary form died in 3–8 days, with severe serofibrinous bronchopneumonia. Cowpox virus, identified by propagation with characteristic cytopathology in chicken embryos, in rabbit skin, and in a pig embryo cell line, and by agar gel double diffusion against specific antisera, was isolated in high titer from pulmonary tissues.

The dermal form of the disease was milder in Felidae but resulted in deaths of both affected anteaters. A virus identical to that from the pulmonary disease was isolated from the skin lesions.

ELEPHANTPOX. Several outbreaks of a pox disease in elephants (*Elephas maximus* and *Loxodonta africana*) have occurred in Germany (Gehring et al. 1972; Gehring and Mayer 1978). In the earliest cases the virus was identified as vaccinia and it was supposed that infection had originated from humans. More detailed virus studies established that the virus was more closely related to cowpox and similar to strains isolated from okapi and wild Felidae (Marennikova et al. 1977). As a prophylactic measure, German zoo elephants are now immunized with smallpox vaccine. Lesions have been severe, the disease greatly debilitating, and mortality has been high (Gehring and Mayer 1978). The early clinical signs included difficulty in chewing and swallowing, excessive salivation, and conjunctivitis and edema of the head, trunk, and abdomen. Typical pox lesions appeared several days after the onset of signs. Multiple or confluent pox lesions occurred on the skin of the feet, legs, perineum, and the underside of the trunk, and also inside the mouth and on the tongue.

Because the initial case of pox has often occurred in only one animal in a group of elephants, the remainder of the group can be protected by immediate vaccination. Pox has occurred also in a black rhinoceros (*Diceros bicornis*) in a zoo in Germany (Grunberg and Burtscher 1968).

Measles

Synonyms: **Rubeola.**

Measles is an acute infectious disease of primates. Generally regarded as a disease of man, it occurs also in monkeys from Asia and Africa when they are imported into North America and Europe for use in medical research. It has occurred commonly in the rhesus and cynomolgous monkeys (*Macaca* spp.) and also in colobus (*Colobus guereza*) and marmosets (*Callithrix* and *Saguinus* spp.) (Hime and Keymer, 1975; Levy and Mirkovik 1971; Potkay et al. 1973; Scott and Keymer 1975).

ETIOLOGY. The causative virus is a member of the distemper-rinderpest-measles group of the Paramyxovirus family (Fenner 1976). Its physiochemical properties are similar to those of the other members of the group.

SIGNS AND PATHOLOGY. Signs of illness commonly occur within a few days of importation (Hime and Keymer 1975). They include ocular and nasal discharge, cough, inappetence, and edema of the face. Skin rash and Koplik's spots are inconsistent. Abortion has occurred in some instances (Renne et al. 1973).

Pathologic lesions are those of a focal giant cell pneumonia, usually accompanied by bronchitis. Encephalomyelitis, enteritis, and endometritis have also been described. Besides the lung, giant cells are commonly found in the lymph nodes and spleen. The giant cells are of two types, as they are in humans. The so-called Warthin-Finkeldey giant cells are believed to be mesenchymal in origin. They have many nuclei, often up to a hundred, bunched together in the center of the syncytia. The other type resembles the Langhans giant cell. It is of epithelial origin, with nuclei arranged around the periphery of the cell, usually in polar orientation (Scott and Keymer 1975). Intracytoplasmic inclusions are rarely found in the Warthin-Finkeldey cells. In the Langhans type, however, acidophilic inclusions are commonly found in nuclei or cytoplasm, sometimes in both locations.

EPIDEMIOLOGY. Surveys for antibodies to measles virus in established monkey colonies have indicated prevalence of past infection of up to 100%. It is apparent, therefore, that the prevalence of infection is much higher than indicated by recognized morbidity and mortality. Since cases reported in the literature have often involved newly imported animals, one might suppose that the stresses of capture, confinement, and shipment may predispose to fatal infections. Serologic studies of free-living monkeys have not produced evidence of infection. It seems, therefore, that measles in captive primates is the result of contact with humans.

TREATMENT AND CONTROL. Vaccination may be feasible but one must bear in mind the variability of species susceptibilities. A virus strain attenuated for man may still be capable of causing disease in another primate species. Any proposal to vaccinate must be preceded by safety tests on the species in question. A highly attenuated Edmonston strain measles vaccine has been used safely on rhesus monkeys, but the same vaccine in marmosets and owl monkeys (*Aotus* spp.) may cause clinical measles and death (D. M. Renquist, personal communication, 1978). For highly sensitive species, Renquist suggested that use of a phenolized vaccine followed in 2–4 weeks by a live vaccine may be a procedure worth considering.

Parainfluenza Virus

Synonyms: **None.**

The role of parainfluenza virus 3 (PI$_3$) virus as a cause of disease is not well defined. The host range of the virus is broad, including man, cattle, horses, and several species of wild animals. Infection occurs in the upper respiratory tract, but the virus may be present without observable disease, or it may occur together with other disease-producing agents, such as *Pasteurella multocida* in bovine shipping fever (Merchant and Packer 1967).

Antibodies to PI$_3$ virus have been found in deer (*Odocoileus* spp.), bighorn sheep (*Ovis canadensis*), and pronghorn antelope (*Antilocapra americana*) in North America and in a wide variety of species in Africa, most of them members of the families Bovidae and Suidae (Hamblin and Hedger 1978). The virus has been isolated from captive bighorn sheep with signs of pneumonia (Parks et al. 1972) and from captive fallow deer (*Dama dama*), captive mule deer (*Odocoileus hemionus*), and free-ranging pronghorns, in which it was not associated with disease (Thorsen et al. 1977). Based partly on what is known about PI$_3$ in humans and domestic animals, it seems safe to conclude that PI$_3$ virus is widespread in many species of wild mammals, that by itself it is not a serious pathogen, but that together with other agents (viral, bacterial, and even helminth) it may contribute to diseases of the respiratory tract.

Bovine Virus Diarrhea

Synonyms: **Mucosal disease.**

Bovine virus diarrhea (BVD) is a viral infection of cattle characterized by acute catarrhal inflammation of the mucous membranes of the gastrointestinal and upper respiratory tracts.

HISTORY AND HOSTS. Richards and coworkers (1956) described a disease of white-tailed deer and mule deer (*Odocoileus* spp.) in North Dakota. The clinical and pathologic signs of this disease resembled, in some respects, mucosal disease of cattle (Schipper et al. 1955). They reported transmission of the disease with bacteria-free blood or tissue suspensions to cattle, deer, and a pronghorn antelope (*Antilocapra americana*). Subsequently, in 1964, Kahrs and associates reported antibody to BVD in white-tailed deer in New York State, and in 1975 Barrett and Chalmers published their findings of antibody to BVD in pronghorn antelope tested in Alberta and Saskatchewan. Other cervid

species with serologic evidence of BVD infection in order of discovery include fallow deer (*Dama dama*) in Australia, moose (*Alces alces*) in Alberta (Thorsen and Henderson 1971), mule deer (*Odocoileus hemionus*) in Idaho (Stauber et al. 1977), red deer (*Cervus elaphus*) in Scotland (McMartin et al. 1977), and Chinese water deer (*C. nippon*) in Britain (Lawman et al. 1978). Romvary (cited in McMartin et al. 1977) reported isolation of BVD virus from a roe deer (*Capreolus capreolus*) in Hungary.

In Kenya, antibody to BVD virus was found in sera of eland (*Taurotragus oryx*) buffalo (*Syncerus caffer*), giraffe (*Giraffa camelopardalis*), and waterbuck (*Kobus defassa*) (Fay 1972).

Brass and his associates (1966) described a BVD-like disease in 11 wild ruminants in the Hanover zoo. The animals affected were seven gazelles (*Gazella dorcas* and *G. granti*), a muntjak (*Muntiacus muntjak*), a gaur (*Bos gauries*), and two bantengs (*B. javanicus*). Virologic studies (unspecified) were negative or inconclusive.

ETIOLOGY. The viruses of BVD and mucosal disease are undoubtedly related etiologically but may not be identical as some suggest (Merchant and Packer 1967). BVD virus is now placed in the family Togaviridae, together with hog cholera virus, with which it cross-reacts antigenically (Fenner 1976).

SIGNS AND PATHOLOGY. The disease in experimentally infected deer and in spontaneous cases was reported to be similar (Richards et al. 1956). Clinical signs included weakness, lack of fear, impaired hearing and vision, dehydration, and emaciation. One of the naturally affected deer had excessive lachrymation and corneal opacity. Feces frequently contained excessive amounts of mucus and sometimes flecks of blood.

Several of the lesions commonly seen in BVD of cattle were found on postmortem examination. These included mucosal erosions of the abomasum and intestines. Other lesions seen in the deer were catarrhal or hemorrhagic inflammation of the trachea, lungs, abomasum, and intestines; cystitis; inflammation of kidneys; and liver necrosis. Petechial or ecchymotic hemorrhages occurred in the turbinates, sinuses, pharynx, trachea, and gastrointestinal tract. Some deer had hemorrhages in the skin, the pillars of the rumen, and the epicardium.

Besides gastrointestinal lesions, some of the Hanover zoo animals had catarrhal inflammation of the mucous membranes of the eyes and nasal passages, edematous swelling of the head, excessive salivation, ulceration of the oral mucosa, and epithelial erosions between the claws and around the coronary bands of the feet.

Although the signs and lesions described by Richards et al. (1956) and by Brass and coworkers (1966) are severe, they cannot with certainty be attributed to the virus of BVD. McMartin et al. (1977) were unable to produce clinical disease in red deer experimentally infected with BVD virus, and a red deer infected spontaneously experienced only subclinical infection.

DIAGNOSIS. Diagnosis may be based on clinical signs and pathology but should be confirmed, if possible, by virus isolation. This is complicated by the fact that some isolates of BVD do not cause cytopathology in cultured cells. Bovine testicular or kidney cells can be used, and noncytopathic strains can be assayed by fluorescent antibody techniques or by virus interference methods (Merchant and Packer 1967). Similarities in clinical signs and pathologic changes require differentiation from malignant catarrhal fever, rinderpest, epizootic hemorrhagic disease, and bluetongue.

REFERENCES

Bankowski, R. A. Vesicular exanthema. *Adv. Vet. Sci.* 10:23–64, 1965.

Barsky, D., Palmer, A. E., London, W. T., and Kerber, W. T. Use of immune serum globulin (human) to reduce mortality in newly imported rhesus monkeys (*Macaca mulatta*). *J. Med. Primatol.* 5(150–159, 1976.

Baxby, D. Poxvirus hosts and reservoirs: Brief review. *Arch. Virol.* 55:169–179, 1977.

Barrett, Morley W., and Chalmers, G. A. A serologic survey of pronghorns in Alberta and Saskatchewan. *J. Wildl. Dis.* 11(2):157–163, 1975.

Blood, D. C., and Henderson, J. A. *Veterinary medicine,* 2nd ed. London: Bailliere, Tindall and Cox, 1963.

Brass, W., Schulz, L. Cl., and Ueberschar, S. Ueber das Auftreten von "Mucosal-Disease" ahnlichen Erkrankungen bein Zooweiderkauern. *Dtsch. Tieraerztl. Wochenschr.* 73:358–362, 1966.

Connell, R. Contagious ecthyma in Rocky Mountain bighorn sheep. *Can. J. Comp. Med.* 18:59, 1954.

Daniel, M. J., and Christie, A. H. C. Untersuchungen ueber Krankheiten der Gemse (*Rupicapra rupicapra*) und des Thars (*Hemitragus jemlaicus*) in der Sudalpen von Neuseeland. *Schweiz. Arch. Tierheilk.* 105(7):399–411, 1963.

Fay, D. Report to the Government of Kenya on Wildlife Disease Research. TA3049. Rome: Food and Agriculture Organization, 1972.

Fenner, F. Classification and nomenclature of viruses: Viruses of vertebrates. *Intervirology* 7(1–2):48–64, 1976.

Gehring, H., Mahnel, H., and Mayer, H. Elefantenpocken. *Zentralbl. Veterinaermed. [B]* 19: 258–261, 1972.

Gehring, H., and Mayer, H. Beitrag zur Diagnostik und Bekampfung der Pockeninfection bein Elefanten. *Prakt. Tieraerztl.* 2:106, 1978.

Grunberg, W., and Burtscher, H. Uber eine pockenartige Erkrankung beim Rhinoceros (*Diceros bicornis*). *Zentralbl. Vet. Med.* 15:649–657, 1968.

Hamblin, C., and Hedger, R. S. Neutralizing antibodies to parainfluenza 3 virus in African wildlife, with special reference to the Cape buffalo (*Syncerus caffer*). *J. Wildl. Dis.* 14:378–388, 1978.

Hanson, R. P. The natural history of hog cholera. *J. Am. Vet. Med. Assoc.* 131:211, 1957.

Hebert, D. M., Samuel, W. M., and Smith, G. W. Contagious ecthyma in mountain goats of coastal British Columbia. *J. Wildl. Dis.* 13(2):399–411, 1977.

Hime, J. M., and Keymer, I. F. Measles in recently imported colobus monkeys (*Colobus guereza*). *Vet. Rec.* 97:392, 1975.

Kahrs, R., Atkinson, G., Baker, J. A., Carmichael, L., Coggins, L., Gillespie, J., Langer, P., Marshall, V., Robson, D., and Sheffy, B. Serological studies on the incidence of bovine virus diarrhea, infectious bovine rhinotracheitis, bovine myxovirus parainfluenza 3 and *Leptospira pomona* in New York State. *Cornell Vet.* 54:360–369, 1971.

Kummeneje, K., and Krogsrud, J. Contagious ecthyma (orf) in the musk ox (*Ovibos moschatus*). *Acta Vet. Scand.* 19:461, 1978.

Lawman, M. J. P., Evans, D., Gibbs, E. P. J., McDiarmid, A., and Rowe, L. A preliminary survey of British deer for antibody to some virus diseases of farm animals. *Br. Vet. J.* 134:85–91, 1978.

Leman, A. D., Glock, R. D., Mengeling, W. L., Penny, R. M. C., Scholl, E., and Straw, B. eds. *Diseases of Swine.* Ames: Iowa State University Press, 1981.

Levy, B. M., and Mirkovic, R. M. An epizootic of measles in a marmoset colony. *Lab. Anim. Sci.* 21:33–39, 1971.

McMartin, D. A., Snodgrass, D. R., and Corrigall, W. Bovine virus diarrhoea antibody in a Scottish red deer. *Vet. Rec.* 100:187, 1977.

Marennikova, S. S., Maltseva, N. N., Korneeva, V. I., and Garanina, N. M. Outbreak of pox disease among carnivora (Felidae) and Edentata. *J. Infect. Dis.* 135(3):358–366, 1977.

Merchant, I. A., and Packer, R. A. *Veterinary Bacteriology and Virology.* Ames: Iowa State University Press, 1967.

Parks, J. B., Post, G., Thorne, T., and Nash, P. Parainfluenza 3 virus infection in Rocky Mountain bighorn sheep. *J. Am. Vet. Med. Assoc.* 161:669–672, 1972.

Potkay, A., Ganaway, J. R., Rogers, N. F., and Kinard, R. An epizootic of measles in a colony of rhesus monkeys (*Macaca mulatta*). *Am. J. Vet. Res.* 27:331, 1973.

Prato, C. M., Akers, T. G. and Smith, A. W. Calicivirus antibodies in wild fox populations. *J. Wildl. Dis.* 13:448–450, 1977.

Renne, R. A., McLaughlin, R., and Jenson, A. B. Measles virus: Associated endometritis, cervicitis, and abortion in a rhesus monkey. *J. Am. Vet. Med. Assoc.* 163:639–641, 1973.

Richards, S. H., Schipper, I. A., Eveleth, D. F., and Shumard, R. E. Mucosal disease of deer. *Vet. Med.* 51:358–362, 1956.

Samuel, W. M., Chalmers, G. A., Stelfox, J. G., Loewen, A., and Thomsen, J. J. Contagious ecthyma in bighorn sheep and mountain goat in western Canada. *J. Wildl. Dis.* 11(1):26, 1975.

Sawyer, J. C., Madin, S. H., Stewart, H., and Skilling, D. E. Isolation of San Miguel sea lion virus from samples of an animal food product produced from northern fur seal (*Callorhinus ursinus*). *Am. J. Vet. Res.* 39:137–139, 1978.

Schipper, I. A., Eveleth, D. F., Shumard, R. F., and Richards, S. H. Mucosal disease of cattle. *Vet. Med.* 50:431–434, 1955.

Scott, G. B. N., and Keymer, I. F. The pathology of measles in Abyssinian colobus monkeys (*Colobus guereza*): A description of an outbreak. *J. Pathol.* 117:229–233, 1975.

Smith, A. W., Akers, T. G., Madin, S. H., and Vedros, N. A. San Miguel sea lion virus isolation, preliminary characterization and relationship to vesicular exanthema of swine virus. *Nature* 244:108–110, 1973.

Smith, A. W., and Latham, A. B., Prevalence of vesicular exanthema of swine antibodies among feral mammals associated with the southern California coastal zones. *Am. J. Vet. Res.* 39:291–296, 1978.

Smith, A. W., Prato, C. and Skilling, D. E. Caliciviruses infecting monkeys and possibly man. *Am. J. Vet. Res.* 39:287–289, 1978.

Stauber, E. H., Nellis, C. H., Magonigle, R. A., and Vaughn, H. W. Prevalence of reactors to selected livestock pathogens in Idaho mule deer. *J. Wildl. Manage.* 41:515–519, 1977.

Thorsen, J., and Henderson, J. P. Survey for antibody to infectious bovine rhinotracheitis (IBR), bovine virus diarrhea (BVD), and parainfluenza 3 (PI₃) in moose sera. *J. Wildl. Dis.* 7:93–95, 1971.

Thorsen, J., Karstad, L., Barrett, M. W., and Chalmers, G. A. Viruses isolated from captive and free-ranging wild ruminants in Alberta. *J. Wildl. Dis.* 13:74–79, 1977.

Wetzel, R., and Rieck, W. *Krankheiten des Wildes.* Hamburg: Verlag Paul Parey, 1962.

Wilson, T. M., Cheville, N. F., and Karstad, L. Sealpox. *Bull. Wildl. Dis. Assoc.* 5:412–418, 1969.

Wilson, T. M., Dykes, R. W., and Tsai, K. S. Pox in young captive harbor seals. *J. Am. Vet. Med. Assoc.* 161(6):611–617, 1972.

Wilson, T. M., and Paglayen-Neuwall, J. Pox in South American sea lions, *Otaria byronia. Can. J. Comp. Med.* 35:174–177, 1971.

Wilson, T. M., and Sweeney, P. R. Morphological studies of seal poxvirus. *J. Wildl. Dis.* 6:94–97, 1970.

Zwart, P., Gispen, R., and Peters, J. C. Cowpox in okapis (*Okapia johnstoni*) at Rotterdam zoo. *Br. Vet. J.* 127:20–24, 1971.

2 Bacterial, Rickettsial, and Mycotic Diseases

18 Tularemia

J. FREDERICK BELL   J. R. REILLY

Synonyms: **Plaguelike disease of rodents, plaguelike lymphadenitis, conjunctivitis tularensis, Francis's disease, deerfly fever, rabbit fever, rabbit disease, cattle-fly fever, Pahvant Valley fever or plague, glandular type tick fever, yato-byo (yato = wild rabbit, byo = disease), Ohara's disease, la Tularemie, and die Tularemie.**

The zoonosis tularemia is primarily a plaguelike disease of wild lagomorphs and rodents, but the host range includes a wide variety of animals. It is an acute, febrile infection caused by the bacterium *Francisella tularensis*. The organism can be transmitted by a variety of ectoparasites, by direct contact with infected animals, and by contact with environmental contamination. It is a three- or four-factor complex, either vertebrate-host-agent-vertebrate-host or vertebrate-host-agent-vector-vertebrate-host. The organism is one of few bacteria capable of reproducing and adapting to the internal environment of arthropods; as a result the arthropods may be considered true biological transmitters (Gelman 1961).

HISTORY. Adaptation of *F. tularensis* to the ectoparasites of lagomorphs and rodents suggests that it is of considerable antiquity and probably has long been enzootic in the New and Old Worlds. Analysis of this adaptation, of the geographic distribution of the organism, and of its transmission in natural nidi indicates that it originated in the Northern Hemisphere at the end of the Miocene or early Pliocene (Olsuf'ev 1965). Additional evidence supporting this postulation may be obtained by review of historical medical descriptions (Barnes 1928; Gelman 1961; Horne 1912; Ohara 1954; Simpson 1929; Sylvest 1936; Thjoetta 1931). These present evidence that tularemia in man may have occurred in the nineteenth century in the United States, Norway, Russia, and Japan before the isolation of the causative organism from California ground squirrels (*Citellus beecheyi*) (McCoy and Chapin 1912).

McCoy (1911) reported a new plaguelike disease in 46 naturally infected California ground squirrels taken in nine counties of California. Subsequently, McCoy and Chapin (1912) were successful in isolating the causative organism, which they named *Bacterium tularense* after Tulare County, California. At the same time they experimentally infected a variety of animals and called attention to the fact that the squirrel flea (*Ceratophyllus acutus*; now *Diamanus montanus*) might be involved in the transmission of disease.

Wherry and Lamb (1914a) first demonstrated presence of the disease in cottontail rabbits (*Sylvilagus floridanus*) found dead in an epizootic in southern Indiana and isolated *B. tularense* from a man thought to have glanders (Wherry and Lamb 1914b). This case, the first diagnosed bacteriologically, was described by Vail (1914). In response to growing evidence that rabbit fever was an occupational disease of market workers who had skinned and dressed cottontail rabbits, Francis (1923a) examined the livers, spleens, and lymph nodes from 914 cottontail rabbits offered for sale in Washington, D.C., markets and demonstrated tularemia.

In 1911, Pearse described six cases of deerfly fever in man and postulated that the infection was due to the bite of the deerfly (*Chrysops discalis*). These constitute the first published human cases to be differentiated clinically. Eight years later Francis (1919) established the etiologic unity of deerfly fever and the plaguelike disease of rodents and established the term tularemia because of the septicemia produced. Subsequently, Francis and Mayne (1921) presented experimental proof that the deerfly could transmit tularemia from rabbit to rabbit and would remain infective for at least 24 days. Wayson (1914) and Francis and Lake (1921, 1922a,b) experimentally transmitted tularemia by other arthropods, including the stable fly (*Stomoxys calcitrans*), the rabbit louse (*Haemodipsus ventricosus*), the bedbug (*Cimex lectularius*), and the mouse louse (*Polyplax serratus*).

Parker et al. (1924) demonstrated transstadial transmission of *F. tularensis* in wood ticks (*Dermacentor andersoni*) and stated that this arthropod was a host and vector of the disease. Transmission to mammals was effected by employing infected wood ticks and rabbit ticks (*Haemaphysalis leporispalustris*). Subsequently, Parker and Spencer (1926) recorded transovarial transmission of the organism in wood ticks and stated that ticks provide a permanent reservoir of the agent. They postulated that this was also true for dog ticks (*D. variabilis*), and rabbit ticks. However, Bell (1945) maintained that transovarial transmission in these species was exceptional. Calhoun and Alford (1955) found the bacterium in unfed larvae of *Amblyomma americanum*.

Infected ticks sometimes suffer greater mortality than uninfected cohorts when kept in the laboratory (Bell and Owen 1953) and there is evidence that a bactericidal principle is present in ticks (Anigstein et al. 1955; Bell 1945; Hopla 1955). Both of these phenomena would act to limit infection in nature.

Japanese workers (Aoki et al. 1925; Ohara 1925, 1926) reported yato-byo, an acute, febrile "new disease in man related to hares," which resulted from contact with wild hares of two subspecies—Japanese hares (*Lepus timidus brachyurus*) and Etigo hares (*L. t. augustidens*). The disease was later identified as tularemia (Francis and Moore 1926).

Parker and Spencer (1925–1926) produced tularemia experimentally in the blue grouse (*Dendragapus obscurus*), demonstrating for the first time that birds were susceptible. Subsequently, a number of birds were experimentally infected or were incriminated as a potential source of infection in man. Green (1943) noted that virulence of *F. tularensis* isolated from grouse (*Bonasa* spp.) was less than that of isolates from hares (*Lepus* spp.) in the same ecosystem, although both hosts were heavily parasitized by *H. leporispalustris*.

A comprehensive review of the history of tularemia in North America can be found in a recent book by Jellison (1974).

DISTRIBUTION. Since its identification in 1911 tularemia has been reported from all the continental United States as well as Alaska, Canada, and Mexico. The disease has also been reported from Japan; Russia; Turkey; Israel; Scandinavia, including Norway, Sweden, and Finland; central Europe, including Austria, Czechoslovakia, and Poland; western Europe, including Belgium, France, Germany, and Italy; and Tunisia (Foshay 1950; Gelman 1961; Shaughnessy 1963). It has not been detected in Australia, the British Isles, or the Iberian Peninsula. In retrospect, a review of medical descriptions would indicate that the disease was probably present in Norway, France, Russia, and Japan during the nineteenth century. (See Tables 18.1, 18.2.)

ETIOLOGY. The causative organism of tularemia has been assigned to several different bacterial genera. Breed et al. (1957) named it *Pasteurella tularensis*, but the systematic assignment to the genus *Pasteurella* is obscure and has often been criticized. Olsuf'ev et al. (1959) reviewed the generic assignment of this organism and indicated that the first available restrictive generic name should be *Francisella* Dorofeev 1947; therefore, they proposed to place the organism between *Brucella* and *Pasteurella* in the family Brucellaceae. Philip and Owen (1961), demonstrating that the organism is not congeneric with other species now assigned to *Pasteurella*, confirmed the designation as the type species of the genus *Francisella* Dorofeev 1947 and assigned the species name *Francisella tularensis* (McCoy and Chapin 1912). The revision has been adopted in the 8th edition of *Bergey's Manual* (Owen 1974). However, the distinguishing criterion of the genus (requirement for cystine to support growth) does not apply to the species *Francisella novicida*. It seems probable that ultimate classification will be based on physicochemical characteristics, that is, on DNA relationships.

Francisella tularensis is a nonspore-forming, gram-negative, aerobic organism. It has an obligate requirement for cystine and grows well on blood glucose cystine agar (Francis 1923b) and on tryptose, thiamine, cysteine, sodium glycolate, and glucose plus 5% defibrinated rabbit blood agar (Gaspar et al. 1961). It is pleomorphic: large or small, coccoid, bacillary, or oval, filamented, bean-shaped, dumbbell-shaped, or bizarre; "involution" forms have been described (Hesselbrock and Foshay 1945). A capsule is demonstrable under certain conditions; it is lost when the organisms are suspended in physiological salt solution (Hood 1977).

TRANSMISSION. Transmission of tularemia is accomplished directly by bloodsucking arthropods, mechanically by means of contaminated mouth parts, or by contamination of the host's skin with arthropod discharges. A variety of bloodsucking arthropods are involved, especially mites, ticks, flies, midges, fleas, mosquitoes, and lice. It is probable that transmission by infected ticks to vertebrate hosts occurs by infectious coxal fluid and feces (Burgdorfer and Owen 1956), as well as by direct inoculation of organisms in saliva of the tick (Hopla 1974). Ingestion of infected ectoparasites during

TABLE 18.1 Wild Mammals Susceptible to and Carriers of *Francisella tularensis*.

Scientific Name	Common Name	Method of Determination	Locale	Reference
ARTIODACTYLA				
Cervidae				
Odocoileus hemionus	mule deer	agglutination	Utah	Thorpe et al. 1965; Vest et al. 1965
		agglutination	Idaho	Shaw 1964
O. virginianus	white-tailed deer	agglutination	Texas	Thorpe et al. 1965
Suidae				
Sus scrofa	European wild boar	contact	France	Mercier 1947
CARNIVORA				
Canidae				
Canis latrans	coyote	experimental infection	...	Parker 1926; Green 1933; Francis 1937; Stagg et al. 1956
		isolation	Utah	Lundgren et al. 1957
		contact	Wisconsin	Guilford 1947
C. l. lestes	coyote	agglutination	Utah	Thorpe et al. 1965; Vest et al. 1965
Vulpes (fulva) vulpes	red fox	contact	New Mexico	Kunkel 1930
		experimental infection	...	Lillie and Francis 1936
V. macrotis	kit fox	isolation	Florida, Georgia	McKeever et al. 1958
		agglutination	Utah	Thorpe et al. 1965
Urocyon cinereoargenteus	gray fox	isolation	Minnesota	Green and Shillinger 1934; Schlotthauer et al. 1934; Schlotthauer et al. 1935
		isolation	Florida, Georgia	McKeever et al. 1958
Felidae				
Lynx rufus	bobcat	agglutination	Florida, Georgia	McKeever et al. 1958
		agglutination	Utah	Thorpe et al. 1965
		agglutination	Florida, Georgia	McKeever et al. 1958
Mustelidae				
Mustela vison	mink	contact	Louisiana	Pullen and Stuart 1945
		contact	Wisconsin	Guilford 1947
		isolation	unknown	Gorham 1949, 1950
		isolation	Wyoming	Nakamura 1950a
M. erminea	ermine	experimental infection	...	Olsuf'ev and Dunaeva 1951
Taxidea taxus taxus	badger	isolation	Wyoming	Nakamura 1950a
		agglutination	Utah	Vest et al. 1965; Thorpe et al. 1965
Spilogale putorius	spotted skunk	agglutination	Florida, Georgia	McKeever et al. 1958

TABLE 18.1 (continued)

Scientific Name	Common Name	Method of Determination	Locale	Reference
Mephitis mephitis	striped skunk	unknown agglutination	unknown Florida, Georgia	Francis 1937 McKeever et al. 1958
Procyonidae *Procyon lotor*	raccoon	unknown agglutination contact	Minnesota Arkansas Louisiana	Green 1933 Calhoun et al. 1956 Pullen and Stuart 1945
HYSTRICOMORPHA *Erethizon dorsatum* *Cavia porcella*	porcupine guinea pig	isolation, contact experimental infection	Wyoming ...	Nakamura 1950b; Kihns et al. 1953 Davis 1935; Lillie and Francis 1936; Lillie and Larson 1945; McCoy 1911; McCoy and Chapin 1912; Olin 1934
ISECTIVORA *Erinaceus europaeus* *Sorex vagrans monticola* not given *Neomys anomalus*	hedgehog wandering shrew mole water shrew	not determined experimental infection isolation contact isolation	Sweden ... Montana USSR Bulgaria	Malmgren 1935 Kamil and Bilal 1938 Kohls and Steinhaus 1943 Miasnikov 1956 Kupenov et al. 1964
LAGOMORPHA *Lepus timidus*	Blue Mountain or varying hare	contact isolation	Sweden Sweden	Thjøetta 1930, 1931 Olin 1934, 1938
L. t. branchyurus	Japanese hare	contact	Japan	Aoki et al. 1925; Ohara 1925a,b, 1926a,b
L. t. augustidens *L. europaeus*	Etigo hare European hare	agglutination, contact isolation isolation contact isolation contact isolation contact isolation isolation isolation isolation	Japan Austria Czechoslovakia France France Belgium Germany, Poland Germany Germany Holland Switzerland Minnesota	Francis and Moore 1926 Tomanek 1937; David 1937 Tomanek 1937; Franek and Wolfov'a 1965; Drbohlav 1937 Girard 1947 Paille 1947; Basset 1949 Nelis et al. 1950 Schoop 1942 Mochmann 1955 Schmidt 1951 Hemmes 1953 Bouvier et al. 1951 Green and Shillinger 1934, 1935; Bell
L. americanus	snowshoe or			

TABLE 18.1 (continued)

Scientific Name	Common Name	Method of Determination	Locale	Reference
L. a. columbiensis	varying hare	isolation	British Columbia	Parker et al. 1931
L. californicus	black-tailed jackrabbit	agglutination	Utah	Parker and Smith 1955
		isolation	Utah	Stoenner et al. 1959
		agglutination, isolation, Utah		Vest et al. 1965; Thorpe et al. 1965
		induced agglutination		
		isolation	Washington	Bacon and Drake 1958; Bacon et al. 1958
L. townsendii	white-tailed jackrabbit	isolation	Montana	Philip et al. 1935
		isolation	Alberta	Gwatkin et al. 1942; Bow and Brown 1943
L. californicus and/or L. townsendii	black-tailed and/or white-tailed jackrabbit	isolation	unknown	Francis 1921
Sylvilagus floridanus	cottontail rabbit	isolation	Indiana	Wherry and Lamb 1914b
		isolation	Minnesota	Green and Shillinger 1932, 1934; Green et al. 1938
		isolation	Virginia	McGinnes 1957
		isolation	Georgia	McKeever et al. 1958
		isolation	South Carolina	McCahan et al. 1962
S. f. mallurus	eastern cottontail	isolation	Virginia	McGuinnes 1964
S. auduboni	desert cottontail	natural infection	New Mexico	Ecke and Holdenried 1952
		isolation, agglutination, induced agglutination	Utah	Thorpe et al. 1965; Vest et al. 1965
S. bachmani	brush cottontail	contact	California	Simons et al. 1953
S. idahoensis	pigmy cottontail	serology	Washington	Bacon and Drake 1958
Oryctolagus cuniculus	European rabbit	isolation	Austria	David 1937
		isolation	Tunisia	Anderson 1938
MARSUPIALIA				
Didelphis (Virginiana) marsupialis	opossum	contact	Florida	Mease 1929
		contact	unknown	Francis 1934, 1937
		contact	Louisiana	Pullen and Stuart 1945
		contact	Missouri	Ossman and Bohrer 1947
		agglutination	Arkansas	Calhoun et al. 1956
		agglutination	Florida, Georgia	McKeever et al. 1958
PRIMATE				
Macaca mulatta	rhesus monkey	experimental infection	...	Coriell et al. 1948; Downs et al. 1947; McCoy 1911; McCoy and Chapin 1912

TABLE 18.1 (continued)

Scientific Name	Common Name	Method of Determination	Locale	Reference
RODENTIA				
Castoridae				
Castor canadensis	beaver	experimental infection	...	Parker 1933; Green 1937
		isolation	Wyoming	Scott 1940
		isolation	Montana	Hammersland and Joneschild 1940
		isolation	Montana, Wyoming	Jellison et al. 1942
		isolation	Montana	Fenstermacher et al. 1949; Parker et al. 1951
		isolation	Ontario	Labzoffsky and Sprent 1952
		isolation	Alberta	Banfield 1954
		isolation	Oregon	Bell et al. 1962
		isolation	Utah	Thorpe et al. 1965
Cricetidae				
Cricetus cricetus frumentarius	field hamster	isolation	USSR	Sarchi 1930
C. auratus	golden hamster	pathology	USSR	Schuller and Erdmann 1943
Reithrodontomys megalotis	western harvest mouse	experimental infection	...	Larson 1945b
		agglutination, induced agglutination	Utah	Vest et al. 1965; Thorpe et al. 1965
Peromyscus maniculatus	deer mouse	agglutination	Utah	Vest et al. 1965
		experimental infection	...	Vest and Marchette 1958
Peromyscus sp.		isolation	California	Stagg et al. 1956; Simons et al. 1953
P. m. (nebrascensis)	Osgood white-footed mouse	isolation	Canada	Ozburn 1944
P. m. artemisiae	white-footed mouse	isolation	Wyoming	Nakamura 1950a
P. m. ribidus	redwood's white-footed mouse	isolation	California	Burroughs et al. 1945
P. m. sonoriensis	sonoran white-footed mouse	experimental infection	...	Stagg et al. 1956
P. crinitus	canyon mouse	experimental infection	...	Vest and Marchette 1958
P. truei	pinyon mouse	experimental infection	...	Vest and Marchette 1958
		agglutination, induced agglutination	Utah	Vest et al. 1965
Neotoma albigula	white-throated wood rat	isolation	Utah	Thorpe et al. 1965
			New Mexico	Ecke and Holdenried 1952
N. fuscipes	dusky-footed wood rat	isolation	California	Burroughs et al. 1945
N. lepida lepida	desert wood rat	experimental infection	...	Stagg et al. 1956; Vest and Marchette 1958

TABLE 18.1 (continued)

Scientific Name	Common Name	Method of Determination	Locale	Reference
Microtus arvalis	continental vole	isolation	Turkey	Oez 1938
		isolation	Belgium	Nelis et al. 1950
		contact	Denmark	Knothe and Zimmermann 1952
		pathology	USSR	Schuller and Erdmann 1943
Microtus sp.				
M. pennsylvanicus	meadow vole	isolation	Montana	Parker et al. 1951
M. p. modestus	Sawatch meadow vole	isolation	Montana	Jellison et al. 1942
M. p. drummondi	Drummond's meadow vole	isolation	Montana	Kohls and Steinhaus 1943
		isolation	Canada	Ozburn 1944
M. californicus	California vole	isolation	California	Burroughs et al. 1945
M. c. aestaurarinus	Tule meadow vole	isolation	California	Perry 1928; Parker 1929
M. montanus	Montana vole	isolation	California, Oregon	Jellison et al. 1958
M. m. montanus	Montana vole	isolation	Oregon, California	Jellison et al. 1959
Arvicola (amphibius) terrestris	water vole	contact, serology, isolation	USSR	Nikanorov 1928; Suvorova et al. 1928; Golov et al. 1928
		pathology	USSR	Schuller and Erdmann 1943
		isolation	USSR	Sarchi 1930
Lagurus lagurus	steppe lemming	isolation	USSR	Kazanzeva and Gorohov 1934
Lemmus lemmus	lemming	isolation	Sweden	Olin 1938
Ondatra zibethicus	muskrat	experimental infection	....	Green et al. 1929
		isolation	Iowa	Green and Shillinger 1933
		isolation	Wyoming, Montana	Jellison et al. 1942
		isolation	Montana	Parker et al. 1943
		isolation	Wisconsin	McDermid 1946
		isolation	Utah	Jellison et al. 1951
		isolation	Alberta	Banfield 1954; Langford 1954
		isolation	Ontario	Labzoffsky and Sprent 1952; Fyvie et al. 1959; Ditchfield et al. 1960
		isolation	Bulgaria	Kupenov et al. 1964
		undetermined	Siberia	Egorova et al. 1964
		contact	Montana	Schwartz 1929
		contact	Ontario	Johns 1933
		contact	Alaska	Williams 1946
		contact	New York	Tartakow 1946; Levy 1952
		contact	Wisconsin	Morgan 1949
		contact	Idaho, Oregon	Parker et al. 1951

TABLE 18.1 *(continued)*

Scientific Name	Common Name	Method of Determination	Locale	Reference
Heteromyidae				
Allactaga sp.	jerboa	experimental infection	...	Kamil and Bilal 1938
Perognathus parvus	Great Basin pocket mouse	isolation, experimental infection	Utah	Thorpe et al. 1965 Vest and Marchette 1958
P. formosus	long-tailed pocket mouse	induced agglutination	Utah	Vest et al. 1965
P. f. incolatus	long-tailed pocket mouse	experimental infection	...	Vest and Marchette 1958
Dipodomys ordii	Ord's kangaroo rat	induced agglutination, isolation	Utah	Vest et al. 1965
		agglutination, isolation, induced agglutination	Utah	Thorpe et al. 1965
D. o. pallidus	Ord's kangaroo rat	experimental infection	...	Vest and Marchette 1958; Stagg et al. 1956
D. microps	chisel-toothed kangaroo rat	agglutination, induced agglutination	Utah	Vest et al. 1965
D. m. bonnevillei	chisel-toothed kangaroo rat	agglutination	Utah	Thorpe et al. 1965
		experimental infection	...	Vest and Marchette 1958
Muridae				
Micromys minutus	harvest mouse	isolation	Turkey	Oez 1938
Rattus norvegicus	Norway rat	experimental infection	...	McCoy and Chapin 1912
		isolation	California	Dieter and Rhodes 1926; Burroughs et al. 1945; Simons et al. 1953
Mus musculus	house mouse	isolation	Turkey	Oez 1938
		pathology	USSR	Schuller and Erdmann 1943
Apodemus agrarius	striped field mouse	contact	USSR	Khatenever 1943
A. sylvaticus	common field mouse	isolation	Belgium	Nelis et al. 1950
Sciuromorpha				
Tamias striatus	eastern chipmunk	isolation	Minnesota	Green 1933
Eutamias sp., probably *minimus*	eastern chipmunk	isolation	Wyoming	Nakamura 1950a; Parker 1945
E. mimus	little chipmunk	experimental infection	...	Vest and Marchette 1958
		agglutination	Utah	Thorpe et al. 1965; Vest et al. 1965
E. dorsalis	cliff chipmunk	agglutination	Utah	Vest et al. 1965; Thorpe et al. 1965
Marmota monax	woodchuck	experimental infection	...	Simpson 1929; Green 1933

TABLE 18.1. (continued)

Scientific Name	Common Name	Method of Determination	Locale	Reference
M. flaviventris	yellow-bellied marmot	experimental infection	...	Lillie and Francis 1936
		serology	Oregon, California	Menges and Galton 1959
Citellus leucurus	antelope ground squirrel	experimental infection	...	Stagg et al. 1956; Vest and Marchette 1958
C. townsendii	Townsend's ground squirrel	isolation	Utah	Vest et al. 1965
		agglutination	Utah	Thorpe et al. 1965
		isolation	Utah	Vest and Marchette 1958
C. t. mollis	Piute ground squirrel	contact	California	Simons et al. 1953
C. richardsonii	Richardson's ground squirrel	culture	unknown	Francis 1919, 1921
		culture	Canada	Ozburn 1944; Brown and Roy 1943; Bow and Brown 1946
C. r. elegans	Wyoming ground squirrel	culture	Montana	Burroughs et al. 1945
C. columbianus columbianus	Columbian ground squirrel	culture	Montana	Burroughs et al. 1945
C. armatus	Uinta ground squirrel	culture	Wyoming	Nakamura 1950a
C. beecheyi	California ground squirrel	isolation	California	McCoy 1911; McCoy and Chapin 1912; Simons et al. 1953
C. v. douglasii	California ground squirrel	isolation	California	Simons et al. 1953
C. b. fisheri	California ground squirrel	isolation	California	Simons et al. 1953
C. pygmaeus	small suslik	isolation	USSR	Kazanzeva and Gorohov 1934
Cynomys leucurus	white-tailed prairie dog	experimental infection	...	Davis 1935
Sciurus carolinensis	gray squirrel	contact	Minnesota	Green 1933
		contact	unknown	Francis 1934
		contact	Ohio	Oosting 1939
S. vulgaris	European red squirrel	contact	Sweden	Olin 1934
S. niger	fox squirrel	contact	Illinois	Kirkwood 1931
		contact	unknown	Francis 1934, 1937
		agglutination	Wisconsin	Morgan 1949
		agglutination	Georgia, Florida	McKeever et al. 1958
Tamiasciurus hudsonicus	red squirrel	contact	unknown	Francis 1934
T. h. ventorum	Wind River pine squirrel	isolation	Wyoming	Nakamura 1950a
Zapoidae				
Zuapus princeps	western jumping mouse	isolation	Wyoming	Nakamura 1950b

TABLE 18.2. Domestic Mammals Susceptible to and Carriers of *Francisella tularensis*.

Scientific Name	Common Name	Method of Determination	Locale	Reference
ARTIODACTYLA				
Capridae				
Ovis aries	domestic sheep	agglutination	Montana	Parker and Dade 1929a,b
		isolation	Idaho, Montana	Parker and Butler 1929
		agglutination, pathology	Montana	Philip et al. 1935
		agglutination, isolation	Canada	Gwatkin et al. 1942
		agglutination, isolation	Idaho	McArthur and Brown 1950; Jellison and Kohls 1950, 1955
		isolation	Wyoming	Ryff et al. 1961
CARNIVORA				
Canidae				
Canis familiaris	dog	contact	United States	Francis 1937
		natural infection	Iowa	Waller 1940
		contact	Austria	Khatenever 1943
		contact	Arkansas	Calhoun 1954
		serology	Arkansas	Calhoun et al. 1956
		natural infection	Alabama	Johnson 1944
		agglutination	Ohio	Ey and Daniels 1941
Felidae				
Felis domesticus	cat	isolation	Minnesota	Green and Wade 1928
		undetermined	United States	Francis 1937
		contact	Indiana	Rudesill 1937
		contact	Connecticut	Jungherr 1942
		contact	Louisiana	Pullen and Stuart 1945
		contact	United States	Miller and Montgomery 1957
		agglutination	Minnesota	Hanson and Green 1929
			Georgia, Florida	McKeever et al. 1958
PERISSODACTYLA				
Equidae				
Equus caballus	domestic horse	isolation, agglutination	Montana	Claus et al. 1959

grooming is another possible source of mammalian infection (Bell 1965; Hopla 1974). The organism may also be transmitted by contact with infected vertebrates (Francis 1937); aerogenically by inhalation of feces-contaminated dust (Burroughs et al. 1945; Maisky 1945); and by ingestion of infected carcasses (Gorham 1949, 1950), insufficiently cooked infected meat (Amoss and Sprunt 1936; Francis 1937), or contaminated water (Jellison et al. 1942, 1950; Maisky 1945; Parker et al. 1951; Schmidt 1948).

In the United States, lagomorphs are the source of infection in 90% of human cases, 70% of which result from contacts with the genus *Sylvilagus* (Jellison and Parker 1945). Jackrabbits (*Lepus* spp.) are important locally (Lane and Emmons 1978) but overall are a minor factor. Infected jackrabbits have been identified as a source of infection in ranch-raised mink (*Mustela vison*) (Gorham 1949, 1950). Snowshoe hares (*L. americanus*) comprise less than 1% of the total as a source of human infection.

Jellison et al. (1961) proposed the hypothesis that two kinds of tularemia can be distinguished by their epidemiologic pattern and the virulence of isolates. The first, type A (*F. tularensis tularensis*), is tickborne tularemia of lagomorphs, is limited to the New World, and is the source of 90% of human infections. This type may also be transmitted by other arthropods to other animals. The second, type B (*F. tularensis palaearctica*), of holarctic distribution, commonly affects rodents and is transmitted among them primarily by contamination of water and by carnivorism, including cannibalism. It is the source of 5–10% of human infections in North America. In spite of the fact that pneumonia with infectious sputum is a common complication of tularemia, the disease is not contagious in man.

SIGNS. In animals clinical manifestations of tularemia are not always evident or clearly recognized. Furthermore, the opportunities to observe these signs in natural outbreaks among wild animal populations are extremely limited and when infected animals are found, they are usually moribund or dead. This may account for the paucity of information in the literature concerning signs of tularemia in wildlife species.

Tularemic hares and cottontails have been observed to behave oddly, to run slowly, and to be captured easily (David 1937). Green (1942) reported that infected rabbits appear to be tame or in a stupor. Infected rabbits do not raise their heads or carry their front feet well; they rub their noses and forefeet into the ground. They have recurrent tonic spasms and stagger a few rods between spasms (Hendrickson 1937). Clinical signs in experimentally infected red foxes (*Vulpes [fulva] vulpes*) were anorexia, diarrhea, and noisy, labored breathing (Lillie and Francis 1936). According to Gorham (1949) infected mink and foxes exhibit anorexia and lassitude.

PATHOGENESIS. Tularemia is an acute infectious disease. The causative organism gains entrance to the bloodstream in a variety of ways, most commonly through the bite of an arthropod vector, or accidentally, through contact with an infected animal carcass. Other routes of infection include ingestion of contaminated flesh of a vertebrate or contaminated water, contact with discharges of arthropods, the inhalation of aerosols of fecal droplets of arthropods (Meyer 1965), or the inhalation of threshing dust contaminated with mouse and vole feces (Apekhtin 1945; Maisky 1945). Lake and Francis (1922) presented evidence that the organism may pass through the intact skin, although infection by this route may be facilitated by the presence of abrasions and lacerations. Experimental evidence of penetration of unbroken skin was presented by Quan et al. (1955), who successfully infected 12 of 21 white mice by applying 7 dex organisms to the abdominal skin.

After gaining entrance to the body or bloodstream, the bacterium multiplies and invades the vascular endothelium, spreading along the superficial and deep lymphatics. Typically, lymphadenitis occurs, and there are scattered foci of necrosis in the spleen, liver, lungs, lymph nodes, and bone marrow (Meyer 1965). The organism may invade the alveolar epithelium, hepatic cells, and reticuloendothelial cells of the spleen and lymph nodes. Bacteria, together with cell debris from the endothelium of capillaries, enhance the development of thrombi which in turn give rise to small necrotic foci in the spleen, liver, and associated lymph nodes (Runnells 1954).

Schricker (1964) reported that in experimental acute tularemia in laboratory rabbits, organisms became established at the site of injection during the first 8 hours. These spread to regional lymph nodes and multiplied rapidly from 8 to 30 hours postinoculation. Clinical disease coincided with generalization of the process. Septicemia was associated with impairment of organ function and progressive pathologic changes. Death occurred 103–145 hours postinoculation. Voles (*Microtus* spp.), which develop acute fatal infection when inoculated parenterally with one organism of type B, can develop chronic nephritis with bacteriuria when large doses of the bacteria are ingested in drinking water (Saito et al. 1978).

PATHOLOGY. In general the gross and histopathologic lesions of tularemia in mammals resemble those of bubonic plague or pseudotuberculosis in rodents. Typical gross lesions are tubercle-like nodules scattered throughout the liver, spleen, and lymph nodes, varying from pinpoint size to large irregular conglomerate foci several millimeters in diameter. The spleen and liver may be dark bluish red and enlarged. There may be small necrotic foci or white plaques on the lungs. Small white nodules may be found in pink solid or red gelatinous bone narrow. These may be so small as to be overlooked readily, and a hand lens or microscope may be required to detect them. The skin of infected animals often has vascular congestion and a plastic consistency.

Histologically, this condition is one of caseous necrosis of focal or diffuse type with intense destruction of cells. Thrombosis of small blood vessels is frequent. The central mass of caseation necrosis is surrounded by a zone of mononuclear and epithelioid cells. The acute form is generally characterized by focal necrosis and suppuration. Lesions of the subacute form are generally granulomatous, and giant cells may be present.

There have been numerous reports concerning the gross pathology and histopathology of tularemia in lagomorphs; the most comprehensive is that of Lillie and Francis (1936), who described these changes in experimentally infected laboratory rabbits (*Oryctolagus cuniculus*). Tularemia in the black-tailed jackrabbit presents a more acute picture and is characterized by parasitization of parenchymal cells of the lung and the reticuloendothelial cells of the spleen and liver.

Pathologic changes in acute experimental tularemia in the opossum are similar to those in the guinea pig. These include well-defined focal caseous necrosis in the spleen and liver with parasitization of the parenchymal and Kupffer's cells of the liver.

Gross pathology and histopathology of experimental and spontaneous tularemia have been described in the California ground squirrel (*Citellus*), the antelope ground squirrel (*Ammospermophilus*), the groundhog (*Marmota*), the southern pocket gopher (*Geomys*), the cotton rat (*Sigmodon*), the hamster (*Mesocricetus*), the house mouse, the Norway rat (*Rattus*), and the guinea pig (*Cavia porcellus*) (Davis 1935; Lillie and Francis 1936; Lillie and Larson 1945; McCoy 1911; McCoy and Chapin 1912; Olin 1934). The most consistent hepatic change in mice is parasitization of parenchymal cells. Pathologic changes in spontaneously infected water voles consist of enlarged inguinal and axillary lymph nodes and splenomegaly with necrotic nodules which can progress to complete diffuse necrosis.

In spontaneously infected beavers, the gross pathologic changes consist of gray and white pinpoint lesions in the liver, spleen, kidneys, and mesenteric lymph nodes; excessive amounts of peritoneal, pleural, and pericardial fluid; hemorrhagic gastritis; and catarrhal enteritis (Hammersland and Joneschild 1940). Muskrats appear to be very susceptible to experimental infection, and the observed lesions are similar to those found in rabbits but are generally more pronounced (Green et al. 1929). Lesions in naturally infected muskrats include excessive, dark serous fluid in the body cavities, petechiae in subcutaneous fat, and congestion of the lungs, liver, and spleen (Banfield 1954; Langford 1954).

In spontaneously infected gray foxes, the gross pathology of tularemia includes enlarged and congested thoracic and abdominal lymph nodes, slight enlargement of the spleen and liver, which are studded with miliary gray necrotic foci, and congested tubercle-like areas in the lungs (Schlotthauer et al. 1934).

Pathologic changes in experimentally infected red foxes include sinus dilation of lymph nodes, exudation of macrophages, caseous necrosis of sinus areas, margination of necrotic areas by vacuolated epithelioid cells, and fibrin exudate (Lillie and Francis 1936). Pneumonic changes consist of diffuse consolidation. Histologically, exudate, monocytes, and macrophages are present in alveoli. The liver is stippled with necrotic foci. The microscopic change is caseation necrosis with or without purulent centers, or margins of vacuolated epithelioid cells. Portal areas are occasionally involved, and some lymphocytic infiltration is observed. The spleen is studded with necrotic foci, with margins of vacuolated eipthelioid cells; karyolytic leukocytes and monocytes are seen.

Gross lesions of experimental tularemia in rhesus monkeys (*Macaca mulatta*) include induration and necrosis of skin at the injection site, multiple petechiae in the skin of the face, shoulders, abdomen, and hind legs (not seen in older animals); enlarged regional lymph nodes, with gross evidence of necrosis and central liquefaction; splenomegaly, with numerous yellow foci of coagulation necrosis; extensive focal hepatitis, with fatty metamorphosis of liver cells; and raised yellowish gray nodules and pleural adhesions on the lungs. Histopathologic changes consist of hyperplastic or necrotic lymph nodes, focal necrosis surrounded by large mononuclear cells, and polymorphonuclear leukocytes. Small foci of necrosis within thickened alveolar walls are evident in the lungs. The alveoli may be filled with an exudate containing mononuclear and polymorphonuclear leukocytes. A few giant cells are seen at the periphery of completely necrotic areas (Coriell et al. 1948; Downs et al. 1947; McCoy 1911; McCoy and Chapin 1912).

DIAGNOSIS. A diagnosis of tularemia must be confirmed by laboratory findings. Isolation of the organism can be effected by inoculating blood glucose cystine agar with blood or organ triturates from suspect material or by subcutaneous inoculation of these into mice, hamsters, or guinea pigs, which usually die in 5–10 days. Recovery of the organism from these, lesions pathognomonic of tularemia, or both are diagnostic.

There are in addition a number of diagnostic procedures used in human medicine that may be applicable to the field of wildlife disease. One of these, the Ascoli, or thermoprecipitin, test, employs a boiled, saline extract of tissues of animals suspected of dying of tularemia and permits early specific diagnosis (Larson 1951). Its greatest value, however, may be the application of this test to populations that decline with no apparent increase in the incidence of discernible disease and to badly decomposed carcasses found during and after epizootics. This test is recommended for use in field studies and has been employed very successfully by Bell et al. (1959) and McDowell et al. (1964); it is applicable even to formalin-fixed tissues. The accelerated slide agglutination test (Vereninova et al. 1962), which uses an antigen prepared from spleens of rodents dead presumably from tularemia, is a modification of this test.

The skin test, which employs a bacterial cell wall antigen, has been used extensively for surveys of tularemia in man (Drobinsky 1946). It is diagnostic for tularemia, specific, and highly reliable in detecting 75–95% of cases.

A hemagglutination test is used to obtain an early diagnosis in man (Wright and Feinberg 1952). Korth (1944) and Tovar (1946) described a "97% accurate" slide agglutination test. Nagle et al. (1943) and Damon and Johnson (1944) proposed a rapid tube agglutination test. In the investigation of tularemia epizootics, particularly those in which the organism is highly virulent, hemagglutinins may be of greater value because they reach diagnostic levels more rapidly than agglutinins (Charkes 1959). The fluorescent antibody test (Franek and Wolfov'a 1965) and fluorescence inhibition (McCahan et al. 1962) have been used successfully for quick diagnosis of tularemia in wild animals. The tube agglutination test (Widal type) is used most commonly in diagnostic laboratories.

PROGNOSIS. Green et al. (1938) reported that agglutinins for *F. tularensis* were never found in sera collected from apparently healthy, wild cottontail rabbits. They interpreted this to mean that cottontail rabbits do not survive the infection. However, seropositive cottontail rabbits of two species (*Sylvilagus* spp.) have since been found in Utah (Ecodynamics 1972). Jackrabbits are frequently found dead of tularemia, and there is little evidence that any survive the infection (Jellison et al. 1961). The prognosis may also be similar in other species—that is, beavers, muskrats, *Microtus* spp., and *Lemmus* spp. However, we have demonstrated nonfatal infection in one naturally infected vole (*Microtus* spp.) and have produced chronic nonfatal infection in this species by feeding large doses of fully virulent type B organisms (Bell and Stewart 1975). Parker et al. (1951) reported that deaths among beavers and muskrats in an epizootic of tularemia in the northwestern United States numbered in the hundreds and thousands, respectively.

Rarity of fatalities among snowshoe hares and the absence of gross tularemic lesions in apparently healthy hares from which the organism had been isolated would seem to indicate that this animal is, ordinarily, rather resistant. The frequent presence of anti-*tularensis* agglutinins in the sera of apparently healthy snowshoe hares, indicating experience with the disease, is additional evidence that tularemia is generally nonfatal in this species. However, there is reason to believe that the hares become more susceptible during the time of cyclic dieoff (Bell 1965), which has been attributed to stress (Christian 1950). Insufficient information is available to speculate on prognosis of this disease in other wild species, such as opossum, fox, skunk, mink, grouse, partridge, and pheasant. Black bears commonly have high serum antibody titers to *F. tularensis*, presumptive evidence of frequent nonfatal exposure to the bacterium (J. Beecham and C. Benninger, personal communication, 1978).

Rabbits made sensitive to ticks by laboratory exposure acquire resistance ("allergic klendusity") to tularemia commonly transmitted by those ticks (Bell et al. 1979).

IMMUNITY. Larson (1945) produced active immunity in white rats against tularemia with a killed vaccine prepared in embryonated chicken eggs and with lysates or acetone extracts of cultures grown in peptone broth. Ether-extracted yolk sac vaccine (Bell et al. 1952) and an antigen derived from cell walls of the organism (Ormsbee and Larson 1955) are highly immunogenic for rats and mice. Significant antibody response was elicited in mice vaccinated with phenolized suspensions of the tularemia organism, but protection was not afforded (Ruchman and Foshay 1949). Bell et al. (1962) reported that ether-extracted cell wall vaccine was not efficacious in protecting mice and beavers.

It has been established that the Russian live tularemia vaccine (American type culture collection no. 29684) evokes a higher degree of immunity and is superior to killed preparations in white mice, guinea pigs, and monkeys against challenge with virulent organisms (Downs and Woodward 1949; Eigelsbach and Downs 1961; Eigelsbach et al. 1958, 1959), particularly if the vaccine is administered aerogenically (Eigelsbach et al. 1961). Bell et al. (1962) believed that live attenuated vaccine was effective in ameliorating the course of a tularemia epizootic in pen-raised beavers.

The transfer of splenic cells or peritoneal leukocytes from donors which had recovered from infections with attenuated *F. tularensis* produced resistance to virulent strains in nonimmune recipient mice (Allen 1962) and rats (Stansberry and Woodward 1962). Therefore it may be postulated that immunity is in some way associated with an altered tissue state.

Reconstituted lyophilized vaccine is used for tularemia control in the Soviet Union (Tigertt 1962); it results in 90–97.5% protection for humans, which lasts for at least 6 years (Karakulov et al. 1957). The potential of aerogenic vaccination of man against tularemia has been recognized by Aleksandrov et al. (1958) and Eigelsbach et al. (1962). Hornick and Eigelsbach (1966) report that 4 dex organisms administered aerogenically ensure the development of antibody; as many as 6 dex or 8 dex may

be administered without undue risk. However, a low-grade febrile disease occurs with more than 90% of the vaccine. High-grade immunity is elicited and protection is afforded against challenge 4 months later. Hornick et al. (1966) have demonstrated the usefulness of the oral route for immunization of man with live attenuated vaccines.

Immunization with live vaccines is quite efficient in preventing tularemia. Therefore, such high-risk populations as residents in enzootic areas, laboratory workers, veterinarians, foresters, wildlife biologists, trappers, and fishermen, who may be exposed to this disease by the nature of their activities, should consider the possibility of prophylactic immunization against tularemia. The lyophilized vaccine is available to physicians from the Bureau of Laboratories, National Center for Disease Control, Department of Health, Education, and Welfare, Atlanta, Georgia 30333. Intradermal inoculation by multiple puncture is the approved method of application in man. Subcutaneous injection is more convenient and quite satisfactory for vaccination of animals.

TREATMENT. Streptomycin, the first effective antibiotic for the treatment of tularemia, has become a universal therapeutic agent of high efficiency (Chapman et al. 1949; Heilman 1944; Tamura and Suyemoto 1947). It is both bacteriostatic and bactericidal and is effective in the treatment of experimental tularemia in mice, rats, and monkeys (Sawyer et al. 1966). Strains resistant to streptomycin (Overholt et al. 1961), but not to tetracycline or chloramphenicol, have been encountered. Sawyer et al. (1966) reported that, unlike streptomycin, tetracycline and other broad-spectrum drugs do not kill *F. tularensis* in vitro or in vivo, but owe their effectiveness to their bacteriostatic action. These drugs check multiplication of the invading organisms until the host defense mechanisms can eliminate them; therefore, withdrawal may result in a relapse (Vosti et al. 1962).

CONTROL. Enzootic tularemia of lagomorphs and rodents cannot be eradicated. Attempts to reduce the numbers of susceptible wild hosts by poisoning may be made on a limited scale but usually at great expense and with the risk of destruction of uninvolved and desirable species. Agricultural practices that minimize food and shelter for rodents coupled with encouragement of raptors is, undoubtedly, the most efficient and safest means of preventing tularemia epizootics. The large-scale use of antitularemia vaccination with living strains in the Soviet Union has effectively reduced the infection in humans (Olsuf'ev and Rudneva 1960). It should be recognized that tularemia serves as a natural control of rodent populations that would otherwise cause enormous damage (Jellison et al. 1958). Furthermore, rapid eradication of excessively high rodent populations by tularemia may prevent epizootics of sylvatic plague in those host species susceptible to both diseases.

Aside from the questionable value of interstate shipment of lagomorphs from one ecosystem into another of different type for wildlife stocking, for example, rabbits from Kansas shipped to Pennsylvania, there is potential danger of exposure of humans to tularemia in the process. In enzootic arees, sportsmen should be cautioned against drinking from streams. Rubber gloves should be worn when dressing lagomorphs, and meat of these animals should be thoroughly cooked to render it harmless.

Other methods of control include avoidance of flies and ticks while in enzootic areas during the seasonal incidence of these arthropods.

Another disease very similar to tularemia, and caused by another species of *Francisella*, has been recognized (Larson et al. 1955). The etiologic agent, *F. novicida*, has been isolated only once, from a water sample collected north of the Great Salt Lake in Utah. It is not known to infect humans. The bacterium does not require cystine in the substrate and, also unlike *F. tularensis*, ferments sucrose.

REFERENCES

Aleksandrov, N. I., Gefen, N. E., Garin, N. W., Gapochko, K. G., Daalberg, I. I., and Sergeyev, V. M. Reactogenicity and effectiveness of aerogenic vaccination against certain zoonoses. *Vopr. Med. Zh.* 12:34–38, 1958.

Allen, W. P. Immunity against tularemia: Passive protection of mice by transfer of immune tissues. *J. Exp. Med.* 115:411–420, 1962.

Allred, D. M., Stagg, G. N., and Lavender, J. F. Experimental transmission of *Pasteurella tularensis* by the tick, *Dermacentor parumapertus. J. Infect. Dis.* 99:143–145, 1956.

Amoss, H. R., and Sprunt, D. H. Tularemia: Review of literature of cases contracted by ingestion of rabbit. *J. Am. Med. Assoc.* 106:1078–1081, 1936.

Anigstein, L., Whitney, D. M., and Micks, D. W. Antibacterial activity of a substance present in ticks (Ixodoidea). *Nature* 166:141–143, 1955.

Aoki, K., Kondo, S., and Tazawa, Y. Bacteriological investigations of a new disease, which is very probably caused by infection from the hare. *Tokyo Iji Shinshi* 2411:1–5, 1925.

Apekhtin, V. N. On epidemiology and parasitology of transmissive outbreaks of tularemia. *Med. Parazitol. (Mosk.)* 14:93–98, 1945. Abstr. *Bull. Hyg.* 21:740, 1946.

Banfield, A. W. F. Tularemia in beavers and muskrats, Waterton Lakes National Park, Alberta, 1952–1953. *Can. J. Zool.* 32:139–143, 1954.

Barnes, W. C. Rabbit fever or tularemia. *Sci. Monthly* 27:463–469, 1928.

Bell, J. F. The infection of ticks (*Dermacentor variabilis*) with *Pasteurella tularensis. J. Infect. Dis.* 76:83–95, 1945.

———. Ecology of tularemia in North America. *J. Jinsen Med.* 11:33–44, 1965.

Bell, J. F., Jellison, W. L., Owen, C. R., and Larson, C. L. Applicability of the Ascoli test to epizootic tularemia in wild rodents. *J. Wildl. Manag.* 23:238–240, 1959.

Bell, J. F., Larson, C. L., Wicht, W. C., and Ritter, S. S. Studies on the immunization of white mice against infections with *Bacterium tularense. J. Immunol.* 69:515–524, 1952.

Bell, J. F., and Owen, C. R. Transovarian transmission of *B. tularense* infection in ticks. Unpublished manuscript, 1953.

Bell, J. F., Owen, C. R., Jellison, W. L., Moore, G. J., and Buker, E. O. Epizootic tularemia in pen-raised beavers and field trials of vaccines. *Am. J. Vet. Res.* 23:884–887, 1962.

Bell, J. F., and Stewart, S. J. Chronic shedding tularemia nephritis in rodents: Possible relation to occurrence of *Francisella tularensis* in lotic waters. *J. Wildl. Dis.* 11:421–430, 1975.

Bell, J. F., Stewart, S. J., and Wikel, S. K. Resistance to tick-borne *Francisella tularensis* by tick-sensitized rabbits: Allergic klendusity. *Am. J. Trop. Med. Hyg.* 28:876–880, 1979.

Breed, R. S., Murray, E. G. O., Smith, M. R., eds. *Bergey's manual of determinative bacteriology,* 7th ed. Baltimore: Williams and Wilkins, 1957.

Burgdorfer, W., and Owen, C. R. Experimental studies of argasid ticks as possible vectors of tularemia. *J. Infect. Dis.* 98:67–74, 1956.

Burgdorfer, W., and Pickens, E. G. A technique employing embryonated chicken eggs for the infection of argasid ticks with *Coxiella burnetii, Bacterium tularense, Leptospira icterohaemorrhagiae* and western equine encephalitis virus. *J. Infect. Dis.* 94:84–89, 1954.

Burroughs, A. L., Holdenreid, R., Longanecker, D. S., and Meyer, K. F. A field study of latent tularemia in rodents with a list of all known naturally infected vertebrates. *J. Infect. Dis.* 76:115–119, 1945.

Calhoun, E. L., and Alford, H. J. Incidence of tularemia and Rocky Mountain spotted fever among common ticks of Arkansas. *Am. J. Trop. Med. Hyg.* 4:310–317, 1955.

Chapman, S. S., Coriell, L. L., and Koval, S. F. Streptomycin studies in tularemia: II. Streptomycin therapy in white rats. *J. Infect. Dis.* 85:39–44, 1949.

Charkes, N. Hemagglutination test in tularemia: Results in 56 vaccinated persons with laboratory acquired infections. *J. Immunol.* 83:213–220, 1959.

Christian, J. J. The adreno-pituitary system and population cycles in mammals. *J. Mammal.* 31:247–259, 1950.

Coriell, L. L., King, E. O., and Smith, M. G. Studies in tularemia: IV. Observations on tularemia in normal and vaccinated monkeys. *J. Immunol.* 58:183–202, 1948.

Damon, S. R., and Johnson, M. B. A rapid agglutination test for the diagnosis of tularemia. *J. Lab. Clin. Med.* 29:976–977, 1944.

David, H. Zhur Diagnose der Tulaeramie des Menschen und der Tiere. *Zentralbl. Bakteriol. [Orig. A]* 140:109–113, 1937.

Davis, G. E. Tularemia: Susceptibility of the white-tailed prairie dog, *Cynomys leucurus*, Merriam. *Public Health Rep.* 50:731–732, 1935.

———. *Bacterium tularense*: Its persistence in the tissues of the argasid ticks *Ornithodoros turicata* and *O. parkeri*. *Public Health Rep.* 55:676–680, 1940.

Dorofeev, K. A. On classification of tularemic bacteriae. *Symp. Res. Workers Inst. Epidemiol. Microbiol.* (Chita, Siberia) 1:177–178, 1947.

Downs, C. M., Coriell, L. L., Pinchot, C. B., Maumentee, E., Klauber, A., Chapman, S. S., and Owens, B. Studies of tularemia: I. The comparable susceptibility of various laboratory animals. *J. Immunol.* 56:217–228, 1947.

Downs, C. M., and Woodward, J. M. Studies on pathogenesis and immunity in tularemia: III. Immunogenic properties of the white mouse to various strains of *Bacterium tularense*. *J. Immunol.* 63:147–163, 1949.

Drobinsky, I. R. The immunobiological diagnosis of tularemia. *Zh. Mikrobiol. Epidemiol. Immunobiol.* 7/8:13–22, 1943. Abstr. *Biol. Abstr.* 20:948, 1946.

Ecodynamics. *Ecology studies in Western Utah, Annual Report.* Ser. 72-1 (May), Salt Lake City, Utah, 1972.

Eigelsbach, H. T., and Downs, C. M. Prophylactic effectiveness of live and killed tularemia vaccines: I. Production of vaccine and evaluation in the white mouse and guinea pig. *J. Immunol.* 87:415–425, 1961.

Eigelsbach, H. T., Downs, C. M., and Herring, R. D. Comparative immunogenicity of live and killed tularemia vaccines for the mouse and guinea pig. *Bacteriol. Proc. 58th General Meeting*, p. 74, 1958.

Eigelsbach, H. T., Tigertt, W. D., Saslaw, S., and McCrumb, F. R., Jr. Live and killed tularemia vaccines evaluation in animals and man. *Proc. Army Sci. Conf.* U.S. Mil. Acad., West Point 1:235–246, 1962.

Eigelsbach, H. T., Tulis, J. J., Overholt, E. L., and Gochenour, W. S., Jr. Immunogenicity of live tularemia vaccine for the monkey. *Bacteriol. Proc., 58th General Meeting*, pp. 87–88, 1959.

Eigelsbach, H. T., Tulis, J. J., Overholt, E. L., and Griffith, W. R. Aerogenic immunization of the monkey and guinea pig with live tularemia vaccine. *Proc. Soc. Exp. Biol. Med.* 108:732–734, 1961.

Foshay, L. Accurate and earlier diagnosis by means of intradermal reaction. *J. Infect. Dis.* 51:286–291, 1932.

———. Tularemia. *Ann. Rev. Microbiol.* 4:313–330, 1950.

Francis, E. Deer-fly fever: A disease of man of hitherto unknown etiology. *Public Health Rep.* 34:2061–2062, 1919.

———. Tularemia in the Washington, D.C., market. *Public Health Rep.* 38:1391–1396, 1923a.

———. The amino-acid cystine in the cultivation of *Bacterium tularense*. *Public Health Rep.* 38:1396–1404, 1923b.

———. Arthropods in the transmission of tularemia. *Trans. 4th Int. Congr. Entomol.* 2:929–944, 1929.

———. Sources of infection and seasonal incidence of tularemia in man. *Public Health Rep.* 52:103–113, 1937.

Francis, E., and Lake, G. C. Experimental transmission of tularemia in rabbits by the rabbit louse *Haemodipsus ventricosus* (Denny). *Public Health Rep.* 36:1747–1753, 1921.

———. Transmission of tularemia by the bedbug, *Cimex lectularius*. *Public Health Rep.* 37:83–95, 1922a.

———. Transmission of tularemia by the mouse louse, *Polyplax serratus* (Brum). *Public Health Rep.* 37:96–101, 1922b.

Francis, E., and Mayne, B. Experimental transmission of tularemia by flies of the species *Chrysops discalis*. *Public Health Rep.* 36:1738–1748, 1921.

Francis, E., and Moore, D. Identity of Ohara's disease and tularemia. *J. Am. Med. Assoc.* 86:1329–1332, 1926.

Franek, J., and Wolfov'a, J. Use of the immunofluorescence method in an epidemic focus of tularemia. *Folia Microbiol.* (Prague) 10:85–92, 1965.

Friedewald, W. F., and Hunt, C. A. The diagnosis of tularemia. *Am. J. Med. Sci.* 197:493–502, 1939.

Gaspar, A. J., Tresselt, H. B., and Ward, M. K. New solid medium for enhanced growth of *Pasteurella tularensis*. *J. Bacteriol.* 82:564–569, 1961.

Gelman, A. C. Tularemia. In J. M. May, ed. *Studies in disease ecology*, pp. 89–108. New York: Hafner, 1961.

Girard, G. *Haemodipus lyriocephalus* Burmeister and *Ixodes ricinus* Linne, ectoparasites of hares, as possible vectors of tularemia in France. *C. R. Soc. Biol.* 144:364–365, 1950.

Gorham, J. R. Mink, fox susceptible to tularemia. *Am. Nat. Fur Market J.* 28:21, 1949.

———. Tularemia kills mink too! *Am. Fur Breeder* 23:15, 1950.

Green, R. G. The occurrence of *Bact. tularense* in the eastern wood tick *Dermacentor variabilis*. *Am. J. Hyg.* 14:600–613, 1931.

———. Tularemia as a hunter's problem. *Conserv. Volunteer* 3:41–45, 1942.

———. Virulence of tularemia as related to animal and arthropod hosts. *Am. J. Hyg.* 38:282–292, 1943.

Green, R. G., Bell, J. F., Larson, C. L., and Evans, C. A. (No title,) *Minn. Wildl. Dis. Invest. Mimeo.* 4:45–51, 1938.

Green, R. G., and Evans, C. A. Role of fleas in the natural transmission of tularemia. *Minn. Wildl. Dis. Invest. Mimeo.* 4:25–28, 1938.

Green, R. G., Wade, E. M., and Dewey, E. T. Experimental tularemia in muskrats. *Proc. Soc. Exp. Biol. Med.* 26:426–427, 1929.

Hammersland, H. L., and Joneschild, E. M. Tularemia in a beaver. *J. Am. Med. Assoc.* 96:96–97, 1940.

Heilman, F. R. Streptomycin therapy in experimental tularemia. *Bull. Hyg.* 19:553–559, 1944.

Hendrickson, G. O. The Mearns' cottontail in Iowa. *Trans. Am. Wildl. Conf.* 2:549–554, 1937.

Hesselbrock, W., and Foshay, L. The morphology of *Bacterium tularense*. *J. Bacteriol.* 49:209–231, 1945.

Hood, A. M. Virulence factors of *Francisella tularensis*. *J. Hyg.* 79:47–60, 1977.

Hopla, C. E. Experimental studies on tick transmission of tularemia organisms. *Am. J. Hyg.* 58:101–118, 1953.

———. The multiplication of tularemic organisms in the lone star tick. *Am. J. Hyg.* 61:371–380, 1955.

———. The ecology of tularemia. *Adv. Vet. Sci. Comp. Med.* 13:25–53, 1974.

Hopla, C. E., and Downs, C. M. The isolation of *Bacterium tularense* from the tick, *Amblyomma americanum*. *J. Kansas Entomol. Soc.* 26:72–73, 1953.

Horne, H. Eine Lemmingpest und eine Meerschweinchenepizootie. Ein Beitrag zur Beleuchtung der Ursachen der Lemmingsterbe in den sogenannten Lemmingjahren. *Zentralbl. Bakteriol.* [*Orig. A*] 69:169–193, 1912.

Hornick, R. B., Dawkins, A. T., Eigelsbach, H. T., and Tulis, J. J. Oral tularemia vaccine in man. In *Antimicrobial agents chemotherapy*, pp. 11–14. Washington, D.C.: American Society of Microbiology, 1966.

Hornick, R. B., and Eigelsbach, H. T. Aerogenic immunization of man with live tularemia vaccine. *Bacteriol. Rev.* 30:532–538, 1966.

Jellison, W. L. *Tularemia in North America, 1930–1974*, monogr. Missoula: University of Montana, 1974.

Jellison, W. L., Bell, J. F., Vertrees, J. D., Holms, M. A., Larson, C. L., and Owen, C. R. Preliminary observations on disease in the 1957–58 outbreak of *Microtus* in western United States. *Trans. North Am. Wildl. Conf.* 23:137–145, 1958.

Jellison, W. L., Epler, D. C., Kuhns, E., and Kohls, G. M. Tularemia in man from a domestic rural water supply. *Public Health Rep.* 65:1219–1226, 1950.

Jellison, W. L., Kohls, G. M., Butler, W. J., and

Weaver, J. A. Epizootic tularemia in the beaver, *Castor canadensis*, and the contamination of stream water with *Pasteurella tularensis*. *Am. J. Hyg.* 36:168–182, 1942.

Jellison, W. L., Owen, C. R., Bell, J. F., and Kohls, G. M. Tularemia and animal populations: Ecology and epizootiology. *Wildl. Dis.* 17 (microcard):1–22, 1961.

Jellison, W. L., and Parker, R. R. Rodents, rabbits and tularemia in North America: Some zoological and epidemiological considerations. *Am. J. Trop. Med.* 25:349–362, 1945.

Jusatz, H. J. Tularemia in Europe, 1926–1951. In E. Rodenwaldt, ed., *Welt-Seuchen Atlas*, vol. I. Hamburg: Falk-Verlag, 1952.

Kamil, S., and Bilal, S. Recherches experimentales sur l'etiologie de la tularemie en Turquie. *Ann. Parasitol. Human Comp.* 16:530–542, 1938.

Karakulov, I. K., Mertsalov, E. M., and Zhokin, A. R. Some results of prophylaxis of infectious disease in the Kazakhstan S.S.R. *J. Microbiol. Epidemiol. Immunobiol.* 28:1384–1387, 1957.

Karpov, S. P., Popov, V. M., Slinkina, A. G., Chernyshev, F. I., and Reazantsov, M. I. Epidemiology of a transmissive outbreak of tularemia. *Zh. Mikrobiol. Epidemiol. Immunobiol.* 7/8:24–28, 1943. Abstr. *Biol. Abstr.* 29:1013, 1946.

Korth, W. Serologische Ergebnisse waehrend einer Tularaemie. *Zentralbl. Bakteriol.* [*Orig. A*] 151:394–399, 1914.

Lake, G. C., and Francis, E. Six cases of tularemia occurring in laboratory workers. *Public Health Rep.* 37:392–413, 1922.

Lane, R. S., and Emmons, R. W. Ecological and epidemiological studies of tularemia in California. *Calif. Vector Views* 24:39–49, 1978.

Langford, E. V. An outbreak of tularemia in beaver and muskrats in Waterton Lakes National Park, Alberta. *Can. J. Comp. Med. Vet. Sci.* 18:28–29, 1954.

Larson, C. L. Immunization of white rats against infection with *Pasteurella tularensis*. *Public Health Rep.* 60:729–734, 1945.

———. Studies on thermostable antigen extracted from *Bacterium tularense* and from tissues of animals dead of tularemia. *J. Immunol.* 66:249–259, 1951.

Larson, C. L., Wicht, W., and Jellison, W. L. A new organism resembling *P. tularensis* isolated from water. *Public Health Rep.* 70:253–258, 1955.

Lillie, R. D., and Francis, E. The pathology of tularemia. *Natl. Inst. Health Bull.* 167:1–217, 1936.

Lillie, R. D., and Larson, C. L. Pathology of experimental tularemia in the golden hamster (*Cricetus auratus*). *Public Health Rep.* 60:1243–1245, 1945.

McCahan, G. R., Moody, M. D., and Hayes, F. A. An epizootic of tularemia among rabbits in northwestern South Carolina. *Am. J. Hyg.* 75:335–338, 1962.

McCoy, G. W. A plague-like disease of rodents. *Public Health Bull.* 43:53–57, 1911.

McCoy, G. W., and Chapin, C. W. Further observations on a plague-like disease of rodents with a preliminary note on the causative agent, *Bacterium tularense. J. Infect. Dis.* 10:61–72, 1912.

McDowell, J. W., Scott, H. G., Stojanovich, C. J., and Weinburgh, H. B. Tularemia. Atlanta: USD-HEW, Public Health Service, Communicable Disease Center, Training Branch, 1964.

Maisky, I. M. Tularemia outbreaks of murine origin. *Zh. Mikrobiol. Epidemiol. Immunobiol.* 7/ 8:32–38, 1945. Abstr. *Bull. Hyg.* 20:612, 1945.

Matheson, R. Ticks and disease with special reference to spotted fever and tularemia in the eastern states. *Cornell Vet.* 30:167–177, 1940.

Meyer, K. F. *Pasteurella* and *Francisella.* In R. J. Dubos and J. G. Hersch, eds., *Bacteria and mycotic infections of man*, 4th ed., pp. 681–697. Philadelphia: Lippincott, 1965.

Nagle, N., Schulze, L., and Willet, J. C. A rapid agglutination test technique. *J. Lab. Clin. Med.* 28:1864–1867, 1943.

Nel'zina, E. W., and Barkov, I. P. The carrying of the microbe of tularemia by certain species of gamasid mites under natural conditions. *Dokl. Akad. Nauk SSSR* 78:829–831, 1951.

Ohara, H. Concerning an acute febrile disease transmitted by wild rabbits: A preliminary report. *Jikken Iho* 11:1, 1925.

———. Experimental inoculation of disease of wild rabbits into human body and its bacteriological study. *Jpn. Med. World* 6:299–304, 1926.

Ohara, S. Studies of yato-byo (Ohara's disease, tularemia in Japan): Report I. *Jpn. J. Exp. Med.* 24:69–79, 1954.

Olin, G. Nouvelles recherches sur la tularemie en Suede. *Bull. Off. Int. Hyg.* 26:890, 1934.

———. Surveys on the origin and mode of propagation of tularemia in Sweden. *Bull. Off. Int. Hyg.* 30:2804–2807, 1938.

Olsuf'ev, N. G. *On the paleogenesis of the causative agent of tularemia.* Proceedings of a symposium: Theoretical questions of natural foci of disease, ed. B. Rosicky and K. Heyberger. *Czechoslovak. Acad. Sci.* pp. 369–378, 1965.

Olsuf'ev, N. G., Emelyanova, O. S., and Dunaeva, T. N. Comparative study of strains of *B. tularense* in the old and new world and their taxonomy. *J. Hyg. Epidemiol. Microbiol. Immunol. (Praha)* 3:138–149, 1959.

Olsuf'ev, N. G., and Rudneva, O. S., eds. *Tularemia.* Moscow: Medgiz, 1960.

Ormsbee, R. A., and Larson, C. L. Studies on *Bacterium tularense* antigens: II. Chemical and physical characteristics of protective antigen preparations. *J. Immunol.* 74:359–370, 1955.

Overholt, E. L., Tigertt, W. D., Kadull, P. J., and Ward, M. K. An analysis of forty-two cases of laboratory-acquired tularemia: Treatment with broad spectrum antibiotics. *Am. J. Med.* 30:785–806, 1961.

Owen, C. R. Part 7. Gram-negative aerobic rods & cocci: Genera of uncertain affiliation. In R. E. Buchanan and N. E. Gibbons, eds. *Bergey's manual of determinative bacteriology*, 8th ed.,

pp. 283–285. Baltimore: Williams and Wilkins, 1974.

Parker, D. D., and Johnson, D. E. Experimental transmission of *Pasteurella tularensis* by the flea, *Orchopeas leucopus* (Baker). *J. Infect. Dis.* 101:69–72, 1957.

Parker, R. R. Recent studies of tick-borne diseases made at the United States Public Health Service Laboratory at Hamilton, Montana. *Proc. 5th Pacific Sci. Congr.* 6:3367–3374, 1933.

Parker, R. R., Bell, J. F., Chalgren, W. S., Thrailkill, F. B., and McKee, M. T. The recovery of strains of Rocky Mountain spotted fever and tularemia from ticks of the eastern United States. *J. Infect. Dis.* 91:231–237, 1952.

Parker, R. R., Brooks, C. S., and Marsh, H. The occurrence of *Bacterium tularense* in the wood tick, *Dermacentor occidentalis*, in California. *Public Health Rep.* 44:1299–1300, 1929.

Parker, R. R., and Spencer, R. R. Tularemia and its occurrence in Montana. *Bien. Rep. Montana Bd. Entomol.* 6:30–41, 1925–1926.

———. Hereditary transmission of tularemia infection by the wood tick, *Dermacentor andersoni*, Stiles. *Public Health Rep.* 41:1403–1407, 1926.

Parker, R. R., Spencer, R. R., and Francis, E. Tularemia infections in ticks of the species *Dermacentor andersoni*, Stiles, in the Bitterroot Valley, Montana. *Public Health Rep.* 39:1057–1073, 1924.

Parker, R. R., Steinhaus, E. A., Kohls, G. M., and Jellison, W. L. Contamination of natural waters and mud with *Pasteurella tularensis* and tularemia in beaver and muskrats in the northwestern United States. *Natl. Inst. Health Bull.* 193:61, 1951.

Pearse, R. A. Insect bites. *Northwest Med.* 3:81, 1911.

Philip, C. B. Tularemia in Alaska. *Proc. 6th Pacific Sci. Congr.* 5:71–75, 1942.

Philip, C. B., Bell, J. F., and Larson, C. L. Evidence of infectious diseases and parasites in a peak population of black-tailed jackrabbits in Nevada. *J. Wildl. Manag.* 19:225–233, 1955.

Philip, C. B., Gill, C. D., and Geary, J. M. Notes on the rabbit tick, *Haemaphysalis leporis-palustris* (Packard), and tularemia in central Alaska. *J. Parasitol.* 40:484–485, 1954.

Philip, C. B., and Hughes, L. E. Disease agents found in the rabbit tick *Dermacentor parumapertus*, in the southwestern U.S. *6th Congr. Int. Microbiol. Riassunti Delle Commun.* 2(sect. 8–16):600, 1953.

Philip, C. B., and Jellison, W. L. The American dog tick, *Dermacentor variabilis*, as a host of *Bacterium tularense. Public Health Rep.* 49:386–392, 1934.

Philip, C. B., and Owen, C. R. Comments on the nomenclature of the causative agent of tularemia. *Int. Bull. Bacteriol. Nomenclature* 11:67–72, 1961.

Philip, C. B., and Parker, R. R. Occurrence of tularemia in the rabbit tick (*Haemaphysalis leporis-palustris*) in Alaska. *Public Health Rep.*

53:574–575, 1938.

Quan, S. F., McManus, A. G., and von Fintel, H. Infectivity of tularemia applied to intact skin and ingested in drinking water. *Science* 123:942–943, 1955.

Romanova, V. P., Bojenko, V. P., and Yakovlev, M. G. Studies of the natural nidus of the water-meadow type of tularemia. In E. N. Pavlovsky, P. A. Petrischeva, D. N. Zasukhin, and N. G. Olsuf'ev, eds. *Natural nidi of human diseases and regional epidemiology*. Leningrad: Medgiz, 1955.

Ruchman, I., and Foshay, L. Immune response in mice after vaccination with *Bacterium tularense*. *J. Immunol.* 61:229–234, 1949.

Runnells, R. A. *Animal pathology*, 5th ed. Ames: Iowa State College Press, 1954.

Saito, T., Yamagata, Y., Ohara, S., Ueno, T., Shiba, H., Bell, J. F., and Stewart, S. Pathology of kidney lesions in experimental shedding tularemia nephritis. *Ann. Rep. Ohara General Hosp. Fukushima* 21:9–18, 1978.

Sawyer, W. D., Jemski, J. V., Hogge, A. L., Jr., Eigelsbach, H. T., Wolfe, E. K. Dangerfield, H. G., Gochenour, W. S., Jr., and Crozier, D. Effect of aerosol age on the infectivity of airborne *Pasteurella tularensis* for *Macaca mulatta* and man. *J. Bacteriol.* 91:2180–2184, 1966.

Schlotthauer, C. F., Olson, C., and Thompson, L. Tularemia in a wild grey fox: Report of a case. *Proc. Mayo Clin.* 9:12–16, 1934.

Schmidt, B. Der Einbruch der Tularaemie in Europa. *Z. Hyg. Infektionskrankh.* 127:139–150, 1947. Abstr. *Bull. Hyg.* 23:855, 1948.

Schricker, R. L. Pathogenesis of acute tularemia in the rabbit. Abstr. of paper presented at the Conference of Research Workers in Animal Diseases, 1964.

Shaughnessy, H. J. Tularemia. In T. C. Hull, *Diseases transmitted from animals to man*, pp. 588–603. Springfield, Ill.: Thomas, 1963.

Simpson, W. M. *Tularemia: History, pathology, diagnosis and treatment*. New York: Hoeber, 1929.

Stansberry, M. H., and Woodward, J. M. Cellular defenses of white rats in immunity to tularemia. *Bacteriol. Proc.*, p. 94, 1962.

Stoenner, H. G., and Waldham, D. Laboratory support of epizootiologic and epidemiologic studies conducted in the Great Salt Lake desert, Utah. In *Symposium on Ecology of Disease Transmission in Native Animals*, Dugway, Utah, pp. 105–111, 1955.

Sylvest, E. Tularemia—disease of lemmings. *Ugeskr. Laeger* 98:307–336, 1936.

Tamura, J. T., and Suyemoto, W. Quantitative aspects of streptomycin therapy on experimental tularemia. *J. Bacteriol.* 54:84, 1947.

Thjoetta, T. Tre tilfelle au tularemia. En i Norge hittil ikke erkjent sykdom. *Norsk Mag. Laegevidensk* 91:224–237, 1930. Abstr. *Biol. Abstr.* 6:2050, 1931.

Tigertt, W. D. Soviet viable *Pasteurella tularensis* vaccines: A review of selected articles. *Bacteriol. Rev.* 26:354–373, 1962.

Tovar, R. M. Bedside agglutination test with whole blood for rapid diagnosis of tularemia. *Proc. Soc. Exp. Biol.* 62:67–69, 1946.

Vail, D. T. A case of "squirrel plague" conjunctivity in man. *Ophthalmol. Rec.* 28:487, 1914.

Vereninova, N. K., Kalacheva, N. F., and Tsareva, S. A. On the problem of the acceleration of the diagnosis of tularemia: I. Detection of tularemia in dead rodents. *Zh. Mikrobiol. Epidemiol. Immunobiol.* 33:107–110, 1962.

Volferz, A., Kolpakova, S., and Flegontova, A. On the epizoology of tularemia: I. The role of ectoparasites in the tularemia epizootic of ground squirrels. *Rev. Microbiol. Sartov.* 13:103–118, 1934.

Vosti, K. L., Ward, M. K., and Tigertt, W. D. Agar gel precipitin analysis in laboratory acquired tularemia. *J. Clin. Invest.* 41:1436–1445, 1962.

Waller, E. F. Tularemia in Iowa cottontail rabbits (*Sylvilagus floridanus mearnsi*) and in a dog. *Vet. Student* 2:54–55, 73, 1940.

Wayson, N. E. Plague and plague-like disease: A report of their transmission by *Stomoxys calcitrans* and *Musca domestica*. *Public Health Rep.* 29:3390–3393, 1914.

———. Tularemia infection found in fleas from prairie dogs in Wyoming. *Public Health Rep.* 56:1521, 1941.

Wherry, W. B., and Lamb, B. H. Discovery of *Bacterium tularense* in wild rabbits and the danger of its transfer to man. *J. Am. Med. Assoc.* 63:2041, 1914a.

———. Infection of man with *Bacterium tularense*. *J. Infect. Dis.* 15:331–340, 1914b.

Woodbury, A. M., and Parker, D. D. Studies of tularemia, *Pasteurella tularensis. Ecology of the Great Salt Lake desert*. Ecol. Res. Spec. Rep. 2. Salt Lake City: University of Utah, 1954.

Wright, G. G., and Feinberg, R. J. Hemagglutination by tularemia antisera: Further observations of agglutination of polysaccharide-treated erythrocytes and its inhibition by polysaccharide. *J. Immunol.* 68:65–71, 1952.

19 *Sylvatic Plague*

PETER F. OLSEN

Synonyms: **Wild rodent plague.**

Plague is an acute infectious disease caused by *Pasteurella pestis* Lehman and Neumann. It is vectored by fleas and primarily affects wild rodents and commensal rats (*Rattus* spp.) in many areas of the world. This zoonosis, listed as one of the six internationally quarantinable diseases, has tremendous public health importance when man becomes a victim of bubonic plague through intervention into the rodent-flea-rodent transmission cycle or from handling infected wild rodents.

HISTORY AND DISTRIBUTION. The causative organism of plague was discovered in 1894 by Yersin in Hong Kong, and in 1897 Ogata tentatively suggested that fleas might be involved in the transmission chain. Reports of the British Plague Research Commission 1905–1906 (Lamb 1908) on its work in India did much to further knowledge about the disease, including the role played by the rat and the rat flea. The actual means by which the bacteria multiply in the stomach of fleas, cause blockage of the proventriculus, and are then regurgitated during a subsequent feeding was worked out in 1914 by Bacot and Martin.

Although commensal rats had long been suspected to be somehow associated with plague, it was not until 1895, when infected tarabagans (*Marmota siberica*) were found in Mongolia and the transbaikalian region of Russia, that it was confirmed that wild rodents were also host to the disease (Meyer 1963). There are now more than 230 species or subspecies of wild rodents which have proved to be naturally plague infected or are strongly incriminated—from western United States, western Canada, Mexico, Argentina, Bolivia, Venezuela, Peru, Ecuador, China, Mongolia, Manchuria, USSR, South Africa, Kenya, Congo, Iran, and India (Meyer 1963; Pollitzer 1954; Pollitzer and Meyer 1961).

In the United States, the first human case of plague was discovered in San Francisco in 1900, and the bacilli were isolated from commensal rats in 1902. It was not until 1908 that wild rodents, California ground squirrels (*Ci-*

tellus beecheyi), were found infected in Costa Contra Country (Eskey and Haas 1940; Link 1955). By 1910 these squirrels had been found infected in nine California counties south of San Francisco Bay. This region remained the only known permanent focus of infection until 1934 when infected Belding's ground squirrels (*C. beldingi*) and bushy-tailed wood rats (*Neotoma cinerea*) were discovered in Modoc County, California, 250 miles north of the nearest known plague focus and east of the Sierra Nevada mountains (Wayson 1947). In this year also, a human case of plague occurred in Oregon and became the first case outside California attributable to association with wild animals. Intensive surveys were undertaken by both state and federal public health agencies, which by 1950 extended through all the Rocky Mountain states to the Great Plains. Plague has now been detected among 57 wild rodent species or their ectoparasites in at least 140 counties of 15 western states as far east as the western portions of Kansas, Oklahoma, and Texas, as well as in Alberta, Saskatchewan, and the state of Coahuila, Mexico (Hubbert et al. 1966; Kartman et al. 1966; Link 1955; Stark et al. 1966).

Whereas it is generally felt that the original home of *P. pestis* was in central Asia or in Africa, the question of how it arrived in North America and became established as an enzootic disease among wild rodents in the western United States is subject to some controversy. It appears from the chronology of the statistics of discovery in the various western states that after an original introduction into West Coast seaports by plague-infected, shipborne *Rattus* spp. and their fleas, an initial commensal rat phase eventually led to wild rodent infection followed by spread in an eastward direction (Eskey and Haas 1940; Link 1955). Other observers (Meyer 1947) feel that plague entered with wild rodents across the Siberian-Alaskan land bridge from central Asia and thus has been a naturally associated ecologic factor since the Pleistocene. Pollitzer (1954) discusses the merits and shortcomings of each theory but does not feel that a conclusion can be made.

That plague is still a significant disease of humans is revealed by the fact that in 1967 there were 5,247 suspected and bacteriologically confirmed cases in South Vietnam, due to contact with commensal rats and their fleas (WHO 1967). Although in the United States a case of human plague acquired from commensal rats has not been recorded since 1924, from 1908 through 1967 there were 119 cases of plague—66 of which were fatal—contracted from wild rodents or rabbits (Kartman et al. 1966; U.S. Public Health Service 1966, 1967). This low case rate belies the fact that there is still a potential danger to public health in this country, since each bubonic plague victim runs the risk of developing the pneumonic form of the disease, with the hazard of aerosol spread to all those with whom he comes in contact. This particular aspect of plague has been explored by Hubbert et al. (1966) and Kartman et al. (1966).

Although there exists a vast literature dating back to 1500 B.C. on human plague infection, this phase has been largely ignored in this discussion and the major emphasis directed to the various manifestations of plague in wild rodents. Since sylvatic plague represents an independent epizootiologic entity from that affecting commensal rats, "classic" rat plague involving *Rattus* spp. and the rat flea *Xenopsylla cheopis* is not discussed to any extent; this is quite thoroughly covered by Pollitzer's monograph (1954) and other standard references dealing with commensal rats, such as Calhoun (1963) and the U.S. Public Health Service (1949). The following are suggested as basic references for those who are commencing work on plague or who wish additional detail: Hirst (1953), Kartman et al. (1958), Kartman et al. (1966), Meyer (1963), Pan American Health Organization (1965), Pollitzer (1954), Pollitzer and Meyer (1961), and Stark et al. (1966).

A summary of the previous year's abstracts of papers dealing with all aspects of plague appears in each year's July issue of *Tropical Diseases Bulletin*.

ETIOLOGY. A vast amount of detail concerning the morphologic and growth characteristics, biochemical properties, resistance, virulence, toxins, and antigenic structure of *P. pestis* has been summarized by Meyer (1965) as well as by Pollitzer (1954, 1960). Only certain aspects of the organism's characteristics which are basic or of special significance will be touched upon in this discussion.

Plague bacilli are gram-negative, nonmotile, bipolar-staining, ovoid rods, $0.5-0.8\mu$ wide by $1.0-2.0\mu$ long in the parasitic stage but characterized by a wide variety of pleomorphic forms, from tissues especially. These organisms grow readily but slowly on ordinary culture media, becoming visible in 24–48 hours at an optimum temperature of 28°C.

Particularly when cultured at 37°C, *P. pistis* is surrounded by an envelope which contains the nontoxic but highly antigenic fraction I (FI) antigen which is believed to protect the cells against phagocytosis (Baker et al. 1952). Pesticin, V, W, and other antigens are elaborated under certain cultural conditions and also seem to be associated with prevention of phagocytosis or the ability to survive and multiply within phagocytic cells. The organism also produces an endotoxin; it is felt that liberation of this toxin from lysed cells is the ultimate cause of death in infected animals, producing effects on the peripheral vascular system which cause hemoconcentration, shock, and parenchymal injury in the liver and kidneys (Rust et al. 1963). The highly variable virulence of wild strains of *P. pestis* is related, among other factors, to the ability to produce certain of these antigenic factors. To be fully virulent, a strain must be highly toxigenic, capable of producing the V and W virulence antigens and the FI envelope antigen, able to synthesize purines, and able to form pigmented colonies on defined media containing hemin (Burrows and Bacon 1956; Meyer 1965; Pollitzer 1960). Other biochemical factors which relate to virulence are discussed by Brubaker et al. (1965) and Surgalla (1960).

The plague bacillus is susceptible to streptomycin, tetracycline, chloramphenicol, and certain other antibiotics but is insensitive to penicillin. It is generally considered a fragile organism, since it can be killed readily by exposure to moderate heat, a variety of chemical agents, and sunlight. It is also readily killed by drying except when protected by organic material. In the latter case *P. pestis* has remained viable in dried sputum for 3 months, in dry flea feces held at room temperature for 5 weeks, and of potential epizootiological importance, in soil for at least 8 weeks and in uninhabited deep rodent burrows for 7–11 months in cold climates (Baltzard et al. 1963; Goldenberg and Kartman 1966; Meyer 1965).

The closely related *P. pseudotuberculosis* resembles *P. pestis* in many respects and has caused problems in diagnosis. Fully specific serologic tests are difficult because of the large number of antigens shared by the two organisms. Differentiation is made on the basis of growth rates in culture, motility, characteristic pathology in laboratory animals, phage lysis, biochemical tests, and fluorescent staining (Baltazard et al. 1956; Quan et al. 1965; Stark et al. 1966).

TRANSMISSION. Although a variety of arthropods other than fleas have been found naturally infected with plague bacilli or have been shown to be susceptible to laboratory infection, none are thought to play a significant role as vectors (Pollitzer 1954; Pollitzer and Meyer 1961). On the other hand, the indispensability of the flea as a vector in the basic plague cycle has been universally acknowledged.

The classic biological transmitting mechanism is that involving the "blocking" phenomenon. Fleas feeding on a septicemic host ingest *P. pestis*, which then undergo multiplication within the stomach. After a variable length of time the proventriculus becomes plugged with a mass of bacilli, and the flea is said to be blocked. In such a state, since blood cannot pass to the ventriculus, the flea becomes starved and avidly seeks a blood meal. In the attempt of the flea to feed, blood filling the esophagus and containing bacteria dislodged from the blocking mass is forced back into the bloodstream of the host due to the elastic recoil of the esophagus walls. There are a number of variations from this general description, characterizing different flea species, and also a great deal of variability as to whether or not blockage occurs at all, length of time before blockage occurs, and so on.

A great volume of literature exists on fleas and flea-plague relationships. Important North American taxonomic works include Hubbard (1947), Jellison and Good (1942), Jellison et al. (1960), and Stark (1958). Lists of fleas which have been shown to be involved with plague naturally and through laboratory experimentation have been compiled by Link (1955), Machiavello (1954), Pollitzer (1952, 1954), Pollitzer and Meyer (1961), and Wayson (1947).

All fleas are not of equal significance in the role they play as vectors. Not only species but also individuals within the same species exhibit profound differences in their potential and actual importance in plague epizootiology. These differences are based on what may be termed ecologic and physiologic factors (Kartman et al. 1958; Kartman et al. 1966; Pollitzer and Meyer 1961; Stark et al. 1966). Some of the known ecologic factors are:

1. Host range and specificity as related to whether these hosts are colonial, gregarious or solitary, or burrowing or surface dwelling and the degree of septicemia they exhibit following infection.
2. Geographic or distributional range of the flea.
3. Prevalence or density on hosts and seasonal occurrence in relation to periods when plague occurs.
4. Feeding habits and whether predominantly a nest or body flea.
5. Resistance to adverse environmental factors, including survival time in the absence of a host.
6. Climate and microclimate with their effects on survival, breeding, and so on.

Physiologic factors which influence the ability of fleas to biologically transmit *P. pestis* include:

1. Proportion that become infected following a meal on a septicemic host.
2. Time between the infecting blood meal and blockage.
3. Whether blockage occurs, the proportion that exhibits it, and whether it is cleared.
4. Survival time following infection or blockage.
5. Inherent ability to transmit when blocked.
6. Presence of *P. pestis* antibodies in the blood meal.

Wheeler and Douglas (1945) devised a method that permits comparison of the relative ability of different flea species to transmit *P. pestis*. The method, as modified by Kartman (1957), combines the results of laboratory transmission experiments and field data into a single numerical value. This value, termed the "flea vector potential," is the product of the infection, blocking, transmission, and blocking-survival potentials and the field infection and field prevalence indexes. The result of studies employing this technique and of others dealing with the relative plague-transmitting efficiency of wild rodent fleas are found in Eskey and Haas (1940), Kartman et al. (1958), and Wheeler and Douglas (1945).

Studies have shown that few wild rodent fleas are efficient as biological vectors. As opposed to *X. cheopis*, many such fleas take a much longer time (2 or more months) to become infective, and some never do block; others do not transmit even when blocked. Also, most wild rodent fleas survive for long periods after infection with some known to harbor *P. pestis* for over a year (Eskey and Haas 1940; Kartman et al. 1966; Pollitzer and Meyer 1961). These and other factors have led some observers to postulate that mechanical transmission may be more important in sylvatic plague epizootiology than previously thought. In this type of transmission, which probably requires the mass attack of a number of fleas to be effective, fleas which have recently fed on a bacteremic rodent may mechanically transmit the organisms via their contaminated mouth parts. Kartman et al. (1958) suggest that mechanical transmission by a highly prevalent flea may be the means by which epizootics among wild rodents flare up once they have been initiated by primary vectors that transmit biologically via the blockage mechanism.

The fact that wild rodent fleas are capable of carrying *P. pestis* for very long periods is a primary reason why most investigators maintain that fleas serve not only as vectors but also as one of the basic mechanisms for the perpetuation of sylvatic plague, especially when in association with microclimatic conditions particularly conducive to long survival such as in deep, cold, rodent burrows (Pollitzer and Meyer 1961; Stark et al. 1966).

One factor which has been little studied, but may affect the ability of fleas to transmit biologically or have an effect on the virulence of strains, is the presence of antibodies to *P. pestis* in blood meals taken by fleas. Bibikova and Gavryushina (1963) showed experimentally that 45% of fleas which fed on plague-immunized gerbils eliminated the infection from their gastrointestinal tract, whereas none of those which fed on normal gerbils did. Fleas fed the immune blood meals also had a longer life span, and there was some indication that a reduction in virulence of the organisms had taken place.

EPIZOOTIOLOGY. Pollitzer and Meyer (1961), commenting on the complexity of plague epizootiology, noted "the infinite variety of manifestations of the disease resulting from the profound differences in hosts, vectors and environmental conditions in different areas." The attempt in this section will be to note some of the ecologic factors which foster or inhibit plague, the concepts which have proved useful in clarifying its many manifestations, and the mechanisms now believed responsible for perpetuation of *P. pestis*.

A salient and apparently universal feature of sylvatic plague is a localized (focal) and discontinuous distribution; this in itself strongly suggests that an interaction of host and environment largely dictates where plague is found. The habitats in which it occurs and the animal

species involved vary tremendously. In the western United States alone, sylvatic plague is maintained in desert and grassland communities, mountain meadows, rock ledges, and fringes of cultivated areas (Eskey and Haas 1940) and involves such diverse wildlife as ground squirrels, wood rats, prairie dogs, chipmunks, marmots, lagomorphs, deer mice, and voles.

An attempt was made by Pavlovsky (1966) nearly 30 years ago to reduce this apparently bewildering complexity to a common denominator for plague and a number of other zoonoses in his concept of the "natural nidality" of disease. This proposes that plague has a natural focal localization within well-defined geographic areas where the pathogen, vectors, and hosts form an ecological association in which, because of certain factors favorable for long-term survival, the organism can circulate for an indefinite period. Here, although epizootics can occur, plague is usually present in a smoldering enzootic form. The interpretation of what constitutes a focus of plague varies with different authors (Stark et al. 1966), but it is probably best thought of as the specific ecological unit in an area where the true reservoiring mechanism perpetuates the organism during interepizootic periods and thus would not include the often much larger area in which plague might be active during an epizootic. In actuality the term is often used much more broadly to include any area where plague evidence is detected, due to the difficulty of delimiting actual boundaries which in themselves may be flexible with time.

In general, conditions favorable for an epizootic of plague are, in addition to the presence of *P. pestis* of sufficient virulence to cause infection, a dense population of susceptible rodents, which upon infection develop a bacteremia, combined with a high index and infestation rate of fleas which are efficient transmitters of the bacillus. But even when these requirements are fulfilled, the disease may not reach epizootic proportions because of the delicate balance between the enzootic and epizootic state. We are actually dealing with a complex interaction of host and parasite within the framework of the environment, creating a dynamic equilibrium wherein minor changes in any of a multitude of influencing factors can tip the balance one way or the other. Some of these factors have been mentioned during the discussion of transmission. Others known or suspected to be influential in plague epizootiology are: the species, subspecies or population of hosts involved, and the age and sex structure of same;

the behavior characteristics of the hosts (degree of sociality, social status within the population, tendency toward and frequency of interspecific contacts); nutritional status with regard to both qualitative and quantitative aspects; movements, mobility, or size of home range of hosts; breeding periods, number of young produced, and rate of population turnover; and fidelity or ubiquity in restriction or choice of habitats and the faunal richness or species diversity of the habitat.

While plague among commensal rats is invariably self-limiting (Pollitzer and Meyer 1961), long-term persistence among wild rodents has been observed by workers all over the world. For instance, Meyer and Eddie (1938) recovered infected ground squirrel fleas from the same burrow systems where diseased ground squirrels were found 20 years before and suggested that sylvatic plague probably persists indefinitely in an area once it has been invaded.

There seems to be consensus that four basic mechanisms are involved in the interepizootic survival and maintenance of *P. pestis* in natural enzootic foci: fleas, soil, hibernating rodents, and association of rodents with a spectrum of susceptibilities to infection. Not all may be operative in any one focus or are all of equal importance.

As noted previously, in many situations fleas are thought to be very important reservoirs as well as vectors due to certain characteristics of wild rodent fleas, especially their ability to retain infection for long periods of time.

Findings in France and Iran (Baltazard et al. 1963) as well as in the United States (Goldenberg and Kartman 1966) indicate that, under the influence of certain microclimatic conditions, the soil itself may serve as a reservoir. It was found that the organism remained viable in soil within unoccupied burrows for many months and could be transmitted to animals coming into contact with this substrate. A hypothesis was forwarded that the remains of dead rodents and fleas and their feces provide the necessary organic material to allow survival of *P. pestis* in deep burrows. This mechanism needs much more investigation before its importance can be assessed, but it is probable that a good potential exists in limited areas where climatic conditions are particularly favorable.

That hibernating rodents may play a role in carrying infection over the winter season was long ago hypothesized and subjected to investigation by workers in several countries (Pollitzer 1954). In various marmots, susliks, and ground squirrels it has been found that if they were infected just before or during the period of torpidity, the infectious process was radically changed, with time to death much prolonged and resistance markedly increased. In many cases the hibernating rodents showed no signs of disease until 4 months later when emerging from hibernation, at which time they sickened and died of typical plague infections. Investigators in the USSR have demonstrated that resistance to plague infection increases in active rodents as the time for hibernation nears (Pavlovsky 1966). While this mechanism is undoubtedly of significance in some plague foci, it is not necessarily essential because there are many areas of entrenched sylvatic plague where hibernating rodents are not part of the community.

Seemingly, the most universal of reservoiring mechanisms is that dependent on the presence in a focus of individuals of varying susceptibility to plague and the circulation of the organism among them (Baltazard 1960; Kartman et al. 1966; Pollitzer and Meyer 1961). The majority of workers (Eskey and Haas 1940) up until the 1950s believed that the primary reservoirs of plague were those species, such as prairie dogs and ground squirrels, which exhibited widespread epizootics and that the occasional finding of *P. pestis* in native mice represented side links in the basic transmission chain. An epizootic among such species, however, often results in a rather complete die-off (Lechleitner et al. 1962) or devastates the population to the point where plague becomes quiescent or absent. Such is not the type of nondestructive, balanced host-parasite relationship that usually evolves between an organism and its maintenance hosts. Neither, however, is the relationship exhibited between plague and completely refractory hosts, since the organisms contacting such hosts meet a dead end because their defense mechanisms do not permit development of a bacteremia which is essential for transmission. Such species may only be indirectly involved in plague perpetuation by providing maintenance blood meals for fleas or by serving as transporters of infected fleas to other susceptible rodents.

Some of the earlier workers in the United States and other countries had noted differences in the relative susceptibility to infection of different populations of the same species of rodents (McCoy 1911; Meyer 1942; Pollizter

1954). Other studies quantitatively assessing the susceptibility of 32 species of native rodents from such widespread geographic areas as New Mexico, Washington, California, and Utah have confirmed that such differences do exist (Bacon and Drake 1958; Holdenried and Quan 1956; Marchette et al. 1962b; Quan and Kartman 1962). These and earlier qualitative studies, summarized in Marchette et al. (1962b), demonstrated not only species variations in susceptibility and differences with regard to sex, age, and season but also differences in the same kind of animal depending on whether they were from areas with or without a previous history of plague. The greater resistance of individuals from populations with previous plague exposure is not believed to be due to active immunity but rather to evolutionary change resulting from natural selection (Quan and Kartman 1962). Another important result of these susceptibility studies was the typically heterogenic response noted among individuals of equivalent experimental groups of animals. Such variation was interpreted by Quan and Kartman (1962) as indicating that the relative susceptibility of populations cannot be applied to individuals, and as a result there will be many resistant individuals in a susceptible population and vice versa.

As a result of the foregoing, emphasis with regard to which rodents constitute vertebrate reservoirs has shifted to those which are resistant to the disease but susceptible to infection with *P. pestis* (Baltazard 1960). In such animals an epizootic could and actually has been shown to sweep through a population without producing clinical disease or excessive mortality and would go completely undetected unless surveys were continually being made and serologic methods used in the diagnosis (Goldenberg et al. 1964; Kartman et al. 1962). These animals, typified by some species of *Peromyscus* and *Microtus* in the United States, while responding with an asymptomatic infection, usually have a transient bacteremia and thus could infect fleas even though their effectiveness in this regard would be less than in rodents dying with terminal septicemia. Whereas persistence of *P. pestis* in the organs of these partially resistant animals for periods of up to 5 weeks after experimental infection and in the field during interepizootic periods has been demonstrated, the significance of this "latent" form of the disease in perpetuation of the organism or in transmission is not clear; only if the bacilli eventually escape the organs and invade the bloodstream

would it have this potential importance (Evans et al. 1943; Holdenried and Quan 1956; Marchette et al. 1962b; Meyer et al. 1943; Quan and Kartman 1962).

It is noteworthy that Payne et al. (1955) as well as other investigators (Pollitzer 1960) found a significant depression of resistance to infection by *P. pestis* in laboratory rats and mice following injection of cortisone or adrenocorticotropic hormone. Death or a generalized infection was observed even from *P. pestis* strains of very low virulence. These findings may have epizootiologic significance in relation to stress induced in wild rodent populations either by adverse environmental factors or sociopsychologically by pathways described by Christian and Davis (1964).

Within a natural focus of plague, survival of *P. pestis* is now generally viewed to depend on the commingling of rodent species of different susceptibilities or of individuals with heterogenic responses within a given species (Kartman et al. 1966; Pollitzer and Meyer 1961). The more resistant individuals infect and maintain fleas and, through ectoparasite exchange, infect susceptible individuals or commensal species; the latter, even though they may succumb, continue the chain by adding to the infected flea population. When the density of susceptibles rises above a certain threshold and other influencing factors are favorable, an epizootic may occur and reduce their numbers; after it has terminated, the infection continues to smolder in the enzootic state in the resistant survivors. A rather clear-cut actual field situation, in which this mechanism is illustrated by a close association of several animal species of variable susceptibilities with transfer of infected fleas from one to another in a mesquite community in southeast New Mexico, is described by Kartman (1960).

Peromyscus maniculatus is a prime example of a rodent species which is capable of acting in this reservoir capacity (Marchette et al. 1962a). In addition to its partial resistance to plague, this species is characterized by a wide geographic distribution, is ubiquitous throughout many habitat types, and is commensal with a variety of other rodent species. Hudson and Kartman (1967) feel that from the consistency with which seropositives are found in this species from many areas, it could be used as an "indicator animal," but they also warn that negative serologic results obtained during a 1-month or one-season sampling period should not be considered evidence that *P. pestis* is absent.

Kartman (1960) aptly sums up the situation concerning which of the reservoiring mechanisms may be operative or more important in a given focus as follows: "In sylvatic plague, mechanisms observed in epizootics cannot be generalized since each focus of the disease constitutes an independent phenomenon and must be investigated as a relatively unique situation. . . . Besides variations in the basic factors, . . . significant differences may occur in the mechanics of sylvatic foci which influence the survival and transmission of the disease in modes peculiar to the given locality at a particular time."

SIGNS, PATHOGENESIS, PATHOLOGY. Relatively few descriptions of the pathologic changes which take place in wild rodents infected with plague have been published. Pollitzer (1960) summarizes the available information for the Asian tarabagans, susliks, and gerbils, and certain of the South American and South African rodents, as well as giving details of the findings in commensal rats and laboratory animals. Pseudotuberculosis and tularemia are the two rodent diseases which might be most readily confused with plague. The gross pathology resulting from both natural and experimentally induced cases in what may be considered a typical species of highly susceptible North American rodent (*Citellus beecheyi*) has been described by McCoy (1911).

McCoy classified the gross pathology observed upon necropsy into three categories:

1. Acute plague: squirrels dying in from 3 to 5 days with one or more hemorrhagic buboes and an enlarged spleen, but no macroscopic lesions in the internal organs.
2. Subacute plague: animals in which death occurred at 6 days or later with caseous buboes without evidence of surrounding hemorrhage and usually with pinpoint, nodular necrotic foci of the spleen, liver, or lungs.
3. Residual (resolving) plague: ground squirrels killed 2–3 weeks following infection in nonlethal cases typically had one or more enlarged lymph glands containing yellow purulent foci.

McCoy called attention to the fact that the lesions of plague are generally quite constant in laboratory animals, but in contrast there is marked diversity, especially in the subacute and resolving form, in the pathology observed among the ground squirrels.

McCoy felt that the variations in pathology reflected variations in the resistance of individual animals and of populations. This has since been confirmed, and workers throughout the world have reported finding an "inapparent" or "latent" form of plague in a variety of species of naturally infected wild rodents characterized by the absence of gross lesions and negative results of direct bacteriologic examination but positive experimental results with the organs of these animals (Pollitzer 1954). Such asymptomatic infections are now believed to be far commoner than previously thought, especially among resistant populations of normally susceptible species or among individuals of species which are typically resistant.

Microtus californicus has been especially well studied in this respect. This species is susceptible to invasion of the organism and its establishment in tissues but usually does not sicken or succumb either in nature or to the experimental inoculation of large numbers of plague bacilli. Although serologic positives may approach 100% in a population, few isolations by either culture or animal inoculation techniques may be made (Goldenberg et al. 1964; Hudson and Kartman 1967; Hudson et al. 1964). It is known that the bacilli persist in *Microtus* for short periods and may resolve into inapparent infections, a situation which has also been noted in other rodent species; in some of these species, however, tissue persistence is quite prolonged (Evans et al. 1943; Holdenried and Quan 1956; Meyer et al. 1943). Goldenberg et al. (1964) stated that the bacilli, after introduction by flea bite, are taken up by the lymphatics, carried to the regional lymph nodes and then to the viscera; after multiplication in these organs, the bacteria appear in the blood. Their isolations of *P. pestis* from the blood and blood-filtering organs in *Microtus* indicate that there is a period of bacteremia. Thus, even in animals with asymptomatic infections, a sporadic or transient bacteremia may provide an opportunity for fleas to become infected (Quan and Kartman 1962). It has been found, however, that some species of resistant rodents (for example, *P. maniculatus* from Utah) often die without a detectable bacteremia (Ecology and Epizoology Research 1963).

DIAGNOSIS. Until 1935 laboratory diagnosis of plague in wild rodents generally consisted of necropsy, with confirmation of gross lesions by microscopic and cultural methods and by inoculation of tissues into guinea pigs. It was not until 1936 that triturated fleas collected from survey animals were routinely inoculated into laboratory animals (Eskey and Haas 1940; Link 1955).

It is impossible to go into all the many facets of plague diagnosis. For additional detail consult American Public Health Association (1963), Baltazard et al. (1956), Goldenberg (1968), Pollitzer (1954, 1960), and Stark et al. (1966).

General diagnostic methods include: culturing of suspect tissue at 25–30°C on blood agar at pH 7.2 or in infusion broth at pH 7.4, microscopic examination of isolated organisms using Gram and Wayson stains, biochemical tests (carbohydrates, urea, desoxycholate-citrate, hydrogen sulfide and indole production, methyl red and methylene blue reduction), specific phage lysis at 25°C, motility tests at 20°C, staining of heat-fixed smears by fluorescent antibody and anti-*pestis* globulin, and subcutaneous inoculation of tissues into white mice and guinea pigs. In the latter, death occurs within 1–5 days with typical pathologic changes: marked infiltration at the site of inoculation, edematous and hemorrhagic buboes in regional lymph nodes, enlargement of the spleen and liver—with both organs often having yellowish, pinpoint, necrotic nodules—and lungs with congestion or areas of consolidation. Smears and impression films made from the heart blood, spleen, liver, and buboes of inoculated guinea pigs usually show great numbers of plague bacilli. The isolation of strains of *P. pestis* which are avirulent for guinea pigs but fully virulent for certain of the native local rodent species (Ecology and Epizoology Research 1963; Marchette 1963) suggests that the latter may be of value as laboratory animals for the isolation of such strains which may be overlooked in a routine survey, when only guinea pigs are employed.

The decayed or mummified carcasses of animals found during field investigations can be tested for the presence of *P. pestis* by use of a modified Ascoli (precipitin) test (Larson et al. 1951) or fluorescent antibody staining techniques (Hudson et al. 1962; Stark et al. 1966). Bone marrow is a useful source of material in such cases.

Goldenberg et al. (1964) have shown that animal inoculation is approximately 3 times more efficient than bacterial culture in obtaining isolations from *Microtus* tissue and have found that approximately 25,000 viable organisms per gram of tissue was the minimum concentration detectable by cultural methods. A similar superiority of animal inoculation techniques has also been shown in detecting plague bacilli in fleas (Quan et al. 1958).

It has only been since the 1960s that highly sensitive and specific serologic methods have been employed with confidence in the retrospective diagnosis of *P. pestis* infection in wild rodents and in detecting natural foci of plague activity. These methods have taken on added importance in view of the difficulty of organism isolation from the relatively resistant rodents now believed to be of primary importance in the maintenance of *P. pestis*. Recent investigators have had considerable success employing the complement fixation and passive hemagglutination tests (Cavanaugh et al. 1965; Hudson and Kartman 1967). Both of these tests employ the FI envelope antigen, recently evaluated by Chen (1966) and prepared according to the method of Baker et al. (1952), and have been adapted to microserologic techniques, so that as little as 0.05 ml or less of serum is required. The majority of investigators feel that the hemagglutination test is superior to the complement fixation test on the basis of sensitivity, ease of performance, and the fact that the frequent occurrence of anticomplementary activity in wild rodent sera often presents difficulties in the complement fixation test. It also has an advantage in detecting enzootic areas since the antibodies detected are more persistent than those determined by complement fixation; the latter appear earlier and disappear more quickly and are thus more indicative of recent infections (Cavanaugh et al. 1965; Hudson and Kartman 1967; Hudson et al. 1964).

Hudson et al. (1964), using the passive hemagglutination test, found positive reactors in from 65–100% of the *M. californicus* trapped during successive plague epizootics in a California study area and present data on average titers, antibody persistence, seasonal incidence, and serologic histories of individual animals. Although this test is quite specific, it is not absolutely so, since antigens of certain *P. pseudotuberculosis* strains may give cross-reactions (Quan et al. 1965). Hudson and Kartman (1967) caution that it is necessary to examine serologic results in the light of known background information concerning the susceptibility of the animal species involved, the previous history of a given area with respect to the occurrence of plague, and concurrent isolation of *P. pestis* from host and vector populations.

It was previously noted that *P. maniculatus* might serve as a sentinel or indicator animal for the presence of plague in an area. Dogs and other carnivores, considered highly resistant to plague, may serve this same function. During the 1965 plague outbreak among prairie dogs on the Navajo Indian Reservation in New Mexico, 13 of 27 dogs tested gave positive results with the passive hemagglutination test; seropositive dogs were associated with 4 of the human cases in this outbreak (Kartman et al. 1967). The only evidence of plague activity in connection with a fatal human case in southeast Utah during 1966 was the finding of positive titers in 2 of the family dogs (Ecology and Epizoology Research, unpublished data, 1966). Hudson and Kartman (1967) note that 3 of 4 dogs associated with a human case in Arizona during 1963 had positive titers, as did dogs from their California plague study area where *Microtus* was primarily involved.

CONTROL. With enzootic plague firmly entrenched in wild rodents over vast areas, control measures are ordinarily undertaken only as emergency steps, with limited objectives in those situations where a high potential exists for transfer of *P. pestis* from sylvatic sources to humans or where a sentinel human case has occurred. In such instances a program combining medical surveillance, publicity and education, flea control, and rodent suppression is most likely to achieve the desired results.

Control measures have almost invariably been directed at the conspicuous, highly susceptible epizootic hosts of the disease such as ground squirrels, marmots, and chipmunks. Such efforts, even if successful, do not lead to elimination of plague from the area, since these animals are not the ones involved in the maintenance function. These efforts can, however, lead to a reduction in the potential for human infection since it is these epizootic hosts rather than the enzootic reservoir mice which have been the principal sylvatic sources of human infections (Murray 1964).

In general, measures taken to reduce the human plague potential in an area should be directed against the flea vectors as well as against the vertebrate hosts; flea control itself has become an important technique in combating plague by interfering with or breaking the normal rodent-flea-rodent transmission chain. If rodent control alone is practiced, the situation may be made worse since large numbers of hungry fleas may remain, which potentially could shift from their normal hosts to man or would attack new rodent hosts as soon as they entered the area; under conditions of high population pressure this might be an immediate influx.

In relatively small areas of high human exposure such as campgrounds and national parks, the insecticide–bait-box method (Barnes and Kartman 1960) of reducing flea infestations on rodents has been effectively employed. The bait box consists of a board, heavily covered with 10% DDT dust or 5% malathion dust, baited with a pan of rolled oats or other attractants in the center, and covered with a tin roof for protection from the weather. Rodents can enter from either end, become dusted with the insecticide and carry some back to their burrows, thereby reducing both body and nest fleas.

For larger areas, 5% malathion at 0.5 pounds per acre, 10% DDT, or other residuals such as dieldrin, aldrin, heptachlor, or benzene hexachloride may be applied by direct dusting of burrows with hand dusters; area application of the insecticides from aircraft or vehicle-mounted power dusters may be effective (Miles and Wilcomb 1953; Ryckman et al. 1953, 1954). Rodent control—when deemed necessary, preferably immediately following or concurrent with flea control—can be achieved by a variety of methods, including fumigation of individual burrows with carbon bisulfide or hydrocyanic gas or burrow or area application of bait containing sodium fluoroacetate (Compound 1080) or other poisons.

The published accounts of the tremendous efforts put forth to eliminate or control sylvatic plague over vast areas in the USSR, by exterminating rodents and fleas in zones where natural foci exist, have been compiled and reviewed by Pollitzer (1966). The unsuccessful attempts in the early 1900s to eliminate plague by eradication of ground squirrels in California are described by Link (1955). Murray (1964) has reviewed the current philosophy of plague suppression in California which embodies a flexible program of rodent and flea control based on zoning of the state according to degrees of epizootic hazard. Tirador et al. (1967) have described the considerations and the methods used to reduce the plague potential during a 1965 outbreak among prairie dogs associated with six human cases on the Navajo Indian Reservation in New Mexico.

REFERENCES

American Public Health Association. *Diagnostic procedures and reagents*. New York: Am. Public Health Assoc., 1963.

Bacon, M., and Drake, C. H. Comparative susceptibility of various species of mice native to Washington to inoculation with virulent strains of *Pasteurella pestis*. *J. Infect. Dis.* 102:14–22, 1958.

Bacot, A. W., and Martin, C. J. Observations on the mechanism of the transmission of plague by fleas. *J. Hyg.* 13 (plague sup. 3):423–439, 1914.

Baker, E. E., Sommer, H., Foster, L. E., Meyer, E., and Meyer, K. F. Studies on immunization against plague: I. The isolation and characterization of the soluble antigen of *Pasteurella pestis*. *J. Immunol.* 68:132–145, 1952.

Baltazard, M. Epidemiology of plague. *WHO Chron.* 14:419–426, 1960.

Baltazard, M., Davis, D. H. S., Devignat, R., Girard, G., Gohar, M. A., Kartman, L., Meyer, K. F., Parker, M. T., Pollitzer, R., Prince, F. M., Quan, S. F., and Wagle, P. Recommended laboratory methods for the diagnosis of plague. *Bull. WHO* 14:457–509, 1956.

Baltazard, M., Karimi, Y., Eftekhari, M., Chamsa, M., and Mollaret, H. H. La conservation inter-epizootique de la peste en foyer invetere. Hypotheses de travail. *Bull. Soc. Pathol. Exot.* 56:1230–1241, 1963.

Barnes, A., M., and Kartman, L. Control of plague vectors on diurnal rodents in the Sierra Nevada of California by use of insecticide bait-boxes. *J. Hyg.* 58:347–355, 1960.

Bibikova, V. A., and Gavryushina, A. I. The multiplication of *P. pestis* in fleas feeding on plague-immune gerbils. Materials from the Scientific Conference on the Natural Nidality and Prophylaxis of Plague (translation), Alma-Ata, pp. 25–26, Feb. 1963.

Brubaker, R. R., Beesley, E. D., and Surgalla, M. J. *Pasteurella pestis*: Role of Pesticin I and iron in experimental plague. *Science* 149:422–424, 1965.

Burrows, T. W., and Bacon, G. A. The basis of virulence in *Pasteurella pestis B. J. Exp. Pathol.* 37:481–493, 1956.

Calhoun, J. B. The ecology and sociology of the Norway rat. U.S. Public Health Service publ. 1008, 1963.

Cavanaugh, D. C., Thorpe, B. D., Bushman, J. B., Nicholes, P. S., and Rust, J. H., Jr. Detection of an enzootic plague focus by serological methods. *Bull. WHO* 32:197–203, 1965.

Chen, T. H. An evaluation of *Pasteurella pestis* Fraction-1-specific antibody for the confirmation of plague infection. *Bull. WHO* 34:911–918, 1966.

Christian, J. J., and Davis, D. E. Endocrines, behavior, and population. *Science* 146:1550–1560, 1964.

Ecology and Epizoology Research. Summary status report on *Pasteurella pestis* 1952–1962. University of Utah, Ecol. Epizool. ser. 92, 1963.

Eskey, C. F., and Haas, V. H. Plague in the western part of the United States. *U.S. Public Health Bull.* 254, 1940.

Evans, F. C., Wheeler, C. M., and Douglas, J. R. Sylvatic plague studies: III. An epizootic of plague among ground squirrels in Kern County, California. *J. Infect. Dis.* 72:68–76, 1943.

Goldenberg, M. I. Laboratory diagnosis of plague infection. *Health Lab. Sci.* 5:38–45, 1968.

Goldenberg, M. I., and Kartman, L. Role of soil in the ecology of *Pasteurella pestis*. *Bacteriol. Proc.* 1966:54, 1966.

Goldenberg, M. I., Quan, S. F., and Hudson, B. W. The detection of inapparent infections with *Pasteurella pestis* in a *Microtus californicus* population in the San Francisco Bay area. *Zoonoses Res.* 3:1–13, 1964.

Hirst, L. G. *The conquest of plague*. London: Oxford Univ. Press, 1953.

Holdenried, R., and Quan, S. F. Susceptibility of New Mexico rodents to experimental plague. *Public Health Rep.* 71:979–984, 1956.

Hubbard, C. A. *Fleas of western North America*. Ames: Iowa State University Press, 1947.

Hubbert, W. T., Goldenberg, M. I., Kartman, L., and Prince, F. M. Public health potential of sylvatic plague. *J. Am. Vet. Med. Assoc.* 149:1651–1654, 1966.

Hudson, B. W., and Kartman, L. The use of the passive hemagglutination test in epidemiologic investigation of sylvatic plague in the United States. *Bull. Wildlife Disease Assoc.* 3:50–59, 1967.

Hudson, B. W., Quan, S. F., and Kartman, L. Efficacy of fluorescent antibody methods for detection of *Pasteurella pestis* in carcasses of albino laboratory mice stored for various periods. *J. Hyg.* 60:443–450, 1962.

Hudson, B. W., Quan, S. F., and Goldenberg, M. I. Serum antibody responses in a population of *Microtus californicus* and associated rodent species during and after *Pasteurella pestis* epizootics in the San Francisco Bay area. *Zoonoses Res.* 3:15–29, 1964.

Jellison, W. L., and Good, N. E. Index to the literature of the Siphonaptera of North America. U.S. Public Health Serv. Natl. Inst. Health Bull. 178, 1942.

Jellison, W. L., Locker, B., and Bacon, R. F. Index to the literature of Siphonaptera of North America. *Wild. Dis. J.* 4:1–201, 1960.

Kartman, L. The concept of vector efficiency in experimental studies of plague. *Exp. Parasitol.* 6:599–609, 1957.

———. The role of rabbits in sylvatic plague epidemiology, with special attention to human cases in New Mexico and use of the fluorescent antibody technique for detection of *Pasteurella pestis* in field specimens. *Zoonoses Res.* 1:169–195, 1960.

Kartman, L., Prince, F. M., Quan, S. F., and Stark, H. E. New knowledge on the ecology of sylvatic plague. *Ann. N.Y. Acad. Sci.* 70:688–711, 1958.

Kartman, L., Quan, S. F., and Stark, H. E. Ecological studies of wild rodent plague in the San Francisco Bay area of California: VII. Effects of plague in nature on *Microtus californicus* and other wild rodents. *Zoonoses Res.* 1:99–119, 1962.

Kartman, L., Goldenberg, M. I., and Hubbert, W. T. Recent observations on the epidemiology of plague in the United States. *Am. J. Public Health* 56:1554–1569, 1966.

Kartman, L., Martin, A. R., Hubbert, W. T., Collins, R. M., and Goldenberg, M. I. Plague epidemic in New Mexico, 1965. Epidemiologic features and results of field studies. *Public Health Rep.* 82:1084–1094, 1967.

Lamb, G. The etiology and epidemiology of plague. A summary of the work of the Plague Research Commission. Supt. Govt. Printing, Calcutta, India, 1908.

Larson, C. L., Philip, C. B., Wicht, W. C., and Hughes, L. E. Precipitin reactions with soluble antigens from suspensions of *Pasteurella pestis* or from tissues of animals dead of plague. *J. Immunol.* 67:289–298, 1951.

Lechleitner, R. R., Tileston, J. V., and Kartman, L. Die-off of a Gunnison's prairie dog colony in central Colorado: I. Ecological observations and description of the epizootic. *Zoonoses Res.* 1:185–199, 1962.

Link, V. B. A history of plague in the United States of America. U.S. Public Health Monograph 26, 1955.

Machiavello, A. Reservoirs and vectors of plague. *J. Trop. Med. Hyg.* 57:45–48, 65–69, 87–94, 1954.

Marchette, M. J. *Pasteurella pestis* of low virulence for mice and guinea pigs isolated from a *Peromyscus* plague focus in Utah. *Am. J. Trop. Med. Hyg.* 12:215–218, 1963.

Marchette, N. J., Bushman, J. B., Parker, D. D., and Johnson, E. E. Studies on infectious diseases in wild animals in Utah: IV. A wild rodent (*Peromyscus* spp.) plague focus in Utah. *Zoonoses Res.* 1:341–361, 1962a.

Marchette, N. J., Lundgren, D. L., Nicholes, P. S., Bushman, J. B., and Vest, D. Studies on infectious diseases in wild animals in Utah: II. Susceptibility of wild mammals to experimental plague. *Zoonoses Res.* 1:225–250, 1962b.

McCoy, G. W. Studies upon plague in ground squirrels. Public Health Bull. 43, 1911.

Meyer, K. F. The known and the unknown in plague. *Am. J. Trop. Med.* 22:9–36, 1942.

———. Relation of diseases in lower animals to human welfare: Prevention of plague in the light of newer knowledge. *Ann. N.Y. Acad. Sci.* 48:429–467, 1947.

———. Plague. In T. G. Hull, ed., *Diseases transmitted from animals to man*, pp. 527–587. Springfield, Ill.: Charles C. Thomas, 1963.

———. *Pasteurella* and *Francisella*. In R. J. Dubos and J. G. Hirsch, eds., *Bacterial and mycotic infections of man*, pp. 659–697. Philadelphia: Lippincott, 1965.

Meyer, K. F., and Eddie, B. Persistence of sylvatic plague. *Proc. Soc. Exp. Biol. Med.* 38:333–334, 1938.

Meyer, K. F., Holdenried, R., Burroughs, A. L., and Jawetz, E. Sylvatic plague studies: IV. Inapparent, latent sylvatic plague in ground squirrels

in central California. *J. Infect. Dis.* 73:144–157, 1943.

Miles, V. I., and Wilcomb, M. J. Control of native rodent fleas with DDT applied to simulate aerial dusting. *J. Econ. Entomol.* 46:255–257, 1953.

Murry, K. F. The evolution of plague control in California. Proc. 2nd Vert. Pest Control Conf., Anaheim, Calif., pp. 143–149, 1964.

Pan American Health Organization. Plague in the Americas. Pan Am. Sanit. Bur., WHO, Washington, D.C., Sci. Publ. 115, 1965.

Pavlovsky, E. N. *Natural nidality of transmissible diseases*. Urbana: Univ. Ill. Press, 1966.

Payne, F. E., Larson, K. F. Studies on immunization against plague: IX. The effect of cortisone on mouse resistance to attenuated strains of *Pasteurella pestis*. *J. Infect. Dis.* 96:168–173, 1955.

Pollitzer, R. Plague studies—7. Insect vectors. *Bull. WHO* 7:231–342, 1952.

———. Plague. WHO Monogr. Ser. 22, Geneva, 1954.

———. A review of recent literature on plague. *Bull. WHO* 23:313–400, 1960.

———. *Plague and plague control in the Soviet Union, history and bibliography through 1964.* Fordham Univ., New York: Institute of Contemporary Russian Studies, 1966.

Pollitzer, R., and Meyer, K. F. The ecology of plague. In J. M. May, ed., *Studies in disease ecology*, pp. 433–590. New York: Hafner, 1961.

Quan, S. F., and Kartman, L. Ecological studies of wild rodent plague in the San Franciso Bay area of California: VIII. Susceptibility of wild rodents to experimental plague infection. *Zoonoses Res.* 1:121–144, 1962.

Quan, S. F., Von Fintel, H., and McManus, A. G. Ecological studies of wild rodent plague in the San Francisco Bay area of California: II. Efficiency of bacterial culture compared to animal inoculation as methods for detecting *Pasteurella pestis* in wild rodent fleas. *Am. J. Trop. Med. Hyg.* 7:411–415, 1958.

Quan, S. F., Knapp, W., Goldenberg, M. I., Hudson, B. W., Lawton, W. D., Chen, T. H., and Kartman, L. Isolation of a strain of *Pasteurella pestis*: An immunofluorescent false positive. *Am. J. Trop. Med. Hyg.* 14:424–432, 1965.

Rust, J. H., Jr., Cavanaugh, D. C., Kadis, S., and Ajl, S. J. Plague toxin: Its effect in vitro and in vivo. *Science* 142:408–409, 1963.

Ryckman, R. E., Ames, C. T., and Lindt, C. C. A comparison of aldrin, dieldrin, heptachlor and DDT for control of plague vectors on the California ground squirrel. *J. Econ. Entomol.* 46:598–601, 1953.

Ryckman, R. E., Ames, C. T., Lindt, C. C., and Lee, R. D. Control of plague vectors on California ground squirrels by burrow dusting with insecticides and the seasonal incidence of fleas present. *J. Econ. Entomol.* 47:604–7, 1954.

Stark, H. E. The Siphonaptera of Utah. U.S. Public Health Serv., Atlanta, Ga., 1958.

Stark, H. E., Hudson, B. W., and Pittman, B. Plague epidemiology. U.S. Public Health Serv., Atlanta,

Georgia, 1966.

Surgalla, M. J. Properties of virulent and avirulent strains of *Pasteurella pestis*. *Ann. N.Y. Acad. Sci.* 88:1136–1145, 1960.

Tirador, D. F., Miller, B. E., Stacy, J. W., Martin, A. R., Kartman, L., Collins, R. N., and Brutsche, R. L. Plague epidemic in New Mexico, 1965. An emergency program to control plague. *Public Health Rept.* 82:1094–1099, 1967.

U.S. Public Health Service. Rat-borne disease prevention and control. Communicable Disease Center, Atlanta, 1949.

———. Morbidity and mortality reports. National Communicable Disease Center, USDHEW, 15:169–453, 1966.

———. Morbidity and mortality reports. National Communicable Disease Center, USDHEW, 16:222–420, 1967.

Wayson, N. E. Plague—field surveys in western United States during ten years (1936–1945). *Public Health Rep.* 67:780–791, 1947.

World Health Organization. Weekly epidemiological reports, no. 20, 1967.

Wheeler, C. M., and Douglas, J. R. Sylvatic plague studies: V. The determination of vector efficiency. *J. Infect. Dis.* 77:1–12, 1945.

20 *Pasteurellosis*

MERTON N. ROSEN

Synonyms: **Hemorrhagic septicemia, shipping fever (cattle), swine plague (swine), snuffles (rabbits), bluebag (sheep), and barbone (buffalo).**

Pasteurellosis is an infectious bacterial disease of wild and domestic animals; the etiologic agent is *Pasteurella multocida*. Clinical manifestations of infection include generalized hemorrhagic septicemia, pneumonia, meningitis, mastitis, and arthritis. Epizootics of pasteurellosis occasionally occur among wild mammals.

HISTORY AND DISTRIBUTION. It is surmised from Bollinger's (1978) descriptions of pathology that he studied epizootics of hemorrhagic septicemia among deer, wild boar, and domestic cattle (Gay 1935). Kitt (1885; quoted in Hagan 1966) described the bacteria in the blood of diseased cattle, and he designated the organism *Bacterium bipolare multicidum*. The classification of this bacterial species changed many times (Topley and Wilson 1931; Trevisan 1887), but finally the name *Pasteurella multocida* Trevisan was accepted and adopted as the type species of the genus *Pasteurella* (Buchanan and Gibbons 1974; Rosenbusch and Merchant 1939).

Generally the term "pasteurellosis" refers to infection of livestock by *P. multocida* or *P. hemolytica*. The isolation of *P. hemolytica* from the blood of a man who was injured while cleaning a deer provided indirect evidence of this organism's occurrence in wildlife (King 1964). Three of five opossums trapped in the wild as part of an experimental survey were found to be infected with *P. hemolytica* and their subsequent death was attributed to this organism. One had lesions in the pericardium, and the other two had lung abscesses (Kaye et al. 1973).

Various wild species have been afflicted with pasteurellosis (Table 20.1). Knowledge of the range of hosts for *P. multocida* has been increased by observations of pasteurellosis among diverse animals in zoos (Table 20.2). A lion (*Felis leo*), panther (*F. pardus*), and opossum (*Didelphis virginiana*) were incriminated as carriers of *P. multocida* when human infec-

tions developed after individuals were bitten by these animals (Hubbert and Rosen 1970).

Schipper (1947) examined 102 wild rats (*Rattus norvegicus*) and found 14 with *P. multocida*. The Norway rat not only carried the organism but also was resistant to intraperitoneal inoculation of 0.5 ml of an undiluted culture. The albino laboratory rat was resistant to a similar experimental exposure, but the cotton rat (*Sigmodon hispidus*) was highly susceptible. In Moscow, Ponomareva and Rodkevich (1964) examined 156,000 rodents and isolated *P. multocida* from 85 rats, 37 house mice, 6 common voles, 8 field mice, 2 moles, and 1 bank vole.

Semiotrochev et al. (1965) reported a human case where the patient acquired infection while cleaning wild hares prior to cooking. An epizootic was present at the time among the wild hares.

Quortrup (1942) fed the liver and other tissues of a mule deer (*Odocoileus hemionus*) that had died of hemorrhagic septicemia to two coyotes (*Canis latrans*) and one bobcat (*Lynx* spp.) without provoking clinical disease. He concluded that the Canidae and Felidae were not susceptible. However, Schipper (1947) shaved the abdomen of a dog and allowed two rats that were carrying the organism to bite through the skin. The dog died 23 days later from pasteurellosis. He also reported that cats have suffered from the disease. As more work is done in the field of wildlife diseases and presumptive diagnoses are confirmed with refined bacteriologic techniques, it probably will be demonstrated the all species of vertebrate animals may either harbor *P. multocida* or have the frank disease caused by this organism.

Pasteurellosis has a worldwide distribution. This has been documented by reports from many countries of domestic and wild animals infected with *P. multocida*, for example, the kangaroo in Australia, water buffalo in Asia, moles of the Soviet Union, cattle of Central Africa (Carter 1967).

ETIOLOGY. *Pasteurella multocida* is a small, occasionally pleomorphic, gram-negative coccobacillus. Typically, it is 0.3–1.25 μ long; is usually single, but may occur in pairs, infre-

TABLE 20.1 Wildlife Reported with Pasteurellosis in the Wild.

Common Name	Scientific Name	Location	Reference
Bighorn sheep	*Ovis canadensis canadensis*	Wyoming	Honess and Frost 1942; Honess and Winter 1956
Bison	*Bison bison*	Yellowstone, Wy.	Gochenour 1924
Black-tailed deer	*O. hemionus columbianus*	California	Rosen 1952; Brunetti 1952
Caribou	*Rangifer* spp.	Canada	Carter and Bain 1960
Chipmunk	*Eutamias* spp.	Canada	Carter and Bain 1960
Deer	species unknown	Germany	Bollinger 1878
Elephant	*Elephas maximus*	Ceylon	DeAlwis and Thambithurai 1965
Elk	*Cervus canadensis*	Jackson Hole, Wy.	Murie 1951
Kangaroo	*Macropus* spp.	Australia	Young 1965
Mink	*Mustela vison*	Germany	Linsert 1940
Mule deer	*O. hemionus hemionus*	Utah	Quortrup 1942
Muskrat	*Ondatra zibethica*	Canada	Carter and Bain 1960
Puma	*Felis concolor*	Poland	Golebrowski et al. 1972
Rabbit	*Lepus europaeus*	Switzerland	Bouvier 1946
Raccoon	*Procyon lotor*	Missouri	Bond et al. 1972
Red fox	*Vulpes vulpes*	Missouri	Bond et al. 1972
Sea lion	*Zalophus californianus*	Washington	Keyes, personal communication, 1968
Wallaby	*Macropus* spp.	Australia	Young 1965
Weasel	*Mustela* spp.	California	Rosen and Morse 1959
White-tailed deer	*Odocoileus virginianus*	Minnesota	Fenstermacher et al. 1943; Erickson et al. 1961
Wild swine	*Sus scrofa*	Germany	Bollinger 1878
		USSR	Mel'nikova and Mel'nikova 1960

TABLE 20.2 Host Range of Captive Wildlife with Pasteurellosis.

Common Name	Scientific Name	Reference
Axis deer	*Axis axis*	Fox 1926
Gazelle	*Gazella* spp.	Fox 1929
Greater kudu	*Strepsiceros strepsiceros*	Fox 1923
Nilgai	*Boselaphus tragocamelus*	Fox 1934
Sable antelope	*Egoceros niger*	Hamerton 1931
Mink	*Mustela vison*	Popovici et al. 1972

Note: Does not include domesticated animals such as reindeer, dromedary, water buffalo of Asia, or species given in Table 20.2.

quently in short chains, and rarely in filaments; and is nonmotile. Wright, Giemsa, methylene blue, or carbol fuchsin stains will demonstrate the characteristic bipolar morphology of the organism which Gram stain tends to obscure.

Pasteurella multocida will grow on ordinary nutrient agar; however, more luxuriant growth is obtained with enriched media such as dextrose starch agar. Serum added to the medium may further enhance growth. The colonies on agar are small, round, and translucent. In broth cultures an even turbidity throughout the medium is evident.

The optimum temperature for *P. multocida* is 37°C, although it will grow from 20–45°C. The organism is aerobic to facultatively anaerobic and has an optimum pH requirement of 7.2 with a range of 6.0–8.5.

Typical biochemical reactions of *P. multocida* and *P. hemolytica* are given in Table 20.3. Some of the biochemical characteristics of different isolates of *P. multocida* may vary (Buchanan and Gibbons 1974). For example, some strains produce traces of sulfide which are detectable only on lead acetate paper, and Gochenour (1924) reported that Yellowstone bison isolates did not reduce nitrates or form indol.

Differentiation of *P. multocida* strains was initially based on fermentation reactions (Khalifa 1954; Rosenbusch and Merchant 1939). Considerable variation exists, so that there may not be a natural grouping derived from selected biochemical reactions (Das 1958; Russa 1939); and Bain (1957) indicated that it is unnecessary

for the biochemical and serologic results to coincide in the grouping of strains. There are many combinations of the fermentation reactions of *P. multocida* strains (Heddleston 1976). All the biochemical actitivies have been compared by electronic computer analysis, and with this technique the isolates may be used to indicate the epizootiology and specific transmission among animal species (Talbot and Sneath 1960).

When isolated from an animal that has recently succumbed to pasteurellosis, *P. multocida* generally is encapsulated. However, after continuous subculture on artificial media the organisms tend to lose their capsules. The loss of capsule is soon followed by autolysis of some strains, so that it is necessary to resort to animal passage if the strain is to be kept viable. Restoration of capsule may be accomplished by serial passage of the bacteria in mice. Lyophilization or suspension of the organisms in normal serum and holding them at −20°C or lower will ensure their viability.

The colonial morphology is influenced by the presence or lack of a capsule and the capsule's size and composition. Carter (1957) standardized the designation of the colonial variants as large mucoid, smooth small iridescent, smooth gray blue noniridescent, and rough. The mucoid colonies are composed of organisms having the largest capsules.

Virulence is related to the colonial morphology of *P. multocida*: smooth iridescent colonies are almost always pathogenic for mice,

TABLE 20.3   Identification of *Pasteurella*.

Reaction	*P. multocida*	*P. haemolytica*	*P. ureae*
Motility	−	−	−
Growth on MacConkey	−	d	−
Potassium cyanide	+	d	−
Glucose (acid) no gas	+	+	+
Xylose (acid) no gas	d	+	−
Lactose (acid) no gas	−	d	−
Sucrose (acid) no gas	(+)	+	+
Glycerol (acid) no gas	−	d	−
Mannitol (acid) no gas	+	+	+
Sorbitol (acid) no gas	d	d	+
Indole	+	−	−
Urease	−	−	+
Lysine decarboxylase	−	−	−
Arginine dihydrolase	−	−	−
Ornithine decarboxylase	+	d	−
Hemolysis	−	+	+

Source: Cowan and Steel 1965.
Legend: + ± 80-100%; d = 21-79%; − = 0-20; ( ) = delayed.

mucoid and noniridescent vary, and rough colonies have a low virulence for mice (Carter 1967).

There is considerable variation in the virulence of the particular strain of organism for different species of animals. For example, my isolate from a black-tailed deer (*Odocoileus hemionus*) would not infect ducks or coots but was pathogenic for laboratory mice. All my isolates from avian cholera epornitics have been extremely virulent for mice.

TRANSMISSION. The means of transmission of pasteurellosis is a matter of speculation. One thesis is that *P. multocida* is an obligate parasite, localized as a potential pathogen in the respiratory tracts of carrier animals. Just prior to an outbreak the carrier rate may rise precipitously (Webster 1924). When physiologic stresses are applied to a herd—such as poor forage conditions, crowding on a deer winter range, or inclement weather—the host's resistance is lowered, possibly the bacteria's virulence increases, and clinical disease ensues. On a mink farm with bad hygienic conditions, transmission occurred by cannibalism (Popovici et al. 1972). The experimental inoculation of cortisone, which is released in greater quantity during times of stress, changed latent infections of *P. multocida* in rats to an acute disease terminating in death (Carter and Bain 1960).

A second theory is that the ubiquitous distribution of this bacterial species in the throats of many varieties of animals, including man, suggests that it is part of the normal flora of the upper respiratory tract (Hubbert and Rosen 1967). The organism would be categorized as an opportunist or secondary invader when infection occurs. This is given support by reports that pneumonia in cattle and swine was initiated by parainfluenza 3 virus followed by *P. multocida* invasion, with subsequent infection (Reisinger 1962).

Regardless of the status of the organism during quiescent periods, when it does multiply it contaminates the environment through the saliva and feces which contain myriads of *Pasteurella* (Hudson 1959). Droplet infection or ingestion are presumed to be the principal means of transmission, despite studies that have been done to incriminate insect vectors (Daubney et al. 1934).

SIGNS. As with most diseases in wildlife, particularly those of an acute or peracute nature, signs are rarely observed. Animals are found dead, or on rare occasion the last agonal stages

of the disease are seen. During an epizootic in California, affected deer were usually found dead, but two prostrate does were observed with nasal and oral mucous discharges.

Signs in bighorn sheep were characteristic of a pleuropneumonia. A bighorn ram, observed 1 week prior to death, was emaciated and barely able to move; when it did walk it had an odd, stiltlike gait. At necropsy there was a mucous discharge from the nostrils (Potts 1937). Other reports of bighorn sheep with pasteurellosis mention the mucous flow from the nose with or without bleeding, coughing, and dyspnea (Marsh 1927, 1938; Post 1962).

PATHOGENESIS AND PATHOLOGY. The portal of entry of *P. multocida* is the respiratory tract. The organism resides in the throats of normal or carrier animals; Bond et al. (1972) swabbed the throats, teeth, and tonsillar fossae of 12 raccoons and 2 red foxes and isolated *P. multocida* from 5 of the raccoons and 1 of the foxes. Opportunity for invasion either follows a period of physiologic stress or is a secondary complication to an initial incitant such as a virus of a nematode. The disease has been endemic among Norwegian reindeer with subclinical carriers. A predisposing factor is lungworm (*Dictyocaulus viviparous*) infection. Spread through the herd is by direct contact, flies, and pastures contaminated with nasal discharges (Kummeneje 1976). Many of the early reports on the disease in bighorn sheep (Post 1962) either attribute the cause of death to occlusion of the bronchioles by lungworms (*Protostrongylus stilesi*) or to a pneumonia-lungworm complex. The latter situation was the case in two instances involving deer in California where *Paraelaphostrongylus odocoilei* was present in great numbers in the lungs and *P. multocida* invaded the parenchyma and established a septicemia (Brunetti 1952). It may be argued that a high lungworm burden is a manifestation of lowered resistance in the animal due to inadequate environmental needs and that under these conditions hemorrhagic septicemia could occur with or without the helminths.

So far as is known, there have been no isolations from wildlife of the myxovirus which in domestic livestock is incriminated, along with *P. multocida*, in the pathogenesis of shipping fever. Parainfluenza 3 virus was eliminated by serologic examination as a contributing pathogen in an outbreak of hemorrhagic septicemia in reindeer (Nordkvist and Karlsson 1962).

Pasteurellosis may assume two separate

but overlapping courses which influence the pathology. The thoracic or respiratory syndrome is a pneumonia with hemorrhages in the lungs, trachea, and, on occasion, the nasal mucosa. Hemorrhagic septicemia is the acute type of disease, wherein the organisms are carried by the general circulation to all of the internal organs; and on occasion the blood-brain barrier is breached, with subsequent central nervous system involvement. The vascular system is engorged and petechial hemorrhages occur in various tissues. Chronic pasteurellosis and snuffles in rabbits may be characterized by necrotic areas or subcutaneous abscesses (Carter 1967).

The pathology in mink appears as a distinctly hemorrhagic condition, with bleeding from the nostrils and trachea, hemorrhages in the lungs, and petechiae on the heart surface. The mink have a catarrhal enteritis (Lewis 1929).

Bison afflicted with pasteurellosis have hemorrhagic lungs, pleura, and pericardium. The musculature of the body is pink and edematous. Although the lumph nodes are swollen and hemorrhagic, the spleen is normal except for hemorrhagic areas beneath the capsule (Gochenour 1924).

At necropsy, black-tailed deer had typical lesions of pneumonia, exudate in the pleural cavity, and red hepatization in the lung. The spleen was apparently normal, although *P. multocida* was isolated from it. Histopathologic examination revealed cloudy swelling in the kidneys and liver, with islands of bacteria in the sinusoids (Brunetti 1967). Fibrinoid degeneration in the glomerular capillaries was observed in reindeer that had died of pasteurellosis (Nordkvist and Karlsson 1962).

DIAGNOSIS. A definite diagnosis of pasteurellosis is based on the pathologic findings, together with isolation of the causative organism and its identification through biochemical reactions.

PROGNOSIS. Recovery from acute or subacute pasteurellosis is unlikely, because the fulminating infection causes death so quickly. The chance for survival is increased if the animal has a chronic form of the disease, especially when the infection is localized (Hudson 1959).

The extent of an outbreak is governed by such predisposing factors as exposure to severe winter conditions, condition of the animals at the time they enter the winter range, the winter range itself, the degree of crowding, and other physiologic stresses. Quortrup (1942) stated that 59 deer died of pasteurellosis on an overcrowded range in Utah, but he did not indicate what portion of the herd succumbed. Murie (1951) suggested that pasteurellosis was not a serious problem in elk. On the other hand, Post (1962) implicated pasteurellosis as a possible contributing factor in the great decline in the bighorn sheep population throughout the Rocky Mountain area. He documented this conclusion by citing Marsh (1927), who claimed that the herd on the Sun River Game Preserve in Montana was reduced from 250 to 65 sheep by a disease that caused coughing and slight bleeding from the nostrils. Later, pneumonia was given as the cause of death of lambs in the National Bison Range, Montana (Marsh 1938). Despite the presence of *P. multocida* and *Corynebacterium pyogenes*, the losses were attributed to nematodes with the bacteria as secondary invaders.

The prognosis must be based on all the above factors, with due consideration given to the virulence of the organism and the presence or absence of lungworms. As with a worm burden, the morbidity is a reflection of forage conditions, and range managers may be able to forecast the extent of the epizootic if all the biological information is available to them. It may be surmised that in most instances outbreaks are sporadic and not likely to recur annually.

IMMUNITY

Serology. The importance of pasteurellosis to the poultry and livestock industry prompted the search for effective immunizing antigens. Failure of some strains to immunize effectively prompted many workers to attempt serologic typing of strains. Practical application of serologic typing for effective vaccine production is not the only important consideration. Another reason for typing is to aid in the investigation of the epizootiology of the disease. Laboratory methods used ran the gamut from the plate and tube agglutination, precipitin, capsular swelling, complement fixation, indirect hemagglutination, fluorescent antibody, mouse serum protection, and Ouchterlony double diffusion tests through bacteriophage and immunoelectrophoresis (Carter 1967; Carter and Bain 1960; Prince and Smith 1966a,b,c; Roberts 1947).

Little and Lyon (1943) separated three serologic types by the plate agglutination test. Carter (1958) refuted their claim on the basis of autoagglutination in saline and interference by the bacterial capsule. Despite his plea to abandon the technique, some workers continued to rely on it (Dorsey 1963a,b; Heddleston 1966; Namioka and Murata 1961a,b,c). Roberts (1947) separated four groups of *P. multocida* by a serum protection test for mice. His groupings were confirmed with a hemagglutination test in which capsular antigen was used to sensitize human O type erythrocytes (Carter 1955). At the present time the recognized grouping of the strain, according to Carter (1963a,b), is A, B, D, and E. Namioka and Murata (1961b) treated the bacteria with normal hydrochloric acid to produce a somatic antigen, and specific serological types were elucidated using cross-absorption tests. Carter (1963b) proposed adoption of the capsular classification and the subtype designations based on somatic antigens of Namioka and Bruner (1963) and Namioka et al. (1964) which included 11 varieties.

The differentiation of strains by either the capsular or somatic designations has been challenged. Bain (1964) tried indirect hemagglutination with a lipopolysaccharide extract (Carter and Rappay 1963) but could find no difference between groups B and E. Prince and Smith (1966a,b,c) used Ouchterlony double diffusion and immunoelectrophoresis and identified 18 soluble antigens of *P. multocida*. They designated two capsular antigens α and β and the more deeply seated antigens *a* through *n* and challenged the assumptions made in current typing techniques for the determination of "capsular" and "O somatic" types.

It may be concluded that there are three ways of looking at the problem. The first is from the viewpoint of the taxonomist who will use all the available methods, including biochemistry and serology and the exacting refinements of each to differentiate the species, groups, types, and subtypes, as has been done with the *Salmonella*. The second is from the more applied aspect of the immunologist who selects strains specifically for the preparation of effective immunizing antigens. This procedure is not always successful, as indicated by "vaccine breaks" (Carter 1967). The third view is that of the epizootiologist who is interested in a facile technique to distinguish strains for studies of the relation among carrier states, transmission, and spread of the etiologic agent. The studies of Carter on capsular antigen and Namioka on somatic antigen are applicable to the field of epizootiology; and further investigations will elucidate more antigenic components, as has been done with the Enterobacteriaceae (Carter 1967).

IMMUNIZATION. Priestly (1936) believed that an effective vaccine could only be prepared with highly virulent encapsulated bacteria. However, Heddleston et al. (1966) disputed this concept with the production of potent vaccines from noncapsulated avirulent *P. multocida*. Rebers et al. (1967) produced antigens from a virulent, capsulated strain which had been isolated from a bison on the National Bison Range in Montana. The antigen was both immunogenic and toxic, to the extent that domestic calves vaccinated with different quantities reacted with signs typical of hemorrhagic septicemia; the higher dose recipients succumbed, whereas those with lower doses established immunity as determined by challenge and mouse protection tests.

Immunization of free-roaming wildlife is impractical. Vaccination of American bison against *P. multocida* serotype 2 without appearance of the disease since 1965 suggests continued immunization to protect the herds (Heddleston and Wessman 1973). Some wildlife workers believe that when deer are yarding or when some herds in the west are on their winter range, they are sufficiently concentrated so that immunization by aerial spray may be effective, but others disagree as to the feasibility of such a procedure.

For captive wildlife—for example, on mink farms or in zoos—not only is there the possibility of carrying out a program of immunization, but it may be that prophylactic vaccination is a necessity if there is a history of recurrent bouts with pasteurellosis. The recently devised oral administration of killed organisms to produce active immunity (Heddleston and Rebers 1967) may simplify vaccination procedures. Hyperimmune serum can provide passive immunity for the immediate protection of animals, but antibiotic medication is preferred (Carter 1967).

TREATMENT AND CONTROL. Treatment with drugs falls into the same category as immunization in the case of wild populations, in that handling of the individual wild animals is an insurmountable task. On the other hand, the prophylactic use of drugs is of value in the case of captive wild animals. According to Stableforth and Galloway (1959), domestic rabbits were given an infective dose of *P. multocida* and then were given 10,000 units of sodium salt penicillin G every 6 hours for 4 days. As long as treatment was continued, the rabbits were healthy; but after it was stopped, they all died. According to the Food and Agriculture Organization of the United Nations (1962) sulfonamides have been successfully used in the therapy of pasteurellosis if started early in the course of the disease and if the dosage is sufficiently large.

Treatment of the environment either chemically by disinfection or physically by removal of the source of infection, such as blockading focal points or picking up infected carcasses, is one possible method for the control of disease in the wild. In addition, the population may be manipulated in several ways. One technique dependent on the nature of the species is herding, although most wildlife species are not sufficiently tractable for this to be feasible. Some may be dispersed, which is just a modification of herding and would tend to dilute the means of transmission or the contacts between carriers and susceptible animals, as well as to thin out the susceptible population. This may be accomplished by special or controlled hunting seasons. Finally, the most drastic approach to a disease control program is slaughter, which should only be used as a last desperate method to prevent such a highly contagious disease as pasteurellosis from being spread from one herd to another.

Chemical disinfection or removal of some environmental source is not feasible in the case of hemorrhagic septicemia in deer or bighorn sheep but is useful on a mink farm. Improving range conditions is warranted and should be employed when dealing with a disease of debility. Herding or dispersal is not practical on winter ranges or where deer are yarding. Limiting the number of animals by adequate harvest is desirable. Slaughter in the case of hemorrhagic septicemia is not a solution to the problem.

Finally, there is an incidental benefit accrued by the rancher who regulates the number of livestock with due regard for his range, tests them regularly, and vaccinates. He lessens the risk of establishing a reservoir of infection in the wild population that lives on or adjacent to the same environment. For the individual whose primary concern is the well-being of wildlife, this might be an indirect method of controlling disease in the wild.

REFERENCES

Bain, R. V. S. A note on some *Pasteurella* types found in Australian animals. *Aust. Vet. J.* 33:119–121, 1957.

——. *Classification of the Pasteurella which causes haemorrhagic septicemia.* Bangkok: South-East Asia Treaty Organization, 1964.

Bollinger, O. *Ueber eine neue Wild-und Rinderseuche.* Muenchen: Finsterlin, 1878.

Bond, R. E., McCune, E. L., and Olson, L. D. Isolation of *Pasteurella multocida* from wild raccoons and foxes: Preliminary report. *J. Wildl. Dis.* 8:296–299, 1972.

Bouvier, G. Observations sur les maladies du givier, de quelques animaux sauvages et des poissons (1942–1945). *Schweiz. Arch. Tierheilk.* 88:268–274, 1946.

Brunetti, O. In W. Longhurst, A. S. Leopold, and R. F. Dasmann, eds. A survey of California deer herds. *Calif. Dept. Fish Game, Game Bull.* 6, 1952.

Buchanan, R. E., and Gibbons, N. E. *Bergey's manual of determinative bacteriology,* 8th ed. Baltimore: Williams and Wilkins, 1974.

Carter, G. R. Studies on *Pasteurella multocida:* I. A hemagglutination test for the identification of serologic types. *Am. J. Vet. Res.* 16(60):481–484, 1955.

——. Studies on *Pasteurella multocida:* II. Identification of antigenic characteristics and colonial variants. *Am. J. Vet. Res.* 18(66):210–213, 1957.

——. Failure of the agglutination test to identify types of *Pasteurella multocida. Nature* 181:1138, 1958.

——. Immunological differentiation of Type B and E strains of *Pasteurella multocida. Can. Vet. J.* 4:61–63, 1963a.

——. Proposed modification of the serological classification of *Pasteurella multocida. Vet. Rec.* 75:1264, 1963b.

——. Pasteurellosis: *Pasteurella multocida* and *Pasteurella hemolytica. Adv. Vet. Sci.* 11:321–379, 1967.

Carter, G. R., and Bain, R. V. S. Pasteurellosis (*Pasteurella multocida*): A review stressing recent developments. *Vet. Rev. Annot.* 6:105–128, 1960.

Carter, G. R., and Rappay, D. E. A haemagglutination test employing specific lipopolysaccharide for the detection and measurement of *Pasteurella* antibodies to *Pasteurella multocida. Br. Vet. J.* 119:73–77, 1963.

Cowan, S. T., and Steel, J. J. *Identification of medical bacteria.* New York: Cambridge University Press, 1965.

Dahlberg, B. L., and Guettinger, R. C. The white-tailed deer in Wisconsin. *Tech. Wildlife Bull.* 14, Game Management Div., Wis. Conserv. Dept., Madison, 1956.

Das, M. S. Studies on *Pasteurella septica* (*Pasteurella multocida*): Observations on some biophysical characters. *J. Comp. Pathol. Ther.* 68:288–294, 1958.

Daubney, R., Hudson, J. R., and Roberts, J. I. Preliminary note on the transmission of bovine haemorrhagic septicemia by the flea *Ctenocephalus felis* Bouche. *J. Comp. Pathol. Ther.* 47:211–213, 1934.

DeAlwis, M., and Thambithurai, V. Hemorrhagic septicemia in a wild elephant in Ceylon. *Ceylon Vet. J.* 13:17–19, 1965.

Dorsey, T. A. Studies on fowl cholera: I. A biochemic study of avian *Pasteurella multocida* strains. *Avian Dis.* 7:386–392, 1963a.

———. Studies on fowl cholera: II. The correlation between biochemic classification and the serologic and immunologic nature of avian *Pasteurella multocida* strains. *Avian Dis.* 7:393–402, 1963b.

Erickson, A. B., Gunvalson, V. E., Stenlund, M. H., Burcalow, D. W., and Blankenship, L. H. The white-tailed deer of Minnesota. *Minn. Dept. of Conserv. Tech. Bull.* 5, 1961.

Fenstermacher, R., Olsen O. W., and Pomeroy, B. S. Some diseases of white-tailed deer of Minnesota. *Cornell Vet.* 33:323–332, 1943.

Food and Agricultural Organization of the United Nations. Rome: F.A.O. Rep. Intern. Meeting on Hemorrhagic Septicemia, Kuala Lumpur, Malaya, 1962.

Fox, H. Special animals (postmortem findings). Rep. Lab. Comp. Pathol., Philadelphia, 1923.

———. Hemorrhagic septicemia in an axis deer. Rep. Lab. Comp. Pathol., Philadelphia, 1926.

———. Infectious disease. Rep. Lab. Comp. Pathol., Philadelphia, 1929.

———. Infectious disease. Rep. Penrose Lab., Philadelphia, 1934.

Gay, F. P. *Agents of disease and host resistance.* Baltimore: Thomas, 1935.

Gochenour, W. S. Hemorrhagic septicemia studies. *J. Am. Vet. Med. Assoc.* 65:433–41, 1924.

Golebrowski, S., Sosnowski, A., and Zuchowska, E. An outbreak of pasteurellosis in pumas (*Felis concolor*). *Med. Weterynaryjna* 28:300–301, 1972.

Hagan, W. A. In D. Bruner and J. Gillespie, eds., *Infectious diseases of domestic animals,* 5th ed. Ithaca, N.Y.: Cornell University Press, 1966.

Hamerton, A. E. Report on the deaths occurring in the Society's gardens during 1930. *Proc. Zool. Soc. London* 1931:527, 1931.

Heddleston, K. L. Immunologic and serologic comparison of three strains of *Pasteurella multocida.* *Cornell Vet.* 56:235–241, 1966.

———. Physiologic characteristics of 1,268 cultures of *Pasteurella multocida.* *Am. J. Vet. Res.* 37:745–747, 1976.

Heddleston, K. L., and Rebers, P. A. Fowl cholera: Active immunity by oral administration of killed *Pasteurella multocida.* *Bacteriol. Proc.* 1967:99, 1967.

Heddleston, K. L., Rebers, P. A., and Ritchie, A. E. Immunizing and toxic properties of particulate antigens from two immunogenic types of *Pasteurella multocida* of avian origin. *J. Immunol.* 96:124–133, 1966.

Heddleston, K. L., Rhoades, K. R., and Rebers, P. A. Experimental pasteurellosis: Comparative studies on *Pasteurella multocida* from Asia, Africa, and North America. *Am. J. Vet. Res.* 28:1003–1012, 1967.

Heddleston, K. L., and Wessman, G. Vaccination of American Bison against *Pasteurella multocida*

serotype 2 infection (hemorrhagic septicemia). *J. Wildl. Dis.* 9:306–310, 1973.

Hine, R. L. *Diseases and parasites in Wisconsin birds and mammals.* Madison: Game Mgt. Div., Wis. Conserv. Dept., 1956.

Honess, R. F., and Frost, N. M. A Wyoming bighorn sheep study. *Wyoming Game and Fish Dept. Bull.* 1, 1942.

Honess, R. F., and Winter, K. Diseases of wildlife in Wyoming. *Wyoming Game and Fish Comm. Bull.* 9, 1956.

Hubbert, W. T., and Rosen, M. N. *Pasteurella multocida* infection due to animal bite. *Am. J. Public Health,* June 1970.

Hudson, J. R. Pasteurellosis. In A. W. Stableforth, and I. A. Galloway, eds., *Infectious diseases of animals,* pp. 413–436. London: Butterworths, 1959.

Kaye, M. D., Mooney, B. F., and Murray R. *Pasteurella hemolytica* in the opossum (*Didelphis marsupialis*). *Lab. Anim. Sci.* 27:118–119, 1973.

Khalifa, I. A. B. In A. W. Stableforth and I. A. Galloway, eds., *Infectious diseases of animals,* p. 433. London: Butterworths, 1954.

King, E. O. *The identification of unusual pathogenic gram-negative bacteria.* Leaflet, Atlanta: DHEW, PHS, CDC, 1964.

Kummeneje, K. Pasteurellosis in reindeer in northern Norway: A contribution to its epidemiology. *Acta Vet. Scand.* 17:488–494, 1976.

Lewis, H. Hemorrhagic septicemia in a mink. *J. Am. Vet. Med. Assoc.* 75:771–773, 1929.

Linsert, H. Pasteurellose beim nerz. *Dtsch. Tieraerztl. Wochenschr.* 48:433–435, 1940.

Little, P. O., and Lyon, B. M. Demonstration of serologic types within the nonhemolytic *Pasteurella. Am. J. Vet. Res.* 4:110–112, 1943.

Marsh, H. General notes. *J. Mammal.* 8:163, 1927.

———. Pneumonia in Rocky Mountain bighorn sheep. *J. Mammal.* 19:214, 1938.

Mel'nikova, T. G., and Mel'nikova, G. V. Pasteurellosis and paratyphoid in wild pigs in Tadzhikistan. *Veterinariya* 7:46, 1960.

Murie, O. J. The elk of North America. Harrisburg, Pa.: Stackpole, 1951.

Namioka, S., and Bruner, D. W. Serological studies on *Pasteurella multocida:* IV. Type distribution of the organisms on the basis of their capsule and O groups. *Cornell Vet.* 53:41–53, 1963.

Namioka, S., and Murata, M. Serological studies on *Pasteurella multocida:* I. A simplified method for capsule typing of the organism. *Cornell Vet.* 51:498–507, 1961a.

———. Serological studies on *Pasteurella multocida:* II. Characteristics of somatic (O) antigen of the organism. *Cornell Vet.* 51:507–521, 1961b.

———. Serological studies on *Pasteurella multocida:* III. O antigenic analysis of cultures isolated from various animals. *Cornell Vet.* 51:522–528, 1961c.

Namioka, S., Murata, M., and Bain, R. V. S. Serological studies on *Pasteurella multocida:* V. Some epizootiological findings resulting from O antigenic analysis. *Cornell Vet.* 54:520–534, 1964.

Nordkvist, M., and Karlsson, K. A. Epizootiskt forlopande infektion med *Pasteurella multocida* hos ren. *Nord. Vet. Med.* 14:1–15, 1962.

Ponomareva, T. N., and Rodkevich, K. V. *Pasteurella multocida* infection among rodents in a large city. *J. Microbiol. Epidemiol. Immunobiol.* 41:144–145, 1964.

Popovici, V., Ungureanu, C., and Paunescu, G. An outbreak of pasteurellosis in mink. *Arch. Vet.* 8:75–83, 1972.

Post, G. Proc. 5th sheep conference. *Wyoming Wildl.* 22:33, 1958.

———. Pasteurellosis of Rocky Mountain bighorn sheep. *Wildl. Dis.* 62:23, 1962.

Potts, M. K. Hemorrhagic septicemia in bighorn sheep of Rocky Mountain National Park. *J. Mammal.* 18:105–106, 1937.

Priestly, F. W. Experiments on immunization against *Pasteurella septica* infection. *J. Comp. Pathol. Ther.* 49:340–347, 1936.

Prince, G. H., and Smith, J. E. Antigenic studies on *Pasteurella multocida* using immunodiffusion techniques: I. Identification and nomenclature of the soluble antigens of a bovine haemorrhagic septicemia strain. *J. Comp. Pathol. Ther.* 76:303–314, 1966a.

———. Antigenic studies on *Pasteurella multocida* using immunodiffusion techniques: II. Relationships with other gram-negative species. *J. Comp. Pathol. Ther.* 76:315–320, 1966b.

———. Antigenic studies on *Pasteurella multocida* using immunodiffusion techniques: III. Relationships between strains of *Pasteurella multocida*. *J. Comp. Pathol. Ther.* 76:321–332, 1966c.

Quortrup, E. R. Hemorrhagic septicemia in mule deer. *North Am. Vet.* 23:34–36, 1942.

Rebers, P. A., Heddleston, K. L., and Rhoades, K. R. Isolation from *Pasteurella multocida* of a lipopolysaccharide antigen with immunizing and toxic properties. *J. Bacteriol.* 93:7–14, 1967.

Reisinger, R. Parainfluenza-3 virus in cattle. *Ann. N.Y. Acad. Sci.* 101:576–582, 1962.

Roberts, R. A. An immunological study of *Pasteurella septica*. *J. Comp. Pathol. Ther.* 57:261–278, 1947.

Rosen, M. N. A survey of California deer herds. In W. Longhurst, A. S. Leopold, and R. F. Dasmann, Calif. Dept. Fish and Game, Game Bull. 6, 1952.

Rosen, M. N., and Morse, E. E. An interspecies chain in a fowl cholera epizootic. *Calif. Fish Game* 45(1):51–56, 1959.

Rosenbusch, C., and Merchant, I. A. A study of the hemorrhagic septicemia Pasteurellae. *J. Bacteriol.* 37:68–69, 1939.

Ruff, F. J. What is "black-tongue" among deer? *Wildl. North Carolina*, June 1950.

Russa, E. Contribuicao ao estudo fermentativo das bacterias do genero "Pasteurella." *Bol. Vet. Ener. Brasil* 6:127–135, 1939. Abstr. *Vet. Bull.* 11:284, 1941.

Schipper, G. J. Unusual pathogenicity of *Pasteurella multocida* isolated from the throats of common wild rats. *Bull. Johns Hopkins Hosp.* 81:333–356, 1947.

Semiotrochev, V. L., Barak, Ts. M., Spitsin, M. P., Pipinyan, I. O., Erusheva, L. F., and Misaleva, O. S. Pasteurellosis in man in the Kazlinsk area of Kzyl'Ordinsk oblast. *Zh. Mikrobiol. Epidemiol. Immunobiol.* 42:143–144, 1965.

Stableforth, A. W., and Galloway, I. A. *Infectious diseases of animals*, 2 vols. London: Butterworths, 1959.

Talbot, J. M., and Sneath, P. H. A. A taxonomic study of *Pasteurella septica*, especially of strains isolated from human sources. *J. Gen. Microbiol.* 22:303–311, 1960.

Topley, W., and Wilson, G. *The principles of bacteriology and immunity*. New York: William Wood, 1931.

Trevisan, V. Sur micrococco della rabbia e sulla possibilita di riconoscere durante il periodo d'incubazione, dall'esame del sangue della persona morsicata, se ha contratta l'infezione rabbica. *Reale Inst. Lombardo Scienze Lettere Rendiconto.* 20(ser. 2):88–105, 1887.

Webster, L. T. Biology of *Bacterium lepisepticum*. *J. Exp. Med.* 39:837–857, 1924.

Young, E. Pasteurellosis in the kangaroo. *Int. Zool. Yearbook* 5:185, 1965.

21 *Pseudotuberculosis*

THEODORE F. WETZLER

Synonyms: **Zoogloeic tuberculosis, rodent pseudotuberculosis, parapest (when the etiologic agent is a gram-negative bacillus), equine ulcerative lymphangitis, caseous lymphadenitis, Preisz-Nocard disease (when the etiologic agent is a gram-positive, diphtheroidal bacterium).**

Pseudotuberculosis is an acute to chronic zoonotic disease, which may be described partially as a regional lymphadenitis or lymphangitis involving many of the visceral organs, especially the spleen, liver, mesenteric lymphatics, lung, and small intestine; occasionally the stomach; and rarely the kidneys. It is characterized by scattered, miliary, or focal necrotic lesions which are granulomas, not tubercles, and which are caseated, not cavitated.

HISTORY. The communicable bacterial disease pseudotuberculosis was first described by Malassez and Vignal (1883, 1884), who isolated a gram-negative coccobacillus which produced a "zoogloeic" tuberculosis in guinea pigs. Eberth (1885) first employed the term *pseudotuberculosis* in describing lesions observed in rabbits and guinea pigs. What were initially descriptive terms of lesions became in time inappropriate terms of disease, resulting in the unfortunate mislabeling of both the etiologic agents and the disease processes which they engender.

The delineation of pseudotuberculosis as a disease of wild animals required an inordinately long period of time after its early description in guinea pigs, laboratory rabbits, and domesticated animals. Of the many explanations offered to excuse the erratic progress of the first 50 years, the following are plausible:

1. There was an early impression that the guinea pig was latently infected with *Pasteurella pseudotuberculosis* and readily stressed into overt disease.
2. There was an impression that *P. pseudotuberculosis* closely resembled a much more important organism, *P. pestis*, the causative agent of plague.
3. The identity of the etiologic agents of both avian pseudotuberculosis and rodent pseudotuberculosis apparently was neither obvious nor pertinent.

Schleifstein and Coleman (1939) described a bacterial pathogen which resembled both *P. pseudotuberculosis* and *Actinobacillus lignieresi*. However, it was not until after the report of Haessig et al. (1949) that attention was focused on the presence of pseudotuberculosislike *Pasteurella*. These bacteria were given the tentative designation, *Yersinia enterocolitica*, by Frederiksen (1964). Most of the natural infections caused by the last-named agents have occurred in chinchillas and, to a lesser extent, in European hares. There are no particularly distinguishing features in the naturally occurring pseudotuberculosis caused by *Y. enterocolitica* as contrasted to disease by *P. pseudotuberculosis*.

An infectious process described by Preisz and Guinard (1891), known as Preisz-Nocard disease, pseudotuberculosis, or caseous lymphadenitis is caused by *Corynebacterium ovis* (syn. *C. pseudotuberculosis rodentium*). Preisz-Nocard disease was not reported in wild ruminants of North America until 1934, when the publications of Shaw et al. revealed this disease in deer (*Odocoileus hemionus*) in Oregon, then it was reported in Montana by Hammersland and Joneschild (1937), in Washington by Seghetti and McKenney (1941), and in British Columbia by Humphreys and Gibbons (1942).

Pseudotuberculosis, whether caused by *P. pseudotuberculosis*, *Y. enterocolitica*, or *C. ovis*, is not rare, merely unnoticed and nondiagnosed. There are great deficiencies both in diagnostic expertise and in accurate reporting.

Consistent with the modern trend to reserve the term "pseudotuberculosis" for only those infectious processes caused by *P. pseudotuberculosis* or *Y. enterocolitica*, this chapter is limited accordingly.

DISTRIBUTION. The geographic distribution of *P. pseudotuberculosis* and *Y. enterocolitica* appears to be predominantly in the Northern Hemisphere and generally north of the 20th parallel. This most likely reflects the loci of the research investigators rather than the foci of the bacterial organisms.

The confirmation of pseudotuberculosis in a wide variety of wild hosts, whether by direct isolation of etiologic agents or by serologic incrimination, has been reported in many countries. *P. pseudotuberculosis* is known to exist in the following continents:

ASIA: India, Vietnam, Mongolia, USSR, and Japan

AFRICA: Belgian Congo, Morocco, and Algeria

AUSTRALIA: (Isolates have been made from sheep and magpies (*Pica pica*), but not from wild animals)

SOUTH AMERICA: Brazil

NORTH AMERICA: Canada, United States, and Mexico

EUROPE: Belgium, Denmark, England, France, Germany, Holland, Hungary, Italy, Latvia, Norway, Poland, Portugal, Romania, Russia, Scotland, and Sweden

Under the stated conditions—that is, direct isolation or serologic incrimination—a number of wild animals have been involved in pseudotuberculosis referable to *P. pseudotuberculosis* (Table 21.1).

At the time of death, the various primates were at zoological gardens or research institutions. It is likely, however, that in some outbreaks the etiologic agents of disease had been acquired by the animal prior to export from the collection site (Mollaret et al. 1963). As an illustration, *P. pseudotuberculosis* exists in the Belgian Congo and has been incriminated by Mollaret (1958) with deaths in damans (rock badgers).

Pseudotuberculosis, referable to *Y. enterocolitica* in wild animals, has been found predominantly in chinchillas (Akkermans and Terpstra 1963; Daniels and Goudzwaard 1963; Frederiksen 1964) and to a lesser extent in hares (Mollaret and Lucas 1965) Several strains of *Y. enterocolitica* have been isolated from feces of apparently healthy deer (*Odocoileus virginianus*) in southern Michigan (Wetzler 1965; Wetzler and Hubbert 1968a; Wetzler et al. 1966).

ETIOLOGY. The etiologic agents of pseudotuberculosis are gram-negative coccobacilli, *P. pseudotuberculosis* and *Y. enterocolitica*. There is considerable confusion in the early pseudotuberculosis literature as to which agent was being described. In at least one instance, the author described a gram-negative bacillus to which he assigned the name, *C. pseudotuberculosis* (Urbain 1942). Reimann (1932) evaluated the old Pribam collection of pseudotuberculosis strains and found that one was a diphtheroid, which corroborated the point that

the isolate was, in fact, *C. ovis* (*B. pseudotuberculosis ovis* Preisz).

Pasteurella pseudotuberculosis. The terms *Bacterium pseudotuberculosis rodentium* or *Bacillus* of Malassez and Vignal were fairly well accepted by the turn of the century. Later with the creation of the family Parvobacteriaceae, this bacterium was called *P. pseudotuberculosis*. Almost from the time that *pseudotuberculosis* and *pestis* were assigned to the genus *Pasteurella* there has been general dissatisfaction with their nomenclature. Since 1946 strong arguments have been made in favor of deleting *P. pestis* and *P. pseudotuberculosis* from the genus. Should official action be taken in this regard, these species will be renamed *Y. pestis* and *Y. pseudotuberculosis*, respectively. It is to be hoped that the ill-advised choice of species epithet for the latter might also be eliminated.

Although *P. pseudotuberculosis* and *P. pestis* are related closely, there are fundamental differences. The former is motile at room temperature, and the latter is not motile at any temperature; the former has an active urease enzyme, the latter usually does not; the former usually does not have the capsular protein antigen called Fraction I, which is highly characteristic of the latter species. There are differences in pathogenesis between the two species: *P. pestis* is usually transmitted by arthropod vector; *P. pseudotuberculosis* is usually transmitted via fecally contaminated foodstuffs or forage.

On the basis of worldwide literature, the bulk of *P. pseudotuberculosis* isolated from or serologically identified with wild animals is about equally divided between rodents or lagomorphs and the subhuman primates.

Yersinia enterocolitica. In 1939 Schleifstein and Coleman proposed the name *Bacterium enterocoliticum* for a pathogenic bacterium which closely resembled *P. pseudotuberculosis* as well as *A. lignieresi*. Dickinson and Mocquot (1961) isolated enteric bacteria from an experimental disease in swine which they called *P. pseudotuberculosis* type B. Knapp and Thal (1963) studied similar organisms which they termed *Pasteurella X* and which Mollaret and Chevalier (1964) called *Bacterium X*. Frederiksen (1964) proposed a new epithet for these organisms, *Y. enterocolitica*.

Until quite recently all the isolates of *Y. enterocolitica* had been isolated from diseased or dead animals, but the agents could rarely be demonstrated to be pathogenic in conventional

TABLE 21.1 *Pasteurella pseudotuberculosis* in Wild Animals. 255

Order	Genus and Species	Common Name
ARTIODACTYLA		boar, wild, nonspecified
	Dama dama	deer, fallow
	Odocoileus hemionus	deer, mule
	Cervus elaphus	deer, red
	Capreolus capreolus	deer, roe
	Odocoileus virginianus	deer, white-tailed
		gazelle, nonspecified
	Ovis aries (syn. *O. musimon*)	sheep, wild (mouflon)
CARNIVORA	*Dendrohydrax* spp.	badger, rock
	Vulpes vulpes	fox
	Vulpes spp.	fox, silver, nonspecified
	Felis leo	lion
	Martes spp.	marten
	Mustela vison	mink
	Felis pardalis	ocelot
	Lutra lutra	otter
	Procyon lotor	raccoon
INSECTIVORA	*Erinaceus europaeus*	hedgehog
		mole, nonspecified
	Suncus murinus	shrew
MARSUPIALIA	*Macropus melanops*	kangaroo, black-faced gray
PRIMATES	*Papio papio*	baboon, dog-faced
	Galago crassicaudatus	bushbaby
	Pan satyrus	chimpanzee
	Hylobates syndactylus	gibbon
	Papio hamadryas	hamadryad
	Happale jacchus	marmoset
		monkeys
	Cercopithecus aethiops	African tree or guenon
	Macaca sylvana	Barbary ape
	Macaca irus	buffoon or crab-eating
	Cebus albifrons	capuchin or sapajous
	Macaca cynomolgus	cynomologous
	Cercopithecus brazzae or *C. neglectus*	De Brazza
	Cercopithecus mona grayi	gray
	Cercopithecus callitrichus	green guenon
	Cercopithecus n. nictitans	large spot-nosed
	Cercocebus cristatus	mangabey
	Erythrocebus patas	patas
	Macaca rhesus, M. mulatta	rhesus
	Cercopithecus leucampyx	silver
	Cercopithecus ascanius	white-nosed African
RODENTIA	*Dasyprocta aguti*	agouti
	Castor canadensis	beaver
	Chinchilla laniger	chinchilla
	Lepus americanus, L. californicus, L. europaeus, L. timidus	hare
	Lemmus lemmus	lemming
	Apodemus spp. *Arvicola* spp., *Clethrionomys* spp. *Mus* spp., *Microtus* (to include *M. mexicanus*), *Pitymus* spp.	mice and voles
	Ondatra zibethica	muskrat
	Myocastor coypus	nutria (rangodin) (coypu)
	Cynomys (either *gunnisoni* or *ludovicianus*)	prairie dog
	Sylvilagus floridanus	rabbit
	Rattus exulans, R. norvegicus, R. rattus	rat
	Citellus leucurus	squirrel, white-tailed antelope

laboratory animals by the usual routes of inoculation. Furthermore, these strains were not susceptible to *P. pseudotuberculosis* bacteriophage, did not ferment rhamnose, did ferment sucrose anaerogenically, and were usually positive for an ornithine decarboxylase. There are other minor biochemical differences between the two agents, *Y. enterocolitica* and *P. pseudotuberculosis*, but the two species are quite closely related (Table 21.2).

Limiting this discussion to wild animals, the majority of *Y. enterocolitica* have been isolated from chinchillas.

TRANSMISSION. Transmission of the agents of pseudotuberculosis in natural disease states is limited apparently to oral-fecal routes.

There have been rather extensive outbreaks of pseudotuberculosis in animals in research institutions, but no epizootics have been reported among animals in their native habitat. When laboratory epizootics occur, they generally are explosive, acute, and often highly fatal. Several instances will suffice to illustrate this point:

1. Paterson and Cook (1963) reported a major epizootic among stock guinea pigs (*Cavia* spp.) at Porton, England, with losses of approximately 1,000 animals. Careful epizo-

otiologic review established that the affected animals were undoubtedly infected by the consumption of field kale that had been fecally contaminated by wood pigeons (*Columba* spp.).

2. Mollaret et al. (1963) described two outbreaks of pseudotuberculosis spaced at a one-year interval at a research institute. One week before the first epizootic occurred, a shipment of 60 dog-faced baboons (*Papio papio*) had been received. Then in February and March 1961, a loss of 71 of 261 animals occurred. Stringent environmental measures were instituted, and the entire population was sacrificed for the production of cell culture systems. A year later in 1962, 33 of 204 dog-faced baboons were lost in another similar epizootic, and all the dead animals were among the new arrivals or were animals which had not been in the colony for any great length of time.

3. Fribourg-Blanc et al. (1963) found, as a result of a serum survey, that 45% of 150 cynomologous monkeys had significant antibody titers to *P. pseudotuberculosis* (>1:150) and to the EV-76 strains of *P. pestis* (>1:150). As circulating antibody titers to *P. pseudotuberculosis* somatic O antigens are not known to persist for any length of time after an infection; one can only surmise that

TABLE 21.2   Biochemical Characterization of Pseudotuberculosis Agents.

Biochemical Reaction	Primary Reactions		Biochemical Reaction	Secondary Reactions	
	P. pseudotuberculosis	*Y. enterocolitica*		*P. pseudotuberculosis*	*Y. enterocolitica*
Aerobic	+	+	acetylmethylcarbinol	—, d	— or +*
Catalase	+	+	amygdalin	—	(+)
Gelatin	—	—	B-D-galactosidase	+	+ or —*
Glucose (acid)	+	+	BCP-milk	NC to Alk	NC to Alk,
Kligler iron	Alk/A	Alk/A			d
Lysine decarboxylase	—	—	cellobiose	—	+
Mannitol	+	+	citrate	—, d	+ or —*
Methyl red	+	+	glycerol	(+), d	(+)
Motility: 37° C	—	—	malonate	(+), d	(+), d
20° C	+	+	melezitose	—, d	—
O-F test	F	F	melibiose	+	—
Oxidase	—	—	nitrate reduction	+, d	+ or —*
Phenylalanine deaminase	—	—	ornithine decarboxylase	—	+, d
Rhamnose	+	—	raffinose	—	—
Sucrose	—	(+)	salicin	(+)	(+), d
Urease	+	+			

ᵃBiochemical subgroups occur, i.e., Franco-Belgian hares (Mollaret and Lucas 1965).

Legend: — = negative in 14 days at 37° C; + = positive in < 2 days at 37° C; (+) = positive in > 2 days at 37° C; d = some strains differ from major reaction; NC = no change; Alk = alkaline; A = acid; O-F = oxidative-fermentative test.

the animals were either recently infected with a subclinical infection or that the animals were latent carriers at the time of serum sampling.

These illustrations point up the possibilities of infection subsequent to ingestion of contaminated foodstuffs, and this possible source of infection gains further support by the fact that a consistent portion of the animal diet is made up of fresh fruits or vegetables.

It is of interest that there have never been pseudotuberculosis outbreaks in managed or wild populations of mice. This is rather difficult to explain satisfactorily.

Much of the reported epizootiology of *Y. enterocolitica* incriminates contaminated forage or water as the likely vehicle of transmission. This is inferred for those outbreaks in herds of chinchillas reported by Wetzler and Hubbert (1968a), since the simple corrective measure of antibiotic treatment of the drinking water and the animal food promptly terminated the outbreaks, and there were no reoccurrences.

In the Leningrad oblast, ixodid ticks were reported to be infected with *P. pseudotuberculosis*. On three occasions Ul'yanova (1961) found this agent in ticks removed from cattle; there was no information on the disease status of the cattle. This is the extent of information in the literature concerning ticks as vectors for transmission of *P. pseudotuberculosis*. Krynski and Becla (1963) report that lice are not suitable transmitting vectors for *P. pseudotuberculosis*, virulent *P. pseudotuberculosis* organisms kill the lice, avirulent populations do not, and the lice do not transmit the avirulent bacteria. Limited studies have been made on the experimental transmission of *P. pseudotuberculosis* by fleas. Most of these attempts have been abortive or fruitless; and where transmission could be attained, it was not particularly efficient or predictable (Blanc and Baltazard 1944).

SIGNS. Very few wild animals become ill or acquire an illness leading to death while under direct observation. As a result little is known about the signs of pseudotuberculosis in wild animals, other than those in zoological gardens or research institutes. Further, populations of wild animals in either of these two loci are highly selected and distort our concepts of natural distribution, susceptibility, resistance, etc. Lastly, there is nothing specific about the signs of animals suffering from pseudotuberculosis.

Signs of *P. pseudotuberculosis* infections have been recorded for some of the Rodentia

and some of the primates. Chapman (1948) and Leader and Baker (1954) observed that affected chinchillas would stop eating, the quantity of feces would diminish, and the animals would demonstrate marked listlessness or depression. Death followed in one or several days. In experimental rodents, mice, and gerbils (*Meriones unguiculatus*), similar syndromes have been noticed; and it may be added that a bimodal febrile reaction occurs at 2–3 days postinoculation, and again sometime after the 5th day. The two major febrile events coincide with bacteremia. Diarrhea is notable with the acute, hemorrhagic syndrome. Chronic infections may lead to substantial weight losses of over 30% before death intervenes (Wetzler 1965).

Mollaret et al. (1963) warn that clinical signs of pseudotuberculosis in primates, such as dog-faced baboons, are deceptive and do not incriminate any one particular disease. During the hours (or rarely, days) preceding death, the affected animals remain immobile in a corner of their cages, heads bent on chests, hair erect, and eyelids apparently swollen. Appetite remains good almost to the time of death which comes without any warning signs.

Nouvel and Rinjard (1949) observed that on the day before death ill baboons suffered marked depression, the fur became dull, and there was a slightly distended abdomen, although the palpable lymphatics were not modified. These authors reported an abundant diarrhea which was virtually a dysentery. They noted that the animals maintained an unimpaired appetite to the time of death.

In terms of signs, pseudotuberculosis of chinchillas caused by *Y. enterocolitica* differs little from that described in the same species by *P. pseudotuberculosis*. Wetzler and Hubbert (1968a) reviewed three outbreaks in North American chinchillas and noted marked depression, inappetence, anorexia, weight loss, diarrhea, and death within several days.

PATHOGENESIS. Mechanisms of pathogenesis of either *P. pseudotuberculosis* or *Y. enterocolitica* in wild animals remain somewhat unstudied in the former agent and purely speculative for the latter.

There has been, however, an intense effort directed toward the various mechanisms of virulence by *P. pestis*. In some instances data were simultaneously amassed for *P. pseudotuberculosis*. Wetzler (1965) reviewed a number of virulence factors associated with both plague and pseudotuberculosis bacteria and reported that the single major virulence antigen of *P. pseu-*

dotuberculosis is the VW complex of Burrows and Bacon (1956, 1960). Such a factor is quite sufficient to account for the acute, rapidly fatal, hemorrhagic syndromes found in rodents or lagomorphs. However, since those conditions in the microenvironment which are necessary to produce or enhance this antigen are those which in time destroy the virulence factor, one must search elsewhere to explain pathogenesis in the chronic death of rodents which is characterized by massive host response. Wetzler (1965) postulated, but did not prove, that death could be the result of a simple physical anorexia at the cellular level secondary to the competition for oxygen by the multiplying microbial population.

Lastly, some Serotype III strains of *P. pseudotuberculosis* possess an exotoxin which, in suitably expressed quality or quantity, leads to a rapidly fulminating hemorrhagic syndrome.

Mechanisms for the pathogenesis, or virulence, of *Y. enterocolitica* are entirely speculative.

Any number of commonly used laboratory animals are suitable for experimental pseudotuberculosis referable to *P. pseudotuberculosis*. Generally, the most suitable routes of injection are subcutaneous or intraperitoneal; and the administered dosage should be realistic—that is, attention given to route, type of host, the production of the virulent culture, and the state of immunity of the challenged host. Wetzler has found the intraperitoneal route to be eminently satisfactory for guinea pigs, rabbits, inbred mice, and gerbils. He agrees that the white rat is refractory (Rowland 1912) and, additionally, has found the Syrian hamster to be completely refractory to any challenge given (Wetzler 1965). Guinea pigs may be latently infected with *P. pseudotuberculosis* but are sensitive reactors when suitably stressed. Gerbils may display an order of sensitivity to either subcutaneous or intraperitoneal challenge analogous to the most virulent of the plague strains—that is, 1–10 viable cells for LD_{50}, 80–135-g animal, in less than 140 hours.

The major virulence antigen or factor of *P. pseudotuberculosis* is the VW antigen (Burrows and Bacon 1956)—in fact, it may be the only virulence factor. However, proper virulence testing of a strain in a suitable animal demands careful attention to the temperature at which the virulent population is cultured. Prolonged holding at 37°C attenuates the VW population and leads to increasing avirulence, reflected in increasing dosages and longer time intervals to death.

The observations summarized by Mollaret (1965) that a worm parasite burden may render the normally quite resistant cat sensitive to experimental pseudotuberculosis, may have its counterpart in natural disease states. An observation was made to the effect that in a recent epizootic in goats the observed animals were carrying many ectoparasites and were heavily parasitized endogenously (Richards 1967).

Yersinia enterocolitica strains have proven to be avirulent for commonly employed laboratory animals by multiple routes and varying dosages (Mollaret and Guillon 1965).

PATHOLOGY. The following gross and microscopic pathologic observations have been made: (1) hypertrophy of the mesenteric lymphatics, which seldom becomes generalized; (2) visceral nodules, primarily of the spleen and liver, frequently in the ileocecal junction, occasionally in the lungs, and quite rarely in the intestine; and (3) serofibrinous peritoneal fluid.

The visceral nodules are miliary abscesses of a gray to yellow color and range up to 3 cm in size. On cut section, these nodules reveal caseated centers made up of the necrotic debris from reticular and histiocytic cells; the outer margins disclose a wide band of histiocytes in active proliferation. The bacteria are most numerous in the outer margins of the nodular wall.

In rodents the gross and microscopic pathology is reminiscent of the findings reported for primates: hypertrophy of spleen (in chronic states this organ is many times its original size and weight); enlarged and friable liver studded with small spherical nodules; and occasionally nodular foci on lungs, diaphragm, and mesenteric lymphatics. Microscopically, the lesions or nodules will be found to have central liquefaction, and the surrounding wall will include a zone of lymphocytes and macrophages. There will be little encapsulation, and no giant cells will be seen. There may be a rarely occurring infiltration of kidney cortices by lymphocytes and mononuclear cells, hyaline and cellular casts in the glomeruli and convoluted tubules, and some necrosis of tubular epithelium. The lungs will usually have an alveolar edema, the interalveolar septa will be thickened by infiltrating mononuclear cells, and there will be numbers of focal areas of neutrophilic infiltration and liquefaction.

The pathology of animals infected with *Y.*

enterocolitica has been described, and these descriptions do not differ substantially from those reported for *P. pseudotuberculosis*. Any intense research directed to this problem is confronted and complicated by the fact that no good laboratory animal has been discovered for experimental pathogenesis. In one outbreak of pseudotuberculosis in chinchillas in North America referable to *Y. enterocolitica*, the gross pathology was similar to that described for *P. pseudotuberculosis*. An exudative inflammation of the nasal passages and edema of the gut has been reported also (Fertig 1968).

DIAGNOSIS. It cannot be overemphasized that pseudotuberculosis caused by *P. pseudotuberculosis* or *Y. enterocolitica* cannot be diagnosed by clinical signs. Diagnosis depends solely upon microbiological laboratory findings, either by the isolation and identification of the agent or the serologic incrimination of a specific serotype.

Serologic identification may be done by whole-cell somatic O agglutination, which is the current practice in Europe (Knapp 1960; Thal 1956), or by the hemagglutination of sensitized, nontanned sheep erythrocytes, which is current practice in the United States (Currie et al. 1966; Wetzler et al. 1968).

A peculiarity of the somatic serology of *P. pseudotuberculosis* lies in the fact that there are five serotypes, three of which are further subdivided. The smooth somatic O antigens which make up each individual serotype are quite independent of all other serotypes. This point is clearly delineated in Table 21.3.

Further complications lie in the fact that: (1) Serotype II of *P. pseudotuberculosis* shares a common antigen with Salmonella type B (Schuetze 1932; Thal 1953); (2) Serotype IV of *P. pseudotuberculosis* shares a common antigen with Salmonella type D (Knapp 1955); (3) Serofactor 1 is a rough somatic antigen of *P. pseudotuberculosis*, which is shared by *P. pestis* (Davies 1956, 1958; Schuetze 1932), *Shigella flexneri*, *Sh. sonnei*, and *Escherichia coli* (Wetzler et al. 1968); and (4) Serofactor 13, which was proposed by Wetzler (1965) as a new, serotype-independent somatic smooth antigen, has been shown to cross with *Y. enterocolitica*, *Flavobacterium meningosepticum*, *Sh. flexneri*, and *Bordetella bronchiseptica* (syn. *Alcaligenes bronchiseptica*), as reported by Wetzler et al. (1968).

We propose, therefore, that considerable attention must be given to the proper identification and interpretation of serologic results, and that many times one will have to perform considerable adsorption of antisera in order to define the etiologic agent with high precision.

The simplest serologic tests of great sensitivity and flexibility are those using the antigen-sensitized, nontanned erythrocyte hemagglutination systems of Currie (1965), Currie et al. (1966), and Wetzler (1965). Multiple antigens may be adsorbed to the erythrocytes at one time.

Fluorescein-isothiocyanate-labeled antibody techniques are suitable under limited circumstances but suffer in sensitivity and are subject to the obvious problems delineated above in the potential, multiple "shared" serofactors (Wetzler 1965).

The definition of *Y. enterocolitica* into serotypes has not been sufficiently studied to date to permit adequate evaluation. It is most likely, however, that there will be at least eight serotypes (Winblad 1968). At the moment, the best evidence which one can amass for diagnosis of this agent is the rather consistent biochemical characterization profile, its lack of inciting pathology in laboratory animals, its nonsensitivity to *P. pseudotuberculosis* bacteriophage, and identification with the various somatic O serofactors which are known at this time (Knapp and Thal 1963; Mollaret and Chevalier 1964; Wetzler and Hubbert 1968b).

PROGNOSIS. Given highly susceptible hosts and suitably virulent strains of the etiologic agent (*P. pseudotuberculosis*, *Y. enterocolitica*), the prognosis is not good.

A virulent inoculum, by any suitable route and in any sensitive host, will lead to death, either by an acute fulminating process or by a

TABLE 21.3 Somatic Antigenic Schema of *Pasteurella pseudotuberculosis*.

Serotype	Subtype	O Antigen
I	I A	1, 2, 3, 13
	I B	1, 2, 4, 13
II	II A	1, 5, 6, 13
	II B	1, 5, 7, 13
III	toxic	1, 8, 13
	nontoxic	1, 8, 13
IV	IV A	1, 9, 11, 13
	IV B	1, 9, 12
V		1, 10, 13

[a]Serofactor 13 occurs irregularly in all serotypes.

chronic syndrome involving massive host response. Based purely on the little information available, it would appear that primates, lagomorphs, and some rodents (gerbils, mice, chinchillas, cavies) are extremely susceptible to *P. pseudotuberculosis*. Chinchillas are apparently highly susceptible to acute infections by *Y. enterocolitica*, and hares only slightly less so.

IMMUNITY. Natural immunity to the gram-negative agents of pseudotuberculosis is cellular, not humoral (Thal and Wellmann 1968).

Such laboratory hosts as white rats (Rowland 1912) and Syrian hamsters (*Mesocricetus auratus*) (Wetzler 1965) are apparently quite refractory to pseudotuberculosis. All experimental laboratory rodents and lagomorphs have quite a high resistance to experimental pseudotuberculosis by *Y. enterocolitica* (Mollaret and Guillon 1965).

TREATMENT. For highly sensitive hosts or valuable animals held in captivity, any broad-spectrum antibiotic may be used with good effect in the treatment of pseudotuberculosis. Streptomycin is less valuable; and penicillin should not be used, for resistant strains may be encountered among the gram-negative agents of the disease (Ippen and Stoll 1959; Joubert and Oudar 1958).

Various sulfonamides might be useful in prophylaxis, and reasonably good results can be anticipated with nitrofurans at suitably high levels of dosage. Wetzler (1965) evaluated a rather comprehensive antibiotic profile of sensitivity-resistance demonstrated by *P. pseudotuberculosis*.

CONTROL. Various control measures have been used during epizootics referable to *P. pseudotuberculosis* and *Y. enterocolitica*. It is uncertain how advantageous some of them have been.

Apparently the use of tetracyclines in medicated feeds or drinking water can prevent the transmission of *P. pseudotuberculosis* and *Y. enterocolitica* in chinchilla herds. For a number of animals who depend upon fresh vegetables or fruit as a major portion of their diets, it would seem more advantageous to prevent fecal contamination of the fresh rations. Should the latter prove impracticable, direct decontamination with various acceptable halogen preparations might be used (hypochlorite, dilute aqueous iodine, and so on).

Although some experimental trials have proved the utility of vaccination (Thal et al. 1964), it is not known how successful this type of acquired immunity would be for wild animal populations. For those institutions using many rare or expensive animals, the use of vaccination warrants greater exploration.

REFERENCES

Akkermans, J. P. W. M., and Terpstra, J. I. Pseudotuberculose bij chinchilla's veroorzaakt door een bijzondere species. *Tijdschr. Diergeneesk.* 88:91–95, 1963.

Blanc, G., and Baltazard, M. Contribution a l'etude du comportement des microbes pathogenes chez les insects hematophages. Premier memoir. *Arch. Inst. Pasteur Maroc* 3:21–49, 1944.

Burrows, T. W., and Bacon, G. A. The basis of virulence in *Pasteurella pestis:* An antigen determining virulence. *Br. J. Exp. Pathol.* 37:481–493, 1956.

———. V and W antigens in strains of *Pasteurella pseudotuberculosis*. *Br. J. Exp. Pathol.* 41:38–44, 1960.

Chapman, M. P. *Pseudotuberculosis rodentium* in chinchilla. A field case. *North Am. Vet.* 29:493–494, 1948.

Currie, J. A. A rapid micro-hemagglutination test for the differentiation of *Pasteurella pseudotuberculosis* types. M.S. thesis, Howard University, 1965.

Currie, J. A., Marshall, J. D., Jr., and Crozier, D. Rapid microhemagglutination test for the detection of *Pasteurella pseudotuberculosis* antibodies. *J. Infect. Dis.* 116:117–122, 1966.

Daniels, J. J. H. M., and Goudzwaard, C. Enkeke stammen von een op *Pasteurella pseudotuberculosis* gelijkend niet geidentificeerd species, geisoleerd bij knaagdieren. *Tijdschr. Diergeneesk.* 88:96–102, 1963.

Davies, D. A. L. A specific polysaccharide of *Pasteurella pestis*. *Biochem. J.* 63:105–216, 1956.

———. The smooth and rough somatic antigens of *Pasteurella pseudotuberculosis*. *J. Gen. Microbiol.* 18:118–128, 1958.

Dickinson, A. B., and Mocquot, G. Studies on the bacterial flora of the alimentary tract of pigs: I. Enterobacteriaceae and other gram-negative bacteria. *J. Appl. Bacteriol.* 24:252–284, 1961.

Eberth, C. J. Zwer mykosen des meerschweinchens. *Virchows Arch. Pathol. Anat. Physiol. Klin. Med.* 100:15–27, 1885.

Fertig, S. Pseudotuberculose animale et humaine en Pologne. Presented at Reunion sur la Pseudotuberculose, Permanent Committee on Biological Standardization, Intern. Assoc. Microbiol. Soc., Inst. Pasteur, Paris, July, 1967. *Symp. Ser. Immunol. Stand.* 9:91–98, 1968.

Frederiksen, W. A study of *Yersinia pseudotuberculosis*-like bacteria (*Bacterium enterocoliticum* and *Pasteurella X*). Proc. 14th Scand. Congr. Pathol. Microbiol., Oslo, Norway. *Abstr. Nr.* 47:103–105, 1964.

Fribourg-Blanc, A., Niel, G., and Mollaret, H. H. Note

sur quelques aspects immunologiques du cyno-cephale africain. *Bull. Soc. Pathol. Exot.* 56:474–485, 1963.

Hammersland, H., and Joneschild, E. M. Pseudotu-berculosis of deer. *J. Am. Vet. Med. Assoc.* 91:186–192, 1937.

Haessig, A., Karrer, J., and Pusterla, F. Ueber Pseu-dotuberkulose beim Muenschen. *Schweiz. Med. Wochenschr.* 79:971–973, 1949.

Humphreys, F. A., and Gibbons, R. J. Some observa-tions on corynebacterial infections with particu-lar reference to their occurrence in mule deer, *Odocoileus hemionus*, in British Columbia. *Can. J. Comp. Med. Vet. Sci.* 6:35–45, 1942.

Ippen, R., and Stoll, L. *Pasteurella pseudotuberculosis* bei einen Virginiahirsch. *Tieraerztl. Wo-chenschr.* 72:439–440, 1959.

Joubert, L., and Oudar, J. La pseudo-tuberculose la-tente du cobaye d'elevage et les erreurs du diag-nostic experimentale. *Bull. Soc. Sci. Vet.* Lyons, 60:119–124, 1958.

Knapp, W. Die diagnostische Bedeutung der antigen-en Beziehungen zwischen *Past. pseudotubercu-losis* und der Salmonella Gruppe. *Zentralbl. Bakteriol.* [*Orig. A*] 164:57–59, 1955.

———. Ueber weitere antigene Beziehungen zwi-schen *Pasteurella pseudotuberculosis* und der Salmonella Gruppe. *Z. Hyg. Infektionskrankh.* 146:315–330, 1960.

Knapp, W., and Thal, E. Untersuchungen ueber die kulturellbiochemischen, serologischen Tierex-perimentellen und immunologischen Eigen-schaften einer vorlaufig *Pasteurella X* bennan-ten Bakterienart. *Zentralbl. Bakteriol.* [*Orig. A*] 190:472–484, 1963.

Krynski, S., and Becla, E. Infection a *P. pseudotuber-culosis* chez le pou. *Ann. Inst. Pasteur* 104:133–136, 1963.

Leader, R. W., and Baker, G. A. A report of two cases of *Pasteurella pseudotuberculosis* infection in the chinchilla. *Cornell Vet.* 44: 262–267, 1954.

Malassez, L., and Vignal, W. Tuberculose zoogleique (forme ou espece de tuberculose sans bacilles). *Arch. Physiol. Norm. Pathol.* 2(ser. 3):369–412, 1883.

———. Sur le microorganisme de la tuberculose zoogleique. *Arch. Physiol. Norm. Pathol.* 4(ser. 3):80–105, 1884.

Mollaret, H. H. Deux cas de pseudo-tuberculose chez le daman. *Bull. Soc. Pathol. Exot.* 51:471–475, 1958.

———. L'infection a bacille de Malassez et Vignal chez le chat: I. La maladie naturelle. II. L'infec-tion experimentale. *Rec. Med. Vet. Exotique* 141:1079–1094, 1187–1201, 1965.

Mollaret, H. H., and Chevalier, A. Contribution a l'etude d'un nouveau groupe de germes proches du bacille de Malassez et Vignal. *Ann. Inst. Pas-teur* 107:121–127, 1964.

Mollaret, H. H. and Guillon, J. C. Contribution a l'etude d'un nouveau groupe de germes (*Yersinia enterocolitica*) proches du bacille de Malassez et Vignal. II. Pouvoir pathogene experimental.

Ann. Inst. Pasteur 109:608–613, 1965.

Mollaret, H. H., and Lucas, A. Sur les particularites biochimiques des souches de *Yersinia enterocoli-tica* isolees chez les lievres. *Ann. Inst. Past.* 108:121–125, 1965.

Mollaret, H. H., Sizaret, Ph., and Vallee, A. A propos d'une epizootie due au bacille de Malassez et Vignal (*Pasteurella pseudotuberculosis*) chez le singe. *Rev. Path. Gen. Physiol. Clin.*, Nr. 750, 753–766, 1963.

Nouvel, J., and Rinjard, J. Pseudotuberculosis in cynocephalid apes (*Papio papio* Desm.) caused by the bacillus of Malassez and Vignal. *Rev. Pathol. Comp. Hyg. Gen.* 49:68–70, 1949.

Paterson, J. S., and Cook, R. A method for the isola-tion of *Pasteurella pseudotuberculosis* from faeces. *J. Pathol. Bacteriol.* 85:241–242, 1963.

Preisz, H., and Guinard, L. Pseudo-tuberculose chez le mouton. *J. Med. Vet. Zootechnic.* 16:563–574, 1891.

Reimann, H. A. Further studies on *B. pseudotuber-culosis. Am. J. Hyg.* 16:206–214, 1932.

Richards, B. Personal communication, 1967.

Rowland, S. Reports on plague investigations in India. LIX. The relation of pseudotubercle to plague as evidenced by vaccination experiments. *J. Hyg.* 12:350–357, 1912.

Schleifstein, J., and Coleman, M. B. An unidentified microorganism resembling *B. lignieri* and *Past. pseudotuberculosis* and pathogenic for man. *N.Y. State J. Med.* 39:1749–1753, 1939.

Schuetze, H. Studies in *B. pestis* antigens. II. The antigenic relationship of *B. pestis* and *B. pseu-dotuberculosis rodentium. Brit. J. Exp. Pathol.* 13:289–293, 1932.

Seghetti, L., and McKenney, F. D. Caseous lymph-adenitis of deer (*Odocoileus hemionus*) in Wash-ington. *J. Am. Vet. Med. Assoc.* 98:129–131, 1941.

Shaw, J. N., Simms, B. T., and Muth, O. H. Some diseases of Oregon fish and game and identifica-tion of parts of game animals. *Oregon Exp. Sta.* Bull. 322, 1934.

Thal, E. Untersuchungen ueber *Pasteurella pseudo-tuberculosis.* Proc. 15th Internationaler Tieraertzlicher Kongress, pp. 1–4, Gernandts Boktrycheriet, Lund, Sweden, 1953.

———. Untersuchungen ueber *Pasteurella pseudotu-berculosis* unter Besonderen Beruecksichtin-gung ihres immunologischen Verhaltens. Ber-lingska Boktrycheriet, Lund, Sweden, 1956.

Thal, E., and Wellmann, G. Weitere Untersuchungen ueber die Waschstumsprobe bei *Yersinia pseu-dotuberculosis.* Presented at Reunion sur la Pseudotuberculose, Permanent Committee on Biological Standardization, Intern. Assoc. Mi-crobiol. Soc., Inst. Pasteur, July 1967, Symp. Ser. Immunol. Standardization 9:211–218, 1968.

Thal, E., Hanko, E., and Knapp, W. Intranasale Vak-zination von Meerschweinchen mit einen aviru-lenten Stamm der *Pasteurella pseudotuberculo-sis. Acta Vet. Scand.* 5:179–187, 1964.

Ul'yanova, N. L. The natural focal occurrence of

pseudotuberculosis. *J. Microbiol. Epidemiol. Immunobiol.* 32:2268–2272, 1961.

Urbain, Ach. Au sujet de la pseudo-tuberculose chez le singe. *C. R. Soc. Biol.* 136:637–638, 1942.

Wetzler, T. F. Antigens and factors affecting virulence of *Pasteurella pseudotuberculosis* and *Yersinia enterocolitica* with a description of a new serofactor and a new strain. Ph.D. thesis, Univ. of Mich., Ann Arbor, 1965.

Wetzler, T. F., and Hubbert, W. T. *Yersinia enterocolitica* in North America. Presented at Reunion sur la Pseudotuberculose, Permanent Committee on Biological Standardization, Intern. Assoc. Microbiol. Soc., Inst. Pasteur, July 1967. Symp. Ser. Immunol. Standardization 9:343–356, 1968a.

Wetzler, T. F., and Hubbard, W. T. *Pasteurella pseudotuberculosis* in North America. Presented at Reunion sur la Pseudotuberculose, Permanent Committee on Biological Standardization, Intern. Assoc. Microbiol. Soc., Inst. Pasteur, July 1967. Symp. Ser. Immunol. Standardization 9:33–44, 1968b.

Wetzler, T. F., Eveland, W. C., and Cowan, A. B. The ecology and epidemiology of *Pasteurella pseudotuberculosis* and *Yersinia enterocolitica*: I. Survey of deer serum for hemagglutination antibody. *Zoonosis Res.*, 1970.

Wetzler, T. F., Eitzen, H. E., Currie, J. A., and Marshall, J. D., Jr. Lipopolysaccharide-like antigens from *Pasteurella pseudotuberculosis* shared by various genera of Enterobacteriaceae as demonstrated by hemagglutination tests. Presented at Reunion sur la Pseudotuberculose, Permanent Committee on Biological Standardization, Intern. Assoc. Microbiol. Soc., Inst. Pasteur, July 1967. Symp. Ser. Immunol. Standardization 9:155–66, 1968.

Winblad, S. Studies on O-antigen factors of *Yersinia enterocolitica*. Presented at Reunion sur la Pseudotuberculose, Permanent Committee on Biological Standardization, Intern. Assoc. Microbiol. Soc., Inst. Pasteur, July 1967. Symp. Ser. Immunol. Standardization 9:337–342, 1968.

22 *Tuberculosis*

CHARLES O. THOEN   ELMER M. HIMES

Synonyms: **Mycobacterial infections.**

For more than a century tuberculosis has been recognized as a serious clinical entity in wild animals maintained in captivity. Although lesions most commonly involve the lung, numerous reports are available on the presence of disease in other organs and tissues including the intestines, liver, spleen, kidney, and reproductive tract. Microscopically the granulomas are usually characterized by a caseous necrotic center bordered by a zone of epithelioid cells, multinucleated giant cells, and lymphocytes. A fibrous connective tissue capsule may be present. *Mycobacterium bovis* is the organism most frequently isolated from hoofed animals; however, nonhuman primates are susceptible to *M. bovis*, *M. tuberculosis*, and *M. avium*.

HISTORY. The dissemination of tuberculosis around the world was probably associated with the spread of civilization. The disease existed and was recognized in ancient civilizations, from which it subsequently spread to the rest of the world. Romans were familiar with tuberculosis and perhaps helped carry the disease throughout the then civilized world. Tuberculosis was probably introduced into Great Britain by Roman invaders (Francis 1958). Denmark and other Scandinavian countries were ap-

parently infected through commerce with Britain in the eighteenth century. European immigrants and their livestock may have brought tuberculosis to the New World.

Some early reports of tuberculosis in wild animals describe the disease as seen in animals in zoological parks. In view of the reduction of tuberculosis in domestic animals and humans, one might expect a decrease in disease in zoo animals. However, this trend has not been observed. There is some evidence that indicates foci of infection persist in wild animal populations for long periods of time. This emphasizes a need for changing the procedures for eliminating tuberculosis from these populations.

There has been an increased interest in tuberculosis in captive exotic species following outbreaks of the disease in animals in zoos, primate centers, animal colonies, and game parks (Thoen et al. 1977). The importance of these occurrences of tuberculosis is emphasized by the difficulty of replacing some rare and endangered exotic animals, by the economic losses, and by the public health hazard.

DISTRIBUTION. Tuberculosis is widely distributed in wild mammals in the United States. Outbreaks of *M. bovis* have been reported in zoos, game parks, and primate colonies in 18 states (Fig. 22.1). The *M. bovis* isolations were from nonhuman primates including baboons as

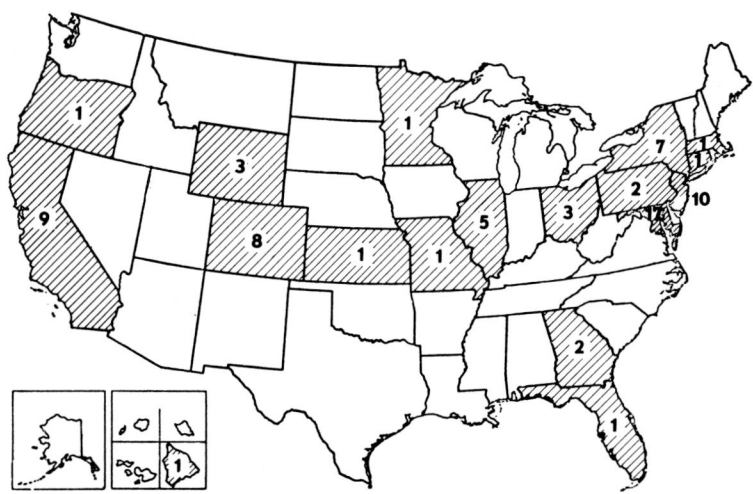

FIG. 22.1 Number of *M. bovis* isolations from wild animals during a 5-year period (July 1, 1976), by state. Reprinted by permission of the *Journal of the American Veterinary Medical Association* 170(9):987–999, 1977.

well as several species of hoofed animals. Tuberculosis has been reported in elephants and giraffes (Nieberle 1938; Thoen et al. 1977). In many instances imported animals were infected and identified as the source of infection, however, in some collections there was evidence that the disease had existed in hoofed animals for several years. At the present time there are no regulations which require the reporting of tuberculosis outbreaks in exotic species to regulatory officials. In many instances necropsies are not conducted. Moreover, there is often a reluctance to publicize the occurrence of tuberculosis in zoo animals because of public relations or maintaining prestige.

Epizootics of *M. bovis* have been reported in exotic animals in other countries. In Germany the disease has been reported in several predacious felines including lions, tigers, leopards, and lynx (Schliesser 1976). No confirmed reports of *M. bovis* infection in exotic felines are available in the United States. Tuberculosis has also been reported in wild mammals in Canada, Africa, South America, and Asia (Costallat et al. 1978; Mandal and Singh 1975; Renner and Bartholomew 1974). Since animals are frequently imported from zoos in other countries, continuous efforts should be made to ascertain their health status before additions are made to established herds or colonies.

Mycobacterium tuberculosis, the human tubercle bacillus, has been reported as the most common cause of tuberculosis in nonhuman primates (Francis 1958). In a recent 5-year study *M. tuberculosis* and *M. avium* were isolated from exotic animals originating in 9 states (Thoen et al. 1977). The widespread occurrence of outbreaks of *M. tuberculosis* are of concern to public health officials, conservation agency officials, and veterinarians responsible for the health status of animals in zoos, animal parks, and primate colonies.

Tuberculosis has not been commonly reported in wild animals except where they have exposure to domestic animals or human beings that have mycobacterial infection (Ruch 1959). *Mycobacterium bovis* infection was reported in wild axis deer in Hawaii and in white-tailed deer in Michigan and New York; infected cattle were considered a possible source of *M. bovis* (Belli 1962; Friend et al. 1963; Quinn et al. 1963; Sawa et al. 1974). Tuberculosis has also been reported in roe deer, red deer, and fallow deer (*Dama dama*) (Hopkinson and McDiarmid, 1964; Jorgensen and Clausen 1976). Gallagher et al. (1972) and Clancy (1977) described outbreaks of tuberculosis in lechwe (marsh antelope) in Zambia where *M. bovis*–infected cattle may have been the reservoir of disease since the lechwe had been feeding in the same area as tuberculous cattle. Similar reports of tuberculosis have been made in African cape buffalo (*Syncerus caffer caffer*) in Uganda and in South African cape kudu (*Strepsiceros* spp.) and cape duiker (*Sylvicapra* spp.) in South Africa (Guilbride et al. 1963; Paine and Martinaglia 1928). Tuberculosis has also been reported in camels in Egypt which had close association with tuberculous cattle (Mason 1917).

Several reports are available on the isolation of tubercle bacilli from wild rodents. In a recent outbreak of bovine tuberculosis in Great Britain, wild badgers in the pasture were infected with *M. bovis* (Murihead et al. 1974). Field voles are suspectible to *M. microti*, a slow-growing, nonchromogenic acid-fast organism (Wells and Oxon 1961). Tuberculosis has been reported in otters (Borg 1964) and in a ferret (Dunkin et al. 1929). Disease has also been reported in ground squirrels (McCoy and Chapin 1911).

ETIOLOGY. Several species of the genus *Mycobacterium* have been isolated from wild animals maintained in captivity. Mycobacteria were isolated from 65% of 261 tissues of wild mammals suspected of having tuberculous lesions on necropsy (Table 22.1). *M. bovis* accounted for the greatest number of isolations (74/166). Of particular interest was the high isolation rate (73%) obtained from tissues of nonhuman primates. Twenty-six *M. bovis* isolates were from monkeys, 13 from deer, 12 from kudus, 8 from llamas, 5 from antelopes, 3 from bisons, 2 from baboons, 2 from sitatungas, and 1 each from an elk, an eland, and a tapir. *M. tuberculosis,* the human tubercle bacilli, was isolated from 28 animals in 9 states; 21 isolates were from monkeys, 4 from oryxes, 2 from addaxes, and 1 from an elephant. *M. avium,* the avian tubercle bacillus, was isolated from 54 exotic mammals; 46 were isolates from monkeys in primate colonies and zoos, and 5 were from hoofed animals. Serotypes 1 and 8 accounted for the greatest number of the *M. avium* isolates from the nonhuman primates.

Although data on the frequency of the mycobacterial isolations is limited, available information indicates that many of the species are susceptible to *M. bovis, M. tuberculosis,* and *M. avium.* The findings may be influenced by the organisms to which the captive animals are exposed. Felines appear to be most susceptible to *M. bovis.* Even in West Germany and Swit-

TABLE 22.1 Mycobacteria Isolated from Wild Mammals during a 5-year Period (July 1, 1971, to June 1, 1976).

	Number of Isolations			
Organism	Nonhuman Primates	Hoofed Animals	Other[a]	Total Number (%)
M. bovis	28	46	−	74 (44.6)
M. avium	46	5	3	54 (32.5)
M. tuberculosis	21	7		28 (16.9)
M. fortuitum	2	1		3 (1.8)
M. chelonei		1	1	2 (1.2)
M. scrofulaceum		2		2 (1.2)
Mycobacterium spp.[b]	2	1		3 (1.8)
Total isolations	99	63	4	166 (65)
Total submissions	135	119	7	261

Source: Isolations made from tissues submitted to National Veterinary Service Laboratories, U.S. Department of Agriculture, Ames, Iowa.

[a]*M. avium* was isolated from 2 tree kangaroos and an opossum; *M. chelonei* was isolated from a manatee.
[b]Rapidly growing mycobacteria.

zerland where bovine tuberculosis has been eradicated since 1961 and 1959 respectively, *M. bovis* infections continue to persist in large cats (Schliesser 1978).

Most clinically significant mycobacteria are slow-growing organisms that usually appear on culture mediums in 2–6 weeks. Microscopically, the mycobacteria usually appear as slender rods, 0.2–0.6 μm in diameter and 1.5–3 μm long. Forms ranging from coccoid to filamentous may be seen in the same culture. The morphology and staining characteristics of pathogenic mycobacteria are similar to those of saprophytes.

An important staining characteristic of mycobacteria is their resistance to acid decolorizing agents. Several staining procedures are available for demonstrating acid-fast bacilli, but the Ziehl-Neelsen or Kinyoun techniques with carbol fuchsin are most widely used (Thoen and Karlson, forthcoming).

TRANSMISSION AND RESISTANCE. The elimination of tuberculosis in wild animals is hampered by the lack of suitable regulations limiting the movement of infected or exposed animals. The problem is further magnified by the inability to detect tuberculous animals early in the course of disease, because clinical signs may not be present until progressive pulmonary disease develops.

In nonhuman primates *M. bovis* and *M. tuberculosis* can produce extensive disease involving the parenchyma of the lung as well as extrapulmonary tissues. The disease may be transmitted in coughs from animals by aerosols or droplets containing tubercle bacilli. Animals may also be infected through feed and water contaminated with urine, fecal material, or exudates from diseased animals shedding tubercle bacilli. Fomites such as thermometers are a definite source of spread, as are cages, masks, and containers used for food and water (Riordan 1943; Ruch 1959).

Among hoofed animals, disease is transmitted through air or through contaminated feed and water. Oryxes and addaxes are examples of hoofed animals which are susceptible to *M. tuberculosis*. These animals may develop extensive pulmonary lesions as well as lesions of the uterus and mammary gland. Therefore, in the young, congenital transmission or transmission by drinking milk from an animal with tuberculous mastitis should be considered (Lomme et al. 1976). Tuberculous humans may also be a source of infection for both susceptible hoofed animals and nonhuman primates.

Crowding appears to be important in the transmission and spread of tuberculosis in animals as in man. In domestic animals, the disease is most common among animals kept in close contact in pens or barns (Thoen and Karlson, forthcoming).

A number of severe outbreaks in fur-bearing animals have resulted from ingestion of contaminated meat. In North America most of the disease reported in mink is caused by *M. avium* and is related to feeding uncooked meat and offal of diseased chickens (Hall and Winkel 1957).

Mycobacteria are relatively resistant to conditions detrimental to other non-spore-forming bacteria. The tubercle bacilli may remain viable for 6 months or more at room temperature if protected from sunlight. It has been demonstrated that some species, such as avian tubercle bacilli, may remain viable in soil and litter for 4 years or more.

PATHOGENESIS. Tubercle bacilli which are inhaled usually locate in alveolar spaces where they are ingested by alveolar macrophages. The reaction of the exotic animals to invasion by mammalian or avian tubercle bacilli is basically similar to that observed in domestic animals (Dannenberg 1978). The development or elimination of disease depends on the microbicidal activities of the ingesting macrophages to destroy the tubercle bacilli. In instances where the organism multiplies within the phagocyte, the host cell may die, resulting in the development of a microscopic tubercle. Initially, the lesion is composed of sensitized leukocytes and specialized macrophages referred to as epithelioid cells. The cellular debris of degenerated macrophages locally sensitizes lymphocytes which may produce lymphokines that attract and immobilize other macrophages. Subsequently, there is a dynamic turnover of engulfment of bacteria and degeneration of phagocytes at the lesion site. As the lesion develops, necrosis occurs and Langhan's giant cells appear in the lesion. As the tubercle progresses, a zone of lymphocytes and mononuclear cells surrounds the site, and there is a proliferation of connective tissue at the periphery, which appears as a capsule. As lesions increase in size, caseation necrosis becomes apparent and mineralization may occur.

No definitive information is available on the subcellular events of mycobacterial infections. However, it has been suggested that the lipid components present in the cell wall interfere with the digestion of acid-fast bacilli by mononuclear macrophages; therefore, the organisms appear to be protected from the hydrolytic enzymes present in the primary and secondary granules of host cells, which are capable of killing and destroying other bacteria (Cheville 1976; Thoen 1979). The ability of a tubercle bacillus to establish a lesion depends on whether the organism can grow intracellularly and the host cells can inhibit its growth.

The success of the host cells in destroying tubercle bacilli probably involves the production and release of microbicidal components. The importance of cell-mediated hypersensitivity by thymic-derived lymphocytes and lymphokines produced by these cells appears to play a major role in attracting macrophages, which are activated and involved in the host resistance to infection and ultimately protect the host from disease.

SIGNS. Clinical signs of tuberculosis in exotic mammals are variable. The kind of disease is often related to virulence of the organism, the route of infection, the stage of infection, and several host-related factors.

In nonhuman primates with pulmonary tuberculosis the animals may exhibit a cough and show some evidence of dyspnea. When visceral lesions are present, an enlarged spleen or liver may be palpated on physical examination. In advanced cases regional lymph nodes may be enlarged and in some instances rupture and drain to the surface. In chronic cases emaciation may result from inappetence. The hair coat may appear rough, and occasionally alopecia is apparent. In acute cases resulting from massive exposure to mammalian tubercle bacilli, the disease may spread so rapidly that no obvious signs develop prior to death.

In outbreaks of *M. avium* infection in monkeys there may be involvement of the digestive tract and associated lymph nodes (Sesline et al. 1975). This disease is usually manifested by a persistent or intermittent diarrhea that fails to respond to therapy. In later stages of disease the animals may appear dehydrated and often have a rough hair coat.

In wild ruminants signs of tuberculosis usually resemble those seen in cattle. The bronchial, mediastinal, and portal lymph nodes are the sites where tubercles are often found. Other tissues that are commonly affected include lung, liver, spleen, and the surfaces of body cavities. When tuberculous lesions are located in the parenchyma of the lung, a productive bronchopneumonia may be present. In severe cases dyspnea, emaciation, and a roughened hair coat are apparent. Lesions have been reported in the genital tract in cases where generalized tuberculosis is present (Lomme et al. 1976). A mucopurulent discharge from the vagina may persist for prolonged periods of time. The report of tuberculous mastitis in an oryx emphasizes the importance of a thorough physical examination supported by adequate laboratory examination.

It is important to emphasize that clinical signs are only rarely apparent in exotic animals. Therefore, it is essential to conduct suitable diagnostic procedures, including delayed type hypersensitivity tests while animals are held in isolation facilities prior to herd addition.

PATHOLOGY

Gross Pathology. Often, wild mammals in which tuberculous lesions have been observed on necropsy have been examined after natural death without prior suspicion of tuberculosis. Gross lesions may extensively involve entire organs of one or both body cavities; however, the anatomic sites of lesions, the extensiveness of pathologic involvement, and consistency of nodular formation with some caseous necrosis are not usually different than that seen in domestic animals (Dannenberg et al. 1978). The obvious difficulties with observations and handling of some wild mammals in managed herds or colonies may contribute to an animal's continued existence with disease progression, although there may be outward appearances of unthriftiness.

Tuberculous tissues observed on necropsy usually have an appearance of yellowish, caseous necrotic areas in nodules of firm white to light gray fibrous tissue (Smith et al. 1972). Tubercles may not appear discrete in instances where lesions become diffuse with existing tissues. Almost invariably there is a multiplicity of other bacteria and other agents present with tuberculous lesions which may affect gross appearance. Some lesions may have purulent consistency, whereas others may be partially dry with caseation or extensive fibrosis. Calcification or caseocalcification may occur in lesions but is often slight in wild mammals. A lung lobe of a greater kudu from which a portion has been removed is shown in Figure 22.2.

Microscopic Pathology. The cellular detail of tuberculous lesions from domestic and wild mammals has been previously described by light microscopy studies (Francis 1958; Smith et al. 1972). Essentially, a tubercle is a granulomatous lesion that is characteristically composed of a caseous, necrotic center bordered by a zone of epithelioid cells, some of which may have formed multinucleated giant cells of lymphocytes and granulocytes and an encapsulation of fibrous connective tissue of varying thickness. Considerable variation exists in the apparent ability of some wild mammals to form tubercles associated with connective tissue and of epithelioid cells to form multinucleated giant cells, which are commonplace in tubercles of domestic bovines. An absence of multinucleated giant cells in tubercles from a lung of an Indian elephant has been reported (Pinto et al. 1973). This may be histologic evidence for species- or animal-associated factors that influence host-parasite relationships. Lung from an Indian elephant with a tuberculous lesion composed of

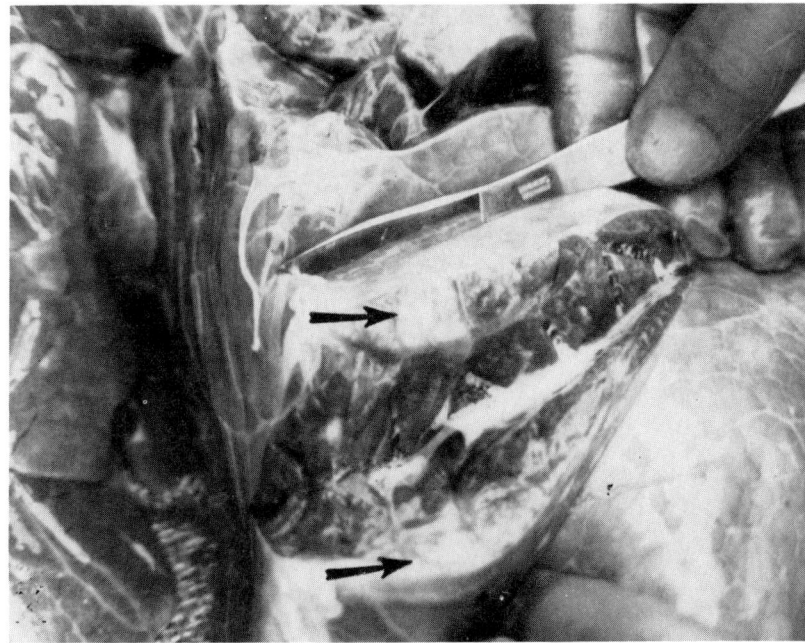

FIG. 22.2 Lung lobe from a greater kudu with tuberculous lesions exposed on cut surface. *M. bovis* was isolated.

a multinucleated giant cell, epithelioid cells, and an area of caseation with no recognizable connective tissue cells is shown in Figure 22.3. Other tuberculous lesions from this elephant lacked connective tissue proliferation. Several lung tubercles examined from another Indian elephant with *M. tuberculosis* had lesions with thick zones of fibrous connective tissue, althrough there was an absence of multinucleated giant cells.

A section of lung from a black rhinoceros with tubercles (Fig. 22.4) is representative of those observed in rhinocerotines and tapirines. Epithelioid cells are numerous throughout the tissue, and some have formed multinucleated giant cells.

Tuberculous lesions from camelines, cervines, and wild bovines closely resemble those of domestic bovines. A lung section from an American bison is shown in Figure 22.5. A central area of caseation and slight calcification is surrounded by a zone of epithelioid cells and lymphocytes and is encapsulated by a thick zone of fibrous tissue. Lesions examined from antelopines such as oryxes, kudus, nilgais, and a sable-horned antelope have been observed to closely resemble other bovines.

Tuberculous lesions examined microscopically from baboons and several species of monkeys have similarities with those in other wild mammals; however, the spleen of a mandrill infected with *M. bovis* exhibited numerous tubercles of uniform size, an absence of multinucleated giant cells, and centers with an appearance of amyloid. Tubercles from nonhuman primates that are infected with *M. bovis* have not been observed to have significant histologic differences to differentiate these from tubercles caused by *M. tuberculosis*.

DIAGNOSIS. Clinical signs are of limited value in establishing a presumptive diagnosis of tuberculosis in exotic animals. Although lesions may involve several organs in the thoracic and abdominal cavity, the animal may not show evidence of disease. Emaciation, dyspnea, and a roughened hair coat may be apparent in some advanced cases; however, these may not be present until a few days or a week before death.

Radiologic examinations have been found to be of value in identifying the occurrence of lesions in tuberculous baboons (Fig. 22.6). In advanced cases in nonhuman primates involving *M. bovis* and *M. tuberculosis*, granulomas

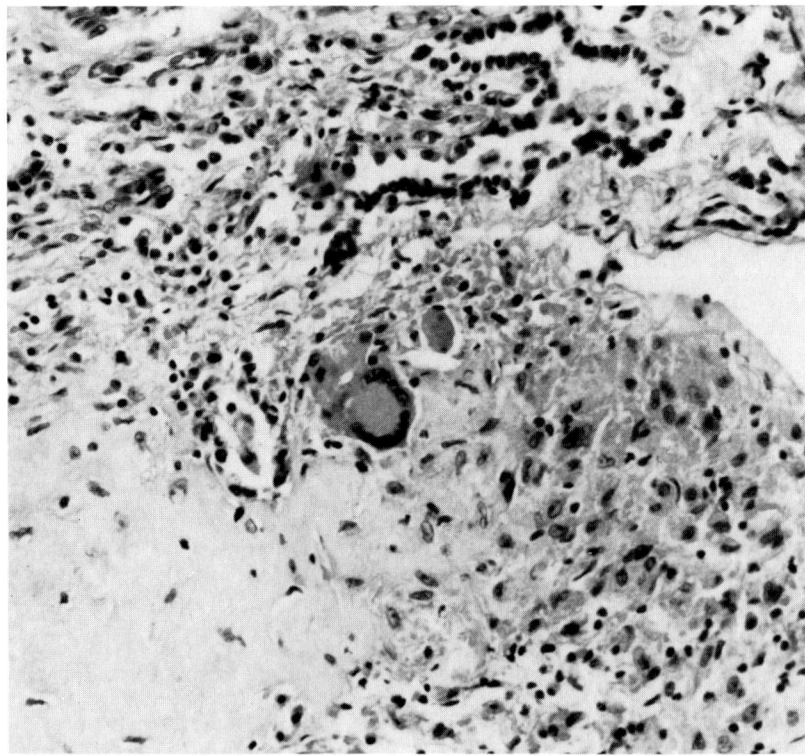

FIG. 22.3 Lung section from an Indian elephant. A multinucleated Langhan's type cell appears along the lesion border in an area that has caseous necrosis. Large vesicular cells and lymphocytes can be observed. *M. tuberculosis* was isolated (HE stain, ×250).

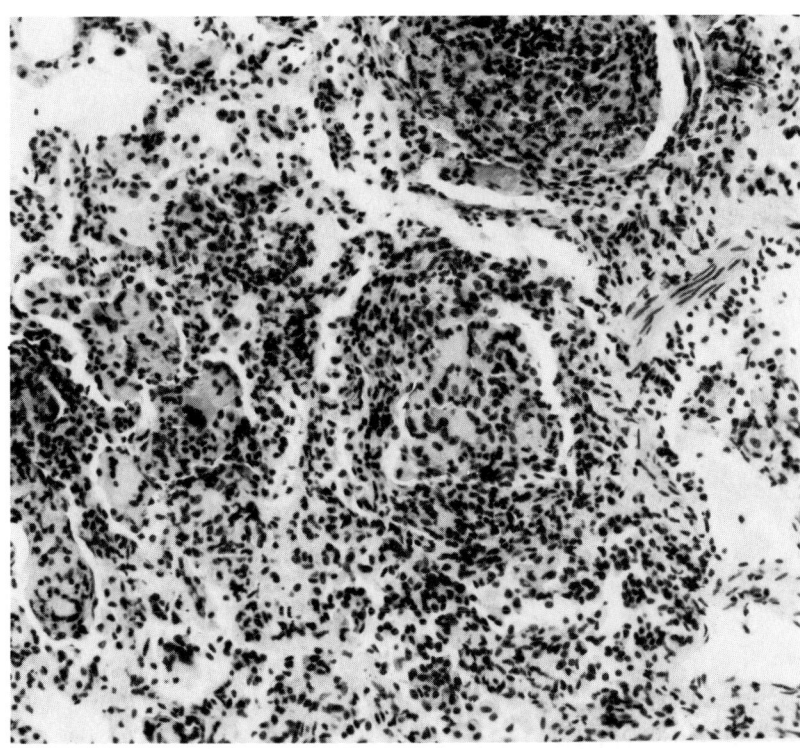

FIG. 22.4 Lung section from a black rhinoceros. Epithelioid cells appear as the predominant type. Several Langhan's giant cells are present. Note a lack of consolidation and encapsulation. *M. bovis* was isolated (HE stain, ×160).

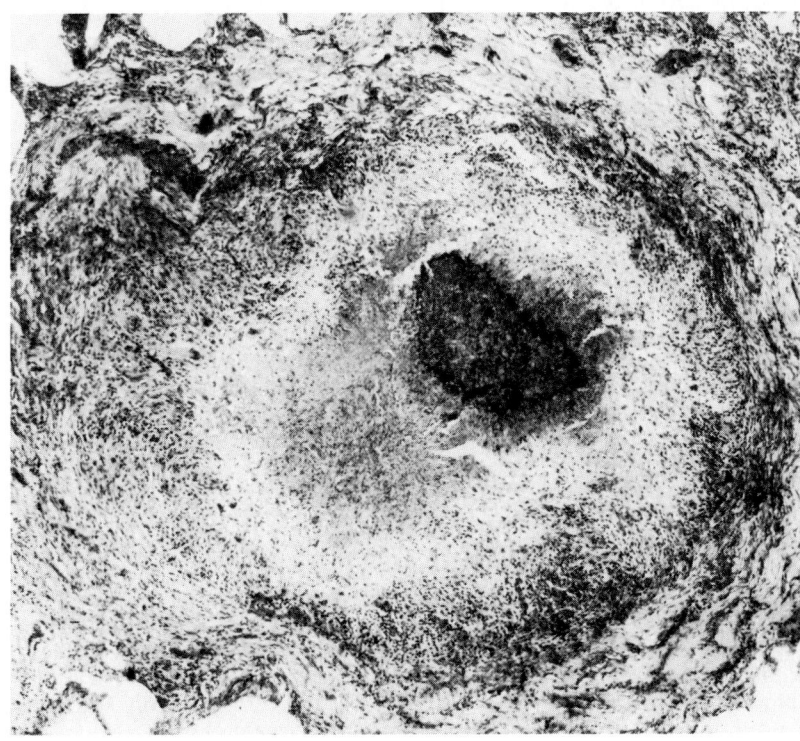

FIG. 22.5 Lung section from an American bison. A central zone of necrosis is surrounded by inflammatory cellular elements and encapsulated by fibrous connective tissue. *M. bovis* was isolated. (HE stain, ×63).

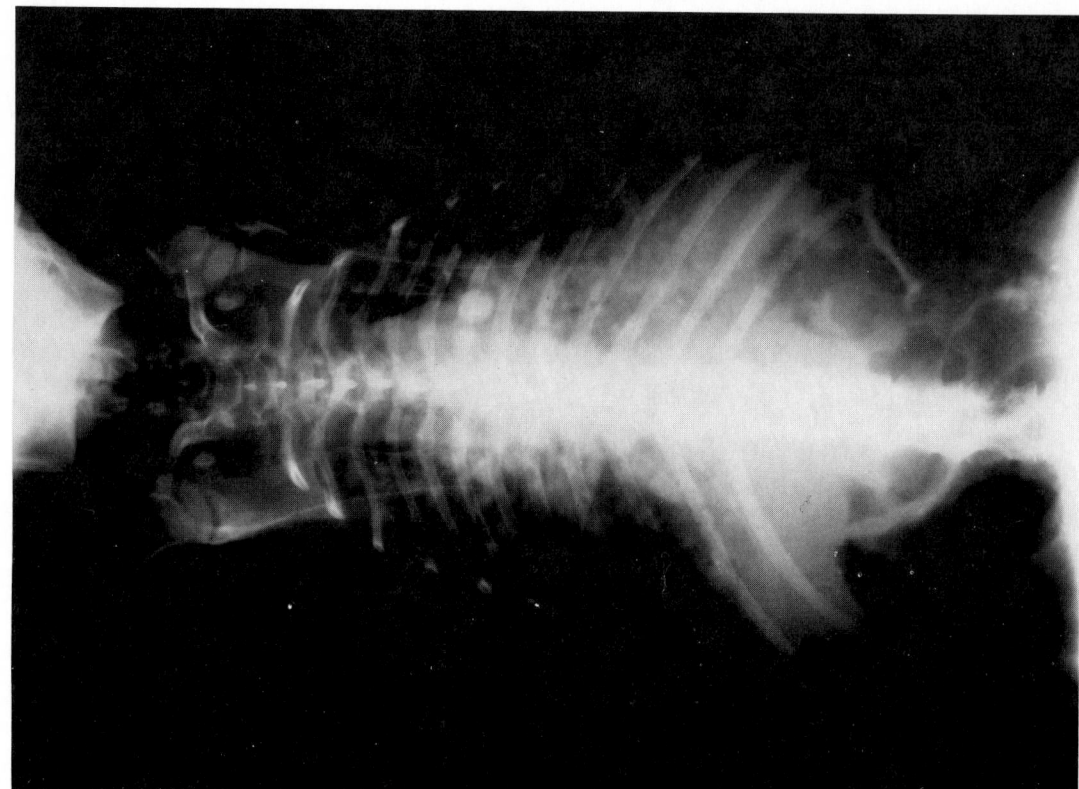

FIG. 22.6 Anterior-posterior chest roentgenogram of a baboon with *M. bovis* infection. Numerous nodular lesions up to 6 mm in diameter and hilar adenopathy are observed. Reprinted by permission of *Archives of Pathology and Laboratory Medicine* 101:291–293, 1977.

usually present in the lung appear as nodular masses. Similar findings have been reported in kudu from which *M. bovis* was isolated on necropsy (Himes et al. 1976).

The tuberculin skin test has been the key to reducing the incidence of tuberculosis in man and cattle. Despite certain limitations, the test is considered the most practical procedure for the diagnosis of tuberculosis in nonhuman primates. However, it is important to recognize that in certain nonhuman primates the test remains negative for several weeks following exposure (Thoen et al. 1977). Factors that may influence tuberculin skin responsiveness in monkeys include isoniazid therapy, desensitization following repeated tuberculin testing, and certain viral infections such as measles (rubeola) that induce anergy (Potkay et al. 1966). Adequate dosage is an important factor in conducting tuberculin tests in nonhuman primates. Tuberculins prepared for human use are unsuitable. Products used in nonhuman primates must be standardized in the species to be tested. Several tuberculins prepared by different methods are in use for testing exotic animals. Koch's old tuberculin (KOT), as originally prepared, was a heat concentrate of glycerol-veal broth in which tubercle bacilli had been grown (Thoen and Karlson 1981). The bacilli were killed by flowing steam and removed; the filtrate was evaporated to 10% of its original volume. In 1934, Dorset produced a tuberculin for veterinary use on a synthetic medium free of animal protein. Three strains of *M. tuberculosis* were used. The test agent was produced in the same general manner as KOT except that it was evaporated to 20% of its original volume and reconstituted to 40% using phosphate buffer, 0.5% phenol, and glycerol. This product is referred to as USDA old tuberculin (UDSA-OT). Recently more refined tuberculins called purified protein derivatives (PPD) have been prepared by precipitation with ammonium sulfate or trichloroacetic acid. Such products have an advantage in that they may be standardized on the basis of nitrogen present in tuberculoprotein.

Studies have been made in nonhuman primates comparing the efficacy of OT and PPD (McLaughlin et al. 1976; Smith and Wolochow 1973). A comparison of several tuberculins in *Macaca mulatta* during a natural outbreak of tuberculosis revealed that either the intrapalpebral or abdominal test sites can be used (McLaughlin et al. 1976). However, it should be noted that either site alone failed to diagnose 10% of the tuberculous monkeys. At the concentrations used, the USDA-OT provided greater accuracy and skin test responses than either KOT or PPD tuberculin. Although local desensitization of the test site as a result of repeated testing has been reported, animals receiving three consecutive tests at 2-week intervals showed strong positive responses on each test. Tuberculin responses should be read at 24, 48, and 72 hours; swelling, erythema, induration, and necrosis at the test site should be recorded.

At present there is no standard procedure for testing great apes. The methods employed vary with respect to the type and concentration of tuberculin and the test site (Kuhn and Selin 1978). Mammalian old tuberculin prepared for veterinary use is usually injected into the upper eyelid, and the site is observed for erythema and induration at 24, 48, and 72 hours. Tests using avian and mammalian tuberculin may provide useful information for differentiating sensitization due to mammalian tubercle bacilli from other acid-fast organisms. Old tuberculins and PPDs have been used for testing the great apes (Haberle 1970).

In some hoofed animals the intradermal tuberculin test is made by injecting 0.2 ml of USDA-OT into the dermal layer of the cervical region of the caudal fold (Himes et al. 1976; Lomme et al. 1976). A positive response is usually apparent by swelling and induration at the site in 72 hours. When skin tests are made in the cervical region, the thickness of skin is measured in millimeters before and at 72 hours after injection; an increase of 3 mm or more is considered a positive response. In some hoofed animals with disseminated disease, the tuberculin test results have been negative. Studies are needed in exotic hoofed animals to evaluate the efficiency of PPD tuberculin in detecting tuberculous animals (Angus 1978). Efforts should be made to establish the optimum dose of PPD, the time for reading responses, and the site of injection in the various species.

Blood tests have not been found to be useful in establishing a diagnosis of tuberculosis in certain animals because of nonspecific reactions and false negative results. However, recently developed techniques involving lymphocyte immunostimulation with specific mycobacterial antigens appear to be of value (Muscoplat et al. 1975). Results of lymphocyte stimulation tests are available within 1 week; this would provide for the rapid removal of infected animals from the population, which is very important in controlling and eliminating the disease. It has the advantage of only handling the animal once as compared to twice for the tuberculin skin tests.

Enzyme immunoassay (EIA) tests have been developed for detecting mycobacterial infections in exotic animals (Thoen et al. 1978, 1980). Studies on sera from monkeys infected with *M. bovis* indicate the rapid EIA test can be useful in the diagnosis of tuberculosis in monkeys and certain other exotic species. Systematic studies are needed in nonhuman primates and hoofed animals to obtain information on the development and persistence of antibodies and EIA reactions in animals at various stages of infection. The soluble antigen fluorescent antibody test is also based on the measurement of circulating antibody (Affronti et al. 1973). Although the test appeared to be of value in identifying experimentally infected animals, it has not come into widespread use.

A comparison of serum lipid and lipoprotein profiles from tuberculin-positive and tuberculin-negative monkeys revealed the presence of a beta component in negative monkeys that was not present in positive monkeys (Thoen et al. 1973). Triglyceride values were significantly higher in the tuberculin-positive monkeys.

Histopathologic examinations of tissues collected at necropsy or on biopsy provide useful information in establishing a diagnosis of tuberculosis. Lesions may vary for different animals; however, typical lesions usually are characterized by the presence of epithelioid cells and multinucleated giant cells. Caseation necrosis and mineralization may be present. Acid-fast bacilli can be demonstrated in the lesions by staining replicate sections with auramine-O (Himes 1978).

Tissues should be collected for bacteriologic studies whenever possible as this is the only procedure available for confirming a diagnosis of tuberculosis (Thoen and Karlson 1980). Specimens for mycobacteriologic examinations should be submitted to the laboratory frozen or in a saturated solution of sodium borate. Tubercle bacilli grow aerobically on in vitro cultivation. The optimal temperature for growth of mammalian strains is 37°C, and for avian strains 43°C; however, some exceptions occur. Sodium hydroxide is usually used to process ground tissue suspensions or other specimens to minimize growth of rapidly growing bacteria or fungi on culture media. Since many of the pathogenic strains of mycobacteria are slowly growing organisms, appropriately prepared cultures should be incubated for 8–10 weeks. Identification of mycobacterial isolates usually is accomplished by conducting appropriate biochemical, drug susceptibility, and supplemental tests. It is recommended that the cultures be submitted to a reference laboratory for final identification.

TREATMENT. Antituberculosis drugs used in man have also been used for treating disease in monkeys and great apes in captivity (Francke 1964; Fremming et al. 1957). Isoniazid (INH) has been effective in controlling clinical disease in monkeys; however, animals may continue to shed tubercle bacilli in secretions or excretions following initiation of therapy. The drug dosage and period for which monkeys and great apes are maintained appears to be very important. In one case, an orangutan on INH therapy developed clinical disease (Haberle 1974). In great apes the recommended dose of INH varies from 25 to 50 mg/kg of body weight per day. Some consideration should be given to using two or more antituberculosis drugs simultaneously when treating nonresponsive animals with signs of progressive disease. Drug sensitivity tests should be conducted in vitro on isolates prior to initiation of long-term therapy; these tests should be redone at periodic intervals on isolates from animals which fail to respond to therapy. Assistance should be obtained from a reference laboratory that is adequately equipped to conduct tests to determine drug sensitivity profiles. No information is available on treatment of animals in their native habitat.

There is evidence that INH is immunosuppressive; therefore, the use of the tuberculin test is of limited value in detecting tuberculous animals receiving INH therapy (Gibson et al. 1971). To obtain a valid test, it is recommended that INH therapy be discontinued 30 days prior to tuberculin skin testing. The risk of infected animals developing fulminating disease is a reason often presented for failure to discontinue drug therapy prior to conducting delayed type tuberculin skin tests.

Isoniazid is an inexpensive drug with minimal side effects; therefore, the drug is presently used prophylactically to control disease in nonhuman primates in many zoological parks and primate colonies. The INH dosage recommended in Old World monkeys ranges from 5 to 20 mg/kg per day for 1 year; however, in New World monkeys a lower dose is recommended (Peters and Gordon 1971). The drug may be added to the food or dissolved in the water. The water intake may vary considerably from one day to another under various environmental conditions; therefore, the addition of INH to food provides for more uniform ingestion. In hoofed animals such as kudu, oryxes, llamas, and rhinoceros, INH should be given at the rate of 15–25 mg/kg per day for 1 year and may be reduced to 10–15 mg/kg per day during the 2nd year of therapy. Peracute deaths have been reported in giraffes treated with INH (Fowler 1978).

Para-amino salicylic acid (PAS), 40–60 mg/kg, and streptomycin are other drugs which may be used in treating animals infected with mammalian tubercle bacilli. Rifampin has been used to treat *M. bovis* infections in mink (Pulling 1952). Antituberculosis drugs are of little value in treating infections caused by *M. avium* or atypical, unclassified mycobacteria unless they are used in combination at a suitable dosage.

CONTROL. Wild animals acquired for addition to a zoo collection, animal park, or primate colony should come from herds with a history free of disease. Quarantines should be imposed on all imports; the period of quarantine should be a minimum of 60 days and preferably 120 days. Tuberculin skin tests can be conducted in nonhuman primates at 14- to 30-day intervals. It is important to use a tuberculin prepared for animal use. Products prepared for human use may not be of suitable potency for animals. When tuberculosis is diagnosed in a monkey colony, it may be necessary to destroy tuberculin-positive animals (Renquist and Whitney 1978). In such instances, the facilities including feeders and watering containers should be thoroughly cleaned and decontaminated using a 5% cresylic compound or a derivative of phenol such as sodium orthophenylphenate. If possible the premises should be disinfected three times at 21-day intervals. Hypochlorites, halides, and benzalkonium chloride, which are commonly used disinfectants, are unsuitable for killing tubercle bacilli.

OTHER MYCOBACTERIAL INFECTIONS. Noncultivatable mycobacteria have been associated with leprosylike disease in wild nine-banded armadillos (*Dasypus novemcinctus*) from several locations in Louisiana (Walsh et al. 1975). Insects and their larvae, as well as soil contaminated with *M. leprae*, have been considered as possible source(s) of the organism. The disease has been transmitted under experimental conditions.

Recently, *M. chelonei*, a rapidly growing acid-fast organism, was isolated from a natterer manatee (*Trichechus inunguis*) with granulomatous lesions in the skin (Boever et al. 1976). The animal failed to respond to antibiotic therapy. The source of the infection was not determined. A similar organism, *M. abscessus*, has been isolated from an owl monkey (*Aetus trivirgatus*) with tuberculosislike lesions (Karlson et al. 1970).

REFERENCES

Affronti, L. F., Fife, E. H., and Grow, L. Serodiagnostic test for tuberculosis. *Am. Rev. Respir. Dis.* 107:882–885, 1973.

Angus, R. D. Production of reference PPD tuberculin for veterinary use in the United States. *J. Biol. Stand.* 6:222–227, 1978.

Belli, L. Bovine tuberculosis in a white-tailed deer (*Odocoileus virginianus*). *Can. Vet. J.* 11:356–358, 1962.

Boever, W. I., Thoen, C. O., Wallach, J. C. *Mycobacterium chelonei* infection in a natterer manatee (*Trichechus inunguis*). *J. Am. Vet. Med. Assoc.* 169:927–929, 1976.

Borg, K. Human tuberculosis in an otter (*Lutra l. lutra*). *5th Int. Symp. Dis. Zoo Anim.* 89:89–90, 1964.

Cheville, N. F. *Cell pathology*. Ames: Iowa State University Press, 1976.

Clancy, J. K. The incidence of tuberculosis in lechwe (marsh antelope). *Tubercle* 58:151–156, 1977.

Costallat, L. F., Simon, F., Giorgi, W. Mycobacteriosis in monkeys: A report of two cases. *Vet. Med.* pp. 651–655, 1978.

Dannenberg, A. M. Pathogenesis of pulmonary tuberculosis in man and animals: Protection of personnel against tuberculosis. In R. J. Montali, ed. *Proceedings of symposium on mycobacterial infections in zoo animals*, pp. 65–75. Washington D.C.: Smithsonian Press, 1978.

Dunkin, G., Laidlaw, P., and Griffith, A. A note on tuberculosis in the ferret. *J. Comp. Pathol. Ther.* 42:46–69, 1929.

Fowler, M. E. Treating giraffes with isoniazid. In R. J. Montali, ed. *Proceedings of symposium on mycobacterial infections of zoo animals*, pp. 185–188, Washington D.C.: Smithsonian Press, 1978.

Francis J. *Tuberculosis in animals and man*. London: Cassell, 1958.

Francke, H. Erfahrungen mit INH-Davertherapie zur Tuberculoseprophylaxe. *5th Int. Symp. Dis. Zoo Anim.* 89:176–180, 1964.

Fremming, B. D., Benson, R. E., Young, R. J., and Harris, M. D. Antituberculosis therapy in *Macaca mulatta* monkeys. *Am. Rev. Tuberc. Pulm. Dis.* 76:225–231, 1957.

Friend, M., Kroll, E., Grust, H. Tuberculosis in a wild white-tailed deer. *N.Y. Fish Game J.* 10:118–123, 1963.

Gallagher, J., Macdam, I., Sayer, J., and Van Lavieren, L. P. Pulmonary tuberculosis in free-living lechwe antelope in Sambia. *Trop. Anim. Health Prod.* 4:204–213, 1972.

Gay, W. Tuberculosis in the eye of a monkey. *J. Am. Vet. Med. Assoc.* 126:225–226, 1955.

Gibson, J. P., Rohovsky, M. W., and Newberne, J. W. Modification of the tuberculin response of rhesus monkeys by isoniazid therapy. *Lab. Anim. Sci.* 21:62–66, 1971.

Guilbride, P., Rollinson, D., McAnulty, E., Alley, J., and Wells, E. Tuberculosis in the free-living African Cape buffalo (*Syncerus caffer caffer*). *J. Comp. Pathol. Ther.* 73:337–348, 1963.

Haberle, A. J. Tuberculosis in an orangutan. *J. Zoo Anim. Med.* 1(2):10–16, 1970.

Hall, R., and Winkel, F. Avian tuberculosis in mink: A case report. *J. Am. Vet. Med. Assoc.* 131:49–51, 1957.

Himes, E. M. Adaption of a fluorescent staining method for the detection of acid-fast bacilli in exotic animals. In R. J. Montali, ed., *Proceedings of symposium on mycobacterial infections in zoo animals*, pp. 103–105, Washington, D.C.: Smithsonian Press, 1978.

Himes, E. M., LyVere, D. B., Thoen, C. O., Essey, M. A., Lebel, J. L., and Freiheit, C. F. Tuberculosis in greater kudu. *J. Am. Vet. Med. Assoc.* 169:930–931, 1976.

Hopkinson, F., and McDiarmid, A. Tuberculosis in a free-living red deer (*Cervus elaphus*) in Scotland. *Vet. Rec.* 76:1251–1522, 1964.

Jorgensen, J. B., and Clausen, B. Mycobacteriosis in a roe deer caused by wood pigeon mycobacteria. *Nord. Vet. Med.* 28:539–546, 1976.

Karlson, A. G., Siebold, H. R., and Wolf, R. H. *Mycobacterium abscessus* infection in an owl monkey (*Aetus trivirgatus*). *Path. Vet.* 7:448–454, 1970.

Kuhn, U. S. G. III, and Selin, M. J. Tuberculin testing in great apes. In R. J. Montali, ed., *Proceedings of symposium on mycobacterial infections of zoo animals*, pp. 129–134. Washington, D.C.: Smithsonian Press, 1978.

Lomme, J. R., Thoen, C. O., Himes, E. M., Vincent, J. W., and King, R. E. *Mycobacterium tuberculosis* infection in two East African oryxes. *J. Am. Vet. Med. Assoc.* 169:912, 1976.

McCoy, G., and Chapin, C. Tuberculosis among ground squirrels (*Citellus beecheyi*). *J. Med. Res.* 25:189–198, 1911.

McLaughlin, R. M., Thoenig, J. R., and Marrs, G. E.,

Jr. A comparison of several intradermic tuberculins in *Macaca mulatta* during an epizootic of tuberculosis. *Lab. Anim. Sci.* 26(1):44–50, 1976.

Mandal, P. C., and Singh, B. Tuberculous metritis in a buffalo (*Bos bubalus*). *Indian J. Anim. Health* 14(2):121–122, 1975.

Mason, F. Tuberculosis in camels. *J. Comp. Pathol. Ther.* 30:80, 1917.

Murihead, R. H., Gallagher, J., and Burn, K. J. Tuberculosis in wild badgers in Gloucestershire: Epidemiology. *Vet. Rec.* 95(24):522–555, 1974.

Muscoplat, C. C., Thoen, C. O., McLaughlin, R. M., Thoenig, J. R., Chen, A. W., and Johnson, D. W. Comparison of lymphocyte stimulation and tuberculin skin reactivity in *Mycobacterium bovis*-infected *Macaca mulatta*. *Am. J. Vet. Res.* 36:699, 1975.

Nieberle, K. Tuberculosis in a giraffe. *Vet. Rec.* 50:1159, 1938.

Paine, R., and Martinaglia, G. Tuberculosis in wild buck living under natural conditions. *J. S. Afr. Vet. Med. Assoc.* 1:87–91, 1928.

Peters, J. H., and Gordon, G. R. Susceptibility of squirrel monkeys to the convulsant action of isoniazid. *Lab. Primate Newsletter* 10:1–3, 1971.

Pinto, M. R. M., Jainudeen, M. R., and Panabokke, R. G. Tuberculosis in a domesticated asiatic elephant (*Elephas maximus*). *Vet. Rec.* 93:622–644, 1973.

Potkay, S., Ganaway, J. R., Rogers, N., and Kinard, R. Epizootic of measles in a colony of rhesus monkeys (*Macaca mulatta*). *Am. J. Vet. Res.* 27:331–334, 1966.

Pulling, F. An outbreak of bovine tuberculosis in mink and treatment with rifampin. *J. Am. Vet. Med. Assoc.* 121:389–390, 1952.

Quinn, J. F., and Towar, D. Tuberculosis problems at a deer park in Michigan. *Proceedings of 100th Ann. Meeting Am. Vet. Med. Assoc.*, pp. 262–264, 1963.

Renner, M., and Bartholomew, W. R. Mycobacteriologic data from two outbreaks of bovine tuberculosis in nonhuman primates. *Am. Rev. Respir. Dis.* 109:11–16, 1974.

Renquist, D. M., and Whitney, R. A. Tuberculosis in nonhuman primates: An overview. In R. J. Montali, ed. *Proceedings of symposium on mycobacterial infections of zoo animals*, pp. 9–16. Washington, D.C.: Smithsonian Press, 1978.

Riordan, J. Rectal tuberculosis in monkeys from the use of contaminated thermometers. *J. Infect. Dis.* 73:93–94, 1943.

Ruch, T. C. *Diseases of laboratory primates*. Philadelphia: Saunders, 1959.

Sawa, T. R., Thoen, C. O., and Nagao, W. T. *Mycobacterium bovis* infection in wild axis deer in Hawaii. *J. Am. Vet. Med. Assoc.* 169:998–999, 1974.

Schliesser, T. Vorkommen and Bedeutung von Mykobakterien bei Tieren *Zentralbl. Bakteriol.* [*Orig A*] 235:184, 1976.

Schliesser, T. A. Prevalences of tuberculosis and mycobacterial diseases in some European zoos. In R. J. Montali, ed. *Proceedings of symposium on mycobacterial infections of zoo animals*, pp. 29–32. Washington, D.C.: Smithsonian Press, 1978.

Sesline, D. H., Schwartz, L. W., Osburn, B. I., Thoen, C. O., Terrell, T., Holmberg, C., Anderson, J. H., and Hendrickson, R. V. *Mycobacterium avium* infection in three rhesus monkeys. *J. Am. Vet. Med. Assoc.* 167:639–645, 1975.

Smith, A. W., and Wolochow, H. Comparison of old tuberculin and purified protein derivative in *Macaca mulatta*. *Lab. Anim. Sci.* 23(3):373–376, 1973.

Smith H. A., Jones, T. C., and Hunt D. H. *Veterinary pathology*, 4th ed., pp. 625–637. Philadelphia: Lea and Febiger, 1972.

Thoen C. O. Factors associated with pathogenicity of mycobacteria. In D. Schliessinger, ed. *Microbiology*, pp. 162–167. Washington, D.C.: American Society of Microbiology, 1979.

Thoen, C. O., Beluhan, E. Z., Himes, E. M., Capek, V., and Bennett, B. T. *Mycobacterium bovis* infection in baboons (*Papio papio*). *Arch. Pathol. Lab. Med.* 101:291–294, 1977.

Thoen, C. O. Eacret, W. G., and Himes, E. M. An enzyme-labeled antibody test for detecting antibodies in chickens infected with *Mycobacterium avium* serotype 2. *Avian Dis.* 22:162–166, 1978.

Thoen, C. O., and Karlson, A. G. The genus *Mycobacterium*. In R. A. Packer, C. J. Mare, and I. A. Merchant, eds. *Veterinary microbiology*, 8th ed. Ames: Iowa State University Press (forthcoming).

Thoen, C. O., Karlson, A. G., and Ellefson, R. D. Comparison of serum lipid and lipoprotein profiles in tuberculin-positive and in tuberculin-negative monkeys (*Macaca* sp.). *Am. Rev. Respir. Dis.* 108:686–687, 1973.

Thoen, C. O., Mills, K., and Hopkins, M. P. Enzyme-linked protein A: An enzyme-linked immunosorbent assay reagent for detecting antibodies in tuberculous exotic aminals. *Am. J. Vet. Res.* 40:833–835, 1980.

Thoen, C. O., Richards, W. D., and Jarnagin, J. L. Mycobacteria isolated from exotic animals. *J. Am. Vet. Med. Assoc.* 170:987–989, 1977.

Walsh, G. P., Storrs, E. E., Burchfield, H. P., Cottrell, E. H., Vidrine, M. F., and Binford, C. H. Leprosy-like disease occurring naturally in armadillos. *J. Reticuloendothel. Soc.* 18:347–354, 1975.

Wells, A., and Oxon, D. Tuberculosis in wild voles. *Lancet* 1:1221, 1961.

23 Johne's Disease (Paratuberculosis)

CHARLES O. THOEN   DONALD W. JOHNSON

Synonyms: **Chronic enteritis.**

HISTORY AND DISTRIBUTION. Johne's disease is caused by *Mycobacterium paratuberculosis* which results in high morbidity and mortality in a variety of wild animals. The importance of Johne's disease in wildlife is emphasized by the occurrence of disease in young animals. The problem is further magnified by the lack of suitable procedures to control and eliminate the disease from captive and wild species. In a recent outbreak of Johne's disease in aoudads and mouflon maintained in a zoological park, it was necessary to eliminate the entire herd (Boever and Peters 1974). Similar action was required in a deer herd kept in an animal park when available control methods failed to eliminate *M. paratuberculosis* infection (Temple et al. 1979).

Johne's disease in wild bighorn sheep and a mountain goat in the Colorado Rocky Mountains caused dehydration and emaciation in animals 2–4 years of age (Williams et al. 1979). The importance of this outbreak remains to be elucidated since many wild hoofed animals that inhabit the same range area are also susceptible to *M. paratuberculosis*. The success or failure of attempts to control or eradicate infections in these wild species will undoubtedly be influenced by the widespread contamination of the range area with feces and by the prolonged survival of *M. paratuberculosis* under environmental conditions (Jorgensen 1977).

Little definitive information is available on the incidence of Johne's disease in wild animals. However, reports have been made on outbreaks of *M. paratuberculosis* infection in animals maintained in captivity and in unconfined herds (Soltys et al. 1967; Thoen et al. 1977; Vance 1961). Since animals are moved freely between zoological parks and animal parks in different areas of the country without testing, it is possible that other foci of infection exist. Veterinarians in charge of wild hoofed animals should consider Johne's disease in differential diagnosis when chronic diarrhea and emaciation are evident. Specimens should be routinely submitted to diagnostic laboratories for cultural examination and a confirmative diagnosis (Thoen and Karlson 1981).

ETIOLOGY. The Johne's bacillus was first identified in 1895 by Johne and Frothingham while studying chronic dysentery in cattle. *Mycobacterium paratuberculosis*, the agent responsible for Johne's disease, grows very slowly on culture media, often requiring 4–16 weeks or more for primary isolation on appropriate media. The bacillus is acid-fast and aerobic and does not form spores or produce toxins. *Mycobacterium paratuberculosis* is mycobactin dependent and grows very slowly at 37°C. The colonies are colorless to white and translucent. Because a prolonged interval is required to isolate this mycobacterium, a presumptive diagnosis may be obtained by preparing appropriately stained smears of feces or mucosa of the rectum. On microscopic examinations acid-fast bacilli can be observed in clumps within macrophages (Fig. 23.1).

Cultures for *M. paratuberculosis* may be made on mycobactin-enriched medium after the specimens (intestinal mucosa or feces) are treated with benzalkonium chloride (USDA, 1974). A tube of mycobactin-free medium is used as a control. A portion of the intestine 3–4 cm anterior to the ileocecal valve and 3–4 cm posterior with associated lymph nodes should be collected on necropsy, washed to remove fecal material, and submitted to the laboratory frozen. The tissues may be ground in 3% trypsin and the sediment decontaminated in 0.1% benzalkonium chloride (Zephiran) for 24 hours. Fecal specimens (about 28 g) collected from the rectum of animals suspected of having Johne's disease should be placed in appropriately identified screw-capped jars or ointment containers. No refrigeration is required. The sample should be transported to the laboratory and processed within 24–36 hours to minimize overgrowth by other microorganisms. An aliquot of the feces is suspended in sterile water and processed with 0.3% Zephiran for 24 hours. Herrold's egg yolk agar slants are inoculated with the treated suspensions (three tubes with mycobactin and one without mycobactin). Inoculated mediums should be incubated at 37°C and examined at 3-week intervals for 20 weeks. Cultures are identified by growth rate, mycobactin dependency, and seroagglutination tests (Jarnagin et al. 1975; Thoen 1979).

TRANSMISSION. *Mycobacterium paratuberculosis* has been isolated from deer, aoudads, mouflon, bighorn sheep, antelope, mountain goats, moose, and camels. Since little or no definitive information is available on the transmission of disease in wild animal species, information will be presented on the transmission of Johne's disease in cattle.

In cattle herds where *M. paratuberculosis* infection persists, animals may be infected when they are very young (less than 3 months old), but they may not develop clinical symptoms until 2 years of age or older (Larsen et al. 1975). A serious problem in controlling spread of Johne's disease is related to the survival of the organisms in certain environments for 6–9 months (Jorgensen 1977; Julian 1975). Because large numbers of organisms may be shed in the feces, it is apparent that animals have considerable exposure when they are maintained in contaminated yards and barns.

Reports of congenital infections and survival of the organism in semen indicate other routes of transmission must be considered when attempts are made to control the spread of Johne's disease. Numerous domestic animals are susceptible to Johne's disease, including cattle, goats, sheep, horses, and swine (Larsen 1972; Thoen et al. 1975). Experimental studies indicate that young calves were more susceptible to *M. paratuberculosis* infection than older animals (Larsen et al. 1975); however, no information was presented on the occurrence of clinical disease. Studies are needed in natural outbreaks of Johne's disease in wildlife to confirm these findings and their importance in the development of clinical disease.

SIGNS. The clinical signs usually seen in wild animals naturally infected with *M. paratuberculosis* may be similar to those observed in domestic animals (Katic 1961). In cattle, Johne's disease is characterized by diarrhea that persists for months. In some cases the diarrhea occurs intermittently and the animal appears to recover. When the enteritis persists, there is a gradual weight loss and the animal becomes emaciated. In advanced stages of disease the animals may have a rough hair coat.

In an outbreak of Johne's disease in Rocky Mountain bighorn sheep and Rocky Mountain goats, diarrhea was often observed (Williams et al. 1979). However, it should be emphasized that clinical signs may not be present. In a recent report of *M. paratuberculosis* infection in deer maintained in captivity, there was no evidence of chronic dysentery.

Since the clinical signs of Johne's disease are variable and in some species may be absent, it is essential to conduct necessary laboratory examinations to confirm a diagnosis.

PATHOLOGY AND PATHOGENESIS. No definitive information is available on the pathogenesis of *M. paratuberculosis* infections in domestic or wild animals. However, in certain mycobacterial infections, it has been suggested that lipid components in the cell wall interfere with digestion of acid-fast bacilli ingested by macrophages (Goren 1977; Thoen 1979). The organisms appear to be protected from hydrolytic enzymes present in lysosomes of host cells that are capable of destroying other bacteria. The role of certain immunologic processes in Johne's disease has been discussed (Merkal et al. 1970).

Mycobacterium paratuberculosis has a predilection for the intestine, which is apparently the site of primary infection and of initial bacterial multiplication. In ruminants, clinical disease usually appears after intestinal lesions develop. The organism may be carried by macrophages to other tissues of the body. The organism has been isolated from the uterus, fetus, and mammary gland of cows and the semen and testes of bulls (Julian 1975; Larsen 1972). However, under natural conditions, *M. paratuberculosis* is usually ingested in water and feed contaminated with feces. Factors that influence the development of clinical disease include age, dose of organism, and stress (Larsen 1972). There is clinical evidence that suggests infection with bovine virus diarrhea may immunosuppress an animal and make it more susceptible to *M. paratuberculosis* infection.

Grossly visible lesions are not always present in the large intestine of many infected cattle. The mucosa may appear reddened as a result of congestion. Similarly, in wild animals there may be few apparent changes indicating an infectious disease. On necropsy the mesenteric lymph nodes may appear swollen and edematous. Microscopic examination of the ileum or cecum or adjacent lymph nodes may reveal the presence of granulomas containing lymphocytes, granulocytes, epithelioid cells, and multinucleated giant cells.

DIAGNOSIS. Numerous diagnostic methods have been developed and evaluated for identifying *M. paratuberculosis*-infected animals. Although some of these methods are highly efficient in detecting experimentally infected animals, few have been found to be of more than limited value in naturally occurring outbreaks of Johne's disease. The slow onset of Johne's disease, and the variability in the course of disease in different animals, as well as variations in age susceptibility, may in part account for the failure of certain serologic tests. Since one test alone may not provide sufficient information to establish a diagnosis of Johne's disease, it is recommended that a diagnostic profile be established by using three or more tests at various time intervals. Isolation and identification of the *M. paratuberculosis* is essential to confirm a diagnosis of Johne's disease (Thoen 1979). Improved methods have been developed for shipping and storing specimens, thereby permitting the collection of large numbers of samples for bacteriologic examination (Richards and Thoen 1977).

Microscopic examination of smear or sections prepared from the jejunum and adjacent lymph nodes or from ileum and cecum on necropsy is a rapid procedure available to the practicing veterinarian (Fig. 23.1). Acid-fast bacilli in clumps can be observed in macrophages in smears fixed with methanol and stained by the Kinyoun method. In animals with Johne's disease, these examinations provide reliable information in making a presumptive diagnosis. Little importance is attached to the finding of single acid-fast bacilli in smears since these may represent saprophytic strains of mycobacteria. Auramine-O staining of duplicate slides should be considered when a microscope with a suitable light source and filter is available. This staining technique allows rapid examination of slides using low-intensity light, which is less tiring when numerous specimens must be examined at one time. Moreover, this technique provides a sensitive method for detecting acid-fast organisms in specimens where only a few bacilli are present because a larger field is visible.

The need for rapid diagnostic tests for identifying *M. paratuberculosis*-infected animals has stimulated the development of in vitro procedures for measuring cell-mediated responses to specific mycobacterial antigens (Alhaji et al. 1974; Thoen et al. 1977). Lymphocyte immunostimulation tests have been made in cattle experimentally infected with *M. paratuberculosis* (Johnson et al. 1978). Calves experimentally infected at 21 days of age with *M. paratuberculosis* were positive on lymphocyte stimulation tests conducted 99 days postinoculation.

Lymphocyte stimulation tests have been evaluated in deer herds where Johne's disease has been diagnosed by isolation of *M. paratuberculosis* from the feces (Temple et al. 1979).

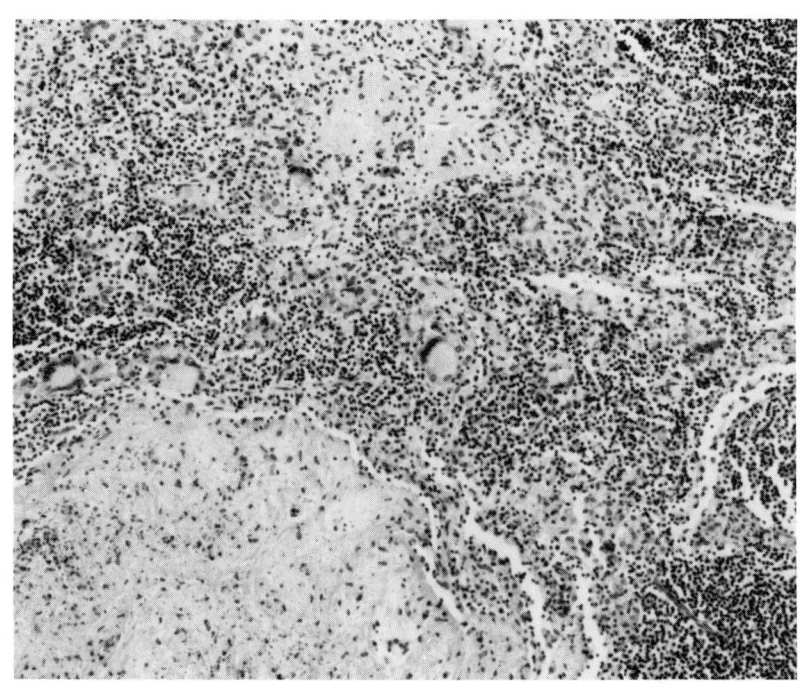

FIG. 23.1 Section of a mesenteric lymph node of an auodad from which *M. paratuberculosis* was isolated. Lesions consisting of epithelioid cells, lymphocytes, and a few granulocytes are present. Several multinucleated giant cells are observed (HE stain, ×125). (The assistance of E. M. Himes, National Veterinary Services Laboratories, Ames, Iowa, in preparation of the photograph is appreciated.)

In adult deer the lymphocyte immunostimulation test appeared to be more efficient than fecal culture technique, a procedure widely used in the diagnosis of paratuberculosis. Although the lymphocyte immunostimulation test offers considerable advantages over the complement fixation test and an agar gel immunodiffusion test, some problems are reported with both false-positive and false-negative results (Buergelt et al. 1977; Johnson et al. 1977). The false-negative responses may be associated with the presence of a humoral immunosuppressive factor which has been demonstrated in the plasma and serum of cattle infected with *M. paratuberculosis* (Davies et al. 1974). It has been reported that when cells were washed and incubated in normal plasma, the mitogen responses returned to normal values. It has been found that lymphocyte blastogenic responses can be potentiated by indomethacin (Muscoplat et al. 1978). Treatment with this drug may be useful in increasing specific antigen responses as reported in some animals infected with *M. paratuberculosis* which appear to be immunosuppressed. The importance of immunosuppressive agents, such as aflatoxin, have been reported (Paul et al. 1977).

Humoral antibodies in *M. paratuberculosis* infections have been demonstrated by several serologic methods (Gilmour 1976; Thoen and Karlson 1980). A common problem with the use of serologic procedures for diagnosis of Johne's disease has been the large numbers of false-positive and false-negative results. The complement fixation test, which is widely requested for the export of cattle, is of limited value because reactions fail to develop early in the infection and disappear soon after clinical symptoms are present. An enzyme-labeled antibody test that was found to be useful in detecting avian tuberculosis has been evaluated in our laboratory using serum from animals experimentally infected with *M. paratuberculosis* (Thoen et al. 1978). Positive responses were observed at 24 weeks postinoculation in each of 6 cattle orally receiving 720 mg viable *M. paratuberculosis* and in 2 cattle receiving 100 mg (Thoen and Muscoplat 1979). No positive reactions were observed in sera of 10 *M. bovis*-infected cattle or in sera of 14 control cows. The significance of these findings needs to be verified in wild animals naturally infected with *M. paratuberculosis*.

The intravenous injection of Johnin produces a temperature increase in sensitized cattle. This test is conducted by recording the rectal temperature immediately prior to and at 4,

6, and 8 hours after the injection of 3 ml Johnin (Larsen 1972). An increase in temperature of 1.5°C is considered a positive reaction. This may be a useful test in wild animals infected with *M. paratuberculosis*.

Delayed type hypersensitivity skin tests are not considered to be reliable for identifying *M. paratuberculosis*-infected animals. The test is not recommended for culling or removing animals from an infected herd because there is usually a high number of false-positive responses (Larsen 1972).

TREATMENT AND CONTROL. Measures for controlling and eliminating Johne's disease in domestic or wild animals should be based on the diagnosis and elimination of infected animals shedding the organism in the feces (Larsen 1973; Moyle 1975).

An important aspect in the control of the disease is to avoid introduction of animals without knowledge of their status of infection with *M. paratuberculosis*. When animals are added to a collection, they should originate from stock known to be free of *M. paratuberculosis* or have passed a series of three negative fecal cultures at 6-month intervals. The possibility of intrauterine transmission should be considered a potential source of infection. Therefore, animals born of known infected dams should be examined annually on fecal culture.

The success of controlling Johne's disease has been limited by the lack of a rapid diagnostic test. Further investigations are needed to develop a practical test with a high degree of specificity and sensitivity. These investigations should include further studies on the use of lymphocyte immunostimulation tests and enzyme immunoassay in detecting animals infected with *M. paratuberculosis*.

REFERENCES

Alhaji, I., Johnson, D. W., Muscoplat, C. C., and Thoen, C. O. Diagnosis of *Mycobacterium bovis* and *Mycobacterium paratuberculosis* infections in cattle by *in vitro* lymphocyte immunostimulation. *Am. J. Vet. Res.* 35:725–727, 1974.

Boever, W. J., and Peters, D. Paratuberculosis in two herds of exotic sheep. *J. Am. Vet. Med. Assoc.* 165:822, 1974.

Buergelt, C. D., Hall, C. E., Merkal, R. S., Whitlock, R. H., and Duncan, J. R. Lymphocyte transformation: An aid in the diagnosis of paratuberculosis. *Am. J. Vet. Res.* 38:1709–1716, 1977.

Davies, D. H., Corbeil, L., Ward, D., and Duncan, J. R. A humoral suppressor of *in vitro* lymphocyte transformation responses in cattle with Johne's disease. *Proc. Soc. Exp. Biol. Med.* 145:1372–1377, 1974.

Gilmour, N. J. L. The pathogenesis, diagnosis and control of Johne's disease. *Vet. Rec.* 99:433–434, 1976.

Goren, M. B. Phagocyte lysosomes: Interactions with infectious agents, phagosomes and experimental perturbations in function. *Ann. Rev. Microbiol.* 31:507–533, 1977.

Jarnagin, J. L., Champion, M. L., and Thoen, C. O. Seroagglutination test for *Mycobacterium paratuberculosis*. *J. Clin. Microbiol.* 2:268–269, 1975.

Johnson, D. W., Muscoplat, C. C., Hoefling, D. C., and Thoen, C. O. The use of lymphocyte transformation for the diagnosis of paratuberculosis (Johne's disease) in infected cattle. In Proceedings of *81st Ann. Meet., U.S. Anim. Health Assoc.*, Minneapolis, October 16, 21, 1977, pp. 467–469, 1978.

Johnson, D. W., Muscoplat, C. C., Larsen, A. B., and Thoen, C. O. Skin testing, fecal culture, and lymphocyte immunostimulation in cattle inoculated with *Mycobacterium paratuberculosis*. *Am. J. Vet. Res.* 38:2023–2026, 1977.

Jorgensen, J. B. Survival of *Mycobacterium paratuberculosis* in slurry. *Nord. Vet. Med.* 29:267–270, 1977.

Julian, R. J. Developments in veterinary science: A short review of some observations of Johne's disease with recommendations for control. *Can. Vet. J.* 16:33–43, 1975.

Katic, I. Paratuberculosis (Johne's disease) with special reference to captive exotic species. *Nord. Vet. Med.* 13:205–214, 1961.

Larsen, A. B. Paratuberculosis: The status of our knowledge. *J. Am. Vet. Med. Assoc.* 161:1539–1541, 1972.

———. Johne's disease: Immunization and diagnosis. *J. Am. Vet. Med. Assoc.* 163:902–904, 1973.

Larsen, A. B., Merkal, R. S., and Cutlip, R. C. Age of cattle as related to resistance to infection with *Mycobacterium paratuberculosis*. *Am. J. Vet. Res.* 36:255–257, 1975.

Larsen, A. B., Moyle, A. I., and Himes, E. M. Experimental vaccination of cattle against paratuberculosis (Johne's disease) with killed bacterial vaccines: A controlled field study. *Am. J. Vet. Res.* 39:65–70, 1978.

Libke, K. G., and Walton, A. M. Presumptive paratuberculosis in a Virginia white-tailed deer. *J. Wildl. Dis.* 11:552–553, 1975.

Merkal, R. S., Kopecky, K. E., Larsen, A. B., and Ness, R. D. Immunologic mechanisms in bovine paratuberculosis. *Am. J. Vet. Res.* 31:475–485, 1970.

Moyle, A. I. Culture and cull procedure for control of paratuberculosis. *J. Am. Vet. Med. Assoc.* 166:689–690, 1975.

Muscoplat, C. C., Rakich, P. M., Thoen, C. O., and

Johnson, D. W. Enhancement of lymphocyte blastogenic and delayed hypersensitivity skin responses by indomethacin. *Infect. Immun.* 20(3):627–631, 1978.

Paul, P. S., Johnson, D. W., Mirocha, C. J., Soper, F. F., Thoen, C. O., Muscoplat, C. C., and Weber, A. F. *In vitro* stimulation of bovine peripheral blood lymphocytes: Suppression of phytomitogen and specific antigen responses by aflatoxin. *Am. J. Vet. Res.* 38:2033–2036, 1977.

Richards, W. D., and Thoen, C. O. Effect of freezing on the viability of *Mycobacterium paratuberculosis* in bovine feces. *J. Clin. Microbiol.* 6:392–395, 1977.

Soltys, M. A., Andress, C. E., and Fletch, A. L. Johne's disease in a moose (*Alces alces*). *Bull. Wildl. Dis. Assoc.* 3:183–184, 1967.

Temple, R. M. S., Muscoplat, C. C., Thoen, C. O., Himes, E. M., and Johnson, D. W. Johne's disease in a captive deer herd. *J. Am. Vet. Med. Assoc.* 175(9):914–915, 1979.

Thoen, C. O. *Mycobacterium*. In G. R. Carter, ed., *Diagnostic procedures in veterinary microbiology*, 3d ed. Springfield, Ill.: Thomas, 1979.

———. Factors associated with pathogenicity of mycobacteria. In R. Brubaker, ed., *Microbiology*. Washington, D.C.: American Society of Microbiology, 1979, pp. 162–167.

Thoen, C. O., Eacret, W. G., and Himes, E. M. An enzyme-labeled antibody test for detecting antibodies in chickens infected with *Mycobacterium avium*. *Avian Dis.* 22:162–166, 1978.

Thoen, C. O., Jarnagin, J. L., and Richards, W. D. Isolation and identification of mycobacteria from porcine tissues: A three year summary. *Am. J. Vet. Res.* 36:1383–1386, 1975.

Thoen, C. O., and Karlson, A. G. The genus *Mycobacterium*. In R. A. Packer, C. J. Mare, and I. A. Merchant, eds., *Veterinary microbiology*, 8th ed. Ames, Iowa: State University Press (forthcoming).

Thoen, C. O., and Muscoplat, C. C. Johne's disease: Recent developments in diagnosis. *J. Am. Vet. Med. Assoc.* 174(8):838–840, 1979.

Thoen, C. O., Muscoplat, C. C., Cram, L. S., Jarnagin, J. L., Johnson, D. W., and Pietz, D. E. Lymphocyte blastogenesis in the diagnosis of tuberculosis in cattle. In *Proceedings of 1st Int. Symp. Vet. Lab. Diag.*, Quanajuato, Mexico, 1:98–109, 1977.

Thoen, C. O., Richards, W. D., and Jarnagin, J. L. Mycobacteria isolated from exotic animals. *J. Am. Vet. Med. Assoc.* 170:987–990, 1977.

U.S. Department of Agriculture. *Laboratory methods in veterinary mycobacteriology*, rev. ed. Ames, Iowa: National Veterinary Services Laboratories, Animal and Plant Health Inspection Service, U.S. Department of Agriculture, 1974.

Vance, H. N. Johne's disease in a European red deer. *Can. Vet. J.* 2(8):305–307, 1961.

Williams, E. S., Spraker, T. R., and Schoonveld, G. G. Paratuberculosis (Johne's diseases) in bighorn sheep and a Rocky Mountain goat in Colorado. *J. Wildl. Dis.* 15(2):221–227, 1979.

24 Brucellosis

J. FRANKLIN WITTER

Synonyms: **Contagious abortion, Bang's disease, Bang's abortion disease; in humans— Malta fever, Mediterranean fever, undulant fever.**

Brucellosis is a highly contagious infection of many animals including man and is caused by bacteria of the genus *Brucella*. Usually this infection begins as a bacteremia, often without clinical signs, and subsequently localizes in the lymph nodes, spleen, reproductive organs, tendon sheaths, joints, and other organs where it persists for long periods.

HISTORY. *Brucella melitensis* was detected in goats and recognized as a cause of illness in humans by Bruce in 1887. *Brucella abortus* was recognized in 1897 by Bang as a cause of abortion in cattle. *Brucella suis* was isolated from aborted swine fetuses by Traum in 1914. In 1918 Evans established the close relationship of *B. melitensis* and *B. abortus*, and in 1920 Meyer and Shaw suggested the generic name *Brucella* for this group of microorganisms (Huddleson, I. F. 1943).

Brucellosis has since been recognized in other domestic animals, including sheep, horses, and dogs, as well as in a large variety of wild animals, notably bison, elk, caribou, reindeer, and carnivores.

Stableforth and Galloway (1959) presented an excellent review of brucellosis in wild animals. It includes information and references on the high incidence of brucellosis in Indian buffalo and Egyptian camels, as well as the potential role of crows (*Corvus brachyrhynchos*), English sparrows (*Passer domesticus*), and rooks as reservoirs of brucellosis.

DISTRIBUTION. Brucellosis has been reported throughout the world and has long been considered an important disease in humans, cattle, goats, and swine. It has been found in bison (*Bison bison*), elk (*Cervus canadensis*) (Choquette et al. 1978; Thorne et al. 1978; Tunnicliff and Marsh 1935), moose (*Alces alces*) (Corner and Connell 1958; Fenstermacher and Olsen 1942; Jellison 1953), Dall sheep (*Ovis dalle*)

(Neiland et al. 1968), caribou (*Rangifer tarandus arcticus*) (Huntley et al. 1963), and reindeer (*R. tarandus*) (Golosov and Zabrodin 1959). *Brucella* infections have been described in several species of deer in Switzerland, Germany, England, the United States, and Canada, in chamois in Switzerland and in antelopes of the Serengeti (Sachs et al. 1966). McDiarmid (1960) and McDiarmid and Mathews (1974) referred to other possible reservoirs of *Brucella* in wildlife.

Brucellosis has been diagnosed as a natural infection in domestic and wild dogs involving three biotypes of *Brucella* (Kimberling et al. 1966; Neiland 1975; Randhawa 1977; Sachs 1979), wild foxes (*Dusicyon gymnocercus antiquues*) (Hoff 1974; Szfres and Tome 1966), wolves (*Canis lupus*) (Neiland 1975), coyotes (*Canis latrans*) (Carmichael 1977; Davis et al. 1979; Hoq 1978; Randhawa et al. 1977), spotted hyena (*Crocuta crocuta*) (Sachs 1979), jackal (*Canis mesomelas*) (Sachs 1979), grizzly bears (*Ursus arctos horribilis*) (Neiland 1975), feral swine (*Sus scrofa*) (Randhawa et al. 1977; Wood et al. 1976), bobcat (*Lynx rufus*) (Carmichael 1977), raccoons (*Procyon lotor*), (Hoff 1974), badgers (*Taxidea taxas*) (Randhawa et al. 1977), hares (*Lepus europaeus* and *L. californicus*) (Kardevan and Kemenes 1961; Thorpe et al. 1965), rabbits (*Sylvilagus floridanus*) (Hoff et al. 1974), mice (*Mus musculus*) (Corey et al. 1964; Thorpe et al. 1965), and wild desert wood rats (*Neotoma lepida*) (Fitch and Bishop 1938; Stoenner and Lackman 1957). It has also been detected in ticks (*Ornithodoros* spp., *Dermacenter* spp.) (Rementsova 1962), and fleas (*Orehopeus sexdentatus*) (Thorpe et al. 1965).

Trainer and Hanson (1960) and Fay (1961) agreed that brucellosis is a comparatively rare disease in deer of the United States and that it is not as important as it is in cattle, bison, and elk.

A 10-year serologic survey for brucellosis by Adrian and Keiss (1977) sampled over 10,000 Colorado mule deer (*Odocoileus hemionus*), elk (*Cervus canadensis*), and antelope (*Antilocapra americana*). All test results were negative.

Thorne, Morton, and Thomas (1978) reported that during a 5-year survey of brucellosis in Wyoming elk, 31% of 1,165 samples were positive. *Brucella abortus* type 1 was isolated from 17 of 45 elk autopsied, and the incidence among mature females was approximately 50%. Thorne and Morton concluded that "no single test should be relied upon to diagnose brucellosis in elk."

Despite their frequently observed intimate relationships with domestic cattle, moose appear to be refractory, judging from the insignificant numbers that have reacted to the brucellosis test. Thorne et al. (1978) stated that the extremely rare occurrence of positive serologic reaction to brucellosis in moose may be due to its usually fatal termination. With only two cases described in the United States (Fenstermacher et al. 1942; Jellison et al. 1953) and two in Canada (Corner and Connell 1958), it is difficult to postulate on the severity of brucellosis in moose.

Camels (*Camelus dromedarius* and *C. bactrianus*) frequently become infected, and herd infections have been reported from Asia as well as North Africa. Abortions occur in pregnant camels; and the organism is excreted in discharges, urine, and milk, as in other ruminants. Human infection from camels is known to occur (FAO 1964).

Hares in Europe apparently have been afflicted with brucellosis for many years. Wetzel and Rieck (1962) referred to "hare syphilis," reported in 1871, and "tuberculosis of the scrotum" in 1900, which was subsequently related to brucellosis. Since 1947 to 1962 they reported that 10–14% of the hares submitted for postmortem examination in Switzerland had brucellosis.

Kardevan and Kemenes (1961) described a survey of 250 hare carcasses in Hungary, 17 of which were infected with an isolate which biochemically and serologically resembled the Danish variety of B. suis. Thorpe et al. (1965) referred to the isolation of B. suis and possibly B. melitensis from black-tailed jackrabbits (*L. californicus*) in Utah. Wetzel and Rieck (1962) reported the isolation of B. abortus from hares (*L. europaeus*) in Switzerland, Czechoslavakia, Denmark, and Germany and B. melitensis from hares in France and Germany. They suggested that brucellosis is spread from sheep and cattle to hares. Kardevan and Kemenes (1961) believed that hares play an unimportant role in maintaining brucellosis in domestic animals except in countries like Denmark where the disease has been eradicated in domestic stock and hares serve as a reservoir of infection. Rementsova (1962) reported brucellosis in hares in Russia and the isolation of *Brucella* organisms from ticks.

Brucella neotomae was reported by Thorpe et al. (1965) to be enzootic in western Utah; it has been isolated from desert wood rats (*Neotoma lepida*) and from the fleas which parasitized them. All areas in Utah where B. neotomae was isolated yielded seropositive animals other than the desert wood rat. All wild animals tested for susceptibility to B. neotomae showed similar susceptibility to B. abortus, B. suis, and B. melitensis.

Although brucellosis has rarely been diagnosed in birds, they have been experimentally infected with *Brucella* spp. There is no documented evidence that birds serve as either reservoirs or disseminators of brucellosis.

These reports make it clear that brucellosis is worldwide and is established in a great variety of species of wild animals, many of which could serve as reservoirs, and in ectoparasites capable of being vectors.

ETIOLOGY. *Brucella* organisms are small, gram-negative, nonmotile, non-spore-forming rods, which are frequently so short as to be mistaken for cocci. They grow on ordinary infusion agar, with or without enrichment, preferably in a 10% carbon dioxide atmosphere. *Brucella* organisms are not resistant to disinfectants, sunlight, drying, or putrefaction. When protected by cold temperatures, they may survive for several months.

The causative agents of brucellosis are strains or species known as B. abortus, B. melitensis, B. suis, B. canis, B. neotomae, and B. rangiferi. The latter species name is used by Russian workers for the strains isolated from reindeer (*Rangifer tarandus*), but American scientists prefer to designate this and other specific *Brucella* isolates from unusual hosts as biotypes of B. abortus, B. melitensis, or B. suis (Meyer 1964, 1966). Meyer (1966) stated that all strains isolated from reindeer are the same and should be classified as B. suis type 4; Neiland et al. (1968) suggested the designation B. suis biotype rangiferi.

Brucella canis is biologically similar to B. suis. However, detailed studies of B. canis by several authors have led to conclusions that B. canis is distinct from other *Brucella* species (Carmichael 1977).

TRANSMISSION. *Brucella* infections are usually transmitted by oral exposure, but susceptible animals can also be infected by contamination of the eyes, wounds, and genital tract. Males can transmit brucellosis during breeding through contaminated semen from their infected genital organs and through genitals contaminated by an infected female. Several Russian reports indicated that male reindeer play an important role in spreading brucellosis. Thorne et al. (1978) concluded that the venereal transmission in elk was unimportant, although it was known to occur.

During bacteremic stages of infection, bloodsucking parasites can serve as vectors. The role of ticks, fleas, and other parasites as vectors can only be conjectured; but the fact that these parasites become contaminated establishes their potential role in the spread of brucellosis.

Edible tissues of infected animals can contaminate humans and predators. Neiland et al. (1968) referred to the close relationship among the Eskimos, their dogs, and the infected caribou as plausible avenues of transmission. This involves the eating of infected caribou meat by both man and dogs and human contact with infected dogs. Dogs are known to spread *Brucella* organisms in their feces and urine.

Milk from *Brucella*-infected udders of cattle and reindeer is a potential source of human infection. Within animal populations, aborted fetuses, placentas, vaginal discharges, and drainage from the joint abscesses of infected animals are all likely agents of dissemination.

One of the first reports of brucellosis in wildlife involved buffalo herds in Yellowstone National Park in 1917. Honess (1956) believed that brucellosis was spread from domestic cattle to buffalo, which in turn transmitted it to elk. He reported that of 110 buffalo tested for brucellosis 58 were positive and 25 suspicious, and of 32 elk using the same range, 3 were positive and 8 suspicious.

Brucellosis has probably existed for a long time in domestic reindeer in Russia, judging from the dates of reports of the occurrence of bursitis and orchitis. There are no sheep, swine, or cattle in this reindeer country; therefore, wild reindeer, which occasionally come in contact with domestic reindeer, are suspected as the source of infection. It is significant that all *Brucella* isolates from all sections of the USSR are similar to one another and to the isolates from the caribou of North America. Meyer (1964) suggested that the transfer of Siberian reindeer to Alaska in 1891 may have provided the opportunity for transfer of brucellosis between the two continents, accounting for the occurrence of *B. suis* type 4 in reindeer from widely separate regions. The incidence of brucellosis reactors in reindeer in the USSR runs as high as 30% (Golosov and Zabrodin 1959).

In certain areas white-tailed deer (*Odocoileus virginianus*) are known to associate with domestic cattle, presenting opportunities for the transmission of brucellosis (Trainer and Hanson 1962). However, Fay (1961) reported that of the 17,000 white-tailed deer and mule deer (*O. hemionus*) tested in various parts of the United States, only 20 white-tailed deer were considered infected, based on the agglutination test interpretation used for cattle. Steen et al. (1955) reported that 996 white-tailed deer tested in Missouri were negative, yet this state has had problems with brucellosis in cattle. Shotts et al. (1958) reported one reactor out of 403 white-tailed deer in the southeastern states. Baker et al. (1962) commented that the low incidence of reactors found in these surveys suggests that either white-tailed deer are not commonly exposed to infection with *Brucella* spp. or that, if exposed, they do not usually become reactors. His report on two deer inoculated with *B. abortus* agrees with the work of others that deer do develop characteristic titers but that the duration of these titers may not be as long as in cattle. There is no evidence to suggest that deer serve as a reservoir or contribute to the spread of brucellosis to domestic stock (Fay 1961).

Meyer (1966) concluded her comprehensive review of host-parasite relationships in brucellosis with this statement: "From the information presented herein, it can be concluded that *Brucella* organisms are not readily transmissible from their preferential host to dissimilar hosts and that no serious or threatening reservoir of infection exists presently in wild animals in the United States."

However, more recent studies suggest that wildlife could act as reservoirs under favorable circumstances. Potentially dangerous carriers in areas of infected livestock are scavengers and predators such as skunks, coyotes, bobcats, and feral swine. A serologic survey of *Brucella* agglutinins in California wildlife conducted by Hoq (1978) indicated that wildlife in the areas sampled were in general free of brucellosis. However, some of the wild mammals were found to have significant *Brucella* agglutinins. Skunks, coyotes, and bobcats trapped around livestock-raising areas had titers of 1:100. According to Hoq, these animals probably picked up brucellosis by feeding on placentas and aborted fetuses of recently calving livestock. The role of these carnivores as reservoirs or disseminators to livestock is yet to be determined.

Swine brucellosis continues to be a problem in the southeastern United States. Domestic swine are reared in outside pens, pastures, and forested lands, creating the opportunity for commingling with feral swine.

Becker et al. (1978) reported that 50,000 feral swine are annually killed by hunters. Swine were the source of brucellosis in man in 39% of the cases in Florida during the period of 1963–1975. Of the 28 confirmed human brucellosis cases during 1974 and 1975, 56% involved swine contact and 22% were in hunters. Several hundred feral swine are translocated annually throughout Florida (Bigler et al. 1976). This movement undoubtedly results in the dissemination of brucellosis. *Brucella suis* biotype 1 was recovered at necropsy from 9 feral swine, and 53% of 95 feral swine were positive to at least 1 of the 4 tests used (Becker et al. 1978). In South Carolina 255 feral hogs were serologically tested for *Brucella* titers; 18% were reactors, and *B. suis* biotype 1 was isolated from 1 boar. In Hawaii 10 of 42 feral hogs had significant *Brucella* titers. There is concern that feral hog populations might function as reservoirs of disease, and this possibility should be considered when implementing disease control programs in domestic swine and in the capture or sale of feral swine to shooting preserves and the use of their meat for food (Wood et al. 1976).

Dogs are susceptible to both natural and experimental infection with *B. abortus*, *B. suis* biotype 4, and *B. canis* without showing clinical signs; yet they can disseminate *Brucella* organisms in their urine and feces (Neiland et al. 1968) and show titers for as long as 10 months.

Rangiferine brucellosis, *B. suis* type 4, commonly produces significant serum titers in sled dogs, wolves, red foxes, and grizzly bears (*Ursus arctos horribilis*) which feed on infected caribou (Neiland 1975).

The prevalence of *Brucella* species, particularly *B. canis*, was determined in 269 wild animals (14 species) in southern Texas by Randhawa et al. (1977). Serologic evidence of brucellosis including *B. canis* infection was detected in coyotes, raccoons, opossums, badgers, jackrabbits, and feral hogs. Man contracts a moderately severe form of brucellosis (Toshach 1955) through contacts with either dogs or caribou and is susceptible in varying degrees to all *Brucella* spp.

Brucellosis in coyotes has been reported from several sources. Davis et al. (1979) reported that 18% of 51 coyotes tested were positive for brucellosis. *Brucella abortus* biotype 1 was isolated from 7 of the 43 coyotes. Congenital transmission was determined. This study indicated that *B. abortus* is commonly disseminated in certain coyote populations in Texas, and this may be a potential public health threat, especially to trappers, wildlife researchers, fur buyers, and veterinarians who handle coyotes. There is a positive correlation between the incidence of brucellosis in livestock and coyotes (Randhawa et al. 1977).

SIGNS. Brucellosis affects many different organs in animals, and consequently, the signs of the disease will be influenced by the nature and extent of the infection and the species involved. For instance, in man the primary effects result from a protracted, undulating febrile condition. Horses occasionally develop *Brucella*-infected abscesses. In ruminants brucellosis commonly induces abortions during the latter half of gestation. Abortions are more common at the onset of an infection in a herd or in young animals in their first pregnancies. Calves are often born immature and weak. Placentas are commonly retained. Corner and Connell (1958) concluded that abortion and birth of nonviable calves are the most frequent signs in cow elk. Neiland et al. (1968) reported seeing "dried-shriveled" afterbirths, signs of "excessive bleeding," and stunted or weak calves in caribou herds. Metritis accompanied by excessive vaginal discharges is a common sign that reflects reproductive failure or breeding difficulties in cattle and possibly in reindeer.

Chronic infections of the bones and joints occur in livestock and reindeer (Golosov and Zabrodin 1959) and elk (Thorne et al. 1978). Cattle and reindeer become lame when the tarsal, carpal, and other joints and their bursae become swollen or sometimes abscessed. Orchitis and epididymitis in one or both testicles of reindeer are evidenced by swelling and, occasionally, abscesses (Golosov and Zabrodin 1959).

Brucellosis is a well-recognized problem in bison herds in North America. Various surveys indicate that as many as 50% of the bison react to the brucellosis test. Choquette et al. (1978) reported that brucellosis in bison causes extended rut and low conception rate. Presumably, like the bovine, infected bison shed *Brucella* in infected uterine discharges and in the placentas which contaminate the water and feed supplies. Animals such as the wolf, coyote, and fox may act as mechanical carriers of the disease by shedding the organism in their excreta after ingesting aborted fetuses and placentas. Corner and Connell (1958) concluded that in males scrotal enlargement and orchitis are the primary signs in bison.

In elk Corner and Connell (1958) and Thorne et al. (1978) concurred that the most important and frequent signs are abortion and birth of nonviable calves. Thorne (1978) reported that the second most important signs in elk are infected hygromata and synovitis in the lower leg areas. The duration of infection extends over several years.

No significant signs have been reported in deer, moose, carnivores, or feral swine.

PATHOGENESIS. The pathogenesis of brucellosis will be influenced by the strain of *Brucella*, its virulence, and the particular host involved. Usually after the organism invades the host, it gains entrance into the circulatory system and subsequently localizes in the uterus, mammary gland, lymph nodes, spleen, liver, bone marrow, bursae of joints, or in the placental tissues of pregnant animals. The endrometrium and associated chorionic tissues become edematous, and the intercotyledonary membranes become thickened and leathery. Eventually fetal circulation is decreased and the pregnancy terminates in abortion. Following abortion in ruminants, *B. abortus* tends to localize in the udder and adjacent lymph nodes. The basic tissue reaction in these organs is that of a granuloma, and such lesions will frequently harbor the infection throughout life.

Brucellosis appears to be primarily a disease of ruminants, but it is not known if it originated in this group of animals. The strains of *Brucella* peculiar to specific animals may have developed by host adaptation. Serologic reactions have been reported in a wide variety of animals, which is evidence of a broad host range.

Brucella canis is a specific pathogen for dogs and its pathogenicity for other domestic animal species is very low. Studies on infection of wildlife species with *B. canis* have been limited. Red foxes (*Vulpes fulva*) that were inoculated orally developed a bacteremia and lesions similar to those seen in dogs, and a persistant positive *Brucella* agglutination titer developed. In a survey by Hoff et al. (1974) significant titers of 1:200 were detected in one bobcat, one red fox, and two coyotes, but not in 766 serums of striped skunks, gray foxes, wolves, and opposums.

PATHOLOGY. *Brucella* infection in ruminants usually localizes in the pregnant uterus, the placentome, and subsequently the intercotyledonary areas of the chorion, producing dull,

thickened leathery areas and edema. This interference with fetal circulation apparently explains the subsequent abortion. Abortions usually occur late in the gestation period and are followed by retained fetal membranes and metritis. Neiland et al. (1968) reported aerial surveys of the Alaskan Arctic herd of 700 caribou in 1963 and 2,000 in 1965 which, respectively, showed 5% and 3.4% with retained placentas and signs of excessive bleeding. Cherchenko (1961) stated that abortions in Siberian reindeer herds occur frequently, but that only 1–5% of the animals at any one time will show bursitis, abortion, metritis, or orchitis. Neiland et al. (1968) detected only occasional caribou with orchitis-epididymitis, bursitis-synovitis, and mastitis. Carpal bursitis ("caribou knees") is most common. In Siberian reindeer serofibrinous bursitis is typical (Cherchenko 1961). Trauma of the carpus probably predisposes it to *Brucella* invasion.

Orchitis and abortions represent the major pathology reported in bison (Corner and Connell 1958). Thorne (1978) reported that brucellosis in moose is different from other animals in that there is a generalized and often fatal infection characterized by emaciation, fibrinous pleuritis, peritonitis, enlarged lymph nodes, and focal necrosis of the liver, kidneys, and spleen. The extent of the sources of these observations was not revealed, but, as previously stated, only four *Brucella*-infected moose have been reported in the literature.

In feral swine the cervical and inguinal lymph nodes are most commonly infected.

Infected hares (Wetzel and Rieck 1962) often appear healthy but have swollen testes that eventually abscess. The penis is usually thickened and dark red. In females abortion is common. The vulva and vagina are swollen, and the surfaces are marked by pustules. The ovaries are often abscessed; lesions occur in the lymph nodes, spleen, liver, lungs, and subcutaneous tissues. Hares may be infected for a year or more before they sicken and die or become vulnerable to predation. Kardevan and Kemenes (1961) described small chronic granulomatous nodules with necrotic centers surrounded by histiocytes and fibrous tissue scattered throughout the spleen, liver, lungs, testicles, uterine wall, and subcutaneous tissues.

DIAGNOSIS. The most common methods for diagnosing brucellosis are the plate and the tube serum agglutination tests. Agglutinins usually develop in animals within 2 weeks after exposure, but occasionally a much longer period is required. The duration of the serum titer is also variable. Cattle may remain seropositive for years, but in other animals serum agglutinins can be transitory (Baker et al. 1962). Nonspecific agglutinins or cross-agglutination with other organisms can, in certain instances, invalidate the test. It is important, therefore, to make isolations of the organism for positive identification. Guinea pig inoculation is standard procedure for assessing the virulence of the isolates (Meyer 1966). Complement fixation, skin allergy, immunofluorescence, and immunodiffusion in agar gel and rivonal precipitation tests are all considered diagnostic aids. No one serologic test is considered adequate for all conditions. *Brucella canis* infections require a special antigen unlike that used for *B. abortus* (Carmichael 1977).

PROGNOSIS. Natural recovery from *Brucella* infections rarely occurs in animals. However, it has been noted over the years that approximately 65% of the cattle that abort following exposure to *B. abortus* do not abort again. The satisfactory reproductive performance of the bison in Yellowstone National Park during 3 years of high incidence of brucellosis (Tunnicliff and Marsh 1935) suggests that this infection "poses no threat to the survival of the population" (Choquette et al. 1978). The effects of brucellosis on reindeer, however, are more disastrous than on other forms of wildlife, and its influence on the future reproductive capacity of this species is yet to be evaluated.

TREATMENT AND CONTROL. Antibiotics, such as the tetracyclines and streptomycin, and sulfonamides have been used with some success to reduce the severity of brucellosis in man and animals. Unfortunately, these treatments cannot be relied on to eliminate infections; hence, they have never been acceptable as a part of the national eradication program for brucellosis in domestic animals in the United States.

Calves and reindeer up to 4 or 5 months of age have higher brucellosis resistance than adults. Orloff (1963) reported experimental work of Russian scientists who vaccinated young reindeer, using one-tenth of the usual bovine dose of Strain 19 vaccine. The vaccinated reindeer developed serum agglutination titers of 1:3,200 in 15 days which began to recede by 3 months. Only 40% of the animals had titers of 1:50 after the 425th day. Eighty percent of the vaccinated reindeer were resistant to challenge with 100,000 organisms of reindeer Strain 010,

but this resistance could be overpowered by more severe exposures. This immunity lasted about 9 months. Vaccination of farm reindeer, therefore, might be as valuable as the vaccination of domestic cattle.

Brucellosis in bison is considered to be a potentially serious impediment to the final phases of the bovine brucellosis eradication program in the United States. It jeopardizes any attempt to raise cattle on a range used by infected bison. Moreover, it is a public health threat in areas where the animals might be hunted (Choquette et al. 1978). Hence, bison have been subjected to federal interstate regulations, similar to those controlling brucellosis in cattle, under the authority of the United States Animal Disease Eradication Division, Title 9, Chapter 1, Subpart E 78.17 to 78.23, which includes official testing, vaccination, and reporting programs. This is the first wild animal to come under a national brucellosis control program. Presently, brucellosis has almost been eradicated from herds of plains bison in Canada's western national parks, where the animals are kept in relative confinement under fence. The disease is still prevalent in the free-roaming bison populations in northern Canada (Choquette et al. 1978). Testing is also being conducted in the controlled reindeer herds, those owned by Eskimos, and those under supervision of the Bureau of Indian Affairs in Alaska.

In summary, the human health hazard of brucellosis associated with contacts with a great variety of wildlife are vividly apparent. Also, the fact that many species of wildlife can carry and spread brucellosis to domestic animals sheds new light on the hazards associated with a nationwide brucellosis control program.

REFERENCES

Adrian, W. J., and Keiss, R. E. Survey of Colorado's wild ruminants for serologic titers to brucellosis and leptospirosis. *J. Wildl. Dis.* 13:429–431, 1977.

Baker, M. F., Dills, G. J., and Hayes, F. A. Further experimental studies on brucellosis in white-tailed deer. *J. Wildl. Manag.* 26:27–31, 1962.

Becker, H. N., Belden, R. C., Breault, T., Burridge, M. J., Frankenberger, W. B., and Nicolletti, P. Brucellosis in feral swine in Florida. *J. Am. Vet. Med. Assoc.* 173:1181–1182, 1978.

Bigler, W. J., Hoff, G. L., and Hemmert, W. H. Trends of brucellosis in Florida: An epidemiologic review. *Am. J. Epidemiol.* 105:245–251, 1976.

Carmichael, L. E. Brucellosis caused by *Brucella canis*. James A. Baker Institute for Animal

Health, New York State College of Veterinary Medicine, Cornell University, Ithaca, 1977.

———. Canine brucellosis: Isolation, diagnosis, transmission. In *Proceedings*. 71st Ann. Meet., U.S. Livestock Sanitary Assoc. 1967:517–527, 1968.

Cherchenko, I. I. Brucellosis in the far north: I. Brucellosis in reindeer. *Zh. Mikrobiol. Epidemiol. Immunobiol.* 32(3):135–139, 1961.

Choquette, L. P. E., Broughton, E., Cousineau, J. G., and Novakowski, N. S. Parasites and diseases of bison in Canada: IV. Serological survey for brucellosis in northern Canada. *J. Wildl. Dis.* 14:329–332, 1978.

Corey, R. R., Paulissen, L. J., and Swartz, D. Prevalence of *Brucellae* in the wildlife of Arkansas. *Wildl. Dis.*, vol. 36 (WD-63-2), 1964.

Corner, A. H., and Connell, R. Brucellosis in bison, elk and moose in Elk Island National Park, Alberta, Canada. *Can. J. Comp. Med.* 22:9–20, 1958.

Davis, D. S., Boeer, W. J., Mains, J. P., Heck, F. C., Adams, L. G. *Brucella abortus* in coyotes: I. A serologic and bacteriologic survey in eastern Texas. *J. Wildl. Dis.* 15:367–372, 1979.

FAO. Agricultural Studies 66. Joint FAO/WHO Expert Committee on Brucellosis, 4th rep., tech. rep. ser. 289, p. 43, Rome, 1964.

Fay, L. D. The current status of brucellosis in white-tailed and mule deer in the United States. Proc. 26th North Am. Wildl. Natl. Resources Conf. Wildlife Management Inst., Washington, D.C., March 6–8, 1961.

Fenstermacher, R., and Olsen, D. W. Further studies of disease affecting moose: III. *Cornell Vet.* 32:241–254, 1942.

Fitch, C. P., and Bishop, L. A. The wild rat as a host of *Brucella abortus*. *Cornell Vet.* 28:304–306, 1938.

Golosov, I. M., and Zabrodin, V. A. Brucellosis in reindeer. *Veterinariya* 36:23–25, 1959.

Hoff, G. L., Bigler, W. J., Trainer, D. O., Debbie, J. G., Brown, G. M., Winkler, W. G., Richards, S. H., and Reardon, M. Survey of selected carnivore and opposum serums for agglutinins to *Brucella canis*. *J. Am. Vet. Med. Assoc.* 165:830–831, 1974.

Honess, R. F. Diseases of wildlife in Wyoming. *Wyoming Game Fish Comm. Bull.* 9, 1956.

Hoq, M. A. A serological survey of Brucella agglutinins in wildlife and sheep. *Calif. Vet.* March: 15–17, 1978.

Huddleson, I. Forest. *Brucellosis in man and animals*, rev. ed., pp. 1, 2. New York: Commonwealth Fund, 1943.

Huntley, B. E., Philip, E. R. N., and Maynard, J. E. Survey of brucellosis in Alaska. *J. Infect. Dis.* 112:100–106, 1963.

Jellison, W. L., Fishel, C. W., and Cheatum, E. L. Brucellosis in a moose, *Alces americana*. *J. Wildl. Manag.* 17:217–218, 1953.

Kardevan, A., and Kemenes, F. A mezei nyulak brucellosisa hazaban. [Brucellosis in hares in Hun-

gary.] *Magy. Allatorv. Lapja* 16:59–61, 1961.

Kimberling, C. V., Luchsinger, D. W., and Anderson, R. K. Three cases of canine brucellosis. *J. Am. Vet. Med. Assoc.* 148:900–901, 1966.

McDiarmid, A. Diseases of free-living wild animals. Animal Health Branch, monogr. 1. Rome: FAO, 1960.

McDiarmid, A., and Mathews, P. R. J. Brucellosis in wildlife. *Vet. Rec.* 94:559, 1974.

Meyer, M. E. The epizootiology of brucellosis and its relationship to the identification of *Brucella* organisms. *Am. J. Vet. Res.* 25:553–557, 1964.

———. Identification and virulence studies of *Brucella* strains isolated from Eskimos and reindeer in Alaska, Canada, and Russia. *Am. J. Vet. Res.* 27:253–358, 1966.

Neiland, K. A. Further observations on rangiferine brucellosis in Alaskan carnivores. *J. Wildl. Dis.* 11:45–53, 1975.

Neiland, K. A., King, J. A., Huntley, B. E., and Skoog, R. O. The diseases and parasites of Alaskan wildlife populations: I. Some observations on brucellosis in caribou. *Bull. Wildl. Dis. Assoc.* 4:27–36, 1968.

Orloff, E. S. Brucellosis in reindeer. Proc. 17th World Vet. Congr., Hanover 1:585–588, 1963.

Pickerill, P. A. Canine brucellosis: Serological host range and epidemiological studies. Ph.D. thesis, Cornell University, 1970.

Randhawa, A. S., Kelly, V. P., and Baker, E. F., Jr. Agglutinins to *Coxiella burnetii* and *Brucella* spp. with particular reference to *Brucella canis*, in wild animals of Southern Texas. *J. Am. Vet. Med. Assoc.* 171:939–942, 1977.

Rementsova, M. M. Brucellosis of wild animals (monogr.). Alma-Ata: Akademiya Nauk Kazakhskoi SSR, 1962.

Sachs, R., and Staak, C. Evidence of brucellosis in antelopes of the Serengeti. *Vet. Rec.* 79:857–858, 1966.

Sachs, R., Staak, C., and Groocock, C. M. Serological investigation of brucellosis in game animals in Tanzania. *Bull. Epizoot. Dis. Afr.* 16:91–100, 1968.

Shotts, E. B., Greer, W. E., and Hayes, F. A. A preliminary survey of the incidence of brucellosis and leptospirosis among white-tailed deer (*Odocoileus virginianus*) of the southeast. *J. Am. Vet. Med. Assoc.* 133:359–361, 1958.

Stableforth, O. O., and Galloway, I. I. *Infectious diseases of animals: Diseases due to bacteria*. New York: Academic Press, 1959.

Steen, M. O., Brohn, A., and Robb, D. A survey of brucellosis in white-tailed deer in Missouri. *J. Wildl. Manag.* 19:320–321, 1955.

Stoenner, H. B., and Lackman, D. B. A new *Brucella* species isolated from the desert wood rat, *Neotoma lepida* Thomas. *Am. J. Vet. Res.* 18:947–951, 1957.

Szyfres, B., and Tome, J. G. Natural *Brucella* infection in Argentina wild foxes. *Bull. WHO* 34:919–923, 1966.

Thorne, E. T., Morton, J. K., and Thomas, G. M.

Brucellosis in elk: I. Serologic and bacteriologic survey in Wyoming. *J. Wildl. Dis.* 14:74–81, 1978.

Thorne, E. T., Morton, J. K., Blunt, F. M., and Dawson, H. A. Brucellosis in elk: II. Clinical effects and means of transmission as determined through artificial infections. *J. Wildl. Dis.* 14:280–291, 1978.

Thorpe, B. D., Sidwell, R. W., Bushman, J. B., Smart, K. L., and Noyes, R. Brucellosis in wildlife and livestock in west central Utah. *J. Am. Vet. Med. Assoc.* 146:225–237, 1965.

Toshach, S. R. *Brucella melitensis* in the Northwest Territories. *Can. J. Public Health* 46:155–157, 1955.

Trainer, D. O., and Hanson, R. P. Leptospirosis and brucellosis serological reactions in Wisconsin deer, 1957–58. *J. Wildl. Manag.* 24:44–52, 1960.

————. The association of white-tailed deer and cattle in Wisconsin. *Cornell Vet.* 52:431–438, 1962.

Tunnicliff, E. A., and Marsh, H. Bang's disease in bison and elk in the Yellowstone National Park and the National Bison Range. *J. Am. Vet. Med. Assoc.* 86:745–752, 1935.

Youatt, W. G., and Fay, L. D. Survey of brucellosis in Michigan wildlife. *J. Am. Vet. Med. Assoc.* 139:677, 1961.

Youatt, W. G., Fay, L. D., Whitehead, G. L., and Newman, J. P. Brucellosis and leptospirosis in white-tailed deer in Michigan. *J. Wildl. Manag.* 23:345–348, 1959.

Wetzel, R., and Rieck, W. *Krankheiten des wildes.* Hamburg: Verlag Paul Parey, 1962.

Wood, G. W., Hendricks, J. B., and Goodman, D. E. Brucellosis in feral swine. *J. Wildl. Dis.* 12:579–582, 1976.

25 *Anthrax*

L. P. E. CHOQUETTE   ERIC BROUGHTON

Synonyms: **Splenic fever, malignant pustule, charbon, sang de rate, milzbrand, miltsiekte.**

Anthrax is an infectious, febrile disease caused by *Bacillus anthracis*. The disease is often characterized by its sudden onset and rapidly fatal course, exudation of tarry blood from the body orifices, enlargement of the spleen, and gelatinous infiltrations of the subcutaneous and subserous tissues.

HISTORY AND DISTRIBUTION. Anthrax is nearly universal in its geographic distribution; very few parts of the world are free of the disease.

Through the ages anthrax has taken a heavy toll in human and animal life. The plague that Moses warned would devastate the cattle of the Egyptians (Exod. 9:3) is generally considered to have been anthrax. Virgil (70–19 B.C.) was probably the first to recognize the infectiousness of anthrax in animals and its transmissibility to humans. Though the manifestations of anthrax were probably known to man in remote times, it is only comparatively recently that its nature has been understood and that workers have been able to differentiate it from other rapidly fatal septicemic diseases.

Berthelemy in 1823, Eilert in 1836, and Brauell in 1857–1858 demonstrated its infectiousness. Between 1838 and 1860 French and German workers saw rod-shaped bodies in the blood of infected animals but failed to recognize their significance. In 1863 Davaine demonstrated that the disease could be transmitted by blood containing these rods which he named *bacterides*. The true cause of anthrax was established in 1876 by Koch, who showed that these rod-shaped bodies could be cultivated outside the body and retain their infectivity. In 1881 Pasteur and his colleagues, Chamberland and Roux, reported on the efficacy of a vaccine against anthrax in animals. This was one of the first infectious diseases against which a bacterial vaccine was shown to be an effective and practical means of prophylaxis.

One of the earliest records of anthrax in wild animals was by Livingstone in 1850 in southern Africa where he encountered a disease which affected antelopes, horses, and cattle and produced a "malignant carbuncle" in humans. The disease is now regarded as having been anthrax (Curasson 1942; Henning 1956). It has since been reported from a wide variety of wild mammals in several parts of Africa. In South Africa, sporadic outbreaks were recorded in zebra (*Equus burchelli*), hartebeest (*Alcelaphus caama*), spring buck (*Antidorcas marsupialis*), black wildebeest (*Connochaetes taurinus*), and kudu (*Strepsiceros strepsiceros*) (de Villiers 1943; Neitz 1965; Thomas and Neitz 1933). In 1959 and 1960 over a thousand fatal cases occurred in Kruger National Park. At that time anthrax also occurred in wildlife in other areas of South Africa and in neighboring Bechuanaland. Wild animals involved were a baboon (*Papio ursinus*), carnivores—civet (*Civettictus civetta*), genet cat (*Genetta felina*), lion (*Leo leo krugeri*), cheetah (*Acinonyx jubatus*), leopard (*Panthera pardus*), honey badger (*Mellivora capensis*), and hyena (species not mentioned)—elephant (*Loxodonta africana*), hippopotamus (*Hippopotamus amphibius*), pigs—warthog (*Phacocoerus aethiopicus*), and bush pig (*Potamochoerus porcus*)—giraffe (*Giraffa camelopardalis*), African buffalo (*Syncerus caffer*), and antelopes—hartebeest, impala (*Aepyceros melampus*), springbuck, sassaby (*Damaliscus lunatus*), waterbuck (*Kobus ellipsiprymnus*), grysbok (*Nototragus sharpei*), roan antelope (*Ozanna equina*), sable antelope (*Ozanna nigra*), eland (*Taurotragus oryx*), nyala (*Nyala angasii*), steenbuck (*Raphicerus campestris*), reedbuck (*Redunca arundinum*), duiker (*Sylvicapra grimmia*), bushbuck (*Tragelaphus scriptus*), and kudu (with the kudu showing the highest incidence) (Neitz 1965; Pienaar 1960, 1961). The disease has also been confirmed in hippopotamus, buffalo, species of antelope, and honey badger or ratel in Uganda and other parts of East Africa (Bere 1959; Curasson 1942; Guilbride et al. 1962; Pienaar 1961).

It is believed that in past centuries anthrax outbreaks in Germany resulted in the death of many wild ungulates. In 1874 in Prussia, 2,000 red deer (*Cervus elaphus*) and fallow deer (*Dama dama*) died of a disease now regarded as having been anthrax (Wetzel and Rieck 1966).

According to Wetzel and Rieck the disease still occurs in Europe in red deer, fallow deer, elk (*Alces alces*), roe deer (*Capreolus capreolus*), and occasionally in the wild boar (*Sus scrofa*), the badger (*Meles meles*), and the hare. It has been reported in elk and hares in the USSR, where elk were thought to have been the source of infection in outbreaks involving livestock (Kryuchkov 1953).

Anthrax has also been reported in wild pigs, wild dogs, and dingoes in Australia (Stein 1954) and in elephants in Asia (Gupta 1928; Howard 1913; McGauchey 1961).

The early history of anthrax in continental North America is not well known. It has been suggested that anthrax was introduced from the valley of the Nile to the plains of the Mississippi Delta by ships from the Old World and that it was spread along the Rio Grande by early Spanish soldiers and adventurers. The disease was already established in Louisiana at the time of its settlement by the French in the early 1700s and was first seen in deer near the mouth of the Mississippi River (Stein 1945). Later the disease appeared in bison roaming the western plains, and contamination persisting in the soil to the present time accounts for outbreaks in livestock in some areas (Stein 1948). It has been suggested that the extermination of mountain sheep in the Bear Paw Mountains of Montana was due to anthrax introduced into the area with domestic sheep (Grinnell 1928). Anthrax has been reported in deer in Florida, Louisiana, California, and Texas and in moose (*Alces a. americanus*) in Wyoming (Good 1956; Stein 1950, 1954; Stein and Stoner 1952; Stein and Van Ness 1954).

The first diagnosed case of anthrax in Canadian wildlife occurred in bison (*Bison bison bison*) in the Northwest Territories in 1962 (Novakowski et al. 1963). Over 1,000 bison died during outbreaks in 1962, 1963, 1964, 1967, and 1971 (Choquette et al. 1972). In 1963 and 1964 the disease was also diagnosed in a few moose in the same general area. It is not known how or when the disease was introduced into northern Canada.

There are several records of the disease from zoological gardens and menageries and in ranch-raised fur-bearing animals (Curasson 1942; Granville et al. 1964; Hoffman 1940; Howarth and Seghetti 1939; Jordan 1964; McNary 1948; Stein 1945, 1954; Stein and Van Ness 1954; Stiles and Davis 1940).

ETIOLOGY. The etiologic agent of anthrax is a large nonmotile bacterium, *Bacillus anthracis*.

It multiplies under aerobic conditions and forms spores when exposed to atmosphere under suitable conditions of humidity and temperature. It is highly virulent; when it gains access to the animal body, it multiplies rapidly, producing septicemia.

In animals that have died of the disease, the vegetative or active stage can be found in the blood, swellings, and tissues. The bacilli are rod shaped, square ended, $1-1.25$ μ thick and $5-8$ μ long. They occur either as single cells or in chains of from two to six elements, each enclosed by a thick capsule demonstrable by certain stains (for example, Wright, Giemsa). In its vegetative stage *B. anthracis* is not very resistant to desiccation, high temperature, or chemical disinfectants. If ingested, anthrax bacilli are destroyed by the gastric juices. In an intact carcass, anthrax bacilli are destroyed within 4 days by putrefaction, except under temperatures of $5-10°C$, when they survive a few weeks (Minnett 1950; Stein 1947a,b).

When material containing bacilli (discharges of a diseased animal, for example) is exposed to air, spores are formed; bacilli within the carcass will not sporulate unless the carcass is opened. The spores are highly resistant to normal environmental temperature, sunlight, prolonged drying, and many of the standard disinfectants; and they are not destroyed by gastric juice. They may retain their viability for many years in the soil (Wilson and Russell 1964); in water; and on hides, hair, and other animal matter. Chemical disinfectants must be used in strong solutions or over long periods of time to be effective. Formalin $(10-20\%)$ or lye (5%) are effective disinfectants, but contaminated objects must be saturated with the disinfectant, which should be allowed to act for at least 24 hours. Iodine at a strength of $0.5-1\%$ will sterilize hides (Stein 1955).

TRANSMISSION. In herbivores anthrax is essentially a soil-borne infection. Soil (and water) contamination is often caused by carcasses of infected animals which have died of the disease or have been dismembered by carrion eaters, as well as by the excreta and discharges of diseased animals. Contamination may originate from the excreta of predators or scavengers that have fed on infected carcasses. Certain scavengers, some seemingly highly resistant, such as hyenas, jackals, coyotes, foxes, vultures, buzzards and crows, as well as some predators, play an important role as disseminators of the disease (Curasson 1942; Dillman 1956; Hayes 1962; Henning 1956; Hutyra et al. 1938; Mollet

1913; Pienaar 1961; Stein and Stoner 1952; Stein and Van Ness 1956).

In northern Canada anthrax spores were found in the cloaca of gulls (*Larus argentatus*) which had fed on bison carcasses. The role of birds in spreading the disease is exemplified by the finding of anthrax spores in the alimentary tracts of sparrows in England (Shrewsbury and Barson 1952).

Animals that wallow in mud or on dry soil can carry contaminated mud or soil from one place to another. Anthrax spores may also be carried by surface drainage or in windborne fragments of disintegrated carcasses.

The occurrence of anthrax is largely influenced by climatic and ecological conditions that determine soil moisture, surface temperature, plant growth, surface water, and evaporation—that is, the suitability of the environment for the survival of the spores.

Conditions under which anthrax outbreaks may occur vary considerably throughout the world. In Europe the disease appears to be confined to low-lying and marshy lands and soils rich in organic matter. In South Africa it occurs as often on dry lands as on marshy veld, and its prevalence is not influenced by the amount of moisture in the soil (Henning 1956). Rainy weather followed by hot days appears to favor the occurrence of the disease, and it often follows in the wake of floods and periodic inundation of low-lying lands. Nevertheless anthrax epizootics frequently occur in hot dry summers, during drought, or in the dry season, when the scant growth of forage forces herbivores to graze close to the soil (Curasson 1942; Stein 1955; Van Ness et al. 1959). In close grazing, contaminated soil may be ingested along with vegetation. During these dry periods, swamps, pools, marshes, and bottomlands dry out and become available for grazing (Stein 1942). In some parts of Africa, infection often originates from marshes that have dried up during the summer; in others the disease is associated with water holes and other bodies of water where animals congregate during the dry season or in times of drought (Curasson 1942; Henning 1956; Pienaar 1961).

In tropical and subtropical regions the disease may occur in all seasons, though it is more prevalent when the weather is hot and humid. In the colder areas of the temperate regions, outbreaks in cattle, originating from soilborne infection, tend to occur when the mean temperature is above 15.5°C (Van Ness 1971).

When outbreaks occur in cattle, they are usually confined to limited areas (Henning 1956; Stein 1942) and are likely to occur there year after year at a more or less predictable time. The same can be said of outbreaks involving wild herbivores. The recurrence of the disease is due to the resistance and viability of the spore of *B. anthracis*. In arid areas where vegetation is of the shrubby type, anthrax is uncommon, if not exceptional, since the lack of pasturage and soil conditions are unfavorable to its maintenance (Curasson 1942).

The persistence of soil contamination is related to the activity of normal soil bacteria. In dry soil where microbial activity is minimal, anthrax spores can live for many years, whereas under the more usual conditions of competition, anthrax contamination may disappear in a few months or rarely persist for more than a few years. This inhibitory effect may be due to antibiotics produced by soil bacteria (Minett and Dhanda 1941) or to other microbial factors (Vasil'va 1958–1959). There are also indications that the type of soil and soil pH affect the survival of anthrax organisms (Curasson 1942; Van Ness and Stein 1956; Zarubkinskii 1958–1959).

Animals usually contract anthrax by ingesting food or water contaminated with spores of *B. anthracis*. However, direct infection is also possible when infected material contaminates wounds on the skin or the mucous membranes. Osteophagia, which is often involved in outbreaks in livestock in South Africa (Sterne 1959), was not an important epizootiologic factor in wild animals in Kruger National Park (Pienaar 1961).

A number of bloodsucking flies, including tabanids or gadflies, stable flies, horn flies, and louse flies, can transmit the disease through inoculation (Curasson 1942; Henning 1956; Rao and Mohiyudeen 1958; Stein and Van Ness 1956). It has also been shown that nonbiting Diptera, such as blowflies and fleshflies, which feed and develop in decaying animal matter, can also play a role in the dissemination of anthrax (Curasson 1942; Sen and Minett 1944). There is reason to believe that in the outbreaks in Kruger National Park in 1960 such insects played a role in the infection of such browsing species as kudu and nyala. When disturbed in their feeding on carcasses, swarms of flies were seen to alight on and contaminate the leaves of trees and shrubs which were later browsed by the herbivores (Pienaar 1961).

SIGNS. The clinical picture of anthrax in wild animals is similar to that exhibited by livestock (Henning 1956; Hutyra et al. 1938; Stein and

Van Ness 1956; Sterne 1959). The incubation period may vary from a few hours to several days, as noted in wild herbivores in South Africa (Pienaar 1961), in bison in northern Canada (Novakowski et al. 1963), and in elephants in Asia (Howard 1913).

The disease may occur in a peracute or fulminant form, the animal developing a rapidly progressing septicemia ending in death. The apparently healthy animal dies a short time after exhibiting signs resembling apoplectic seizures (or without exhibiting signs at all). This form of the disease has been observed in elephants in Asia (Howard 1913) and in zebra, kudu, and other species in South Africa (Pienaar 1961).

Anthrax may also occur in an acute form, running a course of 2−3 days or more and ending in death. Diseased animals may be excited or appear depressed, dull, and indifferent. The latter sign was particularly striking in bison during the rutting season. In bison, rumination ceases and the animal may stop feeding or occasionally may feed voraciously. Walking is difficult; the animal staggers at times and exhibits a stiff-legged gait when forced to run. Bloody discharges from the nostrils and the anus and edematous swellings in various parts of the body are common features (Novakowski et al. 1963). In elephants common signs, in addition to dullness and a disinclination to move, are profuse salivation; watery discharge from the eyes; drooping of head and trunk; pendulous penis; and hot, painful swellings, which may burst open in various parts of the body (Curasson 1942; Gupta 1928; Howard 1913; McGauchey 1961).

The disease may also run a less acute course lasting several days, with some animals of a herd recovering. This is sometimes the case in livestock (Stein and Van Ness 1956; Sterne 1959; Udall 1947) and has been noted in bison in Canada (Novakowski et al. 1963), elephants in Asia (Howard 1913), and ungulates in South Africa (Pienaar 1961).

A cutaneous or localized form of anthrax, characterized by swellings in various parts of the body, may occur in cattle and horses following attack by infected biting insects (Stein and Van Ness 1956). This form may also occur in wild herbivores.

On the basis of observation of captive wild animals, the course of the disease in carnivores is variable also. Animals may die without premonitory signs, within 48 hours of the first signs, or after a longer period. Anorexia dullness, prostration, and inflammation of the lips and tongue are common signs (Hoffman 1940; Urbain 1940; Verge and Placidi 1934). Dyspnea resulting from edematous swellings in the region of the throat is also a common feature. Such local lesions may lead to a fatal septicemia or cause death by suffocation.

PATHOGENESIS. In natural infections early lesions have been seen in the integument and in the alimentary canal (Sterne 1959). Virulent spores gaining access to the host germinate and become enveloped in capsules that protect them against phagocytosis. The developing *B. anthracis* produces a toxin, which has been shown to be composed of three synergistic components, one of them provoking an edema in which the bacilli multiply freely (Lincoln et al. 1964). The toxin emanating from the invasion site interferes with the natural defense mechanisms, thus permitting a very rapid multiplication of bacilli locally and in the organs they may have reached, until a dramatic terminal multiplication in the circulation occurs.

This toxin is probably responsible for the irreversible pathologic changes leading to death that occur as a result of secondary shock (Sterne 1959).

PATHOLOGY. Postmortem appearances in wild animals are essentially the same as in domestic animals. However, it is conceivable that, as in domestic species (Henning 1956; Hutyra et al. 1938; Sterne 1959), great variation occurs.

In animals that have died of anthrax, putrefaction and bloating are rapid. In peracute cases there is no evidence of edematous swellings, though occasionally there is a frothy, bloody discharge from the nostrils. In less acute cases dark, tarry blood or bloodstained fluid oozes from the natural orifices; in some species bloodstained fluid exudes through the skin as a result of subcutaneous hemorrhages. Incomplete or nonexistent rigor mortis and the presence of swellings in various parts of the body are also indicative of anthrax. Such manifestations, although indicative of anthrax, are not restricted to this disease.

Swelling around the throat is a common feature in carnivores (Hoffman 1940; Pienaar 1961; Urbain 1940; Verge and Placidi 1934).

Common necropsy findings are the dark color of the blood and its failure to clot; the presence of yellowish serous fluid in the body cavities; and the presence of blood-tinged, clear, or gelatinous exudates at the site of the swellings. Often the spleen is enlarged, dark, soft, and semiliquid in consistency. The lungs, liver, pancreas, kidneys, and urinary bladder are usually congested and swollen. The urine is often bloodstained. The lymph nodes are enlarged and hemorrhagic. The intestinal mucosa is hemorrhagic and thickened.

DIAGNOSIS. As with domestic species (Elliot et al. 1959) a positive diagnosis of anthrax in wild animals can be made only by microscopic and bacteriologic examinations of material from cadavers. Diagnosis based on signs is difficult. In its peracute form or in less acute cases, anthrax may be mistaken for other diseases; therefore, a tentative clinical diagnosis must be confirmed by a laboratory examination.

In most countries anthrax is a reportable disease. Thus all suspected cases of anthrax must be reported to the appropriate veterinary and public health authorities as stipulated by laws enacted to control and eradicate the disease. Because of the seriousness of the disease, wildlife agencies and personnel should cooperate fully with those responsible for its control and eradication.

Anthrax should be suspected when numerous deaths occur within a short period in populations of herd animals. Bloody discharges from the natural orifices, swellings in parts of the body, abnormal behavior, rapid bloating of the carcass, and absence of or incomplete rigor mortis are also indicative of anthrax.

When anthrax is suspected as the cause of death, it is not advisable to perform a postmortem examination, because opening or skinning the carcass may spread the disease or transmit it to the operator. If a postmortem examination is considered necessary, it should be conducted by an experienced pathologist.

Blood smears on clean glass slides and blood samples from fresh cadavers or moribund animals that have been killed are adequate material for laboratory identification of *B. anthracis*. Smears can be made of blood from small superficial vessels of the ear, limbs, or sternal region. Large blood vessels should not be opened because the flow of uncoagulated blood would result in further contamination of the environment. Blood may be absorbed on small pieces of blotting paper, filter paper, sterile cotton swabs, or gauze; allowed to dry; and then placed in screw type vials. A few drops of blood drawn with a sterile syringe and transferred to a sterile vial should also be collected for culture procedures and inoculation of experimental animals. In cattle, anthrax bacilli are numerous in the blood in the terminal stage of the disease; however, this may not be the case in all wild herbivores.

Anthrax organisms are found in great numbers in the spleen of fresh cadavers. However, the specimens must be properly collected and prepared for shipment and must arrive at the laboratory in satisfactory condition for examination. Collection of such material should not be attempted by inexperienced personnel.

Anthrax bacilli can also be demonstrated in tissue sections and in smears of edema and peritoneal fluid. To distinguish them from saprophytic bacilli, it is necessary to culture material and to assess its pathogenicity in laboratory animals.

As soon as the animal dies, anthrax bacilli in the unopened carcass begin to undergo morphologic changes and are destroyed by the putrefactive processess. As the period after death lengthens, putrefactive organisms invade the blood and tissues, and because some of the invading organisms resemble *B. anthracis*, diagnosis becomes more difficult. A diagnosis of anthrax in decomposed carcasses may be possible by means of a serologic test known as Ascoli's thermoprecipitin reaction (Henning 1956; Hutyra et al. 1938). An extract prepared from an infected organ such as the spleen is tested against an anthrax antiserum. The test was found satisfactory when used for the diagnosis of the disease in putrefied bison and moose carcasses in northern Canada.

Specimens collected for laboratory examination should be placed in clean glass containers, labeled as to their contents, and packed and shipped in unbreakable sealed receptacles. Thermos bottles, in which the containers are packed in sawdust, are satisfactory. Whenever possible the specimens should be frozen and should be shipped in watertight containers packed with ice and sawdust.

Because of the danger of infection, for even a superficial examination of a carcass, rubber gloves and rubber boots should be worn. Gloves, boots, and all instruments that have been used should be properly disinfected or destroyed by fire immediately afterward.

IMMUNITY. All mammalian species are susceptible to anthrax in some degree. Some species are more resistant than others, but apparently no species possesses an absolute immunity. Field observations indicate that among wild herbivores, young animals show greater resistance to the disease than adults. This was noted in outbreaks involving kudus and bison. It was also noted that in both these species the death rate was higher in males than in females; behavioral differences may account for this (Novakowski et al. 1963; Pienaar 1961).

Many types of vaccine are available for the active immunization of animals against anthrax; none, however, confer a long-lasting immunity. An avirulent spore vaccine developed in South Africa is now used in many parts of the world for all species and breeds of domestic animals (Sterne 1959). This vaccine was administered to several thousand bison in northern Canada in 1965 and 1966. Active immunization of many of the free-living species of wildlife is impractical. However, the development of immobilizing drugs and tranquilizers and new techniques for the capture of wild animals now make it possible to vaccinate a significant number of individuals of some species threatened with the disease.

TREATMENT. From a practical standpoint the treatment of free-living animals cannot be considered.

Penicillin alone or penicillin plus streptomycin and other antibiotics such as chlortetracycline and oxytetracycline are effective against anthrax in domestic animals (Lincoln et al. 1964; Sterne 1959). Their use in the treatment of captive wild animals, or prophylactically when it is suspected that animals have been exposed to the disease, is indicated (Jordan 1964; Stein 1954). Supportive therapy should include hydrocortisone. A favorable outcome of the disease is more likely if treatment is instituted early. However, in many species the institution of a course of treatment, especially when the drug is administered parenterally, may prove most difficult and necessitate the use of an immobilizing agent or tranquilizers.

CONTROL. The control of anthrax in free-living animals presents many problems. When involving large numbers of animals over large areas, control becomes a major operation, requiring sufficient personnel, means of rapid transportation from site to site, earth-moving equipment, and aircraft to track the animals and spot the carcasses. Helicopters are useful for the latter purpose. The presence of avian carrion eaters will often indicate where dead animals are to be found. The nature of the terrain and surface features may add to the difficulty, and animal behavioral patterns must be reckoned with.

Control measures rest primarily on the proper and rapid disposal of carcasses by complete incineration or burial at least 2.5 m deep under a layer of quicklime. Whenever possible, disposal should be by cremation using fuel oil and wood. The advantage of cremation over burial is that it eliminates the danger of con-

tamination of water supplies through seepage from the burial pit or mound. It also eliminates the possibility of scavengers gaining access to the carcass.

To prevent dissemination of the disease, every effort should be made to dispose of carcasses before they are dismembered by scavengers. The carcass or remains should be immediately doused with fuel oil to keep flies and scavengers away until disposal can be completed. If the carcass is intact, the natural openings should be plugged with absorbent cotton.

Carcasses should be cremated or buried where found. If a carcass must be dragged to a disposal site, ropes and poles used for this purpose should be burned immediately, and care should be taken to prevent soil contamination. Small animals can be wrapped in polyethylene sheets and carted away for disposal. In Africa large animals such as elephants have been disposed of either by burial or by enclosing them in a corral of thornbrush to decompose before eventual incineration (Pienaar 1961).

Personnel should take care to avoid actual contact with carcasses. Heavy rubber gloves and boots should be worn and disinfected after each disposal operation. In some cases face masks should be worn to prevent inhalation of germ-laden dust. All equipment, including machinery, used in disposing of anthrax-infected cadavers should be thoroughly disinfected or burned.

Removal of healthy individuals and their exclusion from contaminated areas should be undertaken if possible, leaving the obviously sick animals behind. Helicopters or fixed-wing aircraft with a slow cruising speed can be used for this purpose. The burning out of areas to destroy contaminated vegetation and dung has been carried out in Kruger National Park and in northern Canada (Novakowski et al. 1963; Pienaar 1961).

Surface water supplies are often major sources of infection. The closing of infected water holes, attempts to prevent their contamination by scavenging birds, disinfecting them with quaternary ammonium compounds, and the filling of small pools and dry mud holes with earth by bulldozing were measures applied in South Africa's Kruger National Park (Pienaar 1961). Such measures would of course not be applicable in every locality.

In addition to sanitary measures, mass vaccination should be carried out. Experience in South Africa in the control of anthrax in livestock has shown that sanitary measures combined with limited immunization are unlikely to succeed (Sterne 1959). In a heavily contaminated area it is unlikely that sanitary measures and annual mass vaccination will entirely prevent the occurrence of anthrax in a wildlife population. But is is probable that vaccination of a high percentage of the population will prevent explosive outbreaks of anthrax in the non-vaccinated animals by correspondingly reducing the availability and dissemination of inoculum.

For obvious reasons, mass vaccination is limited almost exclusively to herd animals which can be corralled, such as bison. The vaccination of bison in northern Canada serves as an example of the practice of mass vaccination in a free-living population. Helicopters were used to round up and herd animals into an oval corral. From this a funnel led into a chute, which was compartmented by sliding doors. A boardwalk enabled the inoculator to operate safely from above the animals. From this position, animals were vaccinated and branded before their release. In 1965 and 1966, respectively, 4,291 and 4,164 bison were vaccinated. These animals were the bulk of the bison population present in areas where anthrax had occurred during the preceding two or three summers. Since there were no bison deaths attributable to anthrax in the vaccinated or unvaccinated animals in these areas in 1965 or 1966, it is not possible to evaluate the efficacy of the vaccine in bison under field conditions or the effect of mass vaccination on the prevalence of the disease.

Because of a lack of data that can be evaluated statistically, one may question the efficacy of anthrax vaccination in the control of the disease in livestock (Sterne 1959) and, obviously, as a control measure of anthrax in bison or other wildlife species. It is recognized that whenever any large-scale immunization is undertaken without strictly nonimmunized controls, it becomes impossible to show in the statistically accepted form that a gradual decrease in the prevalence of the disease is due to previous immunization (Sterne 1959).

Until routine immunization is possible, control of anthrax in free-living populations will continue to rest essentially on the elimination of sources of infection and on the prevention of infection through management practices. In areas where anthrax has occurred, continued surveillance must be maintained for any signs of outbreaks, so that steps can be taken immediately to minimize losses in wildlife and to prevent the spread of the disease.

ANTHRAX IN HUMANS. Wildlife personnel in-

volved in the control of anthrax, or other such personnel as trappers and hunters active in areas where anthrax is known to occur or to have occurred in wildlife, should be aware of the nature of the disease.

In man the disease may occur in a cutaneous, pulmonary, or intestinal form. The cutaneous form, which is the commonest, is usually acquired by skinning or butchering, or during necropsy examinations of infected livestock carcasses. There are also records of humans contracting anthrax from bison in such circumstances (Pyper and Willoughby 1964; U.S. Public Health Service 1956). A localized lesion, usually on such exposed parts as hands, arms, face, and neck first appears as a small pimple developing rapidly into a large vesicle with a black, necrotic center. It is commonly referred to as malignant pustule (Stein 1955). Death may result if the infection becomes generalized.

The pulmonary form of anthrax (woolsorter's disease) is usually an industrial hazard and is due to the inhalation of spores during the processing of hair or wool (Brachman and Fekety 1958; Stein 1955). It could conceivably occur as a result of inhaling spore-laden dust from the hides of wild animals that have wallowed on contaminated soil or dust raised during the disposal of infected carcasses.

The intestinal form of anthrax sometimes follows the consumption of infected animal products. Both the pulmonary and intestinal forms are considered to be peculiarly deadly, and many cases of this nature may not be recognized during life (Sterne 1959).

Prompt diagnosis and early treatment are of the utmost importance in combating the disease in humans. Some of the sulfonamides and antibiotics such as penicillin, chlortetracycline, and oxytetracycline have proved to be effective (Stein 1955; Sterne 1959).

REFERENCES

Bere, R. M. Queen Elizabeth National Park, Uganda: The hippopotamus problem and experiment. *Oryx* 5:116–124, 1959.

Brachman, P. S., and Fekety, R. R. Industrial anthrax: Animal disease and human health. *Ann. N.Y. Acad. Sci.* 70:574–584, 1958.

Choquette, L. P. E., Broughton, E., Currier, A. A., Cousineau, J. G., and Novakowski, N. S. Parasites and diseases of bison in Canada: III. Anthrax outbreaks in the last decade in northern Canada and control measures. *Can. Field-Naturalist* 86:127–132, 1972.

Curasson, G. *Traite de pathologie exotique veteri-*

naire et comparee, 2d ed. Paris: Vigot Freres, 1942.

de Villiers, S. W. An outbreak of anthrax amongst kodoes. *J. S. Afr. Vet. Med. Assoc.* 14:17–18, 1943.

Dillman, S. B. Vultures as disseminators of anthrax. *Auk* 73:283, 1956.

Elliot, H. B., Twiehaus, M. J., Ward, M. K., Worchester, A. W., and Van Ness, G. B. Laboratory diagnosis of anthrax. *Proc. 63rd meeting, U.S. Livestock Sanitary Assoc.,* pp. 399–405. San Francisco: USLSA, 1959.

Good, G. H. Anthrax in the Wyoming mountains. *J. Am. Vet. Med. Assoc.* 129:470–471, 1956.

Granville, A., Fievez, L., and Kaeckenbeck, A. Une epizootie de charbon bacteridien dans un petit elevage de visons. *Ann. Med. Vet.* 108:170–172, 1964.

Grinnell, G. B. Mountain sheep. *J. Mammal.* 9:1–9, 1928.

Guilbride, P. D. L., Coyle, T. J., McAnulty, E. G., Barber, L., and Lomax, G. D. Some pathogenic agents found in hippopotamus in Uganda. *J. Comp. Pathol. Ther.* 72:137–141, 1962.

Gupta, M. C. Anthrax epidemic in the Minbyin Reserve. *Indian Vet. J.* 4:216–228, 1928.

Hayes, F. A. Vultures: Significant disease carriers? *Virginia Wildl.* 23:12, 1962.

Henning, M. W. *Animal diseases in South Africa; being an account of the infectious diseases of domestic animals,* 3d ed. Johannesburg: Central News Agency, 1956.

Hoffman, E. Anthrax in blue fox. *Scand. Vet. Tidsskr.* 30:161–164, 1940.

Howard, G. G. Anthrax in elephants. *Vet. Rec.* 26:69–71, 1913.

Howarth, C. R., and Seghetti, L. Anthrax in farm-raised mink in Oregon. *J. Am. Vet. Med. Assoc.* 94:433–434, 1939.

Hutyra, F., Marek, J., and Manninger, R. *Special pathology and therapeutics of the diseases of domestic animals,* 4th ed. London: Bailliere, Tindall and Cox, 1938.

Jordan, W. J. An outbreak of acute disease in Chester zoo diagnosed as anthrax. *Vet. Rec.* 76:927–930, 1964.

Kryuchkov, I. I. Anthrax in wild animals. *Veterinariya,* 30:36, 1953.

Lincoln, R. E., Walker, J. S., Klein, F., and Haines, B. W. Anthrax. In C. A. Brandly and E. L. Jungherr, eds., *Advances in veterinary science.* New York and London: Academic Press, 1964.

McGauchey, C. A. The diseases of elephants (p. 1 and 2). *Ceylon Vet. J.* 9:17–21, 41–48, 1961.

McNary, D. C. Anthrax in American bison. *J. Am. Vet. Med. Assoc.* 112:378, 1948.

Minett, F. C. Sporulation and viability of *B. anthracis* in relation to environmental temperature and humidity. *J. Comp. Pathol. Ther.* 60:161–176, 1950.

Minett, F. C., and Dhanda, M. R. Multiplication of *B. anthracis* and *Cl. chauvoei* in soil and water. *Indian J. Vet. Sci.* 11:308–328, 1941.

Mollet, F. Die Bedentung von Kraehe und Fuchs fuer die Verbreitung des Milzbrandes. *Zentralbl. Bakteriol.* 70:19–23, 1913.

Neitz, W. O. A check-list and host-list of the zoonoses occurring in mammals and birds in South and South West Africa. *Onderstepoort J. Vet. Res.* 32:189–374, 1965.

Novakowski, N. S., Cousineau, J. G., Kolenosky, G. B., Wilton, G. S., and Choquette, L. P. E. Parasites and diseases of bison in Canada: II. Anthrax epizooty in the Northwest Territories. *Trans. 28th North Am. Wildl. Natl. Resources Conf.,* pp. 233–239. Washington D.C.: Wildlife Management Institute, 1963.

Pienaar, U. de V. 'n Uitbraak van miltsiekte onder wild in die Nasionale Krugerwildtuin 28.9.50 tot 20.11.59 (English sum.). *Kodoe* 3:238–251, 1960. (Erratum: 28.9.50 should read 28.9.59.)

———. A second outbreak of anthrax among game animals in the Kruger National Park, 5th June to 11th October, 1960. *Kodoe* 4:4–16, 1961.

Pyper, J. F., and Willoughby, L. An anthrax outbreak affecting man and buffalo in the Northwest Territories. *Med. Serv. J. Can.* 20:531–540, 1964.

Rao, K. N. S., and Mohiyudeen, S. Tabanus flies as transmitters of anthrax: A field experience. *Indian Vet. J.* 35:348–353, 1958.

Sen, S. K., and Minett, F. C. Experiments on the transmission of anthrax through flies. *Indian J. Vet. Sci.* 14:149–158, 1944.

Shrewsbury, J. F. D., and Barson, G. F. A bacteriological study of the house sparrow, *Passer domesticus domesticus. J. Pathol. Bacteriol.* 64:605–618, 1952.

Stein, C. D. Anthrax. In *Keeping livestock healthy.* Yearbook of Agriculture, Washington, D.C.: U.S. Department of Agriculture, 1942.

———. The history and distribution of anthrax in livestock in the United States. *Vet. Med.* 40:340–349, 1945.

———. Anthrax in animals and its relationship to the disease in man. *Ann. N.Y. Acad. Sci.* 48:507–534, 1947a.

———. Some observations on the tenacity of *Bacillus anthracis. Vet. Med.* 42:13–22, 1947b.

———. Incidence of anthrax in livestock during 1945, 1946, and 1947 with special reference to control measures in the various states. *Vet. Med.* 43:463–469, 1948.

———. Anthrax in livestock during 1949 and incidence of the disease from 1945 to 1949. *Vet. Med.* 45:205–208, 1950.

———. The incidence of anthrax in livestock during 1953 and the first three quarters of 1954. *Proc., 58th meeting, U.S. Livestock Sanitary Assoc.,* pp. 116–122, Omaha, Nebr., USLSA, 1954.

———. Anthrax. In Thomas G. Hull, ed. *Diseases transmitted from animals to man,* 4th ed. Springfield, Ill.: Thomas, 1955.

Stein, C. D., and Stoner, M. G. Anthrax in livestock during 1951 and comparative data on the disease from 1945 through 1951. *Vet. Med.* 47:315–320, 1952.

Stein, C. D., and Van Ness, G. B. A ten-year survey of anthrax in livestock with special reference to outbreaks in 1954. *Vet. Med.* 49:579–588, 1954.

——. Anthrax. In *Animal diseases*. Yearbook of Agriculture, Washington, D.C.: U.S. Department of Agriculture, 1956.

Sterne, M. Anthrax. In A.W. Stableforth and I.A. Galloway, eds., *Infectious diseases of animals*, 1st ed. London: Butterworths, 1959.

Stiles, G. W., and Davis, C. L. Anthrax in minks. *J. Am. Vet. Med. Assoc.* 96:407–409, 1940.

Thomas, A. D., and Neitz, W. O. The importance of disease in wild animals. *S. Afr. J. Sci.* 30:419–425, 1933.

Udall, D. H. *The practice of veterinary medicine*. Ithaca, N.Y.: D. H. Udall, 1947.

Urbain, A. Receptivite de certains carnivores a la bacteridie charbonneuse. *C. R. Soc. Biol.* 134:8–10, 1940.

U.S. Public Health Service. Anthrax contracted from buffalo. Abstr. *J. Am. Vet. Med. Assoc.* 129:22, 1956.

Van Ness, G. B. Ecology of anthrax. *Science* 172:1303–1307, 1971.

Van Ness, G. B., Plotkin, S. A., Huffaker, R. H., and Evans, W. G. The Oklahoma-Kansas anthrax epizootic of 1957. *J. Am. Vet. Med. Assoc.* 134:125–129, 1959.

Van Ness, G. B., and Stein, C. D. Soils of the United States favorable for anthrax. *J. Am. Vet. Med. Assoc.* 129:7–9, 1956.

Vasil'eva, V. M. Soil bacteria as antagonists of anthrax bacilli. *Sb. Nauchn. Tr. L'vov. Zootekh. Vet. Inst.* 9:149–53, 1958–1959. Abstr. *Vet. Bull.* 30(12):3789, 1960.

Verge, J., and Placidi, L. La fievre charbonneuse chez les animaux de menagerie. *C. R. Soc. Biol.* 116:718–721, 1934.

Wetzel, R., and Rieck, W. *Les maladies du gibier*. Paris: Librairie Maloine, 1966.

Wilson, J. B., and Russell, K. E. Isolation of *Bacillus anthracis* from soil stored 60 years. *J. Bacteriol.* 87:237–238, 1964.

Zarubkinskii, V. S. Self-purification of soil and water from anthrax bacilli. *Sb. Nauchn. Tr. L'vov. Zootekh. Vet. Inst.* 9:51–58, 1958–1959. Abstr. *Vet. Bull.* 30(12):3788, 1960.

26 *Erysipelothrix Infection*

RICHARD L. WOOD   RICHARD D. SHUMAN

Synonyms: **None.**

The bacterium *Erysipelothrix rhusiopathiae* affects a wide variety of animals, both domestic and wild, and causes a septicemia of varying severity. The disease is of economic importance because of its effect on the domestic pig, turkey, sheep, and duck and on pheasants raised in captivity. It is also a source of concern to those responsible for supplying and maintaining captive wild animals and to those involved in problems of public health.

HISTORY AND DISTRIBUTION. Recognition of disease caused by erysipelothrix infection began in 1878 with the discovery by Koch of an organism he called the "bacillus of mouse septicemia." Loeffler, in 1882–1886, and Pasteur and Thuillier, in 1882–1883, subsequently related this organism to *Schweinerotlauf* and *rouget du porc*, respectively, or swine erysipelas. Its relationship to human wound infection, called erysipeloid (not human erysipelas), was recognized by Rosenbach in 1887. Early references associated *E. rhusiopathiae* with the domestic animals already mentioned as well as the horse and cow, such laboratory animals as the mouse and guinea pig, and a variety of captive birds in a zoological garden. The first report of natural infection in wild mammals, however, appears to be that by Wayson (1927) who reported on an epizootic among migrating meadow mice (*Microtus arvalis*) and house mice (*Mus musculus*) in California. *Erysipelothrix rhusiopathiae* has worldwide distribution, and in addition to affecting a wide variety of mammals and birds, it has been associated with marine and freshwater fish, as well as reptiles, amphibians, arthropods, and mollusks. It also has been found in sewage from abattoirs, processed meat, decomposing animal carcasses, soil of swine pens, and streams.

A list of wild mammals, both free and captive, from which isolation of *E. rhusiopathiae* has been reported is given in Table 26.1. Relatively few studies have been made of erysipelothrix infection in other than domestic animals, and information has been obtained generally through reports of investigations that primarily were concerned with human health and incidence reports from diagnostic laboratories. Much of the information in Table 26.1 was obtained from reports of epizootiological surveys in the USSR relative to reservoirs of infectious agents of public health concern, principally the genera *Leptospira*, *Pasteurella*, *Listeria*, *Erysipelothrix*, and *Salmonella*, as well as *Bacillus anthracis*.

Probably the most significant aspect of the

TABLE 26.1   Reports of Natural Infection of Wild Mammals with *Erysipelothrix rhusiopathiae*.

Scientific Name[a]	Common Name	Habitat[b]	Geographic Location	Reference
Insectivora				
Sorex caecutiens	shrew	W	Sakhalin Is., Russia	Surkov et al. 1972; Timofeeva et al. 1975
S. gracillimus	Far Eastern shrew	W	Sakhalin Is., Russia	Timofeeva et al. 1975
S. unguiculatus	long-tailed shrew	W	Sakhalin Is., Russia	Surkov et al. 1972; Timofeeva et al. 1975
Lagomorpha				
Ochotona daurica	pika, mouse hare	W	Transbaikalian region, Russia	Timofeeva and Golovacheva 1959

TABLE 26.1 (*continued*)

Scientific Name[a]	Common Name	Habitat[b]	Geographic Location	Reference
Lepus spp.	hare	H	Alfort, France	Lucas et al. 1960
L. europaeus	hare	H	Hrvatska (Croatia), Yugoslavia	Karlovic and Fras 1971
L. timidus	blue hare	W	Sakhalin Is., Russia	Timofeeva et al. 1975
Rodentia				
Rattus norvegicus	brown rat	W	Denver, Colo.	Stiles 1944
		W	Southeastern Washington	Drake and Hall 1947
		W	Leninakan, Armenian S.S.R.	Ovasapyan et al. 1964
		W	Sakhalin Is., Russia	Surkov et al. 1972; Timofeeva et al. 1975
R. rattus	black rat	W	Sakhalin Is., Russia	Surkov et al. 1972
Micromys minutus	Old World harvest mouse	W	Altai Mts., Russia	Chernukha et al. 1962
Acomys cahirinus	spiny mouse	L	Jerusalem, Israel	Bruchim and Mordohovich 1971
Apodemus speciosus	Old World field mouse, Japanese field mouse	W	Sakhalin Is., Russia	Surkov et al. 1972; Timofeeva et al. 1975
Mus musculus	house mouse	W	Kern County, Calif.	Wayson 1927
		W	Lithuanian S.S.R.	Moteyunas et al. 1974
		W	Sakhalin Is., Russia	Surkov et al. 1972; Timofeeva et al. 1975
Arvicola terrestris	water rat, water vole	W	Altai Mts., Russia	Olsuf'ev et al. 1959
		W	Novosibirsk region, Russia	Gritsenko et al. 1964
		W	Sverdlovsk region, Russia	Zhukova et al. 1966
Ondatra zibethica	muskrat	W	Sakhalin Is., Russia	Timofeeva et al. 1975
Microtus arvalis	meadow mouse, meadow vole	W	Kern County, Calif.	Wayson 1927
		L	Utrecht, Netherlands	Van Dorssen and Jaartsveld 1959
		W	Sverdlovsk region, Russia	Zhukova et al. 1966
M. brandti	Brandt's vole	W	Transbaikalian region, Russia	Timofeeva and Golovacheva 1959
		W	Mongolia	Busoedova et al. 1975
Clethrionomys rutilus	red-backed mouse, northern red-backed vole	W	Sverdlovsk region, Russia	Zhukova et al. 1966
		W	Sakhalin Is., Russia	Surkov et al. 1972; Timofeeva et al. 1975
C. rufocanus	large-toothed red-backed vole, Korean red-backed mouse	W	Sakhalin Is., Russia	Surkov et al. 1972; Timofeeva et al. 1975

TABLE 26.1 (*continued*)

Scientific Name[a]	Common Name	Habitat[b]	Geographic Location	Reference
Cricetus dauricus	daurian hamster	W	Transbaikalian region, Russia	Timofeeva and Golovacheva 1959
Muscardinus avellanarius	dormouse	L	Leicester, England	Blackmore and Gallagher 1964
Sicista caudata	birch mouse	W	Sakhalin Is., Russia	Timofeeva et al. 1975
Marmota bobak	marmot, tarbagan	W	Transbaikalian region, Russia	Timofeeva and Golovacheva 1959
M. sibirica	marmot, woodchuck	W	Mongolia	Peshkov et al. 1975
Citellus dauricus	daurian sousliki, ground squirrel	W	Transbaikalian region, Russia	Timofeeva and Golovacheva 1959
C. undulatus	ground squirrel	W	Mongolia	Peshkov et al. 1975; Busoedova et al. 1975
Sciurus vulgaris	tree squirrel	W	Sakhalin Is., Russia	Surkov et al. 1972
Eutamias minimus borealis	northern chipmunk	W	N.W. Territory, Canada	Connell 1954
Carnivora				
Mustela putorius eversmanni	polecat	W	Mongolia	Peshkov et al. 1975
M. itatsi	weasel	W	Sakhalin Is., Russia	Timofeeva et al. 1975
M. vison	mink	F	Wisconsin	Hartsough 1945
		F	Oregon	Gorham 1949
		F	Poland	Sielicka and Kuprowski 1958
		F	Sakhalin Is., Russia	Surkov et al. 1972; Timofeeva et al. 1975
Martes zibellina	Old World marten, sable	W	Sakhalin Is., Russia	Surkov et al. 1972
		W	Iturup Is., Sea of Okhotsk, Russia	Timofeeva et al. 1975
Lutra lutra	Old World otter	W	Sakhalin Is., Russia	Surkov et al. 1972
Ursus arctos	brown bear	W	Iturup Is., Sea of Okhotsk, Russia	Timofeeva et al. 1975
Canis lupus	wolf	W	N.W. Territory, Canada	Langford and Dorward 1977
Vulpes spp.	fox	W	Slovenia, Yugoslavia	Brglez and Batis 1973
Artiodactyla				
Rangifer tarandus	reindeer	U	Russia	Revnivyka 1939 (cited in Blackmore and Gallagher 1964)
Muntiacus muntjak	muntjac deer	C	Leicester, England	Blackmore and Gallagher 1964
Antilocapra americana	pronghorn antelope	W	Alberta, Canada	Langford and Dorward 1977
Bison bison	buffalo	W	N.W. Territory, Canada	Langford and Dorward 1977

TABLE 26.1 (continued)

Scientific Name[a]	Common Name	Habitat[b]	Geographic Location	Reference
Sus scrofa	wild pig	H	Germany	Wellmann and Liebke 1960
Pinnipedia				
Callorhinus ursinus	fur seal	W	Tyuleniy Is., Sea of Okhotsk, Russia	Timofeeva et al. 1975
Eumetopias jubata	sea lion	W	Tyuleniy Is., Sea of Okhotsk, Russia	Timofeeva et al. 1975
Phoca vitulina	seal	W	Tyuleniy Is., Sea of Okhotsk, Russia	Timofeeva et al. 1975
Cetacea				
Tursiops truncatus	bottle-nosed dolphin	C	Marineland, Fla.	Siebold and Neal 1956; Simpson et al. 1958
		C	Enoshima Marineland, Japan	Nakajima and Takikawa 1961
		C	Philadelphia, Pa.	Geraci et al. 1966
Stenella plagiodon	spotted dolphin	C	Marineland, Fla.	Siebold and Neal 1956
Grampus griseus	Risso's dolphin	C	Enoshima Marineland, Japan	Nakajima and Takikawa 1961
Lagenorhynchus obliquidens	Pacific whitesided dolphin	C	Enoshima Marineland, Japan	Nakajima and Takikawa 1961
Primates				
Saguinus nigricollis	black and red tamarin	C	Davis, Calif.	Hirsch et al. 1975
Cercopithecus diana	diana monkey	C	Memphis, Tenn.	Wallach 1977

[a]Scientific names were not given in some reports.
[b]W = wild; C = captivity; H = hunting preserve, game farm; L = laboratory colony; F = fur farm; U = unknown.

occurrence of erysipelothrix infection in wild mammals is the vast reservoir they provide from which the organism can be transmitted to both human beings and domestic animals. For example, the common brown rat (*Rattus norvegicus*) is a potential carrier, as pointed out by Stiles (1944) and Ovasapyan et al. (1964), who found the organism in rats associated with stockyards and a meat-processing plant, respectively.

Clinical cases of acute erysipelothrix infection in captive wild mammals are uncommon. The organism can cause acute septicemic infection of dolphins, which is considered a serious problem wherever these marine mammals are kept for display or entertainment purposes. Spontaneous epizootics have been reported in laboratory colonies of rodents other than the commonly used laboratory mouse (*Mus musculus*). Heavy losses have been reported in colo-

nies of meadow mice (*Microtus arvalis*) (Van Dorssen and Jaartsveld 1959), Egyptian spiny mice (*Acomys cahirinus*) (Bruchim and Mordohovich 1971), and dormice (*Muscardinus avellanarius*) (Blackmore and Gallagher 1964). Cases of acute erysipelothrix infection in nonhuman primates have been reported. Fatal septicemia attributed to the organism has been described in a black and red tamarin (*Saguinus nigricollis*) (Hirsch et al. 1975) and in diana monkeys (*Cercopithecus diana*) (Wallach 1977). In the latter case, wild mice inhabiting service areas adjacent to the primate cages were strongly implicated as the source of infection, since *E. rhusiopathiae* was isolated from trapped specimens.

Reports of experimental infection of wild mammals with *E. rhusiopathiae* are given in Table 26.2. According to Wellman (1954), specific immunity acquired through prior contact

TABLE 26.2 Reports of Experimental Infection of Wild Mammals with *Erysipelothrix rhusiopathiae.*

Scientific Name[a]	Common Name	Susceptibility	Reference
Rodentia			
Rattus norvegicus	brown rat	low	Wellman 1954
R. rattus	black rat	low	Wellman 1954
Micromys minutus	Old World harvest mouse	high	Wellman 1954
Acomys cahirinus	spiny mouse	high	Bruchim and Mordohovich 1971
Apodemus agrarius	Old World field mouse	low	Wellmann 1954
A. sylvaticus	wood mouse	low	Wellmann 1954
		moderate	Chernukha et al. 1962
A. flavicollis	yellow field mouse	low	Wellmann 1954
Mus musculus	house mouse	high	Wellmann 1954
M. spicilegus	Ahrenmaus	high	Wellmann 1954
Arvicola terrestris	water rat, water vole	low	Wellman 1954
Microtus arvalis	meadow mouse, meadow vole	low	Wellman 1954
		high	Musaev et al. 1968
M. brandti	Brandt's vole	high	Timofeeva and Golovacheva 1959
M. oeconomus	northern burrowing mouse	moderate	Wellmann 1954
M. agrestis	field mouse, earth mouse	low	Wellman 1954
Clethrionomys glareolus	red-backed mouse	high	Wellmann 1954
Cricetus cricetus	common hamster	resistant	Wellmann 1954
Mesocricetus auratus	golden hamster	low[b]	Shuman and Lee 1950
		resistant	Wellmann 1954
Meriones vinogradovi	Vinogradov's gerbil	high	Musaev et al. 1968
Marmota bobak	marmot, tarbagan	moderate	Timofeeva and Golovacheva 1959
Citellus dauricus	daurian sousliki, ground squirrel	low	Timofeeva and Golovacheva 1959
C. xanthroprymnus	small Asian ground squirrel	moderate[c]	Ovasapyan et al. 1965
Carnivora			
Mustela vison	mink	resistant	Hartsough 1945
		resistant	Gorham 1949
Vulpes spp.	fox	resistant	Gorham 1949
Artiodactyla			
Odocoileus virginianus	white-tailed deer	moderate[d]	Sikes et al. 1972
Sus scrofa	wild pig	high	Wellmann and Liebke 1960

[a]Scientific names were not given in some reports.
[b]Susceptibility was enhanced by serial passage.
[c]Susceptible during active season; resistant during hibernation.
[d]Arthritis was induced by intraarticular injection; generalized disease was not reported.

with the organism could be largely responsible for the variations reported in susceptibility of captured rodents. Although Gorham (1949) and Hartsough (1945) isolated *E. rhusiopathiae* from farm-raised mink, neither was able to reproduce disease experimentally in healthy mink; in addition, Gorham exposed foxes without success.

ETIOLOGY. *Erysipelothrix rhusiopathiae* is a gram-positive (but easily decolored) slender bacillus that is nonmotile, non-spore-forming, and non-acid-fast. Filamentous forms resembling mycelia occur but do not form branches. Granules, palisades, and "snapping" division may be seen, suggesting species of coryneforms. Short rods measure $1-2$ μm and the filamentous forms $4-15$ μm or more in length. Colonies are classified into smooth (S), rough (R), and intermediate (S-R) forms. Typical S colonies are circular with entire edges and have a smooth convex surface. Typical R colonies (formed by filamentous bacteria) are also circular but are likely to be irregular with curled edges and to have a flattened rough surface. The S-R colonies have some characteristics of the S and R types and can assume a wide variety of formations. After 24 and 48 hours of growth on solid medium, typical colonies are 0.5 to 0.8 mm in diameter, bluish gray in diffuse transmitted light, and nearly transparent, becoming somewhat opaque as they age. Characteristically, granulelike structures are present, from a few in number to a dense concentration. Young colonies can be easily overlooked, especially when either few in number or mixed with faster growing colonies of other organisms. A hand lens ($7\times$) or a stereoscopic microscope are most useful in this regard.

The organism is a facultative aerobe and grows best at 37°C within a pH range of $7.4-7.8$; the addition of serum to the medium will enhance growth. Useful, but presumptive evidence for its recognition is: (1) the characteristic appearance of colonies, (2) the morphologic appearance of the organism, (3) the characteristic growth at 24 hours in broth culture, aptly described by Smith (1885) as "a faint opalescence . . . , which on shaking was resolved for the moment into delicate rolling clouds," (4) the "test tube brush" appearance in gelatin stab cultures incubated at 20°C, and (5) the production of hydrogen sulfide. Acid production in carbohydrate media can be variable; to avoid confusion, White and Shuman (1961) recommend familiarity with the general pattern of fermentation reactions of known strains

of the organism in a medium routinely used. Relatively uniform results with different strains of the organism can be obtained with a peptone-meat extract broth containing Andrade's indicator and 10% sterile equine serum (Lennette et al. 1974).

TRANSMISSION. It is not specifically known how the disease is transmitted under natural conditions, but it seems reasonable to assume that it can result from ingestion of the organism or from wound infection. *Erysipelothrix rhusiopathiae* may persist in the presence of organic matter, but there is no specific evidence that it can exist indefinitely in the soil. However, there is evidence that it can exist free in nature, at least temporarily. Olsuf'ev et al. (1959) found *E. rhusiopathiae* in samples of stream water in an area where during the summer months the only domestic animals were cows and calves. They also found the organism in the body of a dead water rat (*Arvicola terrestris*) found in the stream, and concluded that rodents inhabiting the banks probably provided a source of continual contamination of the stream. Timofeeva et al. (1975) have reported isolating *E. rhusiopathiae* from fecal droppings of a blue hare (*Lepus timidus*), a red-backed vole (*Clethrionomys rufocanus*), a brown bear (*Ursus arctos*), and a fur seal (*Callorhinus ursinus*), all in wild habitat.

Insects may play a role in the transmission of this disease among wild animals. Kondo and Sugimura (1935) isolated the organism from the common housefly (*Musca domestica*). Korotich et al. (1960) and Olsuf'ev and Dunayeva (Kratokhvil 1954) isolated *E. rhusiopathiae* from the pupa and nymph stage of a tick (*Dermacentor pictus*). Kratokhvil (1954) isolated the organism from this tick as well as from mature *Ixodes ricinus*. Korotich et al. (1960) were able to recover the organism from mites (*Trombicula zachovalkini*) that had fed on experimentally infected mice. Timofeeva and Golovacheva (1959) isolated *E. rhusiopathiae* from various species of fleas inhabiting infected rodents, and Busoedova et al. (1975) isolated the organism from ticks (*D. nuttalli, I. crenulatus*) found on a meadow mouse (*Microtus brandti*) and a ground squirrel (*Citellus undulatus*). Peshkov et al. (1975) reported isolation of *E. rhusiopathiae* from fleas collected on a polecat (*Mustela putorius eversmanni*).

Wellmann (1949) demonstrated that the stable fly (*Stomoxys calcitrans*) could infect susceptible mice and pigs after feeding on a known infected pig. Wellmann (1955) also demonstrated that the common housefly was capable of transmitting infective material. The mouse sucking louse (*Polyplax serrata*) can transmit the infection from sick to healthy mice (Stryszak and Oyrzanowska 1955). Timofeeva et al. (1975) was able to infect laboratory mice experimentally by exposing them to hungry, spontaneously infected female ticks (*I. persulcatus*) collected in the field.

The frequent presence of *E. rhusiopathiae* on the body surfaces of marine and freshwater fish, particularly after they have been stored for a time (Murase et al. 1959), provides a likely source of infection of dolphins and other aquatic mammals that require fish or fish products in their diet. In addition, insects that are attracted to feed preparation areas and skin wounds have been suspected as sources for infection of these animals (Geraci et al. 1966).

SIGNS AND PATHOLOGY. There are no distinct specific signs associated with erysipelothrix infection of wild mammals; one is presented with signs suggestive of an acute illness (rough hair coat, thickened exudate in and around the eyes, prostration) or a history of sudden death. Urticarial lesions, similar to those associated with the acute form of the disease in swine, have been reported on dolphins (Simpson et al. 1958; Sweeney and Ridgway 1975).

An assessment of available information regarding pathologic lesions in wild mammals leads one to the general conclusion that the lesions are those representative of a septicemia; that is, nothing of a strictly pathognomonic nature can be observed.

DIAGNOSIS. Diagnosis depends on isolation of *E. rhusiopathiae*. It is sometimes necessary to examine contaminated material, and the following have proved useful for isolating the organism: (1) subcutaneous injection or inoculation of the scarified ears of mice, (2) intramuscular injection of pigeons, (3) refrigeration of a tissue sample in liquid medium at 4–5°C for 4–5 weeks followed by subculture onto Packer medium (Packer 1943), and (4) use of a liquid antibiotic selective medium coupled with the use of Packer medium (Wood 1970). A serum protection test in mice (Wood 1970) is helpful in confirming the identification of virulent isolates of the organism. Otherwise, the repeated injection of rabbits for subsequent testing of their serum for specific agglutinins can be conducted. Fluorescent antibody testing can be applied to *E. rhusiopathiae* for rapid

tentative identification or confirmation of results of other tests. The methods given by Goldman (1968) are applicable. When performing postmortem examinations, it should be remembered that human infection (erysipeloid) can take place easily through small breaks of the skin.

IMMUNITY. Little information is available concerning immunity in wild animals, although by analogy one can assume that infection (clinical or subclinical) can induce immunity. Vaccination of captive dolphins every 6 months with a commercial aluminum hydroxide adsorbate erysipelothrix bacterin is recommended (Sweeney and Ridgway 1975). Studies to evaluate immunity of dolphins by challenge have not been reported, but serologic studies have been conducted in attempts to evaluate experimentally the stimulation of antibodies (Colgrove 1975; Gilmartin et al. 1971; Gray and Klontz 1974).

TREATMENT AND CONTROL. Specific information is lacking for the treatment of wild mammals. Penicillin, with or without commercial swine erysipelas hyperimmune serum of equine origin, has been used successfully in treating domestic animals and thus probably would be suitable for other animals. A second injection of the antibiotic may be necessary. Sweeney and Ridgway (1975) recommend penicillin or chloramphenicol for treatment of acute disease in dolphins.

In circumstances where captive mammals are involved, strict attention must be given to sanitation of food and quarters and to protection from insects and unconfined rodents. With regard to the use of chemical disinfectants, it should be remembered that disinfectants are generally not effective unless surfaces are first thoroughly cleaned of organic soil. Regular observations must be made for deviations from the usual attitude. Newly acquired specimens from any source should be placed in isolation for at least 30 days.

REFERENCES

Blackmore, D. K., and Gallagher, G. L. An outbreak of erysipelas in captive wild birds and mammals. *Vet. Rec.* 76(42):1161–1164, 1964.

Brglez, I., and Batis, J. *Listeria monocytogenes* and *Erysipelothrix rhusiopathiae* in wild-living foxes. In *Erkrankungen der Zootiere*, XV. Internationalen Symposiums uber die Erkrankungen der Zootiere, Kolmarden, 1973. Berlin, DDR: Akademie-Verlag (1973):271–274.

Bruchim, A., and Mordohovich, D. An outbreak of *Erysipelothrix insidiosa* infection in spiny mice (*Acomys cahirinus*). *Refuah Vet.* 28(4):172–175, 1971. Abstr. *Vet. Bull.* 42(8):4468, 1972.

Busoedova, N. M., Lipaev, V. M., Koslovskaya, O. L., and Shura, N. A combined epizootic of plague and erysipeloid in the foothills of northwestern Khangai. In *International and national aspects of the epidemiological surveillance of plague*, vols. 1 and 2, 1975, Irkutsk, USSR: Ministerstvo Zdravookhraneniya SSSR. Abstr. *Rev. Appl. Entomol.* ser. B 65(4):903, 1977.

Chernukha, Yu. G., Semenova, L. P., Karaseva, E. V., and Dunayeva, T. N. Isolation of a mixed culture of *Leptospira of bataviae type* and *Erysipelothrix rhusiopathiae*. *J. Microbiol. Epidemiol. Immunobiol.* 33(1):118–121, 1962.

Colgrove, G. S. A survey of *Erysipelothrix insidiosa* agglutinating antibody titers in vaccinated porpoises (*Tursiops truncatus*). *J. Wildl. Dis.* 11:234–236, 1975.

Connell, R. *Erysipelothrix rhusiopathiae* infection in a northern chipmunk, *Eutamias minimus borealis*. *Can. J. Comp. Med.* 18(1):22–23, 1954.

Drake, C. H., and Hall, E. R. The common rat as a source of *Erysipelothrix rhusiopathiae*. *Am. J. Public Health* 37(2):846–847, 1947.

Geraci, J. R., Sauer, R. M., Medway, W. Erysipelas in dolphins. *Am. J. Vet. Res.* 27(117):597–606, 1966.

Gilmartin, W. G., Allen, J. F., and Ridgway, S. H. Vaccination of porpoises (*Tursiops truncatus*) against *Erysipelothrix rhusiopathiae* infection. *J. Wildl. Dis.* 7:292–295, 1971.

Goldman, M. *Fluorescent antibody methods*. New York: Academic Press, 1968.

Gorham, J. R. An attempt to infect mink and fox with *Erysipelothrix rhusiopathiae*. *Vet. Med.* 44 (3):136, 1949.

Gray, K. N., and Klontz, G. W. Some serologic aspects of the immune response in the Atlantic bottle-nosed porpoise. *J. Wildl. Dis.* 10:180–186, 1974.

Gritsenko, I. N., Sasov, N. P., and Kozlov, N. A. Isolation and use of pathogenic bacteria for controlling water voles (*Arvicola terrestris*). In N. F. Rostovtseva, ed., pp. 202–211. *Problemy veterinarnoi sanitarii*. Moscow, USSR: IZD. "Kolos", 1964.

Hartsough, G. R. Isolation of *Erysipelothrix rhusiopathiae* from farm-raised mink. *J. Am. Vet. Med. Assoc.* 107(823):242–243, 1945.

Hirsch, D. C., Boorman, G. A., and Jang, S. S. Erysipelas in a black and red tamarin. *J. Am. Vet. Med. Assoc.* 167(7):646–647, 1975.

Karlovic, M., and Fras, A. Izolacija uzrocnika vrbanca iz organa zeca (*Lepus europaeus* Pall.). *Vet. Glasn.* 25(7):525–527, 1971.

Kondo, S., and Sugimura, K. Experimental studies on swine erysipelas bacillus found in fish. *J. Japan. Soc. Vet. Sci.* 14(2):111–138, 1935.

Korotich, A. S., Golota, Y. A., and Guscha, G. I. Mites and ticks as sources of swine erysipelas infection. *Veterinariya*, 37:32–34, 1960.

Kratokhvil, N. I. A case of isolation of the causal agent of erysipeloid from sexually matured ticks (*Ixodes ricinus*). *J. Microbiol. Epidemiol. Immunobiol.* 3:61–63, 1954.

Langford, E. V., and Dorward, W. J. *Erysipelothrix insidiosa* recovered from sylvatic mammals in northwestern Canada during examinations for rabies and anthrax. *Can. Vet. J.* 18(4):101–104, 1977.

Lennette, E. H., Spaulding, E. H., and Truant, J. P., eds. *Manual of clinical microbiology*, 2d ed. Washington, D.C.: American Society for Microbiol., 1974.

Lucas, A., Chauvrat, J., and Laroche, M. Infection du lievre a *Erysipelothrix rhusiopathiae*, bacille du roget du porc. *Rec. Med. Vet.* 136(12): 1207–1208, 1960.

Moteyunas, L. I., Kovaleva, L. I., and Ezerskene, E. P. Spontaneous infection of the population of mouse-like rodents of the Lithuanian S.S.R. with causative agents pathogenic for man. *J. Microbiol. Epidemiol. Immunobiol.* 1974(9):122–123, 1974.

Murase, N., Suzuki, K., Isayma, Y., and Murata, M. Studies on the typing of *Erysipelothrix rhusiopathiae*: III. Serological behaviors of the strains isolated from the body surface of marine fishes and their epizootiological significance in swine erysipelas. *Jpn. J. Vet. Sci.* 21(4):215–219, 1959.

Musaev, M. A., Abushev, F. A., and Yuditskaya, S. K. Sensitivity of Vinogradov's gerbil (*Meriones vinogradovi*) and the common vole (*Microtus arvalis*) to erysipeloid. *Dokl. Akad. Nauk. Azerb. S.S.R.* 24(3):51–54, 1968. Abstr. *Biol. Abstr.* 51:21743, 1970.

Nakajima, M., and Takikawa, I. Swine erysipelas in the dolphin. *J. Jpn. Assoc. Zool. Gardens Aquar.* 3(3):69, 1961.

Olsuf'ev, N. G., Petrov, V. G., and Shlygina, K. N. The detection of the causal organisms of erysipeloid and listerosis in stream water. *J. Microbiol. Epidemiol. Immunobiol.* 30(3):112–119, 1959.

Ovasapyan, O. V., Esadzhanyan, M. M., and Galoyan, V. O. *Rattus norvegicus* as possible carriers of *Erysipelothrix*. *J. Microbiol. Epidemiol. Immunobiol.* 41(12):35–38, 1964.

Ovasapyan, O. V., Galoyan, V. O., and Arakelyan, K. A. Sensitivity of *Citellus xanthoprymnus* to erysipeloid infection. *J. Microbiol. Epidemiol. Immunobiol.* 42(3):151, 1965.

Packer, R. A. The use of sodium azide (NaN_3) and crystal violet in a selective medium for streptococci and *Erysipelothrix rhusiopathiae*. *J. Bacteriol.* 46(4):343–349, 1943.

Peshkov, L. I., Fedorov, V. P., and Bogdanov, A. V. Results of an epizootiological reconnaissance for plague in the Khubsugul region of Mongolia. In *International and national aspects of the epidemiological surveillance of plague*, vols. 1 and 2. 1975, Irkutsk, USSR: Ministerstvo Zdravookhraneniya SSSR. Abstr. *Rev. Appl. Entomol.* ser. B 65(4):891, 1977.

Seibold, H. R., and Neal, J. E. *Erysipelothrix septi-*

cemia in the porpoise. *J. Am. Vet. Med. Assoc.* 128(11):537–539, 1956.

Shuman, R. D., and Lee, A. M. The susceptibility of hamsters to *Erysipelothrix rhusiopathiae. J. Bacteriol.* 60(5):677–678, 1950.

Sielicka, B., and Kuprowski, M. Przypadek rozycy u norki. *Med. Weterynar.* 14(3):141–142, 1958.

Sikes, D., Kistner, T. P., Eve, J. H., and Hayes, F. A. Electrophoretic distribution and serologic changes of blood serum of arthritic (rheumatoid) white-tailed deer (*Odocoileus virginianus*) infected with *Erysipelothrix insidiosa. Am. J. Vet. Res.* 33(12):2545–2549, 1972.

Simpson, C. F., Wood, F. G., and Young, F. Cutaneous lesions on a porpoise with erysipelas. *J. Am. Vet. Med. Assoc.* 133(11):558–559, 1958.

Smith, T. 2nd Ann. Rept. Bur. Animal Ind., p. 187, Washington, D.C., 1885.

Stiles, G. W. Swine erysipelas organisms recovered from a brown rat (*Rattus norvegicus*). *Am. J. Vet. Res.* 5(16):243–245, 1944.

Stryszak, A., and Oyrzanowska, J. Ustalenie drog naturalinego zakazania sie bialych myszy wloskowcem rozycy z uwzglednienieum wplywu temperatury. *Rocz. Nauk Roln.* ser. E 66:549–558, 1955.

Surkov, V. S., Timofeeva, N. S., and Suchkova, N. G. Concerning the natural nidality of erysipeloid in Sakhalin. *J. Microbiol. Epidemiol. Immunobiol.* 1972(7):3–5, 1972.

Sweeney, J. C., and Ridgway, S. H. Common diseases of small cetaceans. *J. Am. Vet. Med. Assoc.* 167(7):533–540, 1975.

Timofeeva, L. A., and Golovacheva, V. Ia. Detection of erysipeloid in rodents in the steppes of the transbaikalian region. *J. Microbiol. Epidemiol. Immunobiol.* 30(3):106–112, 1959.

Timofeeva, A. A., Scherbina, R. D., Evseeva; T. I., Olsufiev, N. G., and Mescheryakova, I. S. Erysipeloid on islands of the sea of Okhotsk: I. Sources and vectors of the pathogen of erysipe-

loid. *J. Microbiol. Epidemiol. Immunobiol.* (9):119–126, 1975.

Van Dorssen, C. A., and Jaartsveld, F. H. J. Spontane infectie van veldmuizen met *Erysipelothrix muriseptica. Tijdschr. Diergeneesk.* 84:593–607, 1959.

Wallach, J. D. Erysipelas in two captive diana monkeys. *J. Am. Vet. Med. Assoc.* 171(9):979–980, 1977.

Wayson, N. E. An epizootic among meadow mice in California, caused by the bacillus of mouse septicemia or of swine erysipelas. *Public Health Rep.* 42:1489–1493, 1927.

Wellmann, G. Die Uebertragung des Schweinerotlauf durch den Saugakt der gemeinen Stechfliege (*Stomoxys calcitrans*) und ihre epidemiologische Bedeutung. *Berl. Muench. Tieraerztl. Wochenschr.*, pp. 39–46, 1949.

———. Rotlaufinfektionsversuche an wilden Mauesen, Sperlingen, Huehnern und Puten. *Tieraerztl. Umschau* 15/16:269–273, 1954.

———. Die Uebertragung der Schweinerotlaufinfektion durch die Stubenfliege (*Musca domestica*). *Zentralbl. Bakteriol. Parasitenk. [Orig. A]* 162:261–264, 1955.

Wellmann, G., and Liebke, H. Nachweis von Rotlaufbakterien (*Erysipelothrix rhusiopathiae*) und deren Antikoerper bei Wildschweinen (*Sus scrofa L.*). *Berl. Muench. Tieraerztl. Wochenschr.* 73 (17):329–332, 1960.

White, T. G., and Shuman, R. D. Fermentation reactions of *Erysipelothrix rhusiopathiae. J. Bacteriol.* 82(4):595–599, 1961.

Wood, R. L. Erysipelothrix. In J. E. Blair, E. H. Lennette, and J. P. Truant, eds., *Manual of clinical microbiology*, pp. 101-105. Bethesda, Md.: American Society for Microbiology, 1970.

Zhukova, L. N., Konshina, T. A., and Popugailo, V. M. Listerosis and erysipeloid infection of rodents in the Sverdlovsk region. *J. Microbiol. Epidemiol. Immunobiol.* 43(7):18–23, 1966.

27 Listeriosis

ROELOF G. DIJKSTRA

Synonyms: **Listeric infection, circling disease.**

Listeriosis is a febrile, infectious, endemic disease, which may be expressed in a number of syndromes. According to its clinical course the disease may be classified as acute to hyperacute, subacute, chronic, and abortive. It may be present also as an inapparent infection.

As a zoonotic disease listeriosis is becoming recognized as one of the more important bacterial diseases of man, domestic animals, and wildlife present on farms and in nearby recreational areas. The disease is caused by the organism *Listeria monocytogenes*, which since 1929 has been the only pathogenic representative of the genus. Larsen and Seeliger (1967) reported the isolation of *L. grayi* spp.n. twice from apparently healthy chinchillas, but the cultures were not pathogenic for laboratory animals. No isolations of the latter have been made from wild animals so that this discussion will be limited to *L. monocytogenes.*

HISTORY. It might be considered significant that the second reported isolation of *L. monocytogenes* was made from wild animals. Only a year after Murray et al. (1926) first described *L. monocytogenes* after isolating it from laboratory rabbits and guinea pigs, Pirie (1927) in South Africa isolated it from the livers of several wild gerbils (*Tatera lobengulae*) during an epizootic of septicemia in the Tiger River district of the then Orange Free State.

In 1964 Gray stated, "The passing of time since Murray et al. (1926) first described the bacterium had added much to our knowledge of the organism. Today it is well known that *L. monocytogenes* is a significant cause of encephalitis in domestic ruminants; of septicemia in monogastric animals and birds; of meningitis in humans, particularly during the perinatal period and in the years beyond 40; of abortion in many mammalian species; and a number of other disorders of lesser significance." Yet many misconceptions are still rampant, for instance, that infections with *L. monocytogenes* are rare, that the organism is always involved in listeric infections, and that the organism is easy to cultivate from infected material. There-

fore, much remains to be determined, including the factors that dictate the pathogenesis of the infection in the various species, the natural reservoir of the organism, and the carriers that perpetuate and transmit the disease.

DISTRIBUTION. The distribution and sources of isolations of *L. monocytogenes* from wild hosts are summarized in Table 27.1; note that the distribution is practically worldwide.

In addition to man, *L. monocytogenes* attacks or may be harbored by at least 43 different mammals and 22 fowls, including domesticated animals; house pets; and zoo, laboratory, fur-bearing, and wild animals. It has been isolated from pond-reared rainbow trout (Stamatin et al. 1957), crustaceans (Shylgina 1959), ticks (Kratokhvil 1953; Mamedov 1957; Olsuf'ev and Emelyanova 1951; Stamatin et al. 1957), houseflies and ticks (Demyancheko et al. 1970; Grebenyuk et al. 1972), activated sewage sludge and soil (Seeliger et al. 1965), clear sewage unchlorinated effluents (Kampelmacher et al. 1974), mud (Bonciu et al. 1956), stream water (Olsuf'ev et al. 1959), silage (Dijkstra 1965; Gray 1960) sand (H. E. Larsen, personal communication, 1962), dust (Odegaard et al. 1952), and plants and fodder from wildlife feeding grounds (Weis and Seeliger 1975). This broad distribution presents a peculiar paradox; that is, *L. monocytogenes* apparently is widely distributed in nature, yet the sporadic occurrence of the disease suggests that it is actually restricted, the organism is pathogenic and recognized only under limited specific conditions, it is often overlooked, or its presence cannot be detected by existing cultural methods. Much remains to be evaluated in the etiology and epizootiology of this disease and the role of wild animals.

ETIOLOGY. *Listeria monocytogenes* is a small, gram-positive, non-spore-forming, extremely resistant, diphtherialike rod with a peculiar tumbling motility at room temperature, but usually nonmotile at 37°C. It is aerobic to microaerophilic. Colonies on blood agar incubated 18–24 hours at 37°C are round, 0.2–0.8 mm in diameter, slightly raised with an entire margin, and usually show a narrow zone of beta hemol-

TABLE 27.1 Isolation of *Listeria monocytogenes* from Wild Hosts.

Species	Country	Reference
Monogastric Mammals		
Baboon		
Baboon	Africa	Pinkerton 1967
Badger	Germany	Weis 1974
Fox		
Silver fox	U.S. (Illinois)	Cromwell et al. 1939
Alopex lagopus	Manitoba	Nordland 1959
Fox	Ontario	Avery and Byrne 1959
Urocyon cinereoargentes	U.S. (Massachusetts)	Reynolds and Smith 1965
	U.S.	Jakowski and Wyand 1971
Fox	U.S. (North Dakota)	McIlwain et al. 1966
	France	Phillippon et al. 1972
	Czechoslovakia	Brglez and Batis 1973
	Germany	Weis 1974
Gerbil		
Tatera lobengulae	South Africa	Pirie 1927
Meriones shawi	Algeria	Balozet 1956
M. meridianus,	USSR (Alma-Ata)	Martinevskii 1961
Rhombomys spp.		
Gopher		
Gopher	U.S. (North Dakota)	McIlwain et al. 1966
Hare		
Lepus timidus	Sweden	Nilsson and Soderlind 1974
	Finland	Stenberg 1961
	Norway	Nordoy et al. 1960
	Denmark	Larsen 1963
	Germany	Weidenmueller 1958;
		Weidlich, 1959;
		Weis 1974
	France	Lucas et al. 1955
	Switzerland	Bouvier et al. 1954
	Poland	Skrodzki and Sokolowska 1953
	USSR (Siberia)	Butko et al. 1972
	USSR (Kazakstan)	Bakulov 1977
	Newfoundland	McKercher and Archibald 1959
Lepus europaeus	Hungary	Kemenes and Vetesi 1977
	Sweden	Nilsson and Soderlind 1974
Hedgehog		
Hedgehog	France	Andre 1966
Lemming		
Lemmus trimucronatus trimucro-	Manitoba, Northwest Territory	Plummer and Byrne 1950;
natus, Dicrostonyx groenlandicus		Barrales 1953; Magus 1955;
groenlandicus, D. g. richardsoni		Nordland 1960
Marten		
Pine marten	Germany	Weis 1974
Mouse		
Apodemus sylvaticus,	Czechoslovakia	Seeman 1957
Clethrionomys glareolus		
A. agrarius	Bulgaria	Manev et al. 1977
A. flavicollis	Bulgaria	Manev et al. 1977
Crocidura suaviolens	Bulgaria	Manev et al. 1977
House mouse	USSR (Mowcow),	Ogneva 1962
	Denmark	Larsen 1963
Mus musculus	U.S. (Illinois)	Killinger 1966
	Bulgaria	Manev et al. 1977
Field mouse	Rhodesia	Hill 1971
Forest/woods mouse	USSR	Zhukova et al. 1966
Raccoon		
Procyon lotor	U.S. (Connecticut)	Gifford and Jungherr 1947

TABLE 27.1 *(Continued)*

Species	Country	Reference
Monogastric Mammals *(continued)*		
Rat		
Wild rat	Brazil	Macchiavello 1942
Rattus norvegicus	Czechoslovakia,	Seeman 1957
	USSR (Moscow)	Malakhov 1962; Ogneva 1962; Ponomareva et al. 1962
	Bulgaria	Manev et al. 1977
Arvicola terrestris	USSR	Olsuf'ev and Emelyanova 1951
Water rat	USSR (Siberia)	Kaplinskii et al. 1962
Muskrat	U.S. (North Dakota)	McIlwain et al. 1966
	France	Philippon et al. 1972
Barn rat	USSR	Zhukova et al. 1966
Sable		
Mustela zibellina	USSR	Eremeev and Stepanenko 1962
Marmot	USSR	Timofeeva and Golovacheva 1962
Shrew		
Neomys fodiens	USSR (Siberia)	Butko et al. 1972
Sorex araneus	Bulgaria	Manev et al. 1977
Skunk		
Mephitis mephitis	U.S. (North Dakota)	Bolin et al. 1955; McIlwain et al. 1966
	U.S. (California)	Osebold et al. 1957
Vole		
Microtus agrestis	England	Levy 1948
	U.S. (North Dakota)	McIlwain et al. 1966
M. arvalis	USSR	Kratokhvil 1953; Glagoleva and Emelyanova 1955
M. montanus	U.S. (Washington)	Bacon and Miller 1958
Red vole	USSR (Moscow)	Ogneva 1962
Vole	Sweden	Nilsson and Karlsson 1959
	USSR (Siberia)	Butko et al. 1972
	USSR (Kirgizia)	Grebenyuk et al. 1973
Ruminants		
Deer		
Deer	Germany	Thamm 1957; Weis 1974; Weis and Seeliger 1975
	U.S. (New York)	Miller and Muraschi 1963
	U.S. (Illinois)	A. H. Killinger, personal communication, 1967
Capreolis capreolis	Sweden	Nilsson and Soderlind 1974
	France	Philippon et al. 1972
	Czechoslovakia	Vasil and Seseviokova 1973
Odocoileus virginianus	U.S. (Michigan)	McCrum et al. 1967
Fallow deer	France	Philippon et al. 1972
Moose		
Moose	Nova Scotia	Archibald 1960
Wapiti		
Cervus canadensis roosevelti	U.S. (California)	Martyny and Botzler 1975
Zoo or Captive Animals		
Ape		
Celebes Black Ape, *Macada niger*	U.S.	McChere and Strozier 1975
Cercopithecus mona	Hungary	Kemenes et al. 1973
Cameroen-goat	Hungary	Kemenes et al. 1970

TABLE 27.1   *(Continued)*

Species	Country	Reference
Zoo or Captive Animals *(continued)*		
Chinchilla	Netherlands	Zwart and Donker-Voet 1959
	Sweden	Nillson and Soderlind 1974
	Hungary	Molnar and Nagy 1974
	Portugal	Da Cunha et al. 1971
	Canada (Alberta)	McDonald et al. 1972
Coyote	Ontario	L. Karstad, personal communication, 1961
Marmoset	Netherlands	Zwart and Donker-Voet 1959
Leopard	Germany	Horter and Hunsteger 1960
Mink	France	Phillippon et al. 1972
Paca	Netherlands	Zwart and Donker-Voet 1959
Serval	France	Lagarde 1958
Squirrel	USSR	Chernousova and Putiato 1956

Source: Modified from Gray 1964.

ysis. Hemolysins and hemagglutinins have been described in pathogenic strains (Jenkins et al. 1964, 1967; Watson and Jenkins 1967).

Cultures are easily confused with hemolytic streptococci and often are mistaken for and discarded as "contaminating diphtheroids." Further distinctive characteristics of the organisms have been described (Wetzler et al. 1968), including Camp phenomenon (Brzin and Seeliger 1974), correlation of several in vitro reactions with pathogenicity (Groves and Welshimer 1977), and use of the chick embryo as a model system for investigating the pathogenicity of strains (Wood and Woodbine 1977).

TRANSMISSION. In view of the seemingly ubiquitous nature of this organism, methods of transmission of the disease would probably be as varied. Suggestions have been made that certain wild animals and birds may have acquired the disease by eating infected animals (Gray 1964; Reed 1955) or by contact with disease in domestic animal species. Apparent associations have been recorded between voles and sheep (Grebenyuk et al. 1972), skunks and abortion in cattle (Osebold et al. 1957), skunks and sheep (Osebold 1963b), deer and sheep (Thamm 1957), partridges and sheep (McDiarmid 1962), rats and sheep (Malakhov 1962), free-living rodents and domestic ruminants (Bakulov 1977), and a pet squirrel and a boy (Chernousova and Putiato 1957).

Soil, grass, and plants can be a source of infection. Weis and Seeliger (1975) isolated the organism from plants, soil, old moldy fodder, and wildlife feeding grounds in the Black

Forest, where Weis (1974) isolated *L. monocytogenes* from wild animals.

The role of ectoparasites or other arthropods as vectors in the transmission of the disease is reported by Demyancheko and Baranekov (1970), who isolated the organism from Hybomitra and Tabanus.

Listeria monocytogenes has been isolated also from *Oestrus ovis* larvae taken from the noses of infected sheep (Gill 1937; Kato and Murakami 1962) and from mice inoculated with suspensions of macerated ticks of several species: *Dermacentor pictus* (Olsuf'ev and Emelyanova 1951), *Ixodes ricinus* (Kratokhvil 1953), *Haemolaelaps glasgowi* (Ogneva 1962), and *I. persulcatus* and lice from a "common vole" (Shylgina 1959); and isolated from mice given infected fleas in their food (Grebenyuk et al. 1972). This subject warrants further study, especially since a woman in Austria who died from a listeric meningitis had a large insect bite on one arm (Schmid 1956) and a deer hunter in Virginia developed the disease after hunting in an area heavily infected with ticks (Welshimer and Winglewish 1959).

SIGNS. The clinical picture in naturally infected wild animals is obscure. When infected animals were observed shortly before death or capture, signs were usually associated with septicemia, but some showed signs of encephalitis (Philippon et al. 1972). Exceptions have been animals that appeared to be rabid (Reynolds and Smith 1965; Scholtens and Brim 1964). Investigators should be aware that rabies and listeric infection may occur in the same animal, as shown in wild fox (Avery and Byrne 1959; Brglez and Batis 1973). Signs may resemble a distemperlike disease (Jakowski and Wyand 1971). *Listeria monocytogenes* may also attack wild ruminants or be harbored by them.

Encephalitis is the predominant manifestation of the disease in domesticated ruminants, while septicemia is seen frequently among wild ruminants. An interesting exception was the isolation of *L. monocytogenes* from the brain of a moose in Nova Scotia thought to be suffering from "moose disease," which clinically mimics listeric encephalitis (Archibald 1960); *L. monocytogenes* was once given serious consideration as the etiologic agent of this disease. However, bacteriologic studies (Gray 1962) failed to detect the organism in the brain of a considerable number of moose with the disease (Benson 1958). Apparently the moose in Nova Scotia either died from a primary listeric infection or was a carrier while ill with moose disease, the etiology of which is now considered to be meningeal worms.

Harboring of *L. monocytogenes* by what appeared to be normal deer (*Odocoileus virginianus*) has been reported (McCrum et al. 1967; Weis 1974). Martyny and Botzler (1975) isolated the organism from fecal samples of 14 of 72 apparently healthy wapiti (*Cervus canadensis roosevelti*) among four herds in northwestern California. Nillson and Karlsson (1959) reported chronic purulent orchitis and subacute fibrinopurulent pericarditis associated with isolation of *L. monocytogenes* from the testicle, liver, and spleen in 1 of 2 deer (*Capreolis capreolis*). The other deer had acute purulent bronchopneumonia and acute septic splenitis; the organism was isolated from the liver and spleen.

The uterine contents of many mammals are highly vulnerable to invasion by *L. monocytogenes*, and what quite likely was listeric abortion has been reported in hares (Larsen 1963; Nilsson and Karlsson 1959; Vallee 1952). Listeric infection should be considered in any animal showing a necrotic metritis. Necrotic purulent placentitis is found in abortions caused by *L. monocytogenes* infection, as Kemenes et al. (1973) reported for a monkey. *Listeria* organisms present in the pregnant uterus of a mammal carrying more than one fetus need not necessarily effect all fetuses (Dijkstra 1965; Kemenes et al. 1970).

Listeria monocytogenes was isolated from the blood of lemmings that had developed a bacteremia. These animals had been shipped from the Arctic Circle to a laboratory in Manitoba, Canada. When they were stressed further by inoculation with *Trichina*, they developed ocular discharge, incoordination, circling, and terminal convulsions (Plummer and Byrne 1950). Since stress seemed to be the inducing or causative factor precipitating the disease, its role in the production of listeriosis in many mammals is not hard to envisage. Moreover, in laboratory studies, stressing healthy animals harboring *L. monocytogenes* might result in a clinical picture quite different from that obtained when animals are exposed by the normal routes of inoculation.

PATHOGENESIS. Little is known about the pathogenesis of these organisms. The oral-fecal route of infection is highly suspected from inferences in the literature and discussions with various researchers in the field, but nervous and tracheal routes of infection are possible (Burdarov and Burdarova 1977). It is possible that the number of organisms, pathogenicity of the strains, host factors, and environmental factors may all, or individually, have a definite role. Excellent reviews of the pathogenesis of listeriosis in domestic animals by Osebold and Inouye (1954) and Osebold (1963a) and studies by Vasil and Sesevickova (1973) and Bakulov (1977) present information that might in many instances apply to wild animals. Gray and Killinger (1966) have stated that the pathogenesis of the disease is not known. Infections resulting in disturbances of the central nervous system appear to have a different pathogenesis from those producing abortion or other disturbances of pregnancy. Further research is definitely needed in this area.

PATHOLOGY. The most characteristic gross lesion of *L. monocytogenes* infection is the presence of varying numbers of well-defined, whitish gray foci on the liver, spleen, lungs, and heart. These are essentially identical to those seen in tularemia or pseudotuberculosis.

Histologically, there are areas of necrosis infiltrated with neutrophils as well as toxic changes in the tissues involved. The organism is usually located at the periphery of the lesion and may be either intracellular or extracellular.

Excellent reviews of the pathology of listeriosis in domestic animals and to some extent in wild animals have been published by Seeliger (1961), Lehnert (1964), Flamm (1955), Osebold and Inouye (1954), Gray and Killinger (1966), and Kemenes et al. (1973).

DIAGNOSIS. The diagnosis of *L. monocytogenes* infections, as with most bacterial diseases, should entail the isolation of the specific organism and its confirmation by biochemical and serologic tests. Although it grows well on most media after isolation, it may be difficult to isolate initially, and isolations are often missed. The bacteria are often confined in the focal lesions of infected tissue, frequently intracellularly; hence, it is necessary to release them by a maceration technique. Diluents for this process should be either distilled water or broth, since salt solution seems to be inhibitory, especially when the organisms are few in number. It has been suggested by certain authors (Solomkin 1959; Suchanova et al. 1958; Sword and Pickett 1961) that L forms of the organism may play a role in the disease process. Other studies have shown that L forms can be induced and isolated (Brem and Eveland 1967; Suchanova and Patocka 1957), so that if the organism is present in that form in the animal body, it would be necessary to use special media for its isolation and conversion to the standard vegetative form.

Suspect tissue should be macerated in a mortar, tissue grinder, or blender with sufficient distilled water or tryptose phosphate broth to cover the material well in the tube or bottle in which it is to be stored. Initial platings should be made on blood agar, tryptose agar, trypticase soy agar, or McBride's agar; the remaining suspension should be incubated at 4°C. Body fluids and swabs should be plated and tryptose phosphate broth added; then they should be stored. Feces should be emulsified in enough tryptose phosphate broth to cover the specimen well and should be stored at 4°C for at least a week before plating. Storage in the cold, besides enhancing the growth of this somewhat psychrophilic organism, tends to destroy most of the gram-negative organisms that might be present in the specimen. Smears or impression smears should be made from the original material for staining by fluorescent antibody methods if specified labeled antiserum is available (Biegeleisen 1963; Eveland 1963; Eveland and Baublis 1967; Smith and Metzger 1963). After 18–24 hours of incubation at 37°C, colonies on the inoculated clear agar are a characteristic and distinctive blue green when examined with a scanning microscope or a hand lens, using obliquely transmitted light with the plate resting on a laboratory tripod. The above schema has been outlined in detail by Gray (1962) and Gray and Killinger (1966).

If the initial culture fails to reveal *L. monocytogenes* after 72 hours of incubation, the refrigerated material should be replated at intervals of several weeks for at least 3 months and possibly as long as 9 months. Evaluations of the cold-storage holding technique by Larsen (1967a) and others have shown that it enhances the probability of isolating *L. monocytogenes* by 31%.

An additional type of enrichment reported by Lehnert (1964) and evaluated by McCrum et al. (1967) has shown the value of a 3.75% potassium thiocyanate broth in early isolations of the organism. A new selective medium, trypaflavine-nalidixicacid serum agar (Ralovich et al. 1971) and enrichment technique using tryptose phosphate broth and Stuart medium (Kampelmacher and Van Noorle Jansen 1969) give better results for heavily contaminated material such as feces. A review of selective and enrichment media to isolate *L. monocytogenes* is reported by Ralovich (1974).

A number of isolations of *L. monocytogenes* have been made by the intraperitoneal inoculation of suspect material into mice (Gray 1960; Olsuf'ev and Emelyanova 1951; Olsuf'ev and Petrov 1959; Solomkin 1959). In this country and in Canada several isolations have been made from mice inoculated intracerebrally with suspended brain tissue (Frappier et al. 1967). It is possible that these techniques may be more effective for initial isolation of the organism than the use of ordinary bacteriologic media.

For detection of carriers of *L. monocytogenes*, the feces, intestinal contents, and in some cases the liver must be cultured. Infected animals can excrete the organism in the feces for long periods. Studies on deer (McCrum et al. 1967; Vasil and Sesevickova 1973), domestic animals (Dijkstra 1965; Larsen 1967b), and man (Bojsen-Moller 1972; Kampelmacher and Van Noorle Jansen 1969) have shown the presence of clinically healthy carriers in these groups. Ponomareva et al. (1962) claim that swabbing the pharynx is an effective method with the common rat. One isolation has been made at the University of Michigan from a pet dog by this technique (Baublis 1980).

Serologic tests have not been a very satisfactory aid to diagnosis of *L. monocytogenes* infections. Standard agglutination and complement fixation tests (Seeliger 1961) and refined antigen agglutination tests (Osebold et al. 1965; Wilkinson and Jones 1974) have been used to determine the presence of antibodies, but care must be exercised in their interpretation because of cross-reactions that occur between *L. monocytogenes* and other organisms such as *Staphylococcus aureus* and *Streptococcus feca-*

lis. Evaluation of the live antigen agglutination test (Potel and Degen 1960) has shown it to be quite sensitive and specific. Further work is needed in this area.

Biological tests as an aid to the identification of *L. monocytogenes* cultures have been discussed by Gray and Killinger (1966). These tests include the production of a monocytosis in rabbits by inoculation of a standardized live culture intravenously and the observation of up to a 30% increase in circulating monocytes, and the conjunctival instillation or Anton test by inoculation of a few drops of an 18- to 24-hour broth culture into the conjunctival sac of a rabbit, guinea pig, or mouse, with the production of a severe conjunctivitis in a few days. Both tests have been used in clinical laboratories in various areas of the world, but these dangerous tests can be replaced by improved bacteriologic examinations.

PROGNOSIS. Since the disease appears to be a self-limiting epizootic among wild animals and isolations of the organism have been made from apparently healthy carriers, little can be said with respect to the prognosis in wild populations. It has been suggested by both Bolin et al. (1955) and Osebold et al. (1967) that listeric infection may have a role in the periodic decline of skunk and raccoon populations.

Thus the disease may be present in wild populations as a single case that dies, recovers, or becomes a carrier or may exist in epizootic proportions in which large numbers of the animals may be decimated, with only a few recovering to become carriers of the organism. Vasil and Sesevickova (1973) reported mortality of roe deer and pheasants when they live together in a small area where the special kind of forest ground and climatological circumstances allow *Listeria* organisms to survive and multiply.

IMMUNITY. Very little is known about the immunity conferred by the organism in wild populations. Studies of normal deer populations have shown fairly high agglutination titers (Wetzler et al. 1967), but is is not known if this has any correlation with protective antibody in the prevention of the disease in these animals. Kemenes and Vetesi (1977) found that 21.7% of 285 hares shot or captured in Hungary had titer values of 1:40 or higher in the blood samples, whereas only 2.6% of rabbit blood showed the same agglutination titers. Hares infected intravenously manifested a lower rate of mortality than rabbits, so it was supposed that hares had a higher natural resistance to listeric in-

fection. This may explain the scarcity of clinical listeriosis in hares.

TREATMENT AND CONTROL. Treatment of listeric infections in man and domestic animals is most effective with use of broad-spectrum antibiotics. It could be inferred that such would be the case with wild mammals.

Many different wild hosts may harbor *L. monocytogenes*, but this does not support the notion that listeric infection is widespread among them. The organism may be distributed among wildlife on their feeding grounds (Weis 1974). Disinfection of the surface soil contributes to control. An efficient control will come only when we have a better understanding of the epizootiology and the enzootiology of this organism.

REFERENCES

Andre, P. Isolement de *Listeria monocytogenes* chez un herisson. *Ann. Inst. Pasteur* 111:225, 1966.

Archibald, R. McG. *Listeria monocytogenes* from a Nova Scotia moose. *Can. Vet. J.* 1:225–226, 1960.

Avery, R. J., and Byrne, J. L. An attempt to determine the incidence of *Listeria monocytogenes* in the brain of mammals. *Can. J. Comp. Med.* 23:296–300, 1959.

Bacon, M., and Miller, N. G. Two strains of *Listeria monocytogenes* (Pirie) isolated from feral sources in Washington. *Northwest Sci.* 32:132–139, 1958.

Bakulov, I. The present status of the study of *Listeria* epizootiology. In *Proceedings of 7th International Symposium on Problems of Listeriosis*, Varna, 1977.

Balozet, L. *Listeria monocytogenes* chez la merion. *Arch. Inst. Pasteur Algerie* 34:349–354, 1956.

Barrales, D. Listeriosis in lemmings. *Can. J. Public Health* 44:180–184, 1953.

Baublis, J. V. Human infections with *Listeria*. In *Brennemann's practice of pediatrics*. Hagerstown, Md.: Hoeber, 1980.

Benson, D. A. Moose "sickness" in Nova Scotia, 1. *Can. J. Comp. Med. Vet. Sci.* 22:244–248, 1958.

Biegeleisen, J. Z. Fluorescent antibody studies on *Listeria monocytogenes*. In M. L. Gray, ed., *2nd Symposium on Listeric Infection*, Aug. 1962, Bozeman, Mont., pp. 183–185, 1963.

Bojsen-Moller, J. Human Listeriosis: Diagnostic, epidemiological and clinical studies. Thesis, University of Copenhagen, 1972.

Bolin, F. M., Turn, J., Richards, S. H., and Eveleth, D. F. Listeriosis of a skunk. *North Dak. Agr. Exp. Sta. Bull.* 18:49–50, 1955.

Bonciu, O., Ungureanu, O., Grecianu, A., Dumitrescu, V. *Studiul unei tulpini de* Listeria monocytogenes *isolata din apa unui lac helioterm*. Bucaresti: Comunicare Inst. Balneol. Fiziolterapie, 1956.

Bouvier, G., Burgisser, H., and Schneider, P. A. *Monographie des maladies du lievre en Suisse*, p. 62. Lausanne: Serv. Vet. Cantonal Inst. Galli-Valerio, 1954.

Brem, A., and Eveland, W. C. Inducing L-forms in *Listeria monocytogenes* types 1 through 7. *Appl. Microbiol.* 15:1510, 1967.

Brglez, I. and Batis, J. *Listeria monocytogenes* and *Erys. rhusiopathiae* in wild living foxes. Verhandlungsbericht des 15. In *International Symposium uber die Erkrankungen der Zootiere*, Kolmarden, p. 271, 1973.

Brzin, B., and Seeliger, H. P. R. A brief note on the Camp phenomenon in *Listeria*. In *Proceedings of 6th International Symposium on Problems of Listeriosis*, p. 34, Leicester: Leicester University Press, 1974.

Burdarov, I., and Burdarova, S. S. On the immunity and pathogenesis of the meningoencephalitic form of listeriosis. In *Proceedings of 7th International Symposium on Problems of Listeriosis*, Varna, 1977.

Butko, M. P., Dyadechko, V. N., Domatskaya, M. D., Kulikovskii, A. V., and Pilipets, Z. I. Isolation and properties of *L. monocytogenes* from wild animals in western Siberia. *Probl. Vet. Sanitar.* 42:86, 1972.

Chernousova, A. V., and Putiato, N. F. The clinical aspects of listeriosis. *Zh. Mikrobiol. Epidemiol. Immunobiol.* 28(3):58–60; 365–367 (Eng. transl.), 1957.

Cromwell, H. W., Sweebe, E. L., and Camp, T. C. Bacteria of the *Listerella* group isolated from foxes. *Science* 89:293, 1939.

Da Cunha, L. P., Arriaga de Aragao, H., Da Assuncao, J. M., and Gaspar, J. P. An outbreak of listeriosis in a chinchilla farm: First isolation in Portugal. *Rev. Port. Ciencas Vet.* 66:21, 1971.

Demyancheko, G. F., and Baranekov, M. A. Transmission of *Listeria monocytogenes* by Tabanidae. *Med. Parazit.* 39:573, 1970. Abstr. *Vet. Bull.* 41:1651, 1972.

Dijkstra, R. G. Een studie over listeriosis bij runderen (A study about listeriosis in cattle). Thesis, University of Utrecht, 1965.

Eremeev, M. N., and Stepanenko, N. D. Listeriosis in Russian sables. *Veterinariya* 39(3):57–58, 1962.

Eveland, W. C. Fluorescent antibody studies on *Listeria monocytogenes*. In M. L. Gray, ed., *2nd Symposium on Listeric Infection*, Aug. 1962, Bozeman, Mont., pp. 186–189, 1963.

Eveland, W. C., and Baublis, M. V. Two case reports of the association of human and canine listeriosis. In *Proceedings of 3rd International Symposium on Listeriosis*, July 1966, Bilthoven, Holland, pp. 269–274, 1967.

Flamm, H. Die patho-histologische Diagnose der Listeriose im Tierversuch. *Schweiz. Z. Allgem. Pathol. Bakteriol.* 18:270–277, 1955.

Frappier, C. L., Becker, M. E., and Heahey, K. K.

Listeriosis in animals submitted for rabies diagnosis. In *Proceedings of 3rd International Symposium on Listeriosis*, July 1966, Bilthoven, Holland, pp. 259–267, 1967.

Gifford, R., and Jungherr, E. Listeriosis in Connecticut with particular reference to a septicemic case in a wild raccoon. *Cornell Vet.* 37:39–48, 1947.

Gill, D. A. Ovine bacterial encephalitis (circling disease) and the bacterial genus *Listerella*. *Aust. Vet. J.* 13:46–56, 1937.

Glagoleva, P. N., and Emelyanova, O. S. Listeriosis in voles caught in meadows and haystacks. *Eksp. Parazitol. Med. Zool.* 9:162, 1955.

Gray, M. L. The isolation of *Listeria monocytogenes* from oat silage. *Science* 132:1767–1768, 1960.

———. *Listeria monocytogenes* and listeric infection in the diagnostic laboratory. *Ann. N.Y. Acad. Sci.* 98:686–699, 1962.

———. Infections due to *Listeria monocytogenes* in wildlife. *Transactions of 29th North American Wildlife and Natural Resources Conference*, pp. 202–214. 1964.

Gray, M. L., and Killinger, A. H. *Listeria monocytogenes* and listeric infection. *Bacteriol. Rev.* 30:309–382, 1966.

Grebenyuk, R. V., Chirov, P. A., Kadyskeva, A. M. *Role of wild animals and blood-sucking arthropods in the epidemiology of listeriosis*. Frunze, Kirgizskaya, USSR: Inst. Biol. Akademija Nauk, 1972. Abstr. *Vet. Bull.* 4397, 1973.

Groves, R. D., and Welshimer, H. J. Separation of pathogenic from apathogenic *Listeria monocytogenes* by three in vitro reactions. *J. Clin. Microbiol.* 5:559, 1977.

Hill, R. R. H. Listeriosis in chinchilla and field mouse. *Rhod. Vet. J.* 1:82, 1971.

Horter, R., and Hunsteger, F. Kasuistischer Beitrag zur Listeriose. *Deut. Tieraerztl. Wochschr.* 67:11–14, 1960.

Jakowski, R. M., and Wyand, D. S. Listeriosis associated with canine distemper in a gray fox (*Urocyon cinereoargenteus*). *J. Am. Vet. Med. Assoc.* 159:626, 1971.

Jenkins, E. M., Adams, E. W., and Watson, B. B. Further investigations on the production and nature of the soluble hemolysins of *Listeria monocytogenes*. In *Proceedings of 3rd International Symposium on Listeriosis*, Bilthoven, Holland, pp. 109–123, 1967.

Jenkins, E. M., Njoku-Obi, A. N., and Adams, E. W. Purification of the soluble hemolysin of *Listeria monocytogenes*. *J. Bacteriol.* 88:418–424, 1964.

Kampelmacher, E. H., and Van Noorle Jansen, L. M. Isolation of *Listeria monocytogenes* from faeces of clinically healthy humans and animals. *Zentralbla. Bakteriol.* [*Orig. A*] 211:353, 1969.

———. Occurrence of *L. monocytogenes* in effluents. In *Proceedings of the 6th International Symposium on Problems of Listeriosis*, p. 66, Leicester: Leicester University Press, 1974.

Kaplinskii, M. D., Burganskii, B. Kh., Kortev, A. I., Malyarchikova, G. S., Ananev, I. T., and Karasev, A. G. On listeriosis in the Urals. In *Material*

Sci. Conf., Tomsk, pp. 105–107, 1962.

Kato, H., and Murakami, T. Isolation of Listeria monocytogenes from an Oestrus ovis larva harvested from a sheep with Listeria encephalitis. Jpn. J. Vet. Sci. 24(1):39–43, 1962.

Kemenes, F., and Vetesi, F. Experimental listeriosis in the hare (Lepus europaeus). In Proceedings of 7th International Symposium on Problems on Listeriosis, Varna, 1977.

Kemenes, F., Vetesi, F., and Balsai, A. Listeriosis bei Kameroen-Ziegen. Verhandlungsbericht des 12. In International Symposium uber die Erkrankungen der Zootiere, Budapest, 1970.

———. Abortion in a Gray's monkey associated with Listeria monocytogenes. Verhandlungsbericht des 15. In International Symposium uber die Erkrankungen der Zootiere, Kolmarden, 1973.

Killinger, A. H. Listeriosis in cattle and sheep. Ill. Res. 8:6–7, 1966.

Kratokhvil, N. I. Excretion of Listeria by field voles and ticks Ixodes ricinus. Zh. Mikrobiol. Epidemiol. Immunobiol, 24(11):60–61, 1953.

Lagarde, E. M. Un cas de listeriose chez un serval du parc zoologique. Bull. Soc. Pathol. Exot. 51:468–470, 1958.

Larsen, H. E. Listeric infection among animals in Denmark. In M. L. Gray, ed., 2nd Symposium on Listeric Infection, Aug., 1962, Bozeman, Mont., pp. 27–29, 1963.

———. Isolation technique for Listeria monocytogenes: Primary cultivation and cold incubation technique. In Proceedings of 3rd International Symposium on Listeriosis. Bilthoven, Holland, pp. 43–49, 1967a.

———. Epidemiology of listeriosis: The ubiquitous occurrence of Listeria monocytogenes. In Proceedings of 3rd International Symposium on Listeriosis, Bilthoven, Holland, pp. 295–303, 1967b.

Larsen, H. E., and Seeliger, H. P. R. A mannitol fermenting Listeria: Listeria grayi sp.n. In Proceedings of 3rd International Symposium on Listeriosis, Bilthoven, Holland, pp. 35–42, 1967.

Lehnert, C. Bakteriologische, serologische und tierexperimentelle Untersuchungen zur Pathogenese, Epizootologie und Prophylaxe der Listeriose. Arch. Exp. Veterinaermed. 18(5):981–1027; (6):1247–1302, 1964.

Levy, M. L. Listeria monocytogenes in voles. Vet. J. 104:310–312, 1948.

Lucas, A., Bouley, G., Quinchon, C., Feugeas, C., Gourdon, J., Gourdon, R., and Toucas, L. Etude sur la listeriose et Listeria monocytogenes dans quelques especes animales. Rec. Med. Vet. Exot. 131:152–170, 1955.

Macchiavello, A. Estudo de una cepa de Listerella monocytogenes aislada de rata. Arq. Hig. Saude Publ. (Sao Paulo) 12:105–108, 1942.

McChere, H. M., and Strozier, L. M. Perinatal listeric septicaemia in a Celebes black ape. J. Am. Vet. Med. Assoc. 167:637, 1975.

McCrum, M. W., Eveland, W. C., Wetzler, T. F., and Cowan, A. B. Listeria monocytogenes in the feces

of white-tailed deer (Odocoileus virginianus). Bull. Wildl. Dis. Assoc. 3:98–101, 1967.

McDiarmid, A. Diseases of free-living wild animals. FAO Agr. Stud. FAO of the U.N. (57):34, 1962.

McDonald, D. W., Wilson, G. S., Howell, J., and Klavano, G. G. Listeria monocytogenes isolations in Alberta, 1951–1970. Can. Vet. J. 13:69, 1972.

McIlwain, P. K., Andrews, M. F., Barnes, R. W., Bolin, F. M., and Eveleth, D. F. Occurrence of Listeria monocytogenes in the brains of wild and domestic animals. Am. J. Vet. Res. 27:1497–1499, 1966.

McKercher, P. D., and Archibald, R. McF. Listeriosis in the Atlantic provinces. Can. J. Comp. Med. 23:274–275, 1959.

Magus, M. Listeriosis in lemmings. Can. J. Public Health 45:27, 1955.

Malakhov, Yu. A. Vection of listeria in rats. Veterinariya 39(2):41–42, 1962.

Mamedov, A. A. Listerellez krupnogo pogatovo skota v Azerbaidzhane. Veterinariya 34(7):38–41, 1957.

Manev, H., Yanakieva, M., Mateva, M., Yaneva, V., Zhelev, G., and Lateva, A. Listeria carriers among the wild animals in Bulgaria. In Proceedings of 7th International Symposium on Problems of Listeriosis, Varna, 1977.

Martinevskii, I. L. Listeriosis in Rhombomys and Meriones meridianus. Zh. Mikrobiol. Epidemiol. Immunobiol. 32(5):85–91; 880–890 (Eng. transl.), 1961.

Martyny, J. W., and Botzler, R. G. Listeria monocytogenes isolated from wapiti (Cervus canadensis roosevelti). J. Wildl. Dis. 11(3):330–335, 1975.

Miller, J. K., and Muraschi, T. F. Human listeriosis in New York State. N.Y. State J. Med. 63:1822–1826, 1963.

Molnar, T., and Nagy, G. Occurrence of listeriosis in a chinchilla farm in Hungary. Magy. Allatorvosok Lopja 29:689, 1974.

Murray, E. G. D., Webb, R. A., and Swann, M. B. R. A disease of rabbits characterized by a large mononuclear leucocytosis, caused by a hitherto undescribed bacillus Bacterium monocytogenes (n.sp.). J. Pathol. Bacteriol. 29:407–439, 1926.

Nilsson, A., and Karlsson, K. A. Listeria monocytogenes isolations from animals in Sweden during 1948 to 1957. Nord. Vet. Med. 11:305–315, 1959.

Nillson, O., and Soderlind, O. L. monocytogenes isolated from animals in Sweden during 1958–1972, Nord. Vet. Med. 26:248, 1974.

Nordland, O. S. Host-parasite relations in initiation of infection: I. Occurrence of listeriosis in Arctic mammals, with a note on its possible pathogenesis. Can. J. Comp. Med. 23:393–400, 1959.

———. Host-parasite relations in initiation of infection: II. Hyperglycemia and stress in experimental infection with L. monocytogenes. Can. J. Comp. Med. 24:57–74, 1960.

Nordoey, S., Torkoldson, D., Jorgensen, W., and Brochmann, A. Listeriose tonyetilfells. Tidsskr. Norske Laegeforen. 80:991–994, 1960.

Odegaard, B., Grelland, R., and Henriksen, S. D. A case of *Listeria* infection in man, transmitted from sheep. *Acta Med. Scand.* 142:231–238, 1952.

Ogneva, N. S. Study on the incidence of listeriosis among rodents in Moscow. In *Material Sci. Conf.,* Tomsk, pp. 107–109, 1962.

Olsuf'ev, N. G., and Emelyanova, O. S. Discovery of *Listerella* infection from wild rodents, insectivores, and *Ixodes* ticks. *Zh. Mikrobiol. Epidemiol. Immunobiol.* 22(6):65–71, 1951.

Olsuf'ev, N. G., and Petrov, V. G. Detection of *Erysipelothrix* and *Listeria* in stream water. *Zh. Mikrobiol. Epidemiol. Immunobiol.* 30:89–94, 1959.

Olsuf'ev, N. G., Petrov, V. G., and Shlygina, K. N. The detection of the causal organisms of erysipeloid and listeriosis in stream water. *Zh. Mikrobiol. Epidemiol. Immunobiol.* (English trans.) 30(3): 112–119, 1959.

Osebold, J. W. Some aspects of the pathogenesis of listeriosis. In M. L. Gray, ed., *2nd Symposium on Listeric Infection*, Aug. 1962, Bozeman, Mont., pp. 109–113, 1963a.

———. Some thoughts on the epidemiology of listeriosis. In M. L. Gray, ed., *2nd Symposium on Listeric Infection*, Aug. 1962, Bozeman, Mont., pp. 140–144, 1963b.

Osebold, J. W., Aalund, O., and Chrisp, C. E. Chemical and immunological composition of surface structures of *Listeria monocytogenes. J. Bacteriol.* 89:84–94, 1965.

Osebold, J. W., and Inouye, T. Pathogenesis of *Listeria monocytogenes* infections in natural hosts: I. Rabbit studies. II. Sheep studies. *J. Infect. Dis.* 95:52–78, 1954.

Osebold, J. W., Shultz, G., and Jameson, E. W., Jr. An epizootiological study of listeriosis. *J. Am. Vet. Med. Assoc.* 130:471–475, 1957.

Philippon, A., Maupas, Ph., and Rioux, J. Cl. Les listeriosis animales. *Econ. Med. Anim.* 13:117, 1972.

Pinkerton, M. E. Bacteremia in wild baboons. *Bacteriol. Proc.* M39:67, 1967.

Pirie, J. H. H. A new disease of veld rodents "Tiger River disease." *Publ. S. Afr. Inst. Med. Res.* 3:163–186, 1927.

Plummer, P. J. G. and Byrne, J. L. *Listeria monocytogenes* in the lemming. *Can. J. Comp. Med. Vet. Sci.* 14:214–217, 1950.

Ponomareva, T. N., Yushchenko, G. V., Rodkevich, L. V., Kovaleva, R. V., and Ogneva, N. S. Comparative data on the isolation of bacterial cultures by means of examination of the tissues of the internal organs and of pharyngeal washings in rodents. *Zh. Mikrobiol. Epidemiol. Immunobiol.* 33(9):116–119, 1962.

Potel, J., and Degen, L. Zur Serologie und Immunobiologie der Listeriose. *Zentralbla. Bakteriol.* [Orig.] 130:61–67, 1960.

Ralovich, B. Selective and enrichment media to isolate *Listeria*. In *Proceedings of 6th International Symposium on Problems of Listeriosis*, p. 286.

Leicester: Leicester University Press, 1974.

Ralovich, B., Forray, A., Mero, E., Malovics, H., and Szazados, I. New selective medium for isolation of *L. monocytogenes. Zentralbla. Bakteriol.* [Orig. A] 216:88, 1971.

Reed, R. W., Gavin, W. F., Crosby, J., and Dobson, P. Listeriosis in man. *Can. Med. Assoc. J.* 73:400–402, 1955.

Reynolds, I. M., and Smith, R. E. Listeriosis of gray foxes in Massachusetts: A case report. *Health Lab. Sci.* 2:250–253, 1965.

Schmid, K. O. Listeriameningitis waehrend der Stillperiode. *Wien. Med. Wochenschr.* 106:665–667, 1956.

Scholtens, R. G., and Brim, A. Isolation of *Listeria monocytogenes* from foxes suspected of having rabies. *J. Am. Vet. Med. Assoc.* 145:466–469, 1964.

Seeliger, H. P. R. *Listeriosis*, pp. 224–251. New York: Hafner, 1961.

Seeliger, H. P. R., Winkhaus, I., Andries, L., and Viebahn, A. Die Isolierung von *Listeria monocytogenes* aus Stuhl-Klaerschlamn und Erdproben. *Pathol. Microbiol.* 28:590–601, 1965.

Seeman, J. *Listeria monocytogenes* in rodents. *Cesk. Epidemiol. Mikrobiol. Immunol.* 6:140–145, 1957.

Shlygina, K. N. Studies of variation in the causative organism of listeriosis. *Zh. Mikrobiol. Epidemiol. Immunobiol.* 30(2):56–61, 1959.

Skrodzki, E., and Sokolowska, B. Isolation of *Listerella monocytogenes* from a hare: Preliminary communication. *Biul. Inst. Marino. Trop. Med. Gdansk.* 5:88–90, 1953.

Smith, C. W., and Metzger, J. F. Identification of *Listeria monocytogenes* in experimentally infected animal tissue by immunofluorescence. In M. L. Gray, ed., *2nd Symposium on Listeric Infection*, Aug. 1962, Bozeman, Mont., pp. 179–182, 1963.

Solomkin, P. A. *Listerellez selskokhozyaistvennikh zhivoltnikh.* Moscow: State Publish. Agr. Lit., 1959.

Stamatin, N., Ungureanu, C., Constantinescu, E., Solnitzky, A., Vasilescu, E. Infectia naturala cu *Listeria monocytogenes* la pastravul curcubeu Salmo irideus. *Anuar. Inst. Patol. Igiena. Anim. Bucuresti* 7:163–180, 1957.

Stenberg, H. Einige Beorbachtungen uber die Listeriose in Finnland 1946–1960. *Zentralbla. Bakteriol.* [Orig. A] 182:485–493, 1961.

Suchanova, M., Mencikova, E., and Patocka, F. Experimentelle Listeriose der Kaninchen. Verlauf der experimentalen Infektion und Studium ihrer Uebertragung von der Mutter auf die Frucht. *Zentralbla. Bakteriol.* [Orig. A] 170:547–564, 1958.

Suchanova, M., and Patocka, F. Pokus o dosazeni L forem *Listeria monocytogenes. Cesk. Epidemiol. Mikrobiol. Immunol.* 6:133–139, 1957.

Sword, C. P., and Pickett, M. J. Isolation and distribution of bacteriophages from *Listeria monocytogenes. J. Gen. Microbiol.* 25:241–248, 1961.

Thamm, H. Listeriose unter Rehwild. *Zentralbla. Bakteriol.* [*Orig. A*] 167:417–418, 1957.

Timofeeva, D. A., and Golovacheva, V. Ya. Characteristics of *Listeria* cultures isolated in Siberia and the Far East. In *Material Sci. Conf.*, Tomsk, p. 104, 1962.

Vallee, A. Un cas de listeriose du lievre en France. *Ann. Inst. Pasteur* 83:832–833, 1952.

Vasil, M., and Sesevickova, A. Epidemiology of listeriosis in roe-deer and pheasants. *Vet. Casopsis* 15:137, 1973.

Watson, B. B., and Jenkins, E. M. Further studies on the heat-stable lipolytic activity associated with Listeria monocytogenes. *Bacteriol. Proc.* M98:77, 1967.

Weidenmueller, H. Listerienfunde beim. *Wildl. Mh. Tierheilk.* 10:66–71, 1958.

Weidlich, N. Ueber Wildkrankheiten im Regierungsbezirk Arnsberg. *Berl. Muench. Tieraerztl. Wochenschr.* 72:21–24, 1959.

Weis, J. The incidence of *Listeria monocytogenes* in domestic and wild animals in Southwest Germany. In *Proceedings of the 6th International Symposium on Problems of Listeriosis*, p. 121. Sutton Bonington: Leicester University Press, 1974.

Weis, J., and Seeliger, H. P. R. Incidence of *Listeria monocytogenes* in nature. *Appl. Microbiol.* 30:29, 1975.

Welshimer, H. J., and Winglewish, N. G. Listeriosis: Summary of seven cases of *Listeria* meningitis. *J. Am. Med. Assoc.* 171:1319–1323, 1959.

Wetzler, T. F., Cowan, A. B., Renkowshi, L., Freeman, N. R., and Carver, O. J. Preliminary studies of *Listeria monocytogenes* in deer from E. S. George Reserve. Abstr. *Bull. Wildl. Dis. Assoc.* 3:93, 1967.

Wetzler, T. F., Freeman, N. R., French, M. L., Renkowski, L. A., Eveland, W. C., and Carver, O. J. Biological characterization of *Listeria monocytogenes* for clinical bacteriology laboratories. *Health Lab. Sci.* 5:46–62, 1968.

Wilkinson, B. J., and Jones, D. Some serological studies on *Listeria* and possible related bacteria. In *Proceedings of 6th International Symposium on Problems of Listeriosis*, p. 251, Sutton: Leicester Univ. Press, 1974.

Wood, L., and Woodbine, M. *L. Monocytogenes*: Low temperature virulence in the chick embryo. In *Proceedings of 7th International Symposium on Problems of Listeriosis*, Varna, 1977.

Zhukova, L. N., Konshina, T. A., and Popugailo, V. M. Listeriosis and erysipeloid infection of rodents in the Sverdlovsk region. *Zh. Mikrobiol. Epidemiol. Immunobiol.* 7:18–23, 1966.

Zwart, P., and Donker-Voet, J. Listeriosis bij in gevangenschap gehouden dieren. *Tijdschrift Diergeneesk.* 84:712–716, 1959.

28 Staphylococcosis in Rabbits and Hares

JOHN W. DAVIS

Synonyms: **None.**

Staphylococcosis of hares and rabbits is an infectious, sometimes fatal disease characterized by pyemia and suppurations; it is usually caused by *Staphylococcus aureus*.

HISTORY AND DISTRIBUTION. Hunters have been aware of this disease for a long time. The first documented loss of hares and cottontails to staphylococcosis was recorded in the late summer of 1903 by Seton (1953) on his estate at Cos Cob, Connecticut, when a hare was found infected with *S. aureus*. Staphylococcal infections were believed to be responsible for the periodic decimation of snowshoe hare populations in the northern MacKenzie River district of the Northwest Territories of Canada (MacFarlane 1905). Later MacLulich (1937) described the frequent occurrence of staphylococcal infections among the varying hares (*Lepus americanus*) and the cottontails (*Sylvilagus floridanus*) in Canada. There were frequent cases of staphylococcal infections in cottontail rabbits of Pennsylvania (Cheatum 1941). *Staphylococcus aureus* was recovered by Bacon and Drake (1958) from cutaneous lesions on the back, abdomen, and lungs of four black-tailed jackrabbits (*L. californicus wallawalla merriam*) from Washington, and Osebold and Gray (1960) described staphylococci infections in the wild jackrabbit (*L. californicus*). A disseminated staphylococcic infection has also been reported by Hagan (1963) in newborn domestic rabbits (*Oryctolagus cuniculus*).

There have been a number of reports of staphylococcosis of hares in Europe: Italy (Spinelli and Penso 1932), Switzerland (Bouvier et al. 1954), England (McDiarmid 1955, 1962), and Germany (Wetzel and Rieck 1962).

ETIOLOGY. There are only two species of the genus *Staphylococcus* listed in the 7th edition of *Bergey's Manual of Determinative Bacteriology*—*S. aureus* and *S. epidermidis*. *Staphylococcus aureus* has been isolated from most cases of staphylococcosis in hares and rabbits (Bouvier et al. 1954; Cheatum 1941; Hagan 1963; McDiarmid 1955, 1962; Osebold and Gray 1960;

Seton 1953). In some cases *S. albus* has been isolated (Bouvier et al. 1954; Corsico and Poggi 1953). White strains of staphylococcus have been considered by some workers to be *S. albus*, but these white strains do not differ from *S. aureus* in physiological or cultural characteristics and currently are considered to be *S. aureus*.

Staphylococcus aureus is gram-positive, and in pus and blood it is usually found in grapelike clusters. When grown in artificial media the cells are grouped irregularly in pairs, and short chains are often seen. The organism does not produce flagella, capsules, or spores; and it is readily stained with ordinary aniline dyes. The organism grows readily in many common laboratory media (Merchant and Packer 1967).

Staphylococcus aureus is worldwide in distribution and is often part of the normal bacterial flora of the skin and mucous membranes of animals and man. It has been called an "opportunist" organism, since it is commonly present on tissues, waiting for appropriate environmental conditions for invasion.

TRANSMISSION. A variety of methods for transmission of staphylococcosis in hares or rabbits exists. Bouvier et al. (1954) stated that the genitalia of the hare may be involved in transmission of the disease, as well as biting and stinging insects. Ingestion has been considered as a method of transmission. Scratch wounds are an additional avenue of infection, particularly among the males who fight more than the females. Hagan (1963) proposed that infection in very young rabbits occurred on the day of birth and that the portal of entry was through the umbilical stump, skin abrasions, or both. Bell and Chalgren (1943) surmised that ticks, especially *Ixodes dentatus*, furnished portals of entry for the organisms.

SIGNS. Sick hares and rabbits become exhausted easily. Abscesses form subcutaneously, often swelling to the size of an orange, especially in the region of the head and the neck. In severe cases, hair may become glued together, and crusts form as a result of drainage from the abscesses. Animals may become emaciated, and males can develop enlargement of the scrotum (Osebold and Gray 1960). Tendovaginitis or purulent arthritis may produce lameness.

PATHOLOGY. MacFarlane (1905) reported swellings in the area of the head and neck of snowshoe hares. Enlargement and necrosis of lymph nodes located in the mandibular and axillary regions was observed in cottontail rabbits (Cheatum 1941). The enlargement and necrosis varied from a single slightly enlarged and partially necrotic mandibular node to a severe bilateral involvement of both mandibular and axillary nodes. Splenic involvement was always accompanied by necrosis of the lymph nodes. Bouvier et al. (1954) noted that during septicemic infection there was an inflammatory process with generalized petechiae and "tumors," or nodular swellings, especially in the spleen. There was hyperemia of lungs with pulmonary edema and hemorrhage of the gastrointestinal mucosa.

In chronic infections, severe multiple abscesses developed in all involved organs. The lungs had numerous abscesses or tubercles, ranging in size from that of a grain of rice to that of a pea. The abscesses were filled with a yellowish white exudate and were often extensive, affecting the entire organ. There were multiple adhesions either serofibrinous or fibrotic, which involved the pleura. The heart and pericardium were often the site of a seropurulent inflammation with numerous adhesions. The spleen was often enlarged and contained necrotic passages or abscesses; the liver and kidneys had multiple abscesses which contained a yellowish white exudate. Often a purulent peritonitis was accompanied by multiple abscesses. Mucoid abscesses filled with a yellowish white exudate sometimes occurred in subcutaneous tissues, and pasty abscesses of varying sizes were often detected in the interstitial spaces of large muscle masses. Swollen leg joints contained a grayish white pus that was characteristic of the disease and often became complicated by necrosis, which resulted in loss of digits. Horny thickening of the epidermis was noted in the area of the external genitalia where small abscesses were followed by ulceration. Of equal importance was a metritis and seropurulent perimetritis.

McDiarmid (1955) reported macroscopic lesions of the heart and lungs of a wild hare. Small, discrete, variable abscesses surrounded by a zone of inflammation occurred in the heart and kidney tissues. There were a slight congestion and petechial hemorrhages in the heart and other organs.

In the jackrabbit, Bacon and Drake (1958) reported caseous nodules in the lungs, and Osebold and Gray (1960) noted massive abscesses in the liver. Spleens were enlarged and dark, and on histologic examination hyperplasia of the red pulp was observed. The lungs contained focal lesions consisting of thickened alveolar walls with fluid and free red blood cells in the collapsed alveolar spaces. Grossly the kidneys appeared normal, but on histologic examination loose aggregates of leukocytes were observed around the tubules in the cortex. The primary lesions in another rabbit involved the epididymis and spermatic cord. Histologically these lesions were encapsulated, and many phagocytized cocci were observed in the exudate. The spleen was enlarged, and the lungs contained several focal areas of atelectasis 3–4 mm in diameter along their margins.

The pathology of a disseminated staphylococci infection in domestic rabbits was described by Hagan (1963). White abscesses were found in the lungs and heart. Microscopically, scattered foci of necrotic areas were observed in the lungs, with varying degrees of degeneration and necrosis. Scattered areas of alveolar emphysema and some collapse and consolidation of the alveoli were noted, but very little serous or cellular exudate was found. Histologically, lesions in the heart appeared necrotic and ischemic, and there were pronounced degenerative changes in muscle fibers; however, inflammatory cells were not observed.

DeDiego et al. (1972) reported one male rabbit with orchitis; two of seven rabbits had generalized abscesses in the internal organs (one rabbit had a few abscesses in the liver and kidneys, and the other had generalized abscesses in all the organs including the liver, heart, kidney, lungs, and spleen).

DIAGNOSIS. A tentative diagnosis of staphylococcosis is based on characteristic signs and gross and microscopic lesions. A positive diagnosis is made by isolation of *S. aureus* from blood or affected tissues.

CONTROL. Information relative to immunity in wild mammals is not available. Control measures are possible only when cases of staphylococcosis are found within borders of a specific area (Wetzel and Rieck 1962). All sick and dead animals found in infected or enzootic areas should be properly disposed of by accepted sanitary measures.

REFERENCES

Bacon, M., and Drake, C. H. Bacterial infection in wild rabbits of eastern and central Washington. *Northwest Sci.* 32:124–131, 1958.

Bell, J. F., and Chalgren, W. S. Some wildlife diseases in the eastern United States. *J. Wildl. Manag.* 7:270–278, 1943.

Bouvier, G., Burgisser, H., and Schneider, P. A. *Monographie des maladies du lievre en Suisse.* Lausanne: Service Veterinaire Cantonal et Institut Galli-Valerio, 1954.

Cheatum, E. L. Lymphadenitis in New York cottontails. *J. Wildl. Manag.* 5:304–308, 1941.

Corscico, G., and Poggi, A. Stafilococcosi delle lepri. *Atti Soc. Ital. Sci. Vet.* 6:212–218, 1953.

deDiego, A. I., Dorta, G. T., and Trumper, S. J. Estafilocacias en liebres. *Rev. Med. Vet.* 53:45–47, 1972.

Hagan, K. W. Disseminated staphylococci infection in young domestic rabbits. *J. Am. Vet. Med. Assoc.* 42:1421–1422, 1963.

McDiarmid, A. Diseases of free-living wild mammals, pp. 5–7, United Nations 57. Rome: FAO, 1962.

———. Staphylococcal pyemia in a wild hare (*Lepus europaeus occidentalis*). *J. Comp. Pathol. Ther.* 65:17–19, 1955.

MacFarlane, R. Notes on the mammals collected and observed in the northern MacKenzie River district, Northwest Territories of Canada, with remarks on explorers and exploration of the Far North. *U.S. Natl. Museum Proc.* 28:673–764, 1905.

MacLulich, D. A. Fluctuations in the numbers of the varying hare (*Lepus americanus*). *Univ. Toronto Stud., Biol. Ser.* 43:80–82, 92–95, 1937.

Merchant, A. I., and Packer, R. A. *Veterinary Bacteriology and Virology*, 7th ed. Ames: Iowa State Univ. Press, 1967.

Osebold, J. W., and Gray, O. M. Disseminated staphylococci infections in wild jackrabbits (*Lepus californicus*). *J. Infect. Dis.* 106:91–94, 1960.

Seton, E. T. *Lives of game animals*, vol. 4, pt. 2, p. 712. Boston: Charles T. Branford, 1953.

Spinelli, A., and Penso, G. Setticopioemia delle lepria a caratere epizootico. *Clin. Vet.* 55:173–189, 1932.

Wetzel, R., and Rieck, W. *Krankheiten des Wildes*. Berlin: Verlag Paul Parey, 1962.

29 *Enterobacterial Disease*

R. M. ROBINSON

Synonyms: **Colibacillosis, dysentery.**

Enterobacterial disease is a term applied to infections caused by bacterial pathogens, alone or in concert with other substances such as toxins, parasites, or enteroviral agents. These pathogens are characterized by destruction of the gastrointestinal lining, producing varying degrees of gastrointestinal disturbance. Diarrhea is the most commonly observed manifestation of these infections, although vomition and dehydration may attend acute infections. Mortality is generally limited to the neonatal mammal, older individuals being more resistant to infection.

HISTORY AND DISTRIBUTION. Bacteria that produce gastrointestinal disease are found worldwide and in all environments. Enterobacterial disease has plagued the mammalian kingdom since time began and still is a common and devastating affliction of neonatal mammals. Early in the history of microbiology, bacteria were thought to be the causative agents of diseases that are now recognized as viral or parasitic. These viral or parasitic pathogens can act as triggering factors to allow invasion and systemic spread by bacteria commonly found in the gastrointestinal tract. As time progresses, more such complex relationships will be defined, linking enterobacterial disease with many viral, parasitic, or toxic agents, each of which may be relatively innocuous by itself but, when combined, may have lethal results.

Salmonella spp. enteritis is common in wild mammals of all species under captive conditions, particularly where adequate sanitation is difficult to achieve. This is also true of other potential enteric pathogens such as *Escherichia coli* and *Proteus vulgaris*. It is difficult to assess the pathogenecity of these latter two potential pathogens, even in captive conditions. However, it may be presumed that these organisms may also be present and constitute a source of neonatal mortality in the wild.

ETIOLOGY. The etiological causes of enterobacterial disease are generally considered to be coliform bacteria: *Salmonella*, *Escherichia*,

Proteus, Klebsiella, and *Arizona*. The most common and significant are *E. coli* and the *Salmonella* spp. Most of these agents are readily found in the gastrointestinal tract of all mammals, which accounts for their ubiquitous occurrence. However, when the enteric bacterial population becomes unbalanced for whatever reason, these agents proliferate and elicit pathologic effects on their host.

Mortality in free-ranging wild animals often goes undetected because of the acute course of the disease. Young mammals that have succumbed disappear rapidly in wild environments, and dead carnivorous species that have not left the den site cannot be observed. Enteric problems are exceedingly common in wild mammals trapped and moved into captivity, and losses in the wild are most likely commensurate with such losses in captivity.

This certainly appears to be the case with *Salmonella* infections in white-tailed deer, which will be used to illustrate the effect of enterobacterial disease in wild populations.

Salmonellosis

TRANSMISSION. *Salmonella* enteritis has been documented in populations of wild white-tailed deer, in which a significant portion of the neonatal population may succumb to this disease (Fig. 29.1) (Debbie 1968; Robinson et al. 1970). These gram-negative bacilli are characterized by their ability to behave as opportunists in the environment. They have been isolated with ease from such poikilothermic hosts as turtles, snakes, and alligators, in which they apparently cause no clinical illness. By this mechanism alone, the bacterium is capable of maintaining a floodplain contamination sufficient to form a source of infection for young mammalian hosts born during a season in which the environment favors bacterial replication. In addition, *Salmonella* spp. are capable of surviving and replicating in organic matter of surface waters, much enhancing their potential as environmental contaminants. The specific type of *Salmonella* appears of minor

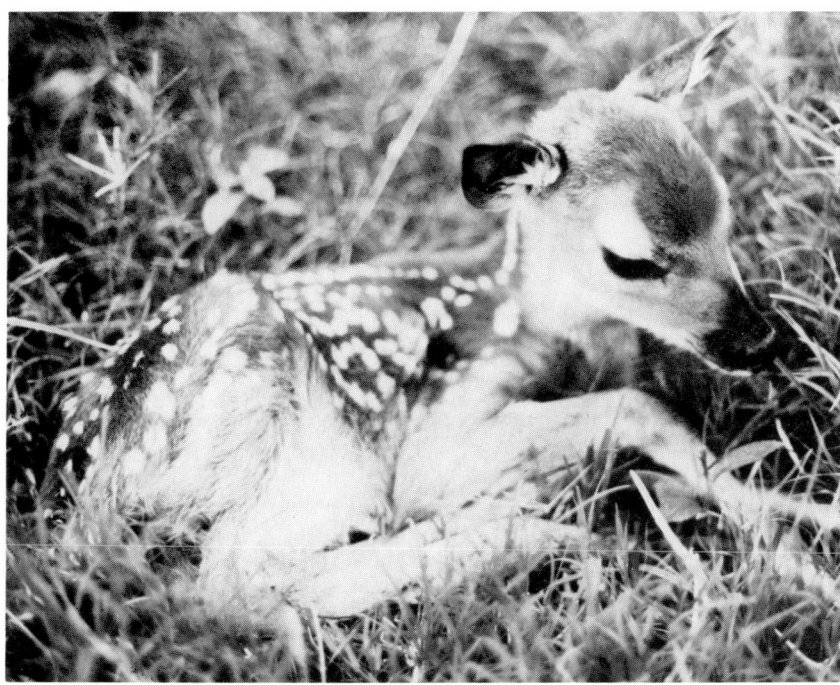

FIG. 29.1 Fawn suffering from acute salmonellosis.

importance. Many serotypes have been documented in white-tailed deer, and all have the potential of producing acute enteritis in neonatal host animals (Cook 1966).

SIGNS AND PATHOLOGY. The disease as observed in white-tailed deer is age dependent, the neonatal host being affected most severely. Fawns that survive a week or more have a prolonged clinical course with the development of external signs of overt enteritis, that is, diarrhea.

In the acute form of the disease, death ensues within 6–12 hours, and dehydration is the only external sign observed. Opisthotonos is seen terminally. Fawns which have died of this form of the disease generally are found in the field with no marks or signs of struggle.

Animals a week of age or older which have contracted the disease develop yellowish mucoid blood-flecked diarrhea, tend to have a more protracted form of the disease, and usually live 2–6 days. These animals generally have coarse, sticky hair coats and tucked-up abdomens and vocalize and wander aimlessly in the field. Weakness and lack of fear are frequently observed. Such animals when consumed by predators are often classed as "predator kills" by field personnel, thus overlooking the initial cause of mortality.

Pathologic lesions in animals dead of the acute form of the disease are not marked. Denudation of the mucosal epithelium with attendant capillary engorgement can occur. This change is difficult to assess unless the time of death is known, because postmortem degenerative change may produce similar changes. Proliferation of reticuloendothelial cells in the sinusoids of the mesenteric lymph nodes is often observed. Small sequestra of neutrophils may be seen in lymph node or liver sections. The more chronic form of the disease may be associated with infiltration of the lamina propria of the intestine with lymphocytes and reticuloendothelial cells and development of edema at that site.

PATHOGENESIS. The gastrointestinal tract is highly subject to injury because of its physical structure; a single cell layer separates the lumen from the internal environment of the organism. Because of its absorptive surface, a relatively small amount of damage is magnified many times in its physiological impact. A variety of substances (abrasion, toxins, or bacterial action) are capable of causing devitalization of the gastrointestinal epithelium.

Below the gastrointestinal epithelium lies a network of blood vessels and lymphatics, whose main function in health is to transport nutrients to the various organs for processing into metabolites. From these the organism may derive substances in proper form for building protein or converting into energy. This capillary bed assumes a great deal of importance when it is exposed to the lumen of the gastrointestinal tract, as it is capable of releasing a tremendous amount of fluid and electrolytes into the gut lumen. Indeed, this is the principal mechanism involved in enteric disease—sudden release of fluids and electrolytes into the lumen, with an inappropriate response by the host in terms of reestablishing an epithelial surface. Enteric disease is then clinically reflected by the degree of damage and the time in which this damage is maintained by the pathogen, toxin, or whatever insult precipitates the enteritis. Host defense against this susceptibility is very rapid mitotic activity of the surface epithelium, with emigration of mucosal epithelium toward the villous tips and contraction of the villous processes to reduce the injured surface areas.

Recovery from enteric disease is dependent on the result of a tenuous balance between epithelial destruction and regeneration. The difficulty of clinical evaluation of this is that it is exceedingly difficult to assess at what point this balance exists. Rapid dehydration without attendant diarrhea is a grave prognostic sign, particularly when followed in a few hours by profuse diarrhea. Mucus and blood in diarrheas may indicate severe enteric damage.

Once the epithelial barrier is passed, hematogenous spread of a pathogen may rapidly ensue. In such cases, secondary pneumonia is frequently seen, with death resulting from the combined effects of enteritis and pneumonia.

DIAGNOSIS. Cultural confirmation is required for a definitive diagnosis, as the gross and microscopic lesions are not pathognomonic. Rectal swabs may be used as a general screen on living subjects; however, because of cultural error, the number of positive cultures must be considered as a minimum number, rather than an actual infection rate. The most reliable source of cul-

tural material on necropsy specimens is the mesenteric lymph nodes, which yield the most consistent results. Rectal swabs should be dampened in sterile saline prior to use and transported to the laboratory in sterile tryptose broth or transport medium for cultural confirmation. Strict adherence to sterile technique is required in taking such samples. Cultural samples are then grown on differential media to isolate the different bacterial genera. Species identification in the Salmonella group is usually done serologically (Ewing 1970).

TREATMENT AND CONTROL. Treatment and control of enterobacterial disease in free-ranging populations of wild mammals is not considered practical at the present time. Habitat alteration and population control probably offer the best approach to control of these groups of diseases.

In captivity, treatment and control are certainly indicated, as these are the most important diseases of neonatal mammals in zoological and private collections. Most therapy should be aimed at reducing electrolyte loss through the injured intestinal mucosa and reestablishing a normal bacterial flora in the gastrointestinal tract. Antibiotic therapy often aggravates the condition by reducing normal intestinal flora.

REFERENCES

Cook, R. L. A study of disease in wildlife of south Texas. Ph.D. dissertation, University of Wisconsin, 1966.
Debbie, J. G. *Salmonella typhimurium* infection in captive white-tailed deer fawns. *Bull. Wildl. Dis. Assoc.* 4:12, 1968.
Ewing, W. H. Differentiation of enterobacteriaceae by biochemical reactions. Atlanta: U.S. Department of Health, Education and Welfare, Center for Disease Control, 1970.
Robinson, R. M., Hidalgo, R., Daniel, W., Rideout D., and Marburger, R. G. Salmonellosis in white-tailed deer fawns. *J. Wildl. Dis.* 6:389–396, 1970.

30 *Leptospirosis*

EMMETT B. SHOTTS, JR.

Synonyms: **None for wild animals. Weil's disease, mud fever, rice paddy disease, autumn fever, seven-day fever, swineherder's disease, black water fever, canicola fever, Fort Bragg fever, Stuttgart disease.**

Leptospirosis is a group of infectious diseases of man and animals, caused by antigenically distinct members of the genus *Leptospira* that are called serovarieties. This group of diseases varies in form from inapparent to fatal, depending on the host involved and the infecting serovar. Leptospiral infections in wildlife are important for several reasons. They may impair the health of wildlife, and certain species are epidemiologically important in that they may serve as a source of infection for other species and for domestic animals and humans.

HISTORY. Japanese workers were the first to show a causal relationship of spirochetes to patients described as having Weil's disease. In 1916 these workers were successful in isolating the organism and named it *Spirochaeta icterohaemorrhagiae*. Later spirochetes were isolated in several areas of the world from jaundiced patients (Alston et al. 1958).

Noguchi (1917) studied spirochetes obtained from workers in Japan and other areas and later gave the generic name *Leptospira* to this group of organisms. *Leptospira interrogans* serovariety *icterohaemorrhagiae* is regarded as the type species representing the pathogenic leptospires. Organisms that were previously given species status are currently given serovariety (serovar) status. *Leptospira biflexa* is considered the type species for the saprophytic leptospires. In 1918 and 1925, respectively, *hebdomadis* and *autumnalis* were described as being causes of seven-day fever in eastern Asia. From Indonesia, *pyrogenes* was first reported in 1923 and *batavieae* in 1926. In 1928, the isolation of *grippotyphosa* was made in the USSR. During the period 1931 to 1937, *andaman*, *canicola*, *australis*, *sejroe*, and *pomona* were reported. The discovery of new serovars continue. By 1954 approximately 50 serovars had been named, and by 1966 the list had grown to almost 100 (Alston et al. 1958; Galton 1966).

Currently there are 184 serovars of leptospires acknowledged (C. R. Sulzer, personal communication, 1979). In North America in 1905 Stimson first observed leptospires in sections of kidney from a patient who died in a New Orleans hospital of an illness believed to be yellow fever. In 1917 *icterohaemorrhagiae* was isolated from rats in Baltimore, and in 1922 the first human infection was documented there (Wadsworth et al. 1922). Leptospirosis in dogs, caused by *canicola*, was recognized in California in 1938 (Meyer et al. 1938).

Histopathologic evidence of leptospiral infection in cattle was reported in 1944, but cultural proof was not obtained until 1948 when *pomona* was isolated (Baker and Little 1948).

For the most part, knowledge of leptospirosis among wild mammals in North America, although incomplete, was gained during the 1960s and 1970s. With the realization of the economic and public health importance of leptospirosis, knowledge concerning leptospiral infections among wildlife became necessary. Most of the information concerning leptospirosis in wild mammals in the United States comes from the studies conducted in Georgia, Pennsylvania, Illinois, Louisiana, North Carolina, Virginia, Washington, Florida, Hawaii, and Canada.

DISTRIBUTION. Leptospirosis enjoys a cosmopolitan distribution. In North America, wherever diligent efforts have been applied, leptospirosis has been reported to occur in man and in domestic and wild animals. The most common serovars in North America associated with disease of domestic animals and man are *icterohaemorrhagiae*, *autumnalis*, *canicola*, *pomona*, *grippotyphosa*, and *hardjo*. Other serovars have a widespread distribution among wild animals but seldom cause disease in man and domestic animals.

Striped skunks (*Mephitis mephitis*) were first found naturally infected with leptospires in Georgia by McKeever et al. (1958a). Ten strains of *pomona* and 5 strains of *ballum* were

The author acknowledges the research and writings of Dr. E. E. Roth who contributed significantly to our knowledge of wildlife leptospirosis.

323

obtained from 132 striped skunks. Additional leptospiral strains were obtained by the same authors and were identified as *mini georgia* and *atlantae* by Galton et al. (1957, 1960). In Louisiana, Roth et al. (1963b) isolated leptospires from 57% of 650 striped skunks examined. The serovars found in the order of their frequency were: *pomona* (21%), *tarassovi* (19%, *ballum* (10%), *canicola* (6%), *icterohaemorrhagiae* (2%), *mini georgia* (1%), *grippotyphosa* (0.2%), and *australis* serogroup (0.2%). Essentially the same serovars were isolated from striped skunks in subsequent studies in Georgia by Gorman et al. (1962), whereas in Pennsylvania (Clark 1961; Clark et al. 1961a), only *pomona* and *ballum* were detected. Striped skunks in Canada were reported as a host for *pomona* (Abdulla et al. 1962b). McKeever et al. (1958a) isolated *ballum* from spotted skunks (*Spilogale putorious*) in Georgia.

Raccoons (*Procyon lotor*) were found to be hosts for leptospires in a number of geographic areas. Of 204 raccoons examined in Louisiana, 22% were found culturally positive for leptospires (Roth 1964). The serovars identified include: *mini georgia, autumnalis, paidjan, canicola, bakeri*, and *grippotyphosa*. Serovars *icterohaemorrhagiae* and *pomona* were detected among the raccoons in Pennsylvania (Clark 1961; Clark et al. 1961a, 1962b), and *pomona* was detected in a raccoon in Canada (Abdulla et al. 1962b). During investigations on leptospirosis among raccoons in Georgia (Gorman et al. 1962; McKeever et al. 1958b) *ballum, pomona, australis, grippotyphosa, autumnalis, hebdomadis, mini georgia*, and *tarassovi* were detected. Subsequent studies in Georgia indicated that the raccoon was a primary host (38% incidence) for *grippotyphosa* (Shotts et al. 1975). Galton et al. (1959) isolated *grippotyphosa* and *australis* from raccoons in North Carolina.

Leptospirosis in opossums (*Didelphis marsupialis*) has been reported from five states. Roth (1964) found 21% of 500 opossums culturally positive. The serovars isolated were *pomona, autumnalis, ballum, paidjan, grippotyphosa, mini georgia, icterohaemorrhagiae, tarassovi*, and *atchafalaya*. In Georgia essentially the same serovars were found by McKeever et al. (1958a) and Gorman et al. (1962). They did not detect *paidjan*, but did detect *atlantae*, which was not found in Louisiana. A subsequent study in Georgia resulted in a 41% isolation rate of *ballum* in opossums (Shotts et al. 1975). Serovar *ballum* was isolated from an opossum in Virginia (Yager et al. 1953), and *icterohaemorrhagiae* was recovered

from an opposum in Maryland (Evans et al. 1962). In Pennsylvania the serovars *ballum* and *pomona* were isolated from opossums (Clark 1961; Clark et al. 1961a, 1962b).

Norway rats (*Rattus norvegicus*) were the first animals found infected with leptospires in the continental United States. Serovar *icterohaemorrhagiae* was recovered from Norway rats in Baltimore by Noguchi (1917), and a carrier rate of 45% was demonstrated. In Louisiana (Roth, unpublished data, 1967) and in Pennsylvania (Clark 1961; Clark et al. 1961a, 1962b), *icterohaemorrhagiae* was isolated frequently, but in Georgia *ballum* was isolated from the roof rat (*R. rattus*) and the cotton rat (*Sigmodon hipidus*) (Brown and Gorman 1960; McKeever et al. 1958a). Rats (*R. norvegicus*) in Canada (McKiel et al. 1961) and Hawaii (Minette 1964) have been identified as hosts principally for *icterohaemorrhagiae*, but infections due to *ballum* were also detected. Two other species of rats (*R. rattus, R. exulans*) in Hawaii were found infected with the same serovars.

Mice are infected with leptospires in many areas of the United States. Serovar *ballum* is the most common leptospire found in house mice (*Mus musculus*) (Clark 1961; Clark et al. 1961a, 1962b; Gorman et al. 1962). Serovar *icterohaemorrhagiae*, in addition to *ballum*, was occasionally isolated from house mice in Pennsylvania and in Hawaii (Minnette 1964). Serovar *pomona* was also detected among mice in Pennsylvania. In Georgia, Gorman et al. (1962) found old field mice (*Peromyscus polionatus*) infected with *ballum*. Later studies in Georgia reported *ballum* in the cotton mouse (*Peromyscus gossypinus*) population (Shotts et al. 1975). The muskrat (*Ondatra zibethica*) was found infected with *grippotyphosa* (Sulzer 1975). Serovars *ballum* and *grippotyphosa* were isolated from the western harvest mouse (*Reithrodontomys megalotis*) in Pennsylvania (Hubbert and Rosen 1966). Diesch et al. (1966) recovered *grippotyphosa* from the western harvest mouse in Iowa.

Of 150 nutria (*Myocastor coypus*), 12 were found positive for leptospires in Louisiana (Roth 1964). The serovars present were *paidjan, zanoni myocastoris, orleans, icterohaemorrhagiae*, and a member of the *australis* serogroup (Roth et al., 1962, 1963a, 1964b).

In Louisiana 8 leptospiral serovars were obtained from 200 armadillos (*Dasypus novencinctus*) by Roth. Serovars *canicola, pomona, louisiana*, and a strain belonging to the *australis* serogroup were identified (Roth, unpublished data, 1964, 1967; Roth et al. 1964b). Two strains of leptospires belonging to the *australis* serogroup were isolated from 35 beavers (*Castor canadensis*) in Louisiana (Roth, unpublished data, 1964, 1967).

The gray fox (*Urocyon cinereoargenteus*) and the red fox (*Vulpes fulva*) have been identified as hosts for leptospires. In Georgia (McKeever et al. 1958a) *ballum* and in North Carolina (Galton et al. 1959) *australis* and *grippotyphosa* were isolated from gray foxes. Serovar *icterohaemorrhagiae* was recovered from gray foxes examined in Pennsylvania (Clark 1961; Clark et al. 1961a, 1962b). In North Carolina (Galton et al. 1959) *grippotyphosa* and in Pennsylvania (Clark 1961; Clark et al. 1960c), *pomona, ballum,* and *icterohaemorrhagiae* were detected among the red fox.

Of 21 muskrats (*Ondatra zibethica*) cultured in Pennsylvania, 1 harbored *icterohaemorrhagiae* (Clark et al. 1961a, 1962b).

The woodchuck (*Marmota monax*) was identified as a host for *pomona* and *icterohaemorrhagiae* in Pennsylvania (Clark et al. 1960a,b). Serovar *pomona* was also recovered from woodchucks in Canada (Abdulla et al. 1962b).

Clark et al. (1961b, 1962a) isolated *ballum* from the meadow vole (*Microtus pennsylvanicus*) and the shrew (*Blarina brevicauda brevicauda*).

In Georgia, the bobcat (*Lynx rufus*) was infected with *pomona, ballum* and *grippotyphosa* (McKeever et al. 1958a; Shotts et al. 1975). Serovar *pomona* was reported from bobcat in Louisiana (Roth 1964).

The cottontail rabbit (*Sylvilagus floridanus*) was infected with *ballum* in Georgia (McKeever et al. 1958a) and Louisiana (Roth, unpublished data, 1967) and with *pomona* in Canada (Galton 1966). Both cottontail rabbit and swamp rabbit (*S. aquaticus*) harbored *grippotyphosa* in Mississippi (Shotts et al. 1971).

The fox squirrel (*Sciurus niger*) was infected with *grippotyphosa* in Minnesota (Diesch et al. 1968). Subsequently in Georgia both the fox squirrel and the gray squirrel (*Sciurus carolinensis*) were found to be infected with *grippotyphosa* and *ballum*, respectively (Shotts et al. 1975).

The mongoose (*Herpestes auropunctatus*) in Hawaii was infected with *icterohaemorrhagiae, canicola,* and *sejroe* (Minette 1964).

Serologic tests have been used advantageously to determine the serologic prevalence of leptospirosis among white-tailed deer (*Odocoileus virginianus*). In Illinois (Ferris et al. 1961a,b) 19% and in Minnesota (Wedman and Driver 1957) 16% of the deer tested were positive for *pomona*. Of 1,256 white-tailed deer in Wisconsin (Trainer and Hanson 1960; Trainer et al. 1963), 26% were found to be reactors for *pomona*. Serologic evidence of infection due to *grippotyphosa* was reported from Illinois (Ferris et al. 1961a,b). Very little definitive serologic work has been done on the white-tailed deer in recent years. The last comprehensive study was of the deer herds of the Southeast, which showed a reactor rate of approximately 20% (Shotts and Hayes 1970). Harrington (1975) reported some titers in deer collected during epidemiological studies of cattle leptospirosis.

Serovar *pomona* was first isolated from naturally infected deer in New York (Reilly et al. 1962a). Subsequently, isolations of *pomona* were made from deer in Pennsylvania (Clark et al. 1962b), Louisiana (Roth et al. 1964a), and Canada (Abdulla et al. 1962a). Another serovar *zanoni zanoni*, was isolated from deer in Louisiana (Roth, unpublished data, 1967).

In Illinois Ferris et al. (1961a,b) reported the isolation of *ballum* from a hog-nosed snake (*Henerodon platyrhimus*). Serovar *tarassovi* was isolated from a turtle (*Psedemus* spp.) in Georgia (J. W. Glosser and J. W. Winkler, personal communication, 1974). A new serovar *ranarum* was isolated in Iowa from a frog (*Rana pipiens*) (Babudieri 1972). Although no natural infections have been reported, goldfish (*Carassius auratus*) have been artifically infected with both *pomona* and *canicola*, and antibodies have been demonstrated in channel catfish (*Ictalurus punctatus*) against *pomona* (Maestrone 1962; E. B. Shotts and C. R. Sulzer, personal communication, 1973). The serovar *pomona* was recovered from the California sea lion (*Zalophus californsonus*) (McIhatten et al. 1971). Additional reports are found in the literature documenting the isolation of leptospires from zoo species which are not included here.

Other species indigenous to other continents have been identified as hosts for leptospires. The reader is referred to more complete works for detailed information (Alston et al. 1958; Galton 1966; Sulzer 1975).

ETIOLOGY. Leptospires are extremely small, coiled, actively motile spirochetes. They are easily killed by disinfectants, heat drying, and pH conditions below 6 and above 8. Special techniques are required to stain and cultivate them in the laboratory.

The members of the genus *Leptospira* are called serovars because their differences are determined by serologic tests. The morphologic and cultural characteristics, except for minor differences, are quite similar. Throughout the world approximtely 184 serovars have been described. In North America 25 have been isolated and more are suspected. With few exceptions every serovar has been isolated from one or more species of wild animal (Galton 1966). The most notable exceptions are the presence of at least 3 serovars of the *hebdomadis* serogroup which cause disease in cattle.

TRANSMISSION. Infective urine constitutes the major source of infection for susceptible wild mammals; urine containing leptospires excreted by carrier animals is generally involved either directly or indirectly in the transmission of leptospirosis. Man and domestic animals may become infected in a similar manner. Environmental conditions that favor the survival of leptospiral organisms outside the body include moist, slightly alkaline soil; stagnant ponds; and slow-moving, slightly alkaline streams. When the above conditions exist in nature, the organisms may survive for several weeks (Gillespie et al. 1957).

Leptospiral organisms usually enter the body through mucous membranes or through abraded skin. Wild animals may become infected by drinking water containing leptospires or by eating infected animals. Probably the most significant mode of spread among carnivorous animals is through the food chain (Reilly et al. 1970).

Current knowledge precludes an accurate assessment of the precise role of wild mammals in the maintenance of leptospires in nature and their role in the transmission of this organism to man and domestic animals. The three most important serovars from the domestic animal and public health standpoint are *icterohaemorrhagiea, autumnalis,* and *canicola.* The norway rat and the roof rat are known reservoirs of *icterohaemorrhagiae,* and infections of this serovar in other wild animals represent side chain or accidental infections. This serovar sometimes causes disease in dogs, and it is an important cause of leptospirosis in man.

Although the fox and raccoon appear to be carriers of *autumnalis,* their role in the epidemiological pattern of this rapidly increasing serovar in humans is not currently known.

The striped skunk may be of secondary importance in the epizootiology of *canicola,* but dogs are considered to be the main source of infection for man.

Mice, especially the house mouse, appears to be the reservoir for *ballum.* Infections of

ballum in other wild mammals are common and may be of secondary importance.

Additional data is necessary from more geographic areas of North America in order to assess the precise importance of certain host-serovar relationships. Raccoons and opossums appear to be an important host for *autumnalis.* Raccoons, opossums, and foxes seem to be the main reservoirs of infection of *grippotyphosa.*

The serovars *zanoni zanoni, zanoni mycocastoris, paidjan, mini georgia, australis, bakeri, atlantae, atchafalaya, louisiana,* and *orleans* have been isolated from only one or two geographic areas; and a high prevalence of these serovars has not been found in any single species of animals.

SIGNS. Very little is known about the signs of leptospirosis in wild mammals. Signs of experimental *pomona* infection in the white-tailed deer include anorexia, weakness, anemia, hemoglobinuria, icterus, fever, and death (Reilly et al. 1962b; Roth, unpublished data, 1967). Abortion has been observed in deer under experimental conditions by Trainer et al. (1961) and most likely occurs occasionally under natural conditions (McGowan et al. 1963). It has not been determined if other species of wild mammals exhibit clinical signs of this disease. Naturally occurring leptospiral infections among wildlife are apparently self-limiting in that animals recover from the initial stages of the disease and remain carriers for varying periods of time. In some instances, however, a chronic carrier state of long duration follows the initial stage of the disease.

Leptospirosis in man is characterized by fever, headache, muscle ache, vomiting, conjunctivitis, weakness, and meningitis; in severe cases icterus is present, and renal failure develops (Kaufmann 1976).

In cattle, infection due to *pomona* produces such signs of disease as fever, loss of weight, anorexia, abnormal milk secretion, anemia, hemoglobinuria, icterus, and abortion (Baker and Little 1948). These signs may vary with outbreaks. Serovars *grippotyphosa* and *hardjo* are more often noted as a causal agent in cattle than *pomona,* and neither serovar produces the classic symptoms of hemoglobinuria and icterus associated with *pomona.* Mortality is rare and inapparent cases are common.

Leptospirosis infections in dogs vary from mild inapparent disease to severe disease and are caused primarily by the serovars *icterohaemorrhagiae* and *canicola* (Alston et al. 1958). Signs of disease when present include fever, anorexia, vomiting, anemia, icterus, and hematuria.

In other domestic animals clinical manifestations are observed less frequently. Most infections in swine are caused by *pomona, grippotyphosa,* or *canicola* and are mild, but abortion is sometimes observed. Leptospirosis in horses is generally a mild, transient disease; but occasionally systemic illness characterized by fever, depression, anorexia, anemia, and icterus is seen.

PATHOGENESIS AND PATHOLOGY. The following generalizations are probably applicable to the majority of leptospiral infections of mammals and man. The organism gains entrance through mucous membranes or broken skin. Leptospiral organisms can be isolated from the blood from the 4th through the 8th day after infection. This precedes the febrile state by several days; and usually at the time fever subsides, leptospiral organisms can no longer be isolated from the blood. Antibodies appear about the 10th day after infection but may appear as early as the 5th day and as late as the 15th day. They reach their peak during the 2nd and 3rd week and may persist at moderate to high levels for several months to several years. In wildlife, however, certain species—particularly the striped skunk—may harbor leptospiral organisms in the kidney but contain no demonstrable agglutinating antibodies in their serum (Roth et al. 1963b). Following infection, rats and mice probably excrete leptospires for the remainder of their lives. It is also important to realize that numerous leptospiral infections among mammalian species, including man, are not characterized by signs or symptoms of disease.

The pathogenesis and pathologic features of leptospiral infections in wild mammals have not received extensive study. Ferris et al. (1960) reported a febrile response in 2 of 4 white-tailed deer following exposure to *pomona.* Trainer et al. (1961) concluded from experiments with unbred white-tailed deer that *pomona* produces an inapparent infection; however, they produced abortion in 4 of 5 pregnant does. They were able to demonstrate leptospires in the urine 25 days after exposure. Reilly et al. (1962b) exposed calves and deer to *pomona* but produced only mild disease in a few animals. The results of studies by Roth (unpublished data, 1967), where calves and deer were experimentally exposed to *pomona,* indicate that the disease may vary from inapparent to fatal. Serovar *pomona* was isolated from the blood of

one deer on 7 consecutive days, but in another it was recovered on only 1 day. Fatal cases in deer were characterized by hemoglobinuria and icterus. Necropsy findings include nephritis, hepatitis, and hemorrhages. Serovar *pomona* was isolated from the kidney tissue of the surviving animals 126 days after inoculation. Interstitial nephritis was reported to be associated with naturally occurring *pomona* infection among white-tailed deer in Canada. In addition *pomona* was isolated from a diseased fetus (McGowan et al. 1963).

On the basis of bacteriologic evidence, the duration of the carrier state in striped skunks was found to be of sufficient length to incriminate them in the epizootiology of leptospirosis (Roth et al. 1963c). Serovar *tarassovi* was isolated periodically from the urine of 5 striped skunks at 774, 499, 418, 371, and 371 days, respectively. Similarly, *pomona* was found in the urine of 4 striped skunks for periods of 321, 303, 299, and 284 days. Two striped skunks were observed to excrete *canicola* in their urine for 400 and 146 days. The number of days leptospires were observed represents minimum periods, because naturally infected animals which were shedders at capture were used in the study. Some of the animals employed excreted two leptospiral serovars simultaneously. The combination of *pomona* and *tarassovi* occurred most often.

Gross lesions of leptospirosis in such species of wild animals as rats, mice, striped skunks, opossums, and raccoons are not very evident. In some instances the cortex of the kidney appears to be pale. Interstitial nephritis, characterized by an abundance of lymphocytic inflammatory exudate, which is easily demonstrated by routine histopathologic methods, is present in varying degrees in chronically infected wild animals (Roth, unpublished data, 1967).

DIAGNOSIS. The commonest means employed for the diagnosis of leptospirosis may arbitrarily be divided into demonstration methods, serologic methods, and bacteriologic methods (Galton et al. 1962; Shotts 1976; Sulzer and Jones 1976). Although darkfield microscopy is an essential tool in leptospiral investigations, it is of little value for the immediate diagnosis of leptospirosis. Any diagnosis of leptospirosis based on darkfield examination should be tentative and supported by other more substantial data. The appropriate application of such special silver strains as the Warthin-Starry can be used for the demonstration of leptospires in tissues of fatal cases and in biopsy material (Bridges and Luna 1957).

The fluorescent antibody procedure has been employed to demonstrate leptospires in the urine and tissues of infected animals (White et al. 1961). Serovar identification cannot be made with this technique.

The microscopic and macroscopic agglutination tests are most commonly employed to detect leptospiral antibodies. The microscopic agglutination test can be employed with either living or formalin-killed organisms as antigen. The miscroscopic agglutination test, using live antigen, is considered to be the reference test. Modifications of the microscopic agglutination test to enable large volume processing has greatly enhanced the ability for serologic evaluation of large numbers of sera (Cole et al. 1973; Galton et al. 1965). Macroscopic agglutination tests have been developed and are used in some laboratories (Galton et al. 1962). The macroscopic methods have served as useful tools for the serologic diagnosis of leptospirosis, but it is not advisable to attach an absolute value to the results obtained. Besides the variable antigenic sensitivity inherent in such tests, the antibody response of the host is even more variable.

The absence of antibodies during the first week of disease prevents an early diagnosis of leptospirosis by serologic means. In some individual animals and man, the antibody titer remains low throughout the disease. Some individual animals retain agglutinating antibodies for several months to years after infection.

When serologic tests are interpreted in the proper perspective, they constitute a valuable laboratory aid for the diagnosis of leptospirosis. The demonstration of a significant rise in antibody titer gives excellent evidence of recent infection when clinical signs of disease commensurate with leptospirosis are present. In domestic animals leptospirosis is generally a herd problem, and the primary concern is a herd diagnosis.

The isolation of leptospires and their subsequent identification provides the most conclusive proof of infection (Galton et al. 1962; Shotts 1976). The choice of tissue or body fluid to be cultured depends on the stage of disease. Organisms can be isolated from a variety of tissue during the first week of infection, but blood commonly is examined from the living animal. In acute fatal cases where tissues are obtained soon after death, leptospires can be isolated from liver and spleen. In chronic cases where death is delayed or where there has been continous antibiotic treatment, the kidney is the tissue of choice (Galton et al. 1962; Shotts 1976).

Leptospires can be isolated from urine by direct culture into semisolid media (Galton et al. 1962; Roth et al. 1963c). The aseptic collection of urine by bladder tap and by employing extended dilutions to avoid and overcome contamination has proved successful. Johnson and Rogers (1964) have suggested the use of 5-fluorouracil as a selective agent for growth of leptospires.

Properly executed bacteriologic procedures are usually as sensitive as laboratory animals for the isolation of leptospires, although occasionally a strain which is difficult or impossible to cultivate is encountered. The results of properly executed bacteriologic examinations are generally most rewarding.

The indirect isolation of leptospires from tissue suspension and body fluids through the use of laboratory animals such as guinea pigs, hamsters, and chinchillas can be used with success (Galton et al. 1962). Laboratory animals are not equally susceptible to all serovars of leptospires; therefore, the choice of animal depends upon the serovar expected.

IMMUNITY. Little is known about the immunologic features of leptospirosis in wild mammals. On the basis of the serovar and prevalence in certain species, a few speculative deductions may be made. Some species of wild mammals, such as rats and mice, generally become infected with *icterohaemorrhagiae* and *ballum*, respectively. They may possess an innate immunity or resistance for other serovars. In the overall picture, however, one would have to consider opportunity of exposure and virulence of the leptospiral serovar. On the other extreme, oppossums and raccoons appear susceptible to numerous leptospiral serovars.

It is not known whether acute leptospirosis, leading to fatalities, occurs regularly among wild mammals. The knowledge accumulated to date deals mainly with chronic leptospirosis. In fact most studies in wild mammals were done to determine their possible role in the maintenance of the disease and its transmission to man and domestic animals. In instances where the chronic infection rate is high, one can deduce that the mortality rate must be low. Furthermore, if the incidence of chronic infection is high, the immunity produced by natural infection is not of sufficient magnitude for the mammalian host to completely rid itself of the organism. In instances where the serologic incidence is low, the natural infection apparently produces a degree of resistance high enough to prevent the development of a permanent carrier state (Roth et al. 1963b).

In man and most domestic animals, recovery from leptospirosis results in a serviceable immunity for the particular serovar that caused the infection. Bacterins of leptospires have played a useful role in reducing the hazard of leptospirosis in man in some areas of the world. In such occupational groups as rice field workers, miners, and military personnel, the bacterins have proved to be safe and provide a serviceable resistance sufficient to reduce the severity of clinical illness. Bacterins for domestic animals appear to be indicated in areas of the world where the problem of leptospirosis is of appreciable magnitude. Leptospiral bacterins are of value in increasing the resistance of cattle, swine, horses, and dogs to leptospirosis. Data accumulated suggest that protection against symptomatic infection is afforded, but documentation is not sufficient to conclude that the bacterins will prevent subclinical infection with subsequent establishment of the carrier state. Repeated vaccinations of animals may cause serologic titers of sufficient magnitude that they cannot be distinguished from titers caused by actual infection; this poses a problem for the diagnostician.

At the present time, vaccination of wild mammals in the natural state is not practical. Neither is it practical to attempt to eradicate leptospirosis from wild mammalian hosts. It does appear that the vaccination of wild mammals kept in captivity may be feasible under certain conditions.

TREATMENT AND CONTROL. There is no information available concerning the treatment of leptospirosis in wildlife. A number of antibiotics—namely, streptomycin, penicillin, and tetracycline—have at one time or another been recommended for the treatment of acute leptospirosis in man and for the alleviation of the carrier state in animals.

The application of efficient sanitary practices will reduce the opportunity for spread of leptospirosis. Protection of drinking water for domestic animals from contamination by urine of other animals lessens the danger of acquiring the disease. Proper drainage of wet, muddy farm areas and maintenance of well-drained feedlots are valuable measures. Swimming in stock ponds or slow-moving streams frequented by wild and domestic animals should be avoided. Workers in high risk occupational groups should be provided with protective gloves and boots where possible and practical. Thorough cleaning with a disinfectant such as sodium hypochlorite solution is effective in eliminating contamination from work areas.

It is highly unlikely that leptospirosis can be eradicated from wild mammals and domestic animals. The basic epidemiologic features of serovar multiplicity, broad host range, and extended carrier state make eradication an extremely difficult, if not an impossible, task.

REFERENCES

Abdulla, P. K., Karstad, L. H., and Fish, N. A. Cultural and serological evidence of leptospirosis in deer in Ontario. *Can. Vet. J.* 3:71–78, 1962a.
———. Investigation of leptospirosis in wildlife in Ontario. *Can. J. Public Health* 53:44–51, 1962b.
Alexander, A. D., Stoenner, H. G., Wood, G. E., and Byrne, R. J. A new pathogenic leptospira, not readily cultivated. *J. Bacteriol.* 83:754–760, 1962.
Alston, J. M., Broom, J. C., and Dougherty, C. J. A. *Leptospirosis in man and animals.* Edinburgh and London: E. and S. Livingstone, 1958.
Babudieri, B. Systematics of a leptospira strain isolated from a frog. *Experimentia* 28:1252, 1972.
Baker, J. W., and Little, R. B. Leptospirosis in cattle. *J. Exp. Med.* 88:295–308, 1948.
Bridges, C. H., and Luna, L. Kerr's improved Warthin-Starry technic (study of the permissible variations) *Lab. Invest.* 6:357–367, 1957.
Brown, R. Z., and Gorman, G. W. The occurrence of leptospiral infections in feral rodents in southwestern Georgia. *Am. J. Public Health* 50:682–688, 1960.
Clark, L. G. Leptospirosis in Pennsylvania: A progress report. *Proceedings of 65th Annual Meeting of U.S. Livestock Sanitary Association*, pp. 140–146. Minneapolis: USLSA, 1961.
Clark, L. G., Kresse, J. I., Carbrey, E. A., Marshak, R. R., and Hollister, C. J. Leptospirosis in cattle and wildlife on a Pennsylvania farm. *J. Am. Vet. Med. Assoc.* 139:889, 1961a.
Clark, L. G., Kresse, J. I., Marshak, R. R., and Hollister, C. J. *Leptospira icterohaemorrhagiae* infection in a woodchuck. *Public Health Rep.* 75:925, 1960a.
———. *Leptospira pomona* infection in a woodchuck. *Public Health Rep.* 75:925, 1960b.
———. *Leptospira pomona* infection in an eastern red fox. *Nature* 188:1040, 1960c.
———. Natural occurrence of leptospirosis in the meadow vole. *Microtus pennsylvanicus. Am. J. Vet. Res.* 22:949, 1961b.
———. *Leptospira ballum* infection in a shrew (*Blarina brevicauda brevicauda*). *Am. J. Trop. Med. Hyg.* 11:664, 1962a.
———. *Leptospira grippotyphosa* infections in cattle and wildlife in Pennsylvania. *J. Am. Vet. Med. Assoc.* 141:710, 1962b.

Cole, J. K., C. R. Sulzer, and A. R. Pursell. Improved microtechnique for the leptospiral microscopic agglutination test. *Appl. Microbiol.* 25:976–980, 1973.

Diesch, S. L., Crawford, R. P., McCulloch, W. F., and Top, F. A. Human leptospirosis acquired from squirrels. *N. Engl. J. Med.* 276:838–842, 1968.

Diesch, S. L., McCullock, W. F., and Braun, J. L. Isolation of *Leptospira grippotyphosa* from a western harvest mouse in Iowa. *Bull. Wildl. Dis. Assoc.* 2:15–17, 1966.

Evans, L. B., Wood, G. E., Flyger, V., Alexander, A. D., Yager, R. H., and Rubin, H. L. Natural occurrence of *Leptospira icterohaemorrhagiae* in an opossum. *Proc. Soc. Exp. Biol. Med.* 110:113–115, 1962.

Ferris, D. H., Hanson, L. E., Alberts, J. O., Calhoun, J. C., and Marlowe, R. Correlative serologic studies on brucellosis and leptospirosis in cattle and deer in Illinois. *Am. J. Public Health* 51:717–722, 1961a.

Ferris, D. H., Hanson, L. E., Hoerlein, A. B., and Beamer, P. D. Experimental infection of white-tailed deer with *Leptospira pomona*. *Cornell Vet.* 50:236–260, 1960.

Ferris, D. H., Hanson, L. E., Rhoades, H. E., and Alberts, J. O. Bacteriologic and serologic investigations of brucellosis and leptospirosis in Illinois deer. *J. Am. Vet. Med. Assoc.* 139:892–896, 1961b.

Galton, M. M. Leptospiral serotype distribution lists. U.S. Department of Health, Education and Welfare, pp. 1–130, 1966.

Galton, M. M., Gorman, G. W., and Shotts, E. B., Jr. A new leptospiral subserotype in the *hebdomadis* group. *Public Health Rep.* 75:917–921, 1960.

Galton, M. M., Hirschberg, N., Menges, R. W., Hines, M. P., and Habermann, R. An investigation of possible wild animal hosts of leptospires in the area of the "Fort Bragg fever" outbreaks. *Am. J. Public Health* 49:1343–1348, 1959.

Galton, M. M., Menges, R. W., Shotts, E. B., Nahmias, A. J., and Heath, C. W., Jr. Leptospirosis: Epidemiology, clinical manifestations in man and animals. U.S. Department of Health, Education and Welfare, publ. 951, pp. 1–70, 1962.

Galton, M. M., Powers, D. K., McKeever, S., and Gorman, G. W. Identification of two leptospiral serotypes new to the United States. *Public Health Rep.* 72:431–435, 1957.

Galton, M. M., Sulzer, C. R., Santa Rosa, C. A., and Fields, M. J. Applications of a microtechnique to the agglutination test for leptospirosis antibodies. *Appl. Microbiol.* 13:81–85, 1965.

Gillespie, R. W. H., Kenzy, S. G., Ringen, L. M., and Bracken, F. K. Studies on bovine leptospirosis: III. Isolation of *Leptospira pomona* from surface waters. *Am. J. Vet. Res.* 18:76–80, 1957.

Gochenour, W. W., Jr., Johnston, R. V., Yager, R. H., and Gochenour, W. S. Porcine leptospirosis. *Am. J. Vet. Res.* 13:158–160, 1952.

Gorman, G. W., McKeever, S., and Grimes, R. D. Leptospirosis in wild mammals from southwest Georgia. *Am. J. Trop. Med. Hyg.* 11:518–524, 1962.

Harrington, R. Leptospiral antibodies in serum from cattle, swine, horses, deer, sheep and goats: 1973 and 1974. *Am. J. Vet. Res.* 36:1367–1370, 1975.

Hubbert, W. T., and Rosen, M. N. Isolation of *Leptospira ballum* from a western harvest mouse (*Reithrodontomys megalotis*). *Bull. Wildl. Dis. Assoc.* 2:18–19, 1966.

Johnson, R. C., and Rogers, P. 5-Fluorouracil is a selective agent for growth of leptospirae. *J. Bacteriol.* 87(2):422–426, 1964.

Kaufmann, A. F. Epidemiologic trends of leptospirosis in the United States 1965–1974. In R. C. Johnson, ed., *The biology of parasitic spirochetes*, pp. 170–190. New York: Academic Press, 1976.

Kenzy, S. G., Gillespie, R. W. H., Ringen, L. M., Okazaki, W., Bracken, F. E., and Keown, G. H. Control of bovine leptospirosis. 61st Annual Meeting of U.S. Livestock Sanitary Association, Nov. 1957.

McGowan, J. E., Karstad, L., and Fish, N. A. Leptospirosis in Ontario Cervidae, isolation of *Leptospira pomona* from a deer fetus. Transactions of 28th North American Wildlife Natural Resources Conference, pp. 199–206. Washington, D.C.: Wildlife Management Institute, 1963.

McIhatten, T. J., Martin, J. W., Wagner, R. J., and Iverson, J. C. Isolation of *Leptospira pomona* from a naturally infected California sea lion. *J. Wildl. Dis.* 7:195–197, 1971.

McKeever, S., Gorman, G. W., Chapman, J. F., Galton, M. M., and Powers, D. K. Incidence of leptospirosis in wild mammals from southwest Georgia with a report of new hosts for 6 serotypes of leptospires. *Am. J. Trop. Med. Hyg.* 7:646–655, 1958a.

McKeever, S., Gorman, G. W., Galton, M. M., and Hall, A. D. The raccoon, *Procyon lotor*, a natural host of *Leptospira autumnalis*. *Am. J. Hyg.* 66:13–14, 1958b.

McKiel, J. A., Cousineau, J. G., and Hall, R. R. Leptospirosis in wild animals in eastern Canada with particular attention to the disease in rats. *Can. J. Comp. Med.* 25:15–18, 1961.

Maestrone, G. Leptospira infection in the goldfish (*Carassius auratus*). *Nature* 195:719–720, 1962.

Meyer, K. F., Eddie B., and Anderson-Stewart, B. Canine, murine, and human leptospirosis in California. *Proc. Soc. Exp. Biol. Med.* 38:17, 1938.

Minette, H. P. Leptospirosis in rodents and mongooses on the island of Hawaii. *Am. J. Trop. Med. Hyg.* 13(6):826–832, 1964.

Noguchi, H. *Spirochaeta icterohaemorrhagiae* in American wild rats and its relation to the Japanese and European strains. *J. Exp. Med.* 25:755, 1917.

Reilly, J. R., Hanson, L. E., and Ferris, D. H. Experimental induced predator–food chain transmission of *L. grippotyphosa* from rodents to wild Marsupialia and Carnivora. *Am. J. Vet. Res,* 31:1443–1448, 1970.

Reilly, J. R., Muraschi, T. F., and Dean, D. J. Leptospirosis in the white-tailed deer, *Odocoileus virginianus. Cornell Vet.* 52:94–98, 1962a.

———. Leptospirosis in the white-tailed deer, *Odocoileus virginianus,* and in cattle. *J. Am. Vet. Med. Assoc.* 140:53–57, 1962b.

Roth, E. E. Leptospirosis in wildlife in the United States. Proceedings of 101st Annual Meeting of American Veterinary Medical Associations, pp. 211–218. Chicago: AVMA, 1964.

Roth, E. E., Adams, W. V., Greer, B., Sanford, G. E., Moore, M., and Newman, K. New leptospiral serotype in the *pyrogenes* serogroup. *Public Health Rep.* 78:727–730, 1963a.

Roth, E. E., Adams, W. V., Sanford, G. E., Greer, B., and Mayerux, P. *Leptospira paidjan (batavieae* serogroup) isolated from nutria in Louisiana. *Public Health Rep.* 77:583–587, 1962.

Roth, E. E., Adams, W. V. Sanford, G. E., Greer, B., Newman, K., Moore, M., Mayeaux, P., and Linder D. The bacteriologic and serologic incidence of leptospirosis among striped skunks in Louisiana. *Zoonoses Res.* 2: 13–39, 1963b.

Roth, E. E., Adams, W. V., Sanford, G. E., Moore, M., Newman, K., and Greer, B. Leptospiruria in striped skunks. *Public Health Rep.* 78:994–1000, 1963c.

Roth E. E., Adams, W. V., Sanford G. E., Newman, K., Moore, M., and Greer, B. Isolation of *Leptospira pomona* from white-tailed deer in Louisiana. *Am. J. Vet. Res.* 104:259–261, 1964a.

Roth, E. E., Greer, B., Moore, M., Newman, K., Sanford, G. E., and Adams, W. V. Serological analysis of two new related leptospiral serotypes isolated in Louisiana. *Zoon. Res.* 3:31–38, 1964b.

Shotts, E. B. Laboratory diagnosis of leptospirosis. In R. C. Johnson, ed., *The biology of parasitic spirochetes,* pp. 209–223. New York: Academic Press, 1976.

Shotts, E. B., Andrews, C. L., and Harvey, T. W. Leptospirosis in selected wild mammals of the Florida Panhandle and Southwest Georgia. *J. Am. Vet. Med. Assoc.* 167:587–589, 1975.

Shotts, E. B., Andrews, C. L., Sulzer, C. R., and Greene, E. Leptospirosis in cottontail and swamp rabbits of the Mississippi Delta. *J. Wildl. Dis.* 7:115–117, 1971.

Shotts, E. B., and Hayes, F. A. Leptospiral antibodies in white-tailed deer of the southeastern United States. *J. Wildl. Dis.* 6:259–298, 1970.

Sulzer, C. R. *Leptospiral serotype distribution lists: July 1966-July 1973.* Atlanta: U.S. Department of Health, Education and Welfare, Center for Disease Control, Public Health Service, 1975.

Sulzer, C. R., and Jones, W. L. *Leptospirosis: Methods in laboratory diagnosis,* publ. no. 76–8275. Atlanta: U.S. Department of Health, Education and Welfare, Center for Disease Control, Public Health Service, 1976.

Trainer, D. O., and Hanson, R. P. Leptospirosis and brucellosis serological reactors in Wisconsin deer, 1957–1958. *J. Wildl. Manag.* 24:44–52, 1960.

Trainer, D. O., Hanson, R. P., Pope, E. P., and Carbrey, E. A. The role of deer in the epizootiology of leptospirosis in Wisconsin. *Am. J. Vet. Res.* 24:159–167, 1963.

Trainer, D. O., Karstad, L., and Hanson, R. P. Experimental leptospirosis in white-tailed deer. *J. Infect. Dis.* 108:278–286, 1961.

Wadsworth, A., Longworthy, H. V., Stewart, F. D., Moore, A. C., and Coleman, M. B. Infectious jaundice occurring in New York State. *J. Am. Vet. Assoc.* 78:1120, 1922.

Wedman, E. E., and Driver, F. C. Leptospirosis and brucellosis titers in deer blood. *J. Am. Vet. Med. Assoc.* 130:513–514, 1957.

White, F. H., Stoliker, H. E., and Galton, M. M. Detection of leptospires in naturally infected dogs, using fluorescein-labeled antibody. *Am. J. Vet. Res.* 22:650–654, 1961.

Yager, R. H., Gochenour, W. S., Jr., Alexander, A. D., and Wetmore, P. W. Natural occurrence of *Leptospira ballum* in rural house mice and an opossum. *Proc. Soc. Exp. Biol. Med.* 84:589–590, 1953.

31 *Necrobacillosis*

MERTON N. ROSEN

Synonyms: **Foot rot, hoof rot, pododermatitis, calf diphtheria, necrotic stomatitis, ulcerative rumenitis, quittor, necrotic rhinitis (in domestic swine), foot abscess, navel ill, grease heel.**

Necrobacillosis is an infectious disease affecting wild ruminants and domestic animals. A purulent necrotic syndrome may affect the feet, throat, and internal organs as a result of invasion by the bacillus. There is a confustion of common names, but it is best called "necrobacillosis" based on the causative organism *Fusobacterium necrophorum* (Buchanan and Gibbons 1974).

HISTORY. Since the beginning of the century, necrobacillosis has been recognized in wildlife. Mohler and Morse (1904) reported isolation of the causative agent from necrotic lesions in the liver of a deer (*Odocoileus hemionus*). Other reports appeared later, and the importance of the malady as a threat to wildlife was emphasized in an editorial that appeared in *California Fish and Game* (Anon. 1925) and by Murie (1930).

During the summer of 1924, hundreds of dead deer were found in Modoc County, California, clustered about mud holes (Anon. 1924). The only source of moisture available to the animals was mud, and examination of the carcasses showed that the deer had ingested large quantities. The condition was given the names "filthy mud disease" and "Modoc deer disease" (Dixon 1934), but judging from the description of the pathology, it was undoubtedly necrobacillosis (McLean 1940).

Murie (1930) reported an epizootic of necrobacillosis among Wyoming elk (*Cervus canadensis*) on the winter feedlots. Rush (1932) confirmed the diagnosis, and during the next 14 years it was estimated that one-tenth of the existing herd succumbed to this disease each winter (Allred et al. 1944; Anderson 1958).

Other reports of necrobacillosis in deer include those of Schilling (1938) and Cass (1947), who described oral abscesses in the white-tailed deer (*O. virginianus*) of North Carolina and Minnesota, respectively; Wobeser et al. (1975), who detected necrobacillosis without foot le-

sions in white-tailed and mule deer in southwestern Saskatchewan; Vogelsang (1946), who described *F. necrophorum* isolated from caseous tumors on the skin of Venezuelan deer (species unknown); Herman and Rosen (1949) and Rosen et al. (1951), who documented epizootics affecting Columbian black-tailed deer and Rocky Mountain mule deer; as well as reports of Carhart (1943), Honess and Winter (1956), Krembs (1939), Martinaglia (1936), Shillinger (1937, 1942), and Winter and Honess (1952). Other species of wildlife have been affected by necrobacillosis (Table 31.1).

Necrobacillosis was described in sheep during the second century B.C. (Barton 1958). Today it is of considerable importance to the livestock industry, affecting horses, cattle, sheep, and swine (Grayson 1947; Hastings 1942; Howarth 1930; Murray et al. 1927, 1928). In addition, the disease has had serious consequences for other domesticated animals, including reindeer (Bergman 1909, cited in Karstad 1964; Borg 1958; Klimontov 1962; Kotov 1936; Nikolaevskii 1944; Rausch 1953) and Asiatic water buffalo (Puchuchuev and Agalarova 1939).

ETIOLOGY. *Fusobacterium necrophorum* is found consistently within the suppurative lesions of foot rot and calf diphtheria. This organism will reproduce the disease in experimental animals, namely, rabbits, hamsters, and mice. In some instances *F. necrophorum* may be a normal saprophyte of the intestinal tract (Bruner and Gillespie 1961; Dack et al. 1937), but it has the ability to generate pathologic processes. This should be sufficient basis to incriminate it as the responsible causative agent despite claims that it is an opportunist (Stableforth and Galloway 1959), a secondary invader, or just incidental to the infectious lesion.

This organism has been given a wide variety of designations, but the last name *Spherophorus necrophorus* had the genus preempted by the botanist Persoon, so in 1974 it was changed to *Fusobacterium necrophorum* (Buchanan and Gibbons 1974).

Beveridge (1936, 1940, 1941, 1959) draws a distinction between necrobacillosis and foot rot of sheep. Necrobacillosis, also termed "foot ab-

TABLE 31.1   Wildlife Reported with Necrobacillosis in the Wild.

Common Name	Scientific Name	Location	Reference
Antelope	*Antilocapra americana*	Saskatchewan	Wobeser et al. 1975
Bighorn sheep	*Ovis canadensis*	Wyoming	Honess and Frost 1942
Caribou	*Rangifer caribou*	Alaska	King 1963
Columbian black-tailed deer	*Odocoileus hemionus columbianus*	California	Herman and Rosen 1949; Rosen et al. 1951
Deer	species unknown	Venezuela	Vogelsang 1946
Eland antelope	*Taurotragus* spp.	Botswana	Kress 1943
Gemsbok	*Oryx gazella*	Africa	Drager 1975
Moose	*Alces americana*	Michigan	Murie 1934
Rocky Mountain mule deer	*Odocoileus hemionus hemionus*	California	Rosen et al. 1951
		Saskatchewan	Winter and Honess 1952; Wobeser et al. 1975
Rocky Mountain elk	*Cervus canadensis*	Wyoming	Murie 1930; Rush 1932; Allred et al. 1944; Anderson 1958
Roosevelt elk	*C. rooseveltii*	California	Brunetti (unpublished)
White-tailed deer	*O. virginianus*	North Carolina	Schilling 1938
		Minnesota	Cass 1947
		Ontario	Debbie 1965
		Saskatchewan	Wobeser et al. 1975

scess" of sheep, is caused by *F. necrophorum*; whereas foot rot of sheep has as its etiology *Fusiformis nodosus*, generally in association with *Spirochaeta penortha*. Calf diphtheria is caused by *F. necrophorum* (Ryff and Lee 1946). There are no records of organisms other than *F. necrophorum* as responsible for foot rot in deer and other wildlife.

Fusobacterium necrophorum is a gram-negative, nonsporulating, nonmotile, filamentous rod (Madin 1949). The long, granulated filaments are $0.75-1.5$ μ wide by $80-100$ μ long. The beaded filaments are characteristic of fresh cultures and material found in lesions, but the organism is highly pleomorphic and may form short rods or even coccoid bodies (Orcutt 1930; Scrivner 1934). It is a strict anaerobe and highly sensitive to oxygen, although under special conditions it may survive and even grow in air (Beveridge 1934a). Broth media should contain 0.01% sodium azide for primary isolation (Forget and Fredette 1962) and growth is enhanced by the addition of serum to the media. The use of methylene blue as an oxidation-reduction indicator is inhibitory to the organism, while resazurin may be used without ill effect. Viability is maintained by frequent transfer. *Fusobacterium necrophorum* has an optimum pH of 7.2 but can survive between 6.0 and 8.4. Several days incubation on solid media may be required before the concave colonies with convex centers appear. If exposed to air at this time, they develop a rough surface and appear cream colored.

The organism forms indole and ammonia and is capable of fermenting glucose, fructose, and maltose with gas formation. It causes hemolysis on blood agar if the red blood cells are human or rabbit, but not if they are horse, sheep, or goat.

Fifteen minutes at 55°C will kill the organism. It will also die after a week at 37°C or 4°C. However, if *Staphylococcus aureus* or *Escherichia coli* are incorporated with *F. necrophorum*, survival is prolonged.

A toxin produced by *F. necrophorum* will kill rabbits following massive intravenous injections, but intracutaneous introduction merely produces an erythematous reaction (Beveridge 1959). The bacteria contain a necrotizing substance that will kill an animal if dead organisms are inoculated in large doses but will cause only local necrosis if inoculated subcutaneously in small doses.

TRANSMISSION. Epizootics of necrobacillosis seem to occur when wildlife are crowded together, as on elk feedlots in winter or when deer congregate about mud holes or seeps during hot weather after prolonged dry periods. Fecal contamination of the environment probably seeds areas of infection for the animals (Anon. 1924). Marsh et al. (1934) were able to isolate the organisms from a pasture 10 months after infected sheep had been on it, but were unable to do so after a second 10-month period. When cultures of the organism were placed in soil, the filaments shortened into rods and coccoid forms within 3 weeks and soon died (Tunnicliff 1938). However, when Beveridge (1934a) repeated this work and mixed *S. aureus* and *E. coli* with *F. necrophorum*, the anaerobe survived. The importance of this apparent symbiotic relationship may be that the normal flora of the skin and intestinal tract includes *S. aureus* and *E. coli*, respectively.

It is believed that the *necrophorum* bacillus does not possess the ability to invade tissues but must await an opportunity that follows abrasions or other injury. Squirreltail grass (Murie 1930), bearded awns (Honess and Frost 1942; Wright 1958), and coarse twigs (Rosen et al. 1951) may puncture the epithelium and permit access of *F. necrophorum*. This theory was questioned by Allred et al. (1944) when they fed corn and second-cutting alfalfa in an effort to reduce the incidence of the disease and found instead that losses increased. Another theory which has been advanced is that mud dries on the feet and cracks, and the resulting fissures allow the organism to enter the deeper tissues. Bleschner (1939) stated that the disease occurs during wet seasons in Australia; however, the worst outbreak occurred during the drought of 1922 when no mud was present.

The appearance of calf diphtheria may occur in domestic species following the shedding of milk teeth and eruption of permanent dentition in young animals (Ryff and Lee 1946). Intestinal forms may gain access following the penetration of the mucous membranes by strongylid larvae (Beveridge 1934b). Whatever portal of entry exists during epizootics in deer, lesions may occur in the feet, the oral cavity and throat, the rumen, the liver, the lungs, or in any combination of these sites.

SIGNS. In deer, necrosis and inflammation of the foot are seen in the acute phase, and arthritis with ankylosis in chronic or healed cases—all of which tend to cause limping. When the deer run, they may only use three feet.

In calf diphtheria or buccal abscesses, deer may appear "bottle jawed." The body temperature is elevated, and the animal loses its appetite (Beveridge 1959). Excessive salivation occurs, and there is a thick, sometimes purulent discharge (Wright 1958). Following spread of the infection to the liver and lungs of deer, death occurs.

PATHOGENESIS AND PATHOLOGY. The *necrophorum* bacillus is a pyogenic organism, and the pathology resulting from its invasion is typically a purulent abscess. The primary lesions may be in the mouth and throat, on one or more feet, or in the rumen or reticulum (Marsh 1944). As with most forms of wildlife diseases in which no medical intervention arrests the pathologic processes, the complete morbid progression follows its natural course until death ensues. As a result, these organisms are not walled off but tend to metastasize, with necrotic nodules appearing in the lungs as an extension of oral involvement, in the liver from either feet or digestive tract infection (Newsom 1938; Smith 1963), and in other areas such as the brain (Debbie 1965).

The purulent abscess has a greenish yellow color and a foul odor. Ulcerated areas may occur on the periodontal membranes extending deeply into the mandibular tissues, inner aspects of the cheeks, tongue, larynx, and pharynx and into the trachea. Croupous membranes may appear, and these have led to terming this syndrome "calf diphtheria." Usually the lungs become involved in the morbid process, and death results from either pneumonia, toxemia, or both.

One or more feet may be infected in cases of foot rot. The foot is swollen (Fig. 31.1), and necrosis may be noted externally about the coronary band or in the interdigital tissues (Beveridge 1941; Flint and Jensen 1951). As the condition progresses, the joints and bones of the foot are affected. Generally the infection does not spread through the leg, but metastases may occur, usually in the liver and on occasion in the lungs.

In ulcerative rumenitis there is accompanying peritonitis, and adhesions may attach the rumen to the diaphragm or other tissues within the peritoneum (Figs. 31.2 and 31.3).

DIAGNOSIS AND PROGNOSIS. As with most diseases, a definite diagnosis of foot rot must be based on recovery and identification of the etiologic agent. The pathology is typical enough to provide a presumptive diagnosis; however, it is important to differentiate calf diphtheria from actinomycosis. The former is indicated by the absence of "sulfur granules" common to actinomycosis. Isolation of *F. necrophorum* may be by culture or inoculation of rabbits (Beveridge 1964) or hamsters.

Because of some difficulty in the isolation of this organism and maintaining its viability, the fluorescent antibody technique is a useful diagnostic tool. Ledbetter and Nelson (1967) developed this method, although there was some cross-reaction with *Streptobacillus moniliformis*.

Infected deer fawns or elk calves usually have a fulminating infection with a high mortality rate (Wright 1958). Older animals can

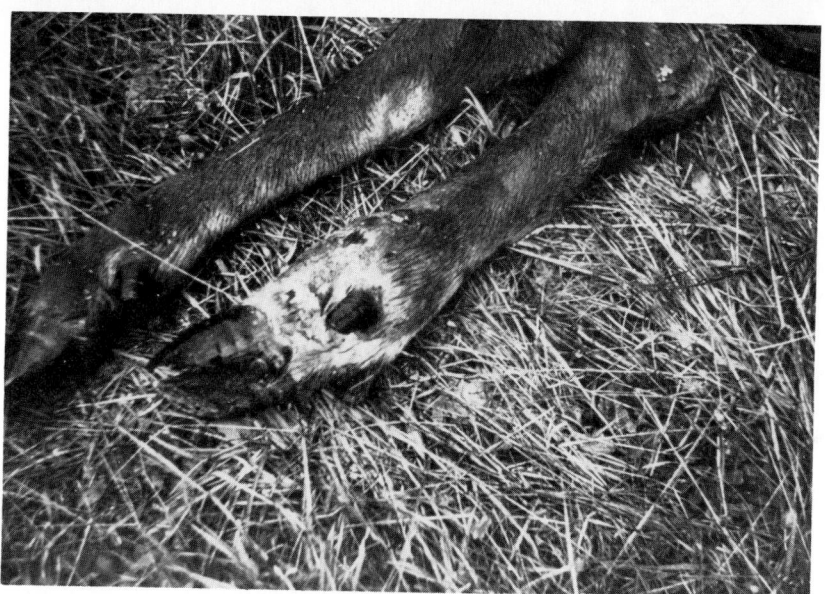

FIG. 31.1 Typical swollen appearance and necrosis of the extremity in foot rot of elk.

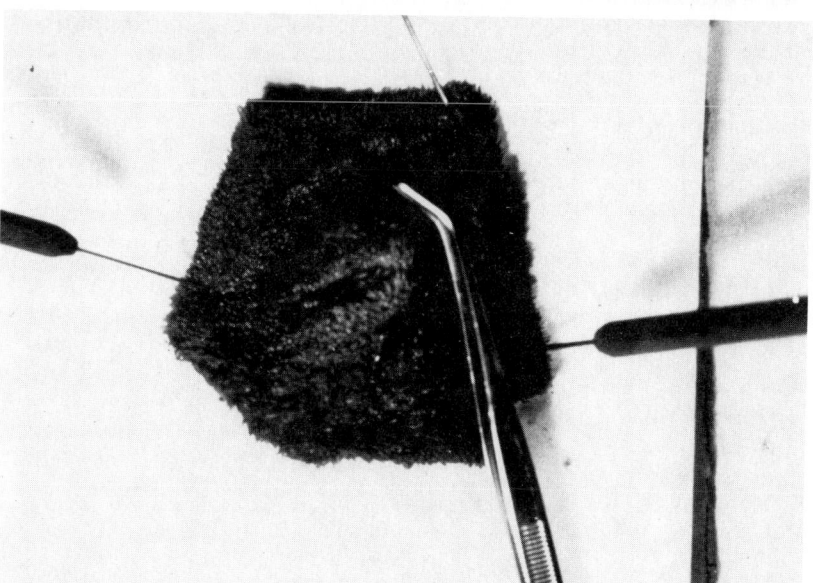

FIG. 31.2 Perforating ulcer of the mucosal aspect of the rumen of a deer with necrobacillosis.

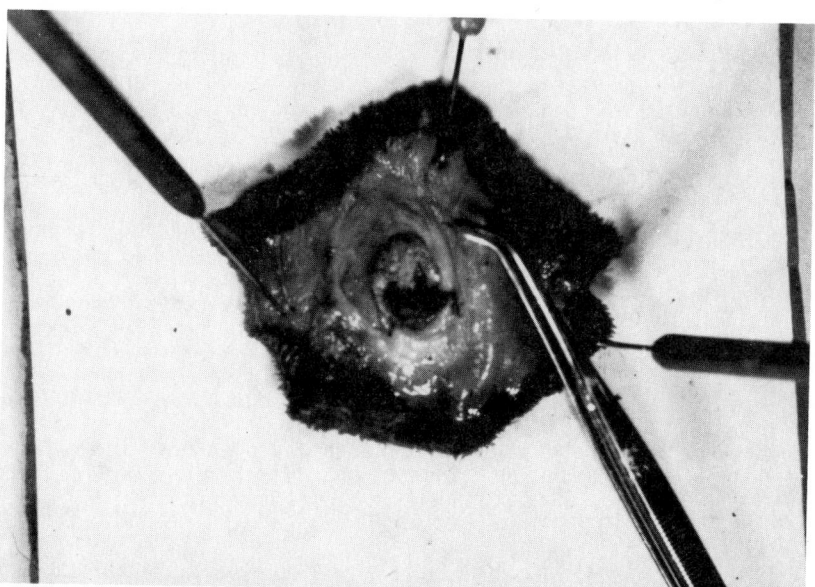

FIG. 31.3 Perforating ulcer on the serosal aspect of the rumen of a deer with necrobacillosis.

335

have lethal infections also but may often have the chronic form of the disease for which they have a better prognosis.

Epizootics of necrobacillosis usually occur in California deer during the late summer and early fall. If the preceding spring has been unusually dry, it is possible to forecast the appearance of foot rot, particularly on overcrowded ranges in the dry parts of the state. Once the disease has appeared in deer herds, it will continue to infect and kill animals until the high temperatures subside and the winter rains appear.

IMMUNITY. Immunity is not produced by infections with *F. necrophorum* (Beveridge 1934a; Orcutt 1930). A natural resistance is evident in the guinea pig, but susceptibility may be increased by vitamin C deprivation (McCullough 1938).

By agglutination tests, Feldman et al. (1936) established four serologic groups containing 14 strains of *F. necrophorum*; there was some cross-reaction between heterologous strains. Their findings that the antibody titer of "normal" horses, cattle, sheep, and swine closely approached that of affected animals of the same species are important in demonstrating that serology is useless for detection of necrobacillosis.

TREATMENT AND CONTROL. The greatest efforts of veterinarians to control foot rot in livestock have been: (1) sanitation and disinfection of premises, (2) surgical treatment of affected feet, and (3) administration of either sulfapyridine, sulfamerazine (Candlin 1947; Forman et al. 1947), or antibiotics. Roberts et al. (1948) found that aureomycin was effective in treatment, but in addition they found that 80% of the affected cattle would recover if no treatment was instituted. The high mortality rate in deer indicates that natural recovery is much lower in this wild species. As of 1981 the only hope for control of this disease in wildlife lay with treatment of the environment.

Concentration of deer around water holes or elk in feedlots only encourages the appearance of necrobacillosis. The herds should be dispersed by providing more water areas for deer and more widely scattered feeding areas for elk (Murie 1951).

Springs should be developed with drains, so that muddy sumps will not be formed. Drying seeps may be disinfected with copper sulfate or calcium hypochlorite. Infectious areas should be closed to the animals by fencing or by piling

brush in a contaminated ravine (Rosen 1962).

If sheep on the range provide the carryover of the *F. necrophorum* bacillus (Fethers 1940) and the area becomes enzootic, the cooperaton of agricultural agencies must be obtained. Working together, the wildlife agency and the agricultural agency can do much toward prevention of necrobacillosis in their respective domains and toward control of interanimal transmission.

REFERENCES

Allred, W. J., Brown, R. C., and Murie, O. J. Disease kills feedground elk. *Wyoming Wildl.* 9:1–8, 27, 1944.

Anderson, C. C. The elk of Jackson Hole. *Wyoming Game Fish Comm. Bull.* 10, 1958.

Anon. Modoc deer disease. *Calif. Fish Game* 11:27–28, 1924.

Anon. Disease makes serious inroads on number of mule deer. *Calif. Fish Game* 12:28–30, 1925.

Barton, A. Diseases of cattle in antiquity. *Vet. Med.* 53:551–553, 1938.

Beveridge, W. I. B. A study of 12 strains of *B. necrophorus* with observations on the oxygen intolerance of the organism. *J. Pathol. Bact.* 38:467–491, 1934.

———. Foot rot in sheep. *Aust. Vet. J.* 10:43–51, 1934b.

———. A study of *Spirochaeta penortha* isolated from foot rot in sheep. *Aust. J. Exp. Biol. Med. Sci.* 14:307–318, 1936.

———. Anaerobic bacteria associated in the etiology of foot rot in sheep. *Rep. Proc. 3rd Int. Congr. Microbiol.* pp. 637–647, 1940.

———. *Fusiformis nodosus. Bull. Council Sci. Ind. Res. Aust.* 140:1–53, 1941.

———. Necrobacillosis, foot rot, etc. In A. W. Stableforth and I. A. Galloway, eds. *Infectious diseases of animals*, vol. 2, pp. 397–412. London: Butterworths, 1959.

———. Differential diagnosis and control of foot rot in sheep. *Bull. Off. Int. Epizoot.* 52:1003–1004, 1964.

Bleschner, H. G. Foot rot in sheep. *Aust. Vet. J.* 15:219–222, 1939.

Borg, K. Untersuchungen an 460 zugrundegegangenen Rehen in Schweden. *Sonderdruck Z. Jagdwiss.* Bd. 4:203–208, 1958.

Buchanan, R. E., and Gibbons, N. E. *Bergey's manual of determinative bacteriology*, 8th ed. Baltimore: Williams and Wilkins, 1974.

Bruner, D. W., and Gillespie, J. H. *Hagan's infectious diseases of domestic animals*. Ithaca: Cornell (Comstock), 1961.

Candlin, F. T. The use of sodium sulfamerazine in foot rot. *J. Am. Vet. Med. Assoc.* 111:278–280, 1947.

Carhart, A. H. Fallacies in winter feeding of deer. *Trans. N. Am. Wildl. Conf.* 8:333–337, 1943.

Cass, J. S. Buccal food impaction in white-tailed deer and *A. necrophorus* in big game. *J. Wildl. Manag.* 11:91–94, 1947.

Dack, G. M., Dragstedt, L. R., and Heinz, T. E. Hepatic liver abscess due to *B. funduliformis. J. Infect. Dis.* 60:335–355, 1937.

Debbie, J. G. Brain abscess in a white-tailed deer (*Odocoileus virginianus*). *Bull. Wildl. Dis. Assoc.* 1:3–4, 1965.

Dixon, J. S. A study of the life history and food habits of mule deer in California. *Calif. Fish Game* 20:182–282, 1934.

Drager, N. A severe outbreak of interdigital necrobacillosis in gemsbok (*Oryx gazella*) in the northern Kalahari. *Trop. Anim. Health Prod.* 7:200, 1975.

Feldman, W. H., Hester, H. R., and Wherry, F. P. The occurrence of *B. necrophorus* agglutinins in different species of animals. *J. Infect. Dis.* 59:159–170, 1936.

Fethers, G. The dangers of foot rot carriers. *Pastoral Rev.* 50:329–330, 1940.

Flint, J. C., and Jensen, R. Pathology of necrobacillosis in the bovine foot. *Am. J. Vet. Res.* 12:5–13, 1951.

Forget, A., and Fredette, V. Sodium azide selective medium for the primary isolation of anaerobic bacteria. *J. Bact.* 83:1217–1223, 1962.

Forman, C. R., Burch, J., Dee, C. E., Kelley, L., Mauw, J. E. Tiegland, M. G., and Yarborough, J. H. The use of sodium sulfonamides as single injection specific treatment in foot rot. *J. Am. Vet. Med. Assoc.* 111:208–214, 1947.

Grayson, A. R. Foot rot in sheep. *J. Agr. Victoria* 45:153–160, 1947.

Hastings, C. C. Foot rot in cattle in relation to diet. *N. Am. Vet.* 23:90–91, 1942.

Herman, C. M., and Rosen, M. N. Disease investigations on mammals and birds by the California Division of Fish and Game. *Calif. Fish Game* 35:193–201, 1949.

Honess, R. F., and Frost, N. M. A Wyoming bighorn sheep study. *Wyoming Game Fish Dept. Bull.* 1:127, 1942.

Honess, R. F., and Winter, K. B. Diseases of wildlife in Wyoming. *Wyoming Game Fish Comm. Bull.* 9:16–20, 1956.

Howarth, J. A. Foot rot in sheep. *Vet. Med.* 25:186–188, 1930.

Karstad, L. Diseases of the Cervidae: A partly annotated bibliography. *Wildl. Dis.* 43:16–22, 1964.

King, J. A. Disease survey trips among caribou herds in Alaska. *J. Am. Vet. Med. Assoc.* 143:887–888, 1963.

Klimontov, M. I. The treatment of early stage necrobacillosis in reindeer. *Veterinariya* 4:52–53, 1962.

Kotov, V. T. Hoof disease of reindeer. *Sov. Vet.* 5:20–23, 1936.

Krembs, J. Fallwilduntersuchungen 1935 mit 1938. *Tieraertzl. Rdsch.* 45:763–766, 773–776, 1939.

Kress, F. Tuberculosis of the lungs, and necrobacillosis of the abomasum of an antelope. *Berl.*

Muench. Tieraerztl. Wochenschr. 24:439–441, 1943.

Ledbetter, E. O., and Nelson, J. D. Immunofluorescence of *Bacteroides funduliformis. Bact. Proc.* 67:86, 1967.

McCullough, N. B. Vitamin C and the resistance of the guinea pig to infection and *B. necrophorus. J. Infect. Dis.* 63:34–53, 1938.

McLean, D. D. The deer of California with particular reference to the Rocky Mountain mule deer. *Calif. Fish Game* 26:139–166, 1940.

Madin, S. H. A bacteriologic study of bovine liver abscess. *Vet. Med.* 44:248–251, 1949.

Marsh, H. Necrobacillosis of the rumen in young lambs. *J. Am. Vet. Med. Assoc.* 104:23–25, 1944.

Marsh, H., Hadleigh, T., and Tunnicliff, E. A. Experimental studies of foot rot in sheep. *Mont. Agr. Expt. Sta. Bull.* 285:3–29, 1934.

Martinaglia, G. Some considerations regarding the health of wild animals in captivity. *S. Afr. J. Sci.* 33:833–844, 1936.

Mohler, J. R., and Morse, G. B. *B. necrophorus* and its economic importance. *21st Rep. Bur. Anim. Ind.,* pp. 21–27, 1904.

Murie, A. The moose of Isle Royal. *Univ. Mich. Mus. Zool. Misc. Publ.* 25:44, 1934.

Murie, O. J. An epizootic disease of elk. *J. Mammal.* 11:214–222, 1930.

———. *The elk of North America.* Harrisburg, Pa.: Stackpole; Washington, D.C.: Wildlife Management Institute, 1951.

Murray, C., Biester, H. E., Burwin, P., and McNutt, S. H. Infectious enteritis of swine. *J. Am. Vet. Med. Assoc.* 72:34–65, 1927.

———. Infectious enteritis of swine. II. *J. Am. Vet. Med. Assoc.* 72:1003–1022, 1928.

Newsom, I. E. A bacteriologic study of liver abscesses of cattle. *J. Infect. Dis.* 63:232–244, 1938.

Nikolaevskii, L. D. Causes of necrobacillus epizootics in reindeer. *Veterinariya* 10:8–13, 1944.

Orcutt, M. L. Study of *B. necrophorus* obtained from cows. *J. Bacteriol.* 20:343–360, 1930.

Pochuchuev, K., and Agalarova, A. Caudal necrosis of buffaloes. *Soviet Vet.* 10/11:94–95, 1939.

Rausch, R. A. On the status of some arctic mammals. *Arctic* 6:91–148, 1953.

Roberts, S. J., Kiesel, G. K., and Lewis, N. F. Foot rot in cattle: A controlled experiment. *Cornell Vet.* 38:122–130, 1948.

Rosen, M. N. Foot rot or calf diphtheria in deer. *Calif. Dept. Fish Game, Game Manag. Leaflet* 7, 1962.

Rosen, M. N., Brunetti, O. A., Bischoff, A. I., and Azevedo, J. A., Jr. An epizootic of foot rot in California deer. *Trans. N. Am. Wildl. Conf.* 16:164–177, 1951.

Rush, W. M. Northern Yellowstone elk study. *Mont. Fish Game Comm.,* 1932.

Ryff, J. F., and Lee, A. M. Etiology of calf diphtheria. *Am. J. Vet. Res.* 7:41–44, 1946.

Schilling, E. A. Management of white-tailed deer on the Pisgah National Game Preserve. *Trans. N. Am. Wildl. Conf.* 3:248–255, 1938.

Scrivner, L. H. The morphology, culture and isolation

of *A. necrophorus*. *J. Am. Vet. Med. Assoc.* 85:360–379, 1934.

Shillinger, J. E. Disease relationship of domestic stock and wildlife. *Trans. N. Am. Wildl. Conf.* 2:298–302, 1937.

———. Diseases of wildlife and their relationship to domestic stock. In *Keeping livestock healthy*, USDA Agr. Yearbook, Washington: USGPO, pp. 1217–1225, 1942.

Smith, L. D. *Spherophorus necrophorus* and liver abscess in cattle. *Bull. Off. Int. Epizoot.* 59:1517–1526, 1963.

Stableforth, A. W., and Galloway, I. A. *Infectious diseases of animals: Diseases due to bacteria*, 2 vols. London: Butterworths, 1959.

Tunnicliff, E. A. *A. necrophorus* in soil cultures. *J. Infect. Dis.* 62:58–65, 1938.

Vogelsang, E. G. Necrobacillosis of domestic and wild animals in Venezuela. *Rev. Med. Vet. Parasit. Caracas* 5:3–11, 1946.

Winter, K. B., and Honess, R. F. Bearded grains cause death of deer. *J. Wildl. Manag.* 16:113–114, 1952.

Wobeser, G., Runge, W., and Noble, D. Necrobacillosis in deer and pronghorn antelope in Saskatchewan. *Can. Vet. J.* 16:3–9, 1975.

Wright, J. F. Necrotic stomatitis in the American elk. *Vet. Med.* 53:520–521, 1958.

32 *Dermatophilosis*

J. L. RICHARD

Synonyms: **Lumpy wool, mycotic dermatitis, cutaneous streptothricosis, strawberry foot rot.**

Dermatophilosis is an exudative dermatitis of man and a variety of other animals, wild and domesticated, caused by the actinomycete, *Dermatophilus congolensis*. Lesions may be present as scaly to scabby areas on any part of an affected animal's body and they may coalesce to form extensive encrustations.

HISTORY AND DISTRIBUTION. The first documentation of determatophilosis was in cattle of the Belgian Congo in 1916 (Van Saceghem 1916). Since that time the disease has been found worldwide in many tropical and temperate regions. The disease was well known in England, Scotland, and Australia before being recognized in the United States in 1961. At this time it was almost simultaneously found to occur in horses, white-tailed deer, and humans in New York and in cattle in Texas (Bentinck-Smith et al. 1961; Bridges and Romane 1961; Dean et al. 1961). The disease has been reported in domestic cattle, horses, sheep, goats, donkeys, pigs, cats, and dogs.

In cattle, horses, and other species where it was manifested as a typical exudative dermatitis, the disease was called "cutaneous streptothricosis," but in sheep where the wool became matted together with exudate, the disease was called "lumpy wool" or "mycotic dermatitis." The disease in sheep involving the feet and distal portions of the leg was called "strawberry foot rot."

Although the disease is frequently diagnosed in domestic animals, wildlife species comprise over two-thirds of the total species

TABLE 32.1   Wildlife Species in Which Dermatophilosis Has Been Reported to Occur.

Species	Reference
Eland (*Taurotragus oryx*)	Hornby 1920
Giraffe (*Giraffa camelopardalis*)	Austwick and Davies 1958
Gazelle (*Gazella thompsonii*)	Austwick and Davies 1958
Deer (*Odocoileus virginianus*)	Dean et al. 1961
Zebra (*Equus* spp.)	Green 1960
Kudu (*Tragelaphus strepsiceros*)	Vandemaele 1961
Cephalophe antelope (*Cephalophus* spp.)	Vandemaele 1961
Hedgehog (*Erinaceus europaeus*)	Kusel'tan 1967
Gerbil (*Gerbillus* spp.)	Kusel'tan 1967
Chamois (*Rupicapra rupicapra*)	Nicolet et al. 1967
Fox (*Vulpes vulpes*)	Austwick 1968
Columbian ground squirrel (*Citellus columbianus columbianus*)	Wobeser and Gordon 1969
Cottontail rabbit (*Sylvilagus floridanus*)	Shotts and Kistner 1970
South American seal (*Otaria bryonia*)	Frese and Weber 1971
Owl monkey (*Aotus trivirgatus*)	McClure et al. 1971; King et al. 1971
Wooly monkey (*Lagothrix lagotrichia*)	Fraser and Garcia 1971
Polar bear (*Thalarctos maritimus*)	Smith and Cordes 1972
Bearded dragon lizard (*Amphibolurus barbatus*)	Simmons et al. 1972; Montali et al. 1975
Raccoon (*Procyon lotor*)	Stone et al. 1975; Salkin et al. 1976
Sable antelope (*Hippotragus niger*)	DeVos and Imes 1976
Roan antelope (*H. equinus*)	DeVos and Imes 1976
Titi monkey (*Callicebus moloch*)	Migaki and Seibold 1976
Marble lizard (*Calotes mystaceus*)	Anver et al. 1976

affected (Richard and Shotts 1976). Some of the reports involved wild species in captivity; others occurred in the wild hosts within their natural habitat. The wild animal species affected and a reference to the first recorded infection in each species is summarized in Table 32.1.

Human infections were acquired from infected deer in one of the first reported cases of dermatophilosis in the United States (Dean et al. 1961).

The isolations of *D. congolensis* from infected polar bears were from bears that had been in captivity for a period of at least 3 or more years (Newman et al. 1975; Smith and Cordes 1972). The disease has not been reported in noncaptive polar bears.

There have been several reports of the occurrence of dermatophilosis in lower vertebrates. Two reports have described dermatophilosis in the bearded dragon lizard from Australia (Montali et al. 1975; Simmons et al. 1972). The disease was also described in 2 of 74 marble lizards from Thailand (Anver et al. 1976).

Dermatophilosis has not been documented in avian species, although a dermatitis in turkeys was described and the causative agent was reported as a "streptothrix" (Soliman and Rollison 1951).

Some of the most recent descriptions of dermatophilosis in wildlife is the finding of the disease in eight raccoons in New York State (Salkin et al. 1976) and in two species of antelope in South Africa (DeVos and Imes 1976). In addition, the disease was recently described in the titi monkey (Migaki and Seibold 1976).

ETIOLOGY. *Dermatophilus congolensis* is a fungallike organism but belongs in the order Actinomycetales in the family Dermatophilaceae. The only other member of the family is *Geodermatophilus*, a noninfectious, soil-inhabiting organism. Past descriptions of some of the diseases caused by *Dermatophilus* will include *D. dermatonomus* as the causative agent of mycotic dermatitis or lumpy wool in sheep and *D. pedis* as the agent of strawberry foot rot in sheep. However, all of these species have been placed in synonymy with *D. congolensis*; therefore, it is the only species within the genus (Gordon 1964).

The fungallike nature of *Dermatophilus* is illustrated by an examination of its life cycle (Fig. 32.1). The spores of the organism are approximately 0.9 μ in diameter and are multiflagellate (Richard et al. 1967). They eventually lose their flagella, enlarge to approximately twice their original diameter, and germinate by a germ tube. The germ tube extends into branching hyphae that are subsequently subdivided by transverse and longitudinal septae, thus transforming the hyphae into multicellu-

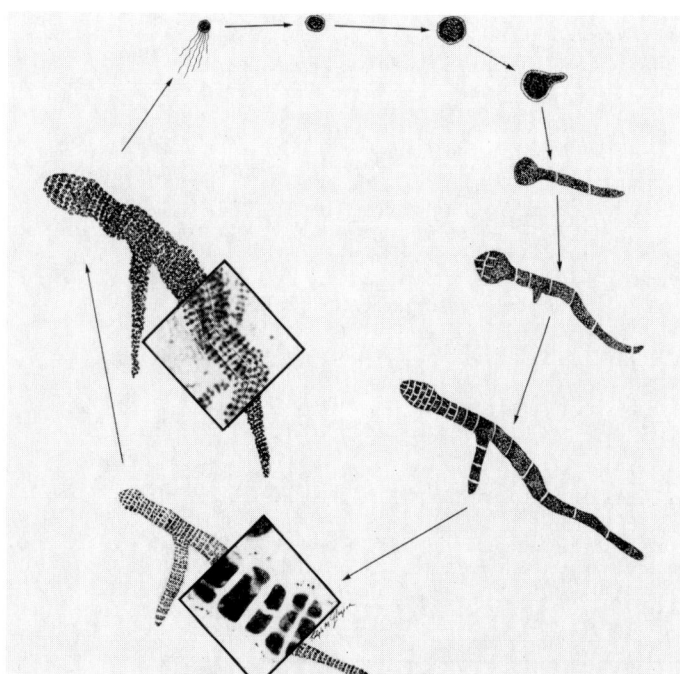

FIG. 32.1 Life cycle of *Dermatophilus congolensis*. (Reprinted courtesy of Iowa State University Press.)

lar bodies, several cells (approximately eight) in width, measuring up to 5 μ. Each individual cell formed in this manner will become a motile zoospore by formation of the spore from the cell cytoplasm and subsequent dissolution of the hyphal cell walls, releasing the motile spores and completing the life cycle. The hyphal elements remain nonseptate near their apices, and branching occurs as in germ tube formation. In some instances the spores will germinate before they are released completely from the hyphae or portions of hyphae (packets of cells).

The organism is gram-positive and non-acid-fast. It is aerobic to facultatively anaerobic and grows best at 37°C. Colonies on enriched medium such as brain heart infusion agar may be smooth or rough, adherent to the medium, and grayish brown to yellowish orange, becoming viscous in some strains, particularly with fresh isolates. No aerial mycelium is produced. *Dermatophilus* is β-hemolytic; however, strains that have been kept in the laboratory may exhibit diminished to no hemolysis. The organism does not grow on Sabouraud dextrose agar, but growth is good on Loeffler's medium, and it is liquefied by most strains. Gelatin is liquefied by most strains, and casein and starch are hydrolyzed. Urease and catalase are produced by *Dermatophilus*. *Dermatophilus* is nonfermentative, but acid is produced from glucose and fructose, transitorily from galactose, and late production from maltose (Gordon 1964).

Although there appear to be differences in species susceptibilities to dermatophilosis, there does not appear to be a wide variation in virulence of different strains of *Dermatophilus*.

TRANSMISSION. An important means of transmission of dermatophilosis from other animals to man and from animal to animal is direct contact. Under moist conditions, the motile zoospores are released from scabs, and through contact with another animal the disease may be spread. This method of transmission was suspected in raccoons, as they den together in small groups (Salkin et al. 1976). The occurrence of the disease in a foal born in an isolation barn is a typical example of the transmission of the disease from an infected mare to her offspring through direct contact (Cheville et al. 1971).

Apparently ticks were active in the transmission of *D. congolensis* infection in cattle, as the disease was controlled by experimental dipping (Plowright 1956). Macadam (1962) established an infection in a rabbit with ticks (*Amblyomma variegatum*) removed from infected

cattle. Other ticks incriminated in the transmission of *D. congolensis* include *A. variegatum* obtained from infected cattle (Oppong 1976) and *Hyalomma asiaticum* (Kusel'tan 1967).

Richard and Pier (1966) successfully transmitted the disease among New Zealand white rabbits by both biting (*Stomoxys calcitrans*) and nonbiting (*Musca domestica*) flies. This type of transmission was mechanical and with fluorescent antibody staining, the organism was observed in the spines on the feet of flies (*S. calcitrans*) that had fed on lesions (Richard and Shotts 1976). In the one report of dermatophilosis in polar bears, Smith and Cordes (1972) incriminated biting flies, *S. calcitrans*.

Dermatophilus congolensis does not survive out of the animal hosts. Unsuccessful attempts have been made to isolate the organism from soil samples of farms where severely infected sheep were located. Also, moist soil did not afford the growth and survival of *D. congolensis* in scab material or as a zoospore suspension (Roberts 1967b).

SIGNS. Early lesions of dermatophilosis may go unnoticed as they may be quite small, involving only a few hair follicles with a slight amount of exudate at the follicle opening. However, this condition usually progresses to form an encrustation matting the hair together. The lesion types may vary depending on the species affected and the type of hair coat or skin condition. Generally, the initial lesions are discrete scabby lesions that may coalesce to form irregular encrusted patches. Frequently, the patches may slough and the new epidermis becomes infected forming dense hyperkeratotic scabs. It is not unusual to find horses or cattle where the entire body is covered with discrete lesions approximately 1–2 cm in diameter with tufts of hair matted together. This is the typical "paint brush" lesion that also may be found in other animal species.

Attempts have been made to classify and characterize the lesions in a variety of domestic animals (Stewart 1972a). This is difficult since the encrustations may be of various forms and several different lesion types may be present on a single animal. The kind of lesions described in wild animal species are usually consistent with those types found in domesticated species. However, in polar bears, one young bear's coat became yellow with an increasing greasiness that subsequently became blackened with "an accumulation of black greasy material in flattened clumps throughout the coat" (Newman et al. 1975). This condition has not been described in other species and may be an additional condition that, in this case, was coincident with dermatophilosis. It is not unusual that such a coincidence occurs, because *D. congolensis* may inhabit or invade lesions caused by other organisms or it may predispose the skin to invasion by other opportunists. *Dermatophilus congolensis* has been found in lesions from cattle presumably caused by bovine mammalitis virus (Yedloutschnig 1971), and simultaneous infections of poxvirus and *D. congolensis* have been described in sheep and goats in Kenya (Munz 1969). This kind of relationship may also be involved in pox-infected South American sea lions (Wilson et al. 1972). Simultaneous infections of *D. congolensis* and stomatitis papulosa virus have been observed in Nigerian cattle (Plowright and Ferris 1959). Simultaneous infection of *D. congolensis* and the mycotic agent *Alternaria alternata* has been described in white-tailed deer, and it was believed that *D. congolensis* predisposed the deer to infection by the opportunistic fungal agent (Salkin et al. 1975).

It is important to realize that *D. congolensis* may cause a chronic or mild occult infection in animals. These animals have a light encrustation around the base of individual or a few hairs, but these encrustations contain an abundance of organisms when smeared on a glass slide stained with Giemsa stain and examined microscopically. These animals are the so-called carrier animal described by Stewart (1972b). Such a situation was described in sheep by Austwick (1958), who found 30 affected flocks whose owners had not noticed any sign of disease. A mare was a carrier animal, and its foal developed the disease with the characteristic exudative dermatitis (Cheville et al. 1971). This same situation may occur in racoons since some of the skins from infected racoons possessed only a dandrufflike appearance and definitive diagnosis was made only by inoculation of infected material onto a rabbit (Salkin et al. 1976). Experimental inoculation of normal skin on white-tailed deer resulted in the lack of clinical evidence of disease; however, hair in the site of inoculation could be epilated with ease at 5 days after inoculation, and the organism could be demonstrated in stained preparations (Richard and Shotts 1976). Similar experimental results were found in dogs (Richard et al. 1973). Deer naturally infected with *D. congolensis* have been observed with no encrustations but with evident areas of alopecia (W. B. Stone, personal communication).

Some unusual forms of dermatophilosis

have been described (Richard and Shotts 1976). Granulomas have been observed to occur on the tongue and on the serosal surface of the bladder in cats (Baker et al. 1972; O'Hara and Cordes 1965), and a granulomatous dermatitis has been described in humans (Albrecht et al. 1974). It should be noted that in these cases the organism was not isolated and the diagnosis was based on histopathologic examination of infected tissues stained with hematoxylin and eosin or with fluorescent antibody stain. Tongue and palate lesions were noted in an unusual case of dermatophilosis in a calf which was suspected to be deficient immunologically based upon a very minimal cellular reaction at the lesion sites (Simpson and Cuming 1976). Similarly, tongue lesions described as hyperplastic nodules of dermatophilosis were reported in a buffalo calf (Kharole et al. 1976). Jones (1976) described a subcutaneous infection of *D. congolensis* in a cat which was characterized as a draining subcutaneous abscess in the region of the right popliteal lymph node. Subcutaneous abscesses were also found in the disease described in the bearded dragon lizard (Simmons et al. 1972). This kind of lesion could be reproduced in the marble lizard with *D. congolensis* (Anver et al. 1976).

PATHOGENESIS AND PATHOLOGY. Roberts (1967b) has thoroughly described infection and pathogenesis of *D. congolensis*. In the typical cases of dermatophilosis, the organism is found within the host epidermis. The motile zoospores of *D. congolensis* are active in establishing the infections within the epidermis; thus, the enhancement or requirement of moisture for infection is understood. In addition to providing a medium for dissemination of the zoospores, moisture can emulsify and disrupt the sebaceous film of the skin, allowing for easier penetration of the disrupted stratum corneum by the hyphae of germinated zoospores. In addition to moisture, mechanical disruption of the skin surface by fly and tick bites, thorn penetration, and other abrasive action leads to easier penetration of the epidermis by the organism. Once the organism has entered the epidermis, the branching hyphae spread through the tissue and invade sheaths of hair and wool follicles. The organism does not invade beyond the basement membrane into the dermis. However, Amakiri (1974) described the organism in the dermis of natural infections in the bovine only in areas where there was disintegration of the basement membrane. In the infectious process the mechanical nature of the hyphal penetration produces an acute inflammatory response; there is cornification of the epidermis and a neutrophilic invasion of the area at the leading edge of the advancing organism. This separates the infected tissue from the dermis. New epidermis is often formed, primarily as outgrowths of follicle sheaths and other adjacent epidermis, beneath the granulocytes. This results in the isolation of the granulocytes between the newly formed epidermis and the infected, cornified epithelium (Roberts 1967b). The process described above is often repeated, resulting in multiple layers of cornified epithelium, debris, and granulocytes. The newly formed epidermis is frequently invaded by lateral growth of the organism existing in follicle sheaths.

DIAGNOSIS. It is obvious from the multiplicity of clinical signs of dermatophilosis that diagnosis must be based on laboratory examination and identification of the organism from infected material. Standardized methods for use in the diagnosis of dermatophilosis have been outlined (Cottral 1978). Clinical specimens should be removed from the infected animal with a sterile forceps to avoid human infection, and the collected specimen should be placed in a dry container for transport to the laboratory. Direct microscopic examination of the clinical specimen can be made by emulsifying a small portion of the scab in a drop of sterile water or saline on a glass slide with a small glass rod. After the suspension is air-dried, the smear can be stained with Giemsa stain and examined under oil at 900× for the typical branched filaments of D. congolensis. These possess longitudinal and transverse septa forming a beaded appearance of the hyphae which may be up to eight coccoid cells in width. These forms are usually readily detected in acute lesions of dermatophilosis; however, in the atypical, chronic, or occult type of lesion, the organism may be present only as cocci or as packets of cocci resembling several other bacteria. An asset to the diagnosis of these types of D. congolensis infections has been the fluorescent antibody test (Pier et al. 1964). The test may also be used to elucidate dual infections where the lesions were assumed to be caused by another recognized agent. The fluorescent antibody test is applicable as a screening procedure, as it may be applied to a large number of smears of exudative crusts.

To culture D. congolensis from clinical specimens, grind approximately 0.06 g of exudative crust in a Ten Broeck tissue grinder with 5 ml of sterile phosphate buffered saline solution (pH 7.4). Allow the tissue suspension to stand at room temperature for 1 hour to settle. Withdraw the supernatant fluid containing the motile zoospores with a syringe and then pass the supernatant fluid through a Millipore Swinney adapter filter (1.2-μ pore size) directly onto the surface of a suitable medium (Pier et al. 1964). A good medium to use is brain heart infusion agar enriched with 5% defibrinated bovine blood. Three drops of filtrate is sufficient inoculum per plate of medium. The inoculum is then streaked for isolation, and the plates are incubated at 37°C. The typical colonies of D. congolensis exhibiting β-hemolysis will usually appear within 48 hours; however, the plates should be retained for examination for 7 days before discarding.

In cases where samples submitted to the laboratory are heavily contaminated, a suspension of the specimen may be applied to a shaved and scarified site on a rabbit. Usually within 7 days lesions will appear on the rabbit, and isolation of D. congolensis can be made from scab material.

Serologic tests may offer some assistance in the diagnostic procedure for dermatophilosis; however, their sensitivity and reliability have not been clearly established. The precipitin test and the passive hemagglutination test have been used to detect chronically infected animals, and the passive hemagglutination test may be sufficiently sensitive to detect carrier animals or animals with occult infections (Bida and Kelley 1976; Pulliam et al. 1967; Richard et al. 1976). Results obtained with these tests applied to cattle serum indicated that many cases of dermatophilosis had gone undetected (Richard et al. 1976).

PROGNOSIS. Domestic animals with dermatophilosis suffer debilitating effects such as poor weight gains or actual weight loss and decreased milk production, but mortality from dermatophilosis is difficult to assess since animals with moderate or severe forms of the disease are usually culled from the herd and sent to slaughter (Lloyd 1976). However, animals with severe cases of dermatophilosis without treatment do become emaciated and die. The actual cause of death may be a secondary cause; nevertheless, dermatophilosis is a major contributing factor. Some animals with mild to moderate acute disease "cure" spontaneously. The possibility remains that some of these cured animals may have developed low-grade chronic infections, some of which are subclinical or occult.

It is even more difficult to assess the prognosis of the disease in wild animals because extensive studies have not been conducted. A number of the cases that have been described in wild animals are from those that have been in captivity and treated. Although the disease may be a rather frequent finding in certain wildlife species within a given locality (Gordon 1976), there do not appear to be widespread epidemics of the disease which significantly reduce the numbers within the species. The finding of the disease in a significant number of species within a given area may be dependent upon wet climatic conditions and other factors such as flies and ticks; therefore, the disease is not necessarily an annual occurrence. Perhaps one reason for the lack of severe outbreaks in the wildlife population is that many infections cure spontaneously. Also, occult or subclinical infections may occur and are not detected.

IMMUNITY. A number of antigenic preparations including whole cell, somatic, and flagellar antigens have been used in producing antibodies to *D. congolensis* in a variety of test animals (Bida and Kelley 1976; Richard et al. 1976; Roberts 1967b). Antibodies produced could be detected using the agglutination test, the agar gel precipitation test and the passive hemagglutination test (Bida and Kelley 1976; Richard et al. 1976). The role of these kinds of circulating antibodies on infection by *D. congolensis* is somewhat varied, but generally there is little or no effect. Resistance to reinfection with *D. congolensis* has been reported following experimental reinoculation (Austwick and Davies 1958; Hudson 1937). Bida and Kelley (1976) found no increased resistance of scarified skin or destruction of *D. congolensis* zoospores in guinea pigs hyperimmunized with whole cell, somatic, or flagellar antigens. Reinfection of rabbits was accomplished at 2-week intervals for a 1-year period with no obvious diminution in the severity of lesions, and there was no apparent resistance to reinfection in deer possessing circulating precipitating antibodies (Richard et al. 1976).

In animals with natural, chronic *D. congolensis* infections precipitating antibodies can be detected with the agar gel precipitin test (Pulliam et al. 1967; Richard et al. 1976; Roberts 1966a).

Vaccination trials have been conducted in cattle using several vaccine preparations (Chamoiseau et al. 1973; Provost et al. 1976); some protection was provided when adjuvant was used with the vaccine (Chamoiseau et al. 1973). Additional work is needed in this area to determine the duration of protection using a variety of vaccine preparations and vaccination regimens.

TREATMENT AND CONTROL. As in many skin disorders of animals, one treatment is the topical application of medicines or the use of dips or spray. Roberts (1962) found that 0.5% zinc sulfate applied to shear cuts prevent infection in sheep. Additional medicaments used have been mercuric chloride solution, 5% formalin ointment, 3% copper sulfate, quarternary ammonia compounds, and dips containing arsenic (Kaplan 1966). However, many of these have proved ineffective because they simply do not penetrate the lesion to provide an effective kill. Some workers have suggested removing the bulk of the encrustations prior to treatment with these topical medicaments.

Although there are many antibiotics that are effective against *D. congolensis* in vitro, only a few are effective in the treatment of dermatophilosis. Roberts (1966b, 1967a) and Roberts and Graham (1966) found streptomycin alone to be fairly effective, but the combination of streptomycin and penicillin given intramuscularly at the rate of 70 mg/kg was most effective in sheep. This combination of antibiotics was also found to be the treatment of choice (parenterally) in naturally infected cattle (Blancou 1976). Blancou also suggested that when the treatment fails on account of resistance, chloramphenicol, the tetracyclines, and spiramycin may be substituted. Extensive experimentation is lacking in the treatment of naturally acquired dermatophilosis in other animals, especially wildlife.

Macadam (1976) recommended that affected animals should remain isolated from other animals during treatment until cure is affected. In many instances animals that are cured develop dermatophilosis when placed back in the herd. Relapses do occur. Other recommendations include keeping the affected animals free of flies, ticks, and other insects, slaughter of animals which do not respond to treatment, dipping, quarantining (for 6 weeks) new animals introduced into existing livestock, and providing shelter to animals during prolonged rainfall.

REFERENCES

Albrecht, R., Horowitz, S., Gilbert, E., Hong, R., Richard, J., and Connor, D. H. *Dermatophilus congolensis* chronic nodular disease in man. *Pediatrics* 53:907–912, 1974.

Amakiri, S. F. Extent of skin penetration by *Dermatophilus congolensis* in bovine streptothricosis. *Trop. Anim. Health Prod.* 6:99–105, 1974.

Anver, M. R., Park, J. S., and Rush, H. G. Dermatophilosis in the marble lizard (*Calotes mystaceus*). *Lab. Anim. Sci.* 26:817–823, 1976.

Austwick, P. K. C. Cutaneous streptothricosis, mycotic dermatitis and strawberry foot rot and the genus *Dermatophilus*, Van Saceghem. *Vet. Rev. Annot.* 4:33–48, 1958.

———. Mycotic infections. *Symp. Zool. Soc. London* 24:249–271, 1968.

Austwick, P. K. C., and Davies, E. T. Mycotic dermatitis in Great Britain 1954–58. *Vet. Rec.* 70:1081–1088, 1958.

Baker, G. J., Breeze, R. G., and Dawson, C. O. Oral dermathophilosis in a cat: A case report. *J. Small Anim. Pract.* 13:649–653, 1972.

Bentinck-Smith, J., Fox, F. H., and Baker, D. W. Equine dermatitis (cutaneous streptothricosis) infection with *Dermatophilus* in the United States. *Cornell Vet.* 51:334–339, 1961.

Bida, S. A., and Kelley, D. C. Immunological studies of antigenic components of *Dermatophilus congolensis*. In D. H. Lloyd, and K. C. Sellers, eds., *Dermatophilus infection in animals and man*, pp. 229–242. New York: Academic Press, 1976.

Blancou, J. M. The treatment of infection by *Dermatophilus congolensis* with particular reference to the disease in cattle. In D. H. Lloyd and K. C. Sellers, eds., *Dermatophilus infection in animals and man*, pp. 246–259. New York: Academic Press, 1976.

Bridges, C. H., and Romane, W. M. Cutaneous streptothricosis in cattle. *J. Am. Vet. Med. Assoc.* 183:153–157, 1961.

Chamoiseau, G., Provost, A., and Touade, M. Recherches immunologiques sur la dermatophilose cutanee bovine: II. Essais d'immunisation de zebu contre la determatophilose naturelle. *Rev. Elev. Med. Vet. Pays. Trop.* 26:7–11, 1973.

Cheville, N. F., Cysewski, S. J., and Richard, J. L. Dermatophilosis in a foal. *Iowa State Vet.* 33:128–131, 1971.

Cottral, G. E., ed. *Dermatophilus*. In *Manual of standardized methods for veterinary microbiology*, pp. 559–561. Ithaca, N. Y.: Cornell University Press, 1978.

Dean, D. J., Dordon, M. A., Severinghause, C. W., Kroll, E. T., and Reilly, J. R. Streptothricosis: A new zoonotic disease. *N.Y. State J. Med.* 61:1283–1287, 1961.

DeVos, V., and Imes, G. D. An outbreak of dermatophilosis in sable (*Hippotragus niger*) and roan (*Hippotragus equinus*) antelope in the Kruger National Park. *Koedoe* 19:1–15, 1976.

Fraser, C. E. P., and Garcia, F. G. Cutaneous streptothricosis (dermatophilosis) in a wooly monkey. *Primate Zoonosis Surveillance*, rep. no. 5, Jan.-March 1971. Atlanta: Department of Health, Education and Welfare, Public Health Service, U.S. Health Services and Mental Health Administration, Center for Disease Control, 1971.

Frese, Von K., and Weber, A. Eine dermatitis bei mahnenrobber (Otaria Bryoni Blainville) hervorgerufen durch *Dermatophilus congolensis*. *Berl. Muench. Tieraerztl. Wochenschr.* 3:60–54, 1971.

Gordon, M. A. The genus *Dermatophilus*. *J. Bacteriol.* 88:509–522, 1964.

———. The disease in America: Discussion. In D. H. Lloyd and K. C. Sellers, eds., *Dermatophilus infection in animals and man*, p. 125. New York: Academic Press, 1976.

Green, H. F. Streptothricosis in zebra and donkeys and demodectic mange in eland in Kenya. *Vet. Rec.* 72:1098, 1960.

Hornby, H. E. A contagious impetigo of cattle. *Vet. J.* 76:210–216, 1920.

Hudson, J. R. Cutaneous streptothricosis. *Proc. R. Soc. Med.* 30:1457–1460, 1937.

Jones, R. T. Subcutaneous infection with *Dermatophilus congolensis* in a cat. *J. Comp. Pathol.* 86:415–421, 1976.

Kaplan, W. Dermatophilosis: A recently recognized disease in the United States. *Southwest. Vet.* 20:14–19, 1966.

Kharole, M. U., Gupta, P. P., Singh, B., and Dhingra, P. N. Dermatophilosis (streptothricosis) in a buffalo calf (*Bubalus bubalis*). *Zentralbla. Vet. Med. B.* 23:604–608, 1976.

King, N. W., Fraser, C. E. O., Garcia, F. G., Wolf, L. A., and Williamson, M. E. Cutaneous streptothricosis (dermatophilosis) in owl monkeys. *Lab. Anim. Sci.* 21:67–74, 1971.

Kusel'tan, I. V. Nocardiosis of lambs in the Tadzhik S.S.R. *Vet. Bull.* 38:590, 1967. (Abstr.)

Lloyd, D. H. The economic effects of bovine streptothricosis. In D. H. Lloyd and K. C. Sellers, eds., *Dermatophilus infection in animals and man*, pp. 274–291. New York: Academic Press, 1976.

Macadam, I. Bovine streptothricosis: Production of lesions by the bites of the tick (*Amblyomma variegatum*). *Vet. Rec.* 74:643–646, 1962.

———. Some observations on *Dermatophilus* infection in the Gambia with particular reference to the disease in sheep. In D. H. Lloyd and K. C. Sellers, eds., *Dermatophilus infection in animals and man*, pp. 33–40. New York: Academic Press, 1976.

McClure, H. M., Kaplan, W., Bonner, W. B., and Keeling, M. E. Dermatophilosis in owl monkeys. *Sabouraudia* 9:185–190, 1971.

Migaki, G., and Seibold, H. R. Dermatophilosis in a titi monkey (*Callicebus moloch*). *Am. J. Vet. Res.* 37:1225–1226, 1976.

Montali, R. J., Smith, E. E., Davenport, M., and Bush, M. Dermatophilosis in Australian bearded lizards. *J. Am. Vet. Med. Assoc.* 167:553–555, 1975.

Munz, E. Gleichzeitiges auftratan von orf und streptothricose bei ziegen und schafen in Kenya. *Berl.
Muench. Tieraerztl. Wochenschr.* 82:221–226,
1969.

Newman, M. S., Cook, R. W., Appelhof, W. K., and
Kitchen, H. Dermatophilosis in two polar bears.
J. Am. Vet. Med. Assoc. 167:561–564, 1975.

Nicolet, J., Klingler, K., and Fey, H. *Dermatophilus
congolensis,* agent of streptothricosis in chamois.
Pathol. Microbiol. 30:831–837, 1967.

O'Hara, P. J., and Cordes, D. O. Granulomata caused
by *Dermatophilus* in two cats. *N.Z. Vet. J.*
11:151–154, 1965.

Oppong, E. N. W. Epizootiology of *Dermatophilus*
infection in cattle in the Accra plains of Ghana.
In D. H. Lloyd and K. C. Sellers, eds., *Dermatophilus infection in animals and man.* pp.
17–32. New York: Academic Press, 1976.

Pier, A. C., Richard, J. L., and Farrell, E. F. Fluorescent antibody and cultural techniques in cutaneous streptothricosis. *Am. J. Vet. Res.*
25:1014–1020, 1964.

Plowright, W. Cutaneous streptothricosis of cattle: I.
Introduction and epizootiologic features in Nigeria. *Vet. Rec.* 68:350–355, 1956.

Plowright, W., and Ferris, R. D. Papular stomatitis of
cattle in Kenya and Nigeria. *Vet. Rec.*
71:717–723, 1959.

Provost, A., Touade, M. P., Guillame, M., Peleton, H.,
and Damsou, F. Vaccination trails against bovine dermatophilosis in southern Chad. In D. H.
Lloyd and K. C. Sellers, eds., *Dermatophilus
infection in animals and man,* pp. 260–268.
New York: Academic Press, 1976.

Pulliam J. D., Kelley, D. C., and Coles, E. H. Immunologic studies of natural and experimental cutaneous streptothricosis infections in cattle. *Am.
J. Vet. Res.* 28:447–455, 1967.

Richard, J. L., and Pier, A. C. Transmission of *Dermatophilus congolensis* by *Stomoxys calcitrans*
and *Musca domestica. Am. J. Vet. Res.*
27:419–423, 1966.

Richard, J. L., Pier, A. C., and Cysewski, S. J. Experimentally induced canine dermatophilosis.
Am. J. Vet. Res. 34:797–799, 1973.

Richard, J. L., Ritchie, A. E., and Pier, A. C. Electron
microscopic anatomy of motile-phase and ger-
minating cells of *Dermatophilus congolensis. J.
Gen. Microbiol.* 49:23–29, 1967.

Richard, J. L., and Shotts, E. B. Wildlife reservoirs of
dermatophilosis. In L. A. Page, ed., *Wildlife diseases,* pp. 205–214. New York: Plenum, 1976.

Richard, J. L., Thurston, J. R., and Pier, A. C. Comparison of antigens of *Dermatophilus congolensis* isolates and their use in serological tests in
experimental and natural infections. In D. H.
Lloyd and K. C. Sellers, eds., *Dermatophilus
infection in animals and man,* pp. 216–228. New
York: Academic Press, 1976.

Roberts, D. S. An approach to the control of mycotic
dermatitis. *Wool Tech. Sheep Breed.* 9:101–103,
1962.

————. The influence of delayed hypersensitivity on
the course of infection with *Dermatophilus congolensis. Br. J. Exp. Pathol.* 47:9–16, 1966a.

————. The treatment of lumpy wool. *Wool Tech.
Sheep Breed.* 13:65–67, 1966b.

————. Chemotherapy of epidermal infection with
Dermatophilus congolensis. J. Comp. Pathol.
77:129–136, 1967a.

————. *Dermatophilus* infection. *Vet. Bull.* 37:
513–521, 1967b.

Roberts, D. S., and Graham, N. P. H. Control of ovine
cutaneous actinomycosis. *Aust. Vet. J.* 42:74–78,
1966.

Salkin, I. F., Gordon, M. A., and Stone, W. B. Dual
infection of a white-tailed deer by *Dermatophilus congolensis* and *Alternaria alternata. J. Am.
Vet. Med. Assoc.* 167:571–573, 1975.

————. Dermatophilosis among wild raccoons in New
York state. *J. Am. Vet. Med. Assoc.* 169:949–
951, 1976.

Shotts, E. B., and Kistner, T. Naturally occurring
cutaneous streptothricosis in a cottontail rabbit.
J. Am. Vet. Med. Assoc. 157:667–670, 1970.

Simmons, G. C., Sullivan, N. D., and Greer, P. E.
Dermatophilosis in a lizard (*Amphibolurus bar-
batus*). *Aust. Vet. J.* 48:465–466, 1972.

Simpson, B. H., and Cuming, G. An unusual case of
dermatophilosis in a calf. *N.Z. Vet. J.* 24:21–22,
1976.

Smith, C. F., and Cordes, D. O. Dermatitis caused by
Dermatophilus congolensis infection in polar
bears (*Thalactos maritimus*). *Brt. Vet. J.*
128:366–371, 1972.

Soliman, K. N., and Rollinson, D. H. L. Mycotic infection of the skin of the turkey. *Vet. Rec.*
63:20–24, 1951.

Stewart, G. H. Dermatophilosis: A skin disease of
animals and man (pt. I). *Vet. Rec.* 91:537–544,
1972a.

————. Dermatophilosis: A skin disease of animals
and man (pt. II). *Vet. Rec.* 91:555-561, 1972b.

Stone, W. B., Salkin, I. F., and Gordon, M. A. Dermatophilosis in wild raccoons (*Procyon lotor*). *Abstr.
Annu. Meet. Am. Soc. Microbiol.* p. 93, 1975.

Vandemaele, F. P. Enquete sur la streptothricose
cutanee en Afrique. *Bull. Epizoot. Dis. Afr.*
9:251–258, 1961.

Van Saceghem, R. Etude complimentaire sur la der-
matose contagieuse (impetigo contagieux). *Bull.
Soc. Pathol. Exot.* 10:290–293, 1916.

Wilson, T. M., Dykes, R. W., and Tsai, K. S. Pox in
young captive harbor seals. *J. Am. Vet. Med.
Assoc.* 161:611–617, 1972.

Wobeser, G., and Gordon, M. A. *Dermatophilus* infection in Columbian ground squirrels. *Bull. Wildl.
Dis. Assoc.* 5:31–32, 1969.

Yedloutschnig, R. J., Breese, S. S., Hess, W. R., Dar-
dairi, A. H., Taylor, W. D., Barnes, D. M., Page,
R. W., and Reubke, H. J. Bovine herpes mam-
millitis-like disease diagnosed in the United
States. *Proc. U.S. Anim. Health Assoc.*
74:208–212, 1971.

33 *Tyzzer's Disease*

G. WOBESER

Synonyms: **Errington's disease, hemorrhagic disease of muskrats, megaloileitis of rats, wet-tail of hamsters, focal bacterial hepatitis of foals.**

Tyzzer's disease (TD), caused by a pleomorphic spore-forming, gram-negative, intracellular bacterium (*Bacillus piliformis*), produces enterocolitis and focal hepatic necrosis in a wide range of laboratory, domestic, and wild mammals. Epizootics can occur as well as inapparent infections that may result in clinical disease when such animals are stressed.

HISTORY AND DISTRIBUTION. Tyzzer (1917) described an acute, fatal, epizootic disease of Japanese waltzing mice (*Mus musculus*) characterized by the occurrence of unusual intracellular bacteria within hepatocytes and intestinal epithelial cells surrounding foci of necrosis. The disease is now known to occur in laboratory mice throughout the world. It was reported in laboratory rabbits by Allen et al. (1965), and cases have since been reported in a wide variety of laboratory rodents as well as cats, dogs, horses, and rhesus monkeys. The first report of TD in a wild mammal was by Karstad et al. (1971), who identified the disease in muskrats (*Ondatra zibethica*) in Ontario and described similarities between the disease and Errington's disease of muskrats. TD has subsequently been diagnosed in muskrats in Connecticut (Hall and Van Kruiningen 1974), British Columbia (Chalmers and MacNeil 1977), and Saskatchewan (Wobeser et al. 1978), and in captive coyotes (*Canis latrans*) in Kansas (Marler and Cook 1976). Ganaway et al. (1976) detected antibody to *B. piliformis* in wild cottontail rabbits (*Sylvilagus floridanus*) in Maryland and were able to infect cottontails with *B. piliformis* of domestic rabbit origin. Takagaki et al. (1966) produced TD experimentally in the red mouse (*Clethrionomys glareolus*) with material from laboratory mice.

Errington (1946) reported an epizootic disease in Iowa muskrats characterized by hemorrhagic enteritis and focal hepatic necrosis; he termed the condition "hemorrhagic disease." Epizootics attributed to this disease (Errington's disease) have been recognized in Iowa, Maryland, Michigan, Wisconsin, Ohio, Oregon, Montana, Idaho, Wyoming, Ontario, Manitoba, Saskatchewan, British Columbia, and the McKenzie delta of the Northwest Territories (Errington 1963). The etiology of Errington's disease was unknown, although Errington suspected a virus and Lord et al. (1956) suggested that a *Clostridium* spp. was involved. Karstad et al. (1971) proposed that Tyzzer's and Errington's diseases were synonymous, a hypothesis supported by Wobeser et al. (1978). When histologic material from muskrats found dead in Iowa in 1947 by Errington was reexamined, lesions typical of TD were found (Wobeser et al. 1979).

It has been proposed that TD is the cause of wet-tail in hamsters (Nakayama et al. 1975) and megaloileitis in rats (Jonas et al. 1970), and that an acute enteritis of captive cottontails described by Richter and Hendren (1969) might be due to TD (Van Kruiningen and Blodgett 1971).

ETIOLOGY. The name *Bacillus piliformis*, applied to the agent seen in mice by Tyzzer (1917), has been used for the bacteria seen in TD of all species; however, the taxonomic status and the relationships among the organisms seen in various species require further study. The vegetative form of *B. piliformis* is highly unstable, and despite vigorous attempts at isolation, there is no good evidence that the organism has been cultured in cell-free media. The reported isolation by Kanazawa and Imai (1959) has not been confirmed by others (Ganaway et al. 1971a), and the identity of the organism isolated by Simon (1977) was not confirmed by animal inoculation.

The agent can be cultivated in embryonated eggs and transmitted by serial animal inoculation. The vegetative form is a slender bacillus approximately 0.5 μ by 8–10 μ, with occasional forms up to 40 μ long (Ganaway et al. 1971a), arranged in parallel or criss-cross bundles within host cells. The organisms are difficult to detect in routine histologic preparations as they stain only faintly basophilic, if at all, with hematoxylin and eosin and are either nonreactive or faintly gram-negative with

Gram stain. The organism is stained by strongly basic aniline dyes (Giemsa, thionine, methylene blue) and is periodic acid Schiff positive, but silver impregnation techniques (Warthin-Starry, Warthin-Faulkner, Gomori methenamine silver, Levaditi) are best for the demonstration of organisms in tissue. The organism often appears beaded or irregularly stained in tissue, and occasionally larger cells with subterminal swelling are seen. Spores are recognized infrequently in tissue. The organism is motile by peritrichous flagellae (Craigie 1966a; Fujiwara et al. 1968). The ultrastructure of the organism has been described (Goto et al. 1974; Fujiwara et al. 1963; Kuroshina and Fujiwara 1972; McLeod et al. 1977; Pulley and Shivelly 1974).

EPIZOOTIOLOGY. The original description of TD in mice was of a highly fatal epizootic disease, and similar epizootics have been reported in other species. However, inapparent enzootic infection is probably more common than overt epizootic disease. The occurrence of subclinical infection is indicated by the high prevalence of antibodies to *B. piliformis* in laboratory animal colonies in the absence of detectable disease (Fries 1977, 1978; Fujiwara 1967). The presence of latent infection is implied by the occurrence of clinical disease among animals stressed by poor environmental conditions or by the administration of corticosteroids (Takagaki et al. 1967). Based on field observations, Errington (1963) suggested that changes in the prevalence of hemorrhagic disease were due to changes in the resistance of the muskrat population; the occurrence of TD in muskrats shortly after capture suggests activation of a latent infection by stress (Chalmers and MacNeil 1977; Karstad et al. 1971).

Natural transmission likely occurs through the ingestion of spores from an environment contaminated by the feces of infected animals. Bedding contaminated during an epizootic in mice remained infectious for 1 year at room temperature (Tyzzer 1917), and material collected from a natural focus of TD in muskrats (Wobeser et al. 1978) was infective after 16 months at −10°C. Errington (1954) reported that some hot spots (foci of infection) retained infectiousness for at least 5 years in the total absence of muskrats. The outcome of peroral infection depends upon the number of spores ingested, the pathogenicity of the organism, and the resistance of the host as influenced by immunity from prior exposure (Fujiwara et al. 1965) and less specific factors such as nutritional state and diet (Maejima et al. 1965), age, genetic factors, and the presence of intercurrent disease or various stressors. Errington (1946) believed the incubation period of hemorrhagic disease to be 7–8 days, and muskrats died 5–10 days after intragastric inoculation of contaminated bedding material (G. Wobeser, unpublished data). Usually TD is a disease of young or weanling animals; however, all ages of muskrat are affected. Any stressful factor may predispose the animals to the disease, and simultaneous administration of corticosteroids is often required for reliable experimental transmission.

Transmission by cannibalism has been suggested (Fujiwara et al. 1973), and transplacental infection has been documented in experimentally infected mice (Fries 1978). Although interspecies spread can be accomplished experimentally, there are no reports of natural interspecific spread.

SIGNS. In most species clinical TD occurs as an acute disease, and no premonitory signs are seen. If, during the short clinical course, signs are seen, they include diarrhea, depression, anorexia, and a rough hair coat. Melena, uncommon in laboratory animals, occurs in both cottontail rabbits (Ganaway et al. 1976) and muskrats (Chalmers and MacNeil 1977; Wobeser et al. 1978).

PATHOGENESIS AND PATHOLOGY. TD is primarily an enteric infection with spread to the liver via the portal system (Tyzzer 1917). The combination of enteric and hepatic lesions is a feature of the spontaneous disease in all species, although the severity and prevalence of the lesions may vary. Enteric lesions may occur without hepatic involvement (Mullink 1968; Nakayama et al. 1975; Takagaki et al. 1966). The location and extent of enteric lesions varies among species, but the cecum, colon, and terminal ileum are affected most commonly. Nakayama et al. (1976) reported hepatic lesions following inoculation of *B. piliformis* into the ligated cecal sac of hamsters. Myocardial lesions have been reported in mice (Craigie 1966b), domestic rabbits (Allen et al. 1965), hamsters (Zook et al. 1977), rats (Fries and Svendsen 1978), horses (Whitwell 1976), and cottontail rabbits (Ganaway et al. 1976). Allen et al. (1965) suggested that involvement of intestinal lymphatics could lead to direct extension to the heart. A terminal bacteremia occurs, probably as a result of release of organisms from the liver (Takagaki and Fujiwara 1968).

The gross lesions are variable among species, but enteritis is usually present. In muskrats there is an ulcerative necrotizing colitis and typhlitis with extensive intramural and subserosal edema and hemorrhage. The content may be fluid and usually contains fresh blood. Hepatic lesions are similar in all species with variable numbers of discrete white foci, 1–3 mm in diameter, within the hepatic parenchyma. In those species having cardiac involvement, gross lesions appear as white streaks or foci within the myocardium. The lungs are congested and pneumonia may be present. The mesenteric lymph nodes may be swollen, hyperemic, and edematous, but focal necrosis, which is common in diseases such as tularemia, is not found in either the lymph nodes or spleen. Muskrats dead of TD usually have food in the stomach.

Histologically there may be epithelial necrosis and ulceration in the intestine with necrosis, hemorrhage, and edema of the underlying lamina propria, submucosa, and muscular layers. Organisms may be found in epithelial and muscle cells. The hepatic lesions vary with chronicity from foci of acute coagulation necrosis with only a few attendant granulocytes to fibrotic scars surrounded by histiocytes and occasional giant cells. Organisms are found in apparently viable hepatocytes about the margin of acute lesions but may be absent in more chronic cases (Ganaway et al, 1971a). The number of bacteria evident in cells seems to vary among species; for example, large numbers are seen in horses, but relatively few are found in muskrats.

DIAGNOSIS. The definitive diagnosis of TD depends upon the histologic demonstration of *B. piliformis* within host cells, in association with suitable lesions. As the organism is not readily visible with ordinary stains, appropriate techniques must be used for diagnosis. The location, morphology, and tinctorial properties of the organism are all important for identification, and the ultrastructural morphology, particularly the presence of peritrichous flagellae, is also useful.

Hepatic tissue is routinely used for examination; however, not all animals develop hepatic lesions, so intestinal tissue should also be examined. Routine techniques for the isolation of other agents should be conducted to rule out concurrent infection.

The organism may be cultivated in the yolk sac of embryonated eggs (Craigie 1966a; Ganaway et al. 1971b; Zook et al. 1977), and the disease has been transmitted to susceptible animals by peroral and parenteral routes (Ganaway et al. 1971a). Transmission attempts may be complicated by the unstable nature of the vegetative form of *B. piliformis* and by the occurrence of either immunity to, or subclinical infection with, *B. piliformis* in the experimental animals.

Fluorescent antibody techniques have been developed for the diagnosis of TD in laboratory animals (Fries 1977, 1978; Savage and Lewis 1972), and a number of techniques are available for the demonstration of serum antibodies (Fries 1977; Fujiwara 1967, 1971; Ganaway et al. 1976).

TREATMENT AND CONTROL. No suitable measures exist for the control of TD in wild animals, and Fujiwara (1971) has indicated the problems involved in controlling the disease in laboratory animal colonies. Ganaway et al. (1971a) suggested that cesarean-derived animals should be free of the disease; however, Fries (1978) and Fries and Svendsen (1978) have demonstrated widespread occurrence of TD in specific pathogen-free laboratory animal colonies and have shown that transplacental infection can occur.

The antibiotic sensitivity of *B. piliformis* has been highly variable, but there is general agreement that the tetracyclines are effective for treatment (Shoenbaum and Kariv 1976; Takagaki et al. 1964; Van Kruiningen and Blodgett 1971; Yokoiyama and Fujiwara 1971), whereas chloramphenicol is ineffective (Ganaway et al. 1971a; Karstad et al. 1971) or effective only at high dosage (Yokoiyama and Fujiwara 1971). Various sulfa drugs are either ineffective (Yokoiyama and Fujiwara 1971) or may potentiate the disease (Chalmers and MacNeil 1977; Ganaway et al. 1971a).

REFERENCES

Allen, A. M., Ganaway, J. R., Moore, T. D., and Kinard, R. F. Tyzzer's disease syndrome in laboratory rabbits. *Am. J. Pathol.* 46:859–882, 1965.

Chalmers, G. A., and MacNeil, A. C. Tyzzer's disease in wild-trapped muskrats in British Columbia. *J. Wildl. Dis.* 13:114–116, 1977.

Craigie, J. "*Bacillus piliformis*" (Tyzzer) and Tyzzer's disease of the laboratory mouse: I. Propagation of the organism in embryonated eggs. *Proc. R. Soc. Lond. [Biol.]* 165:35–60, 1966a.

———. "*Bacillus piliformis*" (Tyzzer) and Tyzzer's disease of the laboratory mouse: II. Mouse pathogenicity of *B. piliformis* grown in embryonated eggs. *Proc. R. Soc. Lond. [Biol.]* 165:61–77, 1966b.

Errington, P. L. Special report on muskrat diseases. *Iowa Coop. Wildl. Res. Unit Q. Rep.* 1946.

———. The special responsiveness of minks to epizootics in muskrat populations. *Ecol. Monogr.* 24:377–393, 1954.

———. *Muskrat populations.* Ames: Iowa State University Press, 1963.

Fries, A. S. Studies on Tyzzer's disease: Application of immunofluorescence for detection of *Bacillus piliformis* and for demonstration and determination of antibodies to it in sera from mice and rabbits. *Lab. Anim.* 11:69–73, 1977.

———. Demonstration of antibodies to *Bacillus piliformis* in SPF colonies and experimental transplacental infection by *Bacillus piliformis* in mice. *Lab. Anim.* 12:23–26, 1978.

Fries, A. S., and Svendson, O. Studies on Tyzzer's disease in rats. *Lab. Anim.* 12:1–4, 1978.

Fujiwara, K. Complement fixation reaction and agar gel double diffusion test in Tyzzer's disease of mice. *Jpn. J. Microbiol.* 11:103–117, 1967.

———. Problems in checking inapparent infections in laboratory mouse colonies: An attempt at serological checking by anamnestic response. In *Defining the laboratory animal.* Washington, D.C.: National Academy of Science, 1971.

Fujiwara, K., Fukuda, S., Takagaki, Y., and Tajima, Y. Tyzzer's disease in mice: Electron microscopy of the liver lesions. *Jpn. J. Exp. Med.* 33:203–212, 1963.

Fujiwara, K., Hirano, N., Takenaka, S., and Sato, K. Peroral infection in Tyzzer's disease of mice. *Jpn. J. Exp. Med.* 43:33–42, 1973.

Fujiwara, K., Kurashina, H., Maejima, K., Tajima, Y., Takagaki, Y., and Naiki, M. Actively induced immune resistance to the experimental Tyzzer's disease of mice. *Jpn. J. Exp. Med.* 35:259–275, 1965.

Fujiwara, K., Kurashina, H., Matsunuma, N., and Takahashi, R. Demonstration of peritrichous flagella of Tyzzer's disease organism. *Jpn. J. Microbiol.* 12:361–363, 1968.

Ganaway, J. R., Allen, A. M., and Moore, T. D. Tyzzer's disease. *Am. J. Pathol.* 64:717–730, 1971a.

———. Tyzzer's disease of rabbits: Isolation and propagation of *Bacillus piliformis* (Tyzzer) in embryonated eggs. *Infect. Immun.* 3:429–437, 1971b.

Ganaway, J. R., McReynolds, R. S., and Allen, A. M. Tyzzer's disease in free-living cottontail rabbits (*Sylvilagus floridanus*) in Maryland. *J. Wildl. Dis.* 12:545–549, 1976.

Goto, N., Oghiso, Y., Lee, Y. -S., Takahashi, R., and Fujiwara, K. Fine structure of the Tyzzer's organism in the feline liver. *Jpn. J. Exp. Med.* 44:373–378, 1974.

Hall W. C., and Van Kruiningen, H. J. Tyzzer's disease in a horse. *J. Am. Vet. Med. Assoc.* 164:1187–1189, 1974.

Jonas, A. M., Percy, D. H., and Craft, J. Tyzzer's disease in the rat: Its possible relationship with megaloileitis. *Arch. Pathol.* 90:516–528, 1970.

Kanazawa, K., and Imai, A. Pure culture of the pathogenic agent of Tyzzer's disease of mice. *Nature* 184:1810–1811, 1959.

Karstad, L., Lusis, P., and Wright, D. Tyzzer's disease in muskrats. *J. Wildl. Dis.* 7:96–99, 1971.

Kuroshina, H., and Fujiwara, K. Fine structure of the mouse liver infected with Tyzzer's organism. *Jpn. J. Exp. Med.* 42:139–142, 1972.

Lord, G. H., Todd, A. C., Kabat, C., and Mathiak, H. Studies on Errington's disease in muskrats: II. Etiology. *Am. J. Vet. Res.* 17:307–310, 1956.

McLeod, C. G., Stookey, J. L., Harrington, D. G., and White, J. D. Intestinal Tyzzer's disease and spirochetosis in a guinea pig. *Vet. Pathol.* 14:229–235, 1977.

Maejima, K., Fujiwara, K., Takagaki, Y., Naiki, M., Kurashina, H., and Tajimas, Y. Dietetic effects on experimental Tyzzer's disease of mice. *Jpn. J. Exp. Med.* 35:1–10, 1965.

Marler, R. J., and Cook, J. E. Tyzzer's disease in two coyotes. *J. Am. Vet. Med. Assoc.* 169:940–941, 1976.

Mullink, J. W. M. A. Tyzzer's disease: Intestinal lesions in both S.P.F. and conventional mice, 2. *Versuchstierk. Bd.* 10:271–284, 1968.

Nakayama, M., Machii, K., Goto, Y., and Fujiwara, K. Typhlohepatitis in hamsters infected perorally with the Tyzzer's organism. *Jpn. J. Exp. Med.* 46:309–324, 1976.

Nakayama, M., Saegusa, J., Itoh, K., Kiuchi, Y., Tamura, T., Ueda, K., and Fujiwara, K. Transmissable enterocolitis in hamsters caused by Tyzzer's organism. *Jpn. J. Exp. Med.* 45:33–41, 1975.

Pulley, L. T., and Shively, J. N. Tyzzer's disease in a foal: Light- and electron-microscopic observations. *Vet. Pathol.* 11:203–211, 1974.

Richter, C. B., and Hendren, R. L. The pathology and epidemiology of acute enteritis in captive cottontail rabbits (*Sylvilagus floridanus*). *Pathol. Vet.* 6:159–175, 1969.

Savage, N. L., and Lewis, D. H. Application of immunofluorescence to detection of Tyzzer's disease agent (*Bacillus piliformis*) in experimentally infected mice. *Am. J. Vet. Res.* 33:1007–1011, 1972.

Shoenbaum, M., and Kariv, N. An outbreak of Tyzzer's disease in a commercial rabbitry in Israel. *Refuah Vet.* 33:26–30, 1976.

Simon, P. C. Isolation of *Bacillus piliformis* from rabbits. *Can. Vet. J.* 18:46–48, 1977.

Takagaki, Y., and Fujiwara, K. Bacteremia in experimental Tyzzer's disease of mice. *Jpn. J. Microbiol.* 12:129–143, 1968.

Takagaki, Y., Ito, M., Fujiwara, K., Maejima, M., Naiki, M., and Tajima, Y. Effets d'antibiotiques et de sulfamides sur la maladie de Tyzzer chez la souris experimentalement infectee. *C. R. Soc. Biol.* 158:414–418, 1964.

Takagaki, Y., Ito, M., Naiki, M., Fujiwara, K., Okugi, M., Maejima, K., and Tajimia, Y. Experimental Tyzzer's disease in different species of laboratory animals. *Jpn. J. Exp. Med.* 36:519–534, 1966.

Takagaki, Y., Naiki, M., Ito, M., Noguchi, G., Fujiwara, K. Checking of corynebacteriosis and Tyzzer's disease in mice by cortisone treatment. *Exp. Anim.* 16:12–19, 1967.

Tyzzer, E. E. A fatal disease of the Japanese waltzing mouse caused by a spore-bearing bacillus (*Bacillus piliformis*, n.sp.). *J. Med. Res.* 37:307–338, 1917.

Van Kruiningen, H. J., and Blodgett, S. B. Tyzzer's disease in a Connecticut rabbitry. *J. Am. Vet. Med. Assoc.* 158:1205–1212, 1971.

Whitwell, K. E. Four cases of Tyzzer's disease in foals in England. *Equine Vet. J.* 8:118–122, 1976.

Wobeser, G., Hunter, D. B., and Daoust, P. -Y. Tyzzer's disease in muskrats: Occurrence in free-living animals. *J. Wildl. Dis.* 14:325–328, 1978.

Wobeser, G., Barnes, H. J., and Pierce, Kay. Tyzzer's disease in muskrats: Re-examination of specimens of hemorrhagic disease collected by Paul Errington. *J. Wildl. Dis.* 15:525–527, 1979.

Yokoiyama, S., and Fujiwara, K. Effect of antibiotics on Tyzzer's disease. *Jpn. J. Exp. Med.* 41:49–57, 1971.

Zook, B. C., Huang, K., and Rhorer, R. G. Tyzzer's disease in Syrian hamsters. *J. Am. Vet. Med. Assoc.* 171:833–836, 1977.

34 Epizootic Chlamydiosis of Muskrats and Snowshoe Hares

JOSIP SPALATIN   J. O. IVERSEN

Synonyms: **Generic and vernacular synonyms for the genus name Chlamydia are Miyagawanella Brumpt, Bedsonia Meyer, psittacosis-lymphogranuloma venereum agents, psittacosis-lymphogranuloma venereum-trachoma agents.**

Epizootic chlamydiosis is a fatal septicemic disease of muskrats (*Ondatra zibethicus*) and snowshoe hares (*Lepus americanus*) caused by an organism of the genus *Chlamydia* (Page 1966). The only recorded epizootic of the disease occurred during 1959–1961 in the province of Saskatchewan, Canada (Spalatin et al. 1966).

HISTORY. According to Connell (Spalatin et al. 1966), the populations of snowshoe hares and muskrats in north central Saskatchewan appeared to be approaching peak densities in 1959. An excessive number of dead, sick, and malnourished muskrats were found during the winter of 1959–60. Muskrat deaths continued to occur the following winter. By February 1961 sick and dead snowshoe hares were found, and a decline in the hare population was obvious.

During the winter of 1961, 25 carcasses of muskrats and snowshoe hares were collected and examined for the cause of the fatalities, and the causative agent was isolated and identified.

In addition to the muskrats and snowshoe hares, experimental infections with the chlamydial agent were established in other wild species—cottontail rabbits (*Sylvilagus floridanus*), Franklin ground squirrels (*Citellus franklini*), deer mice (*Peromyscus maniculatus*), and mallard ducklings (*Anas platyrhynchos*) (Spalatin, unpublished data, 1969). The broad range of host and tissue pathogenicity of the chlamydial agent suggests it is possible that other wildlife may be involved.

DISTRIBUTION. Epizootic chlamydiosis of muskrats and snowshoe hares has been reported only in Saskatchewan, but there is serologic evidence of the infection in muskrats in the Canadian Arctic and Wisconsin (Iversen et al. 1970).

ETIOLOGY. Chlamydial agents were isolated from both the blood and spleens of the snowshoe hares and muskrats examined. Four isolates were recovered in both embryonating eggs and albino mice. They were considered to be identical on the basis of neutralization tests using the mouse as the test animal. One of the muskrat isolates (strain designated M56) was selected as a prototype and studied in detail. It was identified as a member of the *Chlamydia* on the basis of morphologic and tinctorial properties and on the possession of the group-specific antigen (Spalatin et al. 1966). Although it shared group-specific antigen with the *Chlamydia*, it had unique type-specific cell wall antigens (Fraser 1966).

Further studies have shown that the inclusion bodies are diffuse and glycogen free. The M56 strain is insusceptible to sulfadiazine and d-cycloserine (Spalatin, unpublished data, 1969). Therefore, the M56 strain can be placed in the Gordon and Quan (1965) subgroup type B according to Lin and Moulder (1966) and may be designated *C. psittaci* (Page 1968).

Evidence that chlamydial agents caused the fatalities of muskrats and snowshoe hares in Saskatchewan in 1961 was: (1) recovery of chlamydial agents from the blood of animals found dead of acute disease in areas where the die-off was occurring, (2) demonstration of antibodies in naturally infected muskrats and snowshoe hares, (3) susceptibility of the muskrat and the snowshoe hare to experimental infections with the M56 strain, (4) similarity of lesions in naturally and experimentally infected animals, and (5) reisolation of cultures of *Chlamydia* from naturally and experimentally infected animals. The experimental studies suggest an enzootic infection of muskrats and an epizootic infection of snowshoe hares (Iversen et al. 1970).

TRANSMISSION. Although the method of transmission of the chlamydial agent in nature is unknown, several possible routes merit consideration. Contamination of marsh habitats with the excretions and carcasses of infected animals could provide an efficient means of transmission to marsh dwellers. Experimental infections of muskrats resulted in the shedding of the agent from the intestinal tract. Muskrat houses, nesting sites of birds, or food and water might be sources of infection of susceptible hosts. In connection with the intermingling of various animal species inhabiting marshes, it is interesting to point out certain facts related to the 1942 epidemic of fatal human pneumonitis that occurred in Louisiana (Olson and Treuting 1944). The first person to become diseased earned a living by the trapping and pelting of muskrats from the marshes of coastal Louisiana. Although muskrats were not incriminated as the source of this index case, numerous muskrat fatalities had occurred just preceding the illness of the muskrat trapper. Seven years later it was shown by Rubin (1953) that egrets in the marshes of Louisiana were infected with an agent very similar to that causing the human pneumonitis episode.

When there are peak populations of muskrats and snowshoe hares, contacts could be high enough to ensure transmission. The experimental establishment of oral infections in muskrats and hares suggests a possible means of transmission during epizootics (Iversen et al. 1970). The tendency of both species to consume flesh is well documented (Errington 1963; Seton 1929).

The recovery of the agent from ticks engorging on experimentally infected hares suggests the possibility of the involvement of ticks in the transmission of the M56 strain (Iversen et al. 1970). Meyer (1967) postulates a more widespread involvement of arthropods in the transmission of *Chlamydia* than has been previously suspected.

SIGNS

Muskrat. Muskrats infected by various routes with the M56 strain develop a mild febrile response (1°C rise), malaise, anorexia, and cachexia. The course of the disease may be cyclic, with apparent recovery followed by regression. Erratic behavior may occur (nonresponsiveness to stimuli, hyperexcitability, uncontrolled movements), and nasal discharge and diarrhea were observed. The outcome was dependent on the route of infection. Of 20 muskrats 6 died from the 6th to the 18th day postexposure (Iversen, et al. 1970).

Snowshoe Hare. Snowshoe hares infected by various routes develop a biphasic febrile response (>2°C rise). The fever persists in the hare until shortly before death. With the marked febrile response, the hares become passive but remain alert. Rapid weight loss occurs, although the hares continue to eat. Some animals develop icterus and diarrhea. Lethargy, inappetence, and a marked drop in body temperature occur just before death. The terminal features of the syndrome are opisthotonos and convulsions associated with hypoglycemia. Of 20 hares, 19 died from the 2nd to the 13th day postexposure (Iversen et al. 1970).

PATHOGENESIS

Muskrat. Generalized infection occurred in more than one-half the experimentally infected muskrats, as indicated by the recovery of the M56 strain in high titers from a variety of tissues including the brain, liver, spleen, and small intestine. In animals surviving 90 days or more, the agent was commonly recovered from the brain, although it had disappeared from the liver and spleen. It was also recovered in the contents of the small intestine at that time (Iversen et al. 1970).

Snowshoe Hare. The snowshoe hare almost invariably succumbed to experimental M56 infection whether inoculated by the intravenous, subcutaneous, or oral routes. Intravenous infection of the hares with less than 10 mouse intracerebral LD_{50} was fatal. *Chlamydia* were present in the bloodstream in low titer, beginning as early as 48 hours, rose to peak titers of 10_6 mouse $ICLD_{50}$, and remained in the blood until death. By the 3rd day postinfection the agent was found to be widespread in the tissues of the reticuloendothelial system (Iversen et al. 1970).

PATHOLOGY

Muskrat. During the epizootic the gross lesions of the 14 muskrats varied considerably and fell into two categories: (1) well-nourished, fat carcasses with full gastrointestinal tracts but with congested livers, slightly to greatly enlarged spleens, and reddish fluid in the serous cavities, and (2) emaciated carcasses with empty gastrointestinal tracts, livers showing small necrotic areas (0.5–1.5 mm in diameter), spleens of normal size, and fluid in the peritoneal cavity. The first category probably represented acute, rapidly fatal infections, and the second category probably consisted of chronically infected individuals (Iversen et al. 1970).

In experimentally infected muskrats, widely disseminated hepatic necrosis was the most common lesion. Livers were tannish red with white to yellow foci. The foci were 1−4 mm in diameter and irregularly circumscribed. Microscopically, the necrotic foci were characterized by degenerating hepatic cells and leukocytes. Occasionally, fibrinous pericarditis and fibrinous pneumonia were also observed. Granular inclusion bodies were most easily seen in the cytoplasm of inflammatory cells of the alveoli. No lesions were observed in the organs of muskrats sacrificed 30−96 days postexposure (Iversen et al. 1970).

Snowshoe Hare. During the epizootic, the necropsies of 11 snowshoe hares revealed the following: (1) livers congested, with some showing small yellowish necrotic foci on the surface; (2) slight to marked splenomegaly; (3) normal serous fluids; (4) empty stomachs; and (5) severe enteritis (Spalatin et al. 1966).

In experimentally infected snowshoe hares, the striking lesions were hepatomegaly and splenomegaly. Livers were tan to brown and friable. White to yellow foci were scattered on the surface and within the parenchyma of the liver. There was a marked destruction of the parenchyma, and necrosis was evident throughout the lobules. In liver sections taken immediately after death and stained with periodic acid Schiff's stain, glycogen was either absent or greatly reduced. The spleens were at least three times as large as the spleens of controls. They were black and friable, and the pulp bulged from the cut surface. Microscopically, it could be seen that the enlargement was due to an augmentation of the pulp. Many macrophages were seen to contain blood pigment (Iversen et al. 1970).

DIAGNOSIS. Diagnosis of epizootic chlamydiosis in muskrats and snowshoe hares is based primarily upon isolation of the etiologic agent. In natural infections the agent is obtained from the blood and spleens of dead animals. In experimentally induced latent infections the best sources of the agent are the brain, the iris and ciliary body of the eye, and the joints (Iversen, unpublished data, 1969). The unfrozen tissues should be ground as 10% suspension in a suitable medium such as tryptone broth. Streptomycin or kannamycin may be added to the suspension; however, penicillin must be avoided. If it is necessary to store tissues before attempting an isolation, the tissues should be kept at either +4 or −60°C due to the relative stability of the M56 agent at these temperatures. Suspensions should be inoculated intracerebrally into 18-day-old to 21-day-old weanling albino mice. The use of antibiotics is to be avoided in the food and water of the mice. The mice should be observed for at least 21 days. Seven-day-old chick embryos may also be inoculated via the yolk sac with suspensions. Eggs should be observed for at least 10 days (Spalatin, unpublished data, 1969). If mortality is observed in the mice or eggs, a standard procedure for identification of *Chlamydia* should be followed (Page 1968). The sections of infected yolk sacs or impression smears of tissues could be stained and then examined microscopically for the specific inclusions.

The hepatic lesions produced by the chlamydial agent could present a problem of differential diagnosis. In muskrats similar lesions are caused by *Eimeria* spp., *Salmonella typhimurium*, and *Francisella tularensis*. Liver necrosis is also found in Errington's disease, along with intestinal and pulmonary hemorrhages (Errington 1963). Although liver necrosis was observed in muskrats experimentally infected with the M56 strain, the hemorrhagic element of Errington's disease was not produced (Iversen et al. 1970).

There are similarities between the syndrome and pathology produced by the M56 strain and other diseases reported in snowshoe hares. Similarities between the chlamydiosis of the hare and shock disease of the hare are emaciation, liver necrosis, and terminal hypoglycemia with opisthotonos and convulsions. However, shock disease is nontransmissible and is accompanied by atrophy of the liver and spleen (Green and Larson 1938). When liver necrosis is observed in the hare, differentiation of the chlamydiosis from listeriosis or tularemia requires cultivation and identification of the etiologic agent (Iversen 1968).

IMMUNITY. Little is known of the natural immunity to chlamydial agents in wild populations of muskrats and snowshoe hares. However, there is evidence that specific complement fixing and serum neutralizing antibodies existed in muskrats in locations where the epizootics occurred. The virulence of this agent for snowshoe hares could partially explain the absence of antibodies in the hare. Specific immunologic responses were obtained regularly in most of the experimentally exposed muskrats. The detection of specific antibody could serve as an indicator of previous and/or current infection (Iversen et al. 1970).

TREATMENT AND CONTROL. The use of tetracycline compounds is most effective for the treatment and prevention of chlamydial infections in man and domestic animals, and it could be inferred that such would be the case in wild animals. Protracted treatment with large doses may be required to eliminate chronic infections.

The incompleteness of epizootiologic information on chlamydiosis in nature makes it impossible at this time to propose control measures (Spalatin, unpublished data, 1969).

REFERENCES

Errington, P. L. *Muskrat populations.* Ames: Iowa State University Press, 1963.

Fraser, C. E. O. Ph.D. thesis, University of Wisconsin, 1966.

Gordon, F. B., and Quan, L. L. Occurrence of glycogen in inclusions of psittacosis-lymphogranuloma venereum-trachoma agents. *J. Infect. Dis.* 115:186–196, 1965.

Green, R. G., and Larson, C. L. A description of shock disease in the snowshoe hare. *Am. J. Hyg.* 28:190–212, 1938.

Iversen, J. O. Ph.D. thesis, University of Wisconsin, 1968.

Iversen, J. O., Spalatin, J., Fraser, C. E. O., Hanson, R. P., and Berman, D. T. The susceptibility of muskrats and snowshoe hares to experimental infection with a chlamydial agent. *Can. J. Comp. Med.* 34:80–89, 1970.

Lin, H., and Moulder, J. W. Patterns of response to sulfadiazine, d-cycloserine, and d-alanine in members of the psittacosis group. *J. Infect. Dis.* 116:372–376, 1966.

Meyer, K. F. The host spectrum of psittacosis-lymphogranuloma venereum (PL) agents. *Am. J. Ophthalmol.* 63:1225–1246, 1967.

Meyer, K. F., and Eddie, B. Psittacosis-lymphogranuloma venereum group (Bedsonia infections). In *Diagnostic procedures for virus and rickettsial diseases,* 3d ed., pp. 603–639. New York: Am. Public Health Assoc., 1964.

Olson, B. J., and Treuting, W. L. An epidemic of a severe pneumonitis in the bayou region of Louisiana: I. Epidemiological study. *Public Health Rep.* 59:1299–1311, 1944.

Page, L. A. Revision of the family Chlamydiaceae Rake (rickettsiales): Unification of the psittacosis-lymphogranuloma venereum-trachoma group of organisms in the genus *Chlamydia* Jones, Rake and Stearns, 1945. *Int. J. System. Bacteriol.* 16:223–253, 1966.

———. Proposal for the recognition of two species in the genus *Chlamydia* Jones, Rake and Stearns, 1945. *Int. J. System, Bacteriol.* 18:51–66, 1968.

Rubin, H. A disease in captive egrets caused by a virus of the psittacosis-lymphogranuloma venereum group. *J. Infect. Dis.* 94:1–8, 1953.

Seton, E. T. *Lives of game animals,* vol. 4. New York: Doubleday, 1929.

Spalatin, J., Fraser, C. E. O., Connell, R., Hanson, R. P., and Berman, D. T. Agents of psittacosis-lymphogranuloma venereum group isolated from muskrats and snowshoe hares in Saskatchewan. *Can. J. Comp. Med. Vet. Sci.* 30:64–69, 1966.

35 *Histoplasmosis*

VANCE L. SANGER

Synonyms: **Darling's disease, reticuloendo-theliosis, reticuloendothelial cytomycosis.**

Histoplasmosis is a mycotic infection caused by *Histoplasma capsulatum*. The reticuloendothelial system is primarily involved even when the infection is generalized. Wild and domestic animals as well as humans are susceptible to infection. Birds are less readily infected or not at all. The organism lives as a saprophyte in soil, from which most infections occur.

HISTORY. Histoplasmosis was first reported in a man from the Panama Canal Zone by Darling (1906). He recognized that the organism in the tissues was different from any other he had seen, but he was not certain of its classification. He proposed the name *Histoplasma capsulata*. Between 1906 and 1934, several other human cases were recognized as being the same disease. In 1934, DeMonbreun isolated the causative organism, cultivated it on laboratory media, and reproduced the disease in two monkeys. DeMonbreun (1939) isolated the organism for the first time from a dog, in 1949 it was recovered for the first time from soil (Emmons et al. 1949), and since then it has been recovered many times from soil (Emmons et al. 1955; Menges et al. 1967; Murdock et al. 1962; Taylor and Shacklette 1962; Zeidberg et al. 1952). The first reports of its isolation from wild animals were by Emmons et al. (1947) and Olson et al. (1947). They cultured *Histoplasma* from house mice (*Mus musculus*) and from 10 of 222 wild rats (*Rattus norvegicus*) (Emmons et al. 1947). In this study by Emmons et al. (1947) a total of 1,620 animals, mostly rodents, were examined.

DISTRIBUTION AND HOST RANGE. The distribution of *H. capsulatum* is worldwide and is found in both temperate and tropical zones. A large and diverse number of species, both wild and domestic, have been detected with the disease (Kaplan 1973). Birds and bats are responsible for transmitting or introducing the organism to an area (Schwarz and Kauffman 1977). Bats are the only known mammal to

excrete the organism in a medium in which it can propagate itself (Isbister et al. 1976). One report suggested that tornadoes help disseminate the organism.

Histoplasmosis is endemic in the central United States, and many cases have been reported from Central America and South America. In Mexico, *H. capsulatum* was found primarily in caves, abandoned mines, and houses where bat guano was found (Velasco-Castrejon and Gonzalez-Ochoa 1977). Altogether, it has been reported from more than 30 countries (Conant et al. 1971; Negroni 1965; Smith et al. 1972). Kreske and Swieconek (1971) have published a comprehensive bibliography on *H. capsulatum* and *H. duboisii*.

The host range of *H. capsulatum* includes a wide variety of mammals. In some investigations large numbers of the same species have been examined; in others a single member of a species may be listed. For example, some reports included large numbers of rats, mice, and bats, because these three species were trapped and examined extensively in efforts to find natural hosts and reservoirs. A report on a single member of a species frequently represents an accidental finding. In addition to a wide variety of wild animals, dogs, cats, humans, horses, and cows are susceptible (Conant et al. 1971; Menges and Kintner 1951; Menges et al. 1963; Richman 1948; Smith et al. 1972).

Histoplasma capsulatum has been recovered from a variety of wild or captive animals (Table 35.1).

A captive ferret which had been used for hunting rats and rabbits had parasitic organisms in liver, spleen, and lung cells. Levine et al. (1938) did not identify the organism as *H. capsulatum*, but based on its appearance in cells in the photomicrograph, Negroni (1965) suggested it might be spontaneous histoplasmosis. However, in the same study, 18 reptiles and 48 birds were negative. Oels et al. (1969) tested serums from 127 wild mammals and birds for antibodies to *H. capsulatum*. Of 96 geese and 12 bats 22 and 7, respectively, were positive for hemagglutinating antibody to *H. capsulatum*. Reports of natural infections in wild birds were not found, although Murdock et al. (1962) re-

TABLE 35.1 Wild and Captive Animals from which *H. capsulatum* Was Recovered.

Common Name	Scientific Name	Number Positive	Number of Animals Examined from Same or Multiple Species	Reference
House mouse	*Mus musculus*	1	936	Emmons et al. 1947
Wild rat	*Rattus norvegicus*	10	222	
Rat	*R. norvegicus*	16	565	Emmons and Ashburn 1948
Brown rat	*R. norvegicus*	7	459	Emmons et al. 1949
Roof rat	*R. rattus*	4	855	
Spotted Skunk	*Spilogale putorius*	5	6	
Rat	*R. norvegicus*	75	2,149	Emmons et al. 1955
Opposum	*Didelphis virginiana*	3	95	
Skunk	*Mephitis mephitis*	2	18	
Mouse	*Mus musculus*	1	988	
Fox	*Urocyon cinereoargenteus*	1	30	
Woodchuck	*Marmota monax*	1	37	
Raccoon	species not given	4	4	Menges et al. 1954
Rat	species not given	3	545	
Skunk	species not given	1	7	
Monkey	species not given	34	1,187	Menges et al. 1967
Bat	*Tadarido brasiliensis mexicana*	8	555	Di Salvo et al. 1969
Bat	*Leptonycteris sanborni*	7	555	
Bat	*Myotis austroriparius*	80	170	Di Salvo et al. 1970
Bat	*Pteronotus rubiginosa* *Carollia perspicillata* *Phyllostomus hastatus*	57	109	Hasenclever et al. 1969
Bat	*C. perspicillata* *Glossophaga soricina* *Molossus* *Phyllostomus hastatus* *Pteronotus rubiginosa* *Tadarida yucatanica*	some animals positive	. . .	Hasenclever et al. 1972
Bat	*Chilonycterus rubiginosa fuscal*	9	30	Shacklette et al. 1962[a]
Bat	*Glossophaga sorcina sorcina*	1	135	Marinkelle and Grose 1965
Bat	*Myotis myotis*	1	. . .	Ajello et al. 1977[b]
Bat	*M. austroriparius*	83	190	Johnson et al. 1970
Bat	*Brachyphylla cavernarum*	1	30	Carvajal Zamora 1977
Bat	*Eptesicus fuscu* *M. austroriparius* *M. grisescens* *M. lucifugus* *M. sodalis* *Nycticeuis humeralis*	154	1,120	Tesch and Schneidau 1967
Bat	*Carollia perspiculata* *Chilonycteris rubiginosa* *Micronycteris megalotis* *Mollosus major* *Glossophaga soricina* *Phyllostomus hastatus*	62	623	Klite and Diercks 1965
Baboon	*Papio papio*	1	. . .	Walker and Spooner 1960
Monkey	*Cynocephalus babuin*	5	. . .	Mariat and Segretain 1956
Monkey	species not given	3	. . .	Courtois et al. 1955
Spring rat	*Proechimys semispinosus*	12	143	Taylor and Schacklette 1962
Common opossum	*Didelphis marsupialis*	7	81	
Four-eyed opossum	*Philander o. fuscogriseus*	4	18	
Rodent	*Proechimys guyanensis*	4	314	Lainson and Shaw 1975
Sloth	*Choloepus didactylus*	1	314	
Mouse	*Mus musculus*	1	886	Olson et al. 1947
Badger	*Meles meles*	1	. . .	Burgisser et al. 1961

[a]Tissues were pooled to facilitate testing; the infection may not have been present in all animals.
[b]Ajello and co-workers included a critical review of all reports concerning the occurrence of *H. capsulatum* and histoplasmosis in the Middle East.

covered *H. capsulatum* from droppings under a starling roost. They did not capture and examine any birds.

A limited amount of research has been conducted on domestic chickens (*Gallus domesticus*) and it will be reviewed briefly because of possible application to other avian species. Zeidberg et al. (1952) tested two groups of domestic chickens intradermally with histoplasmin. The 12 hens in one group did not react serologically, and cultures of their organs were negative. Of a second group of 89 birds, 2 were positive to the intradermal test, but cultures from organs were negative. Menges (1951) tested 98 hens intradermally with histoplasmin and found 1 positive. In addition to chickens, some investigators have used pigeons as experimental animals or have examined them as possible carriers of the organism. Chickens and pigeons can be experimentally infected with *H. capsulatum*. If the organism is given via the intraocular route a severe ophthalmitis develops. Later the organism can be recovered from internal organs by culture (Schwarz and Sethi 1969).

Schwarz et al. (1957) injected 44 pigeons and ten 2-day-old chicks intravenously with about 50,000 viable *H. capsulatum* cells. Another 10 chickens were inoculated intraperitoneally. Organisms were recovered from organs of 5 of 10 chicks injected intravenously, but none from the other group. Of the 44 pigeons 20 were positive.

According to Ajello et al. (1960) domestic fowl do not excrete spores of *H. capsulatum* in their feces. They do not seed soil with fungus, and there is no basis for saying that *H. capsulatum* is carried by birds.

Menges et al. (1954) tested serums for antibodies from 4 chickens, 69 pigeons, 4 crows, 1 quail, and 2 sparrows and all were negative.

Apparently the relationship of *H. capsulatum* to soil mixed with bird droppings is one of a favorable environment for the organism rather than direct contamination from birds.

ETIOLOGY AND DIAGNOSIS. Negroni (1965) listed the name of the causative organism as *H. capsulatum* Darling 1906. It is a fungus with both a mycelial and a yeast phase. In a culture at room temperature, it has a typical moldlike filamentous phase (Conant et al. 1971). Within the cytoplasm of a tissue cell it appears as a small, oval, yeastlike body, $1-5$ μ in diameter; few to many may be present. In hematoxylin-eosin-stained tissue sections the organism ap-

pears as a central, spherical basophilic body, surrounded by an unstained zone and a thin cell wall. The clear halolike zone is part of the wall (Smith et al. 1972). In tissue sections *Histoplasma* must be differentiated from *Toxoplasma* organisms seen in pseudocysts.

Incubation of the organism on 5% rabbit blood agar at 30°C produces a mycelial growth which is thick, dirty white, and moist in consistency. Incubation at 28°C on Sabouraud dextrose agar produces aerial mycelia which are abundant, cottony white, and without a fluffy border. The reverse side is uncolored (Negroni 1965).

Suspected material should be cultured on brain-heart infusion glucose blood agar at 37°C or on Sabouraud glucose agar slants at room temperature. The latter should have antibiotics added (Beneke and Rogers 1970). In tissue sections the organism can be stained with hematoxylin and eosin, Gomori methenamine silver nitrate, periodic acid-Schiff, or Gridley fungus stain (Smith et al. 1972). Slide mounts can be made of either the mycelial or yeast phase to be examined under the microscope, and fresh touch preparations can be prepared from suspected tissue and stained with Wright or Giemsa stain (Beneke and Rogers 1970). Organisms have been cultured regularly from liver, spleen, and lung of infected bats and animals.

Laboratory animals—including guinea pigs, rats, white mice, dogs, and monkeys—are susceptible to infection with either the yeast phase or the filamentous phase (Beneke and Rogers 1970).

Antibodies appear in the serum a few weeks after infection in both man and animals. Serologic tests have been developed which are useful as an aid in diagnosis (Negroni 1965). For a discussion of these tests and cross-reactions that occur with other disease agents see Kaufman (1966).

TRANSMISSION. The infection occurs by inhalation, by ingestion, or by skin contact with infective spores of *H. capsulatum* (Kirk 1977). The infection does not spread from animal to animal or from animal to humans (Ajello et al. 1963). However, the disease may appear in animals and humans from the same vicinity because of their contact with the same environmental source of the organism, that is, the soil (Menges et al. 1967; Negroni 1965; Smith et al. 1972). *Histoplasma capsulatum* occurs naturally and exists as a saprophyte in the soil (Ajello et al. 1963). Organisms have been found in the soil around an animal burrow, and animals which lived in the burrow were positive for *H. capsulatum*.

SIGNS. *Histoplasma* has been recovered from many species of wild animals, but based on the percentage of recoveries of the organism from examinations of thousands of animals, the incidence is remarkably low. Almost without exception, clinical evidence of disease and gross lesions of the infection were absent. *Histoplasma capsulatum* was recovered only because a search was made for the organism.

Commenting on numerous reports of histoplasmosis in a large number of animals, Negroni (1965) stated that in all those animals, there were no macroscopic or microscopic lesions, and the parasite was revealed by the microscopic studies and by cultures. The dog is the only one that develops a progressive and fatal form comparable to human histoplasmosis.

TREATMENT AND CONTROL. Sulfonamides and amphotericin B have been found useful in the treatment of histoplasmosis in man and experimental infections in laboratory animals (Hildick-Smith et al. 1964; Negroni 1965). However, currently, only amphotericin B is recommended (Ausherman 1973; Goodman and Gilman 1970; Kirk 1977).

Since *H. capsulatum* is a natural inhabitant of the soil, is of minor importance in wild mammals, and does not occur in wild birds, control measures do not seem to be urgent and perhaps would not be practical except under limited circumstances, such as in animal quarters or under wild-bird roosts.

REFERENCES

Ajello, L., Briceno-Maaz, T., Campins, H., and Moore, J. C. Isolation of *Histoplasma capsulatum* from an oil bird (*Steatornis caripensis*) cave in Venezuela. *Mycopathol. Mycol. Appl.* 12:199–206, 1960.

Ajello, L., Georg, L. K., Kaplan, W., and Kaufman, L. *Laboratory manual for medical mycology.* Atlanta: Department of Health, Education and Welfare, Communicable Disease Center, 1963.

Ajello, L., Kuttin, E. S., Beemer, A. M., Kaplan, W., and Padhye, A. Occurrence of *Histoplasma capsulatum* Darling, 1906 in Israel, with a review of the current status of histoplasmosis in the Middle East. *Am. J. Trop. Med. Hyg.* 26:140–147, 1977.

Ausherman, R. J. Treatment of blastomycosis and histoplasmosis in the dog. *J. Am. Vet. Med.*

Assoc. 163:1048–1049, 1973.

Beneke, E. S., and Rogers, A. L. *Medical mycology manual*, 3d ed. Minneapolis: Burgess, 1970.

Burgisser, H. von, Fankhauser, R., Kaplen, W., Klingler, K., and Scholer, H. J. Mykose bei einem Dachs in der Schweiz: Histologisch Histoplasmose (Mycosis in a badger in Switzerland: Histological histoplasmosis). *Pathol. Microbiol.* 24:794–802, 1961.

Carvajal Zamora, J. R. Isolation of *Histoplasma capsulatum* from tissues of bats captured in the Aquas Buenos caves, Aquas Buenos, Puerto Rico. *Mycopathologia* 60:167–169, 1977.

Conant, N. F., Smith, D. T., Baker, R. D., and Callaway, J. L. *Manual of clinical mycology*, 3d ed. Philadelphia: Saunders, 1971.

Courtois, G., Segretain, G., Mariat, F., and Levaditi, J. C. Mycose cutanee a corps levuriformes observe chez des singes africains en captivite (Cutaneous mycosis in captive African monkeys caused by a yeast-shaped organism). *Ann. Inst. Pasteur* 89:124–127, 1955.

Darling, S. T. A protozoon general infection producing pseudotubercles in the lungs and focal necrosis in the liver, spleen and lymph nodes. *J. Am. Med. Assoc.* 46:1283–1285, 1906.

DeMonbreun, W. A. The cultivation and cultural characteristics of Darling's *Histoplasma capsulatum*. *Am. J. Trop. Med.* 14:93–125, 1934.

―――. The dog as a natural host for *Histoplasma capsulatum*. *Am. J. Trop. Med.* 19:565–587, 1939.

Di Salvo, A. F., Ajello, L., Palmer, J. W., Jr., and Winkler, W. J. Isolation of *Histoplasma capsulatum* from Arizona bats. *Am. J. Epidemiol.* 89:606–614, 1969.

Di Salvo, A. F., Bigler, W. J., Ajello, L., Johnson, J. E., III, and Palmer, J. Bat and soil studies for sources of histoplasmosis in Florida. *Public Health Rep.* 85:1063–1069, 1970.

Emmons, C. W. Isolation of *Histoplasma capsulatum* from soil. *Public Health Rep.* 64:892–896, 1949.

Emmons, C. W., and Ashburn, L. L. Histoplasmosis in wild rats: Occurrence and histopathology. *Public Health Rep.* 63:1416–1422, 1948.

Emmons, C. W., Bell, J. A., and Olson, B. J. Naturally occurring histoplasmosis in *Mus musculus* and *Rattus norvegicus*. *Public Health Rep.* 62:1642–1646, 1947.

Emmons, C. W., Morlan, H. B., and Hill, E. L. Histoplasmosis in rats and skunks in Georgia. *Public Health Rep.* 64:1423–1430, 1949.

Emmons, C. W., Rowley, D. A., Olson, B. J., Mattern, C. F. T., Bell, J. A., Powell, E., and Marcey, E. A. Histoplasmosis: Proved occurrence of inapparent infection in dogs, cats and other animals. *Am. J. Hyg.* 61:40–44, 1955.

Goodman, L. S., and Gilman, A., eds. *The pharmacological basis of therapeutics*, 4th ed. New York: Macmillan, 1970.

Hasenclever, H. F. Histoplasmosis in bats. *Health Lab. Sci.* 9:125–132, 1972.

Hasenclever, H. F., Shaklette, M. H., Hunter, A. W., George, E., and Schwarz, J. The use of culture and histologic methods for the detection of *Histoplasma capsulatum* in bats:Absence of a cellular response. *Am. J. Epidemiol.* 90:77–83, 1969.

Hildick-Smith, G., Blank, H., and Sarkany, I. *Fungus diseases and their treatment*. Boston: Little, Brown, 1964.

Isbister, J., Elliott, M., and Nogrady, S. Histoplasmosis: An outbreak occurring among young men who visited one cave. *Med. J. Aust.* 2:243–248, 1976.

Johnson, J. E., III, Radimer, G., Di Salvo, A. F., Ajello, L., and Bigler, W. Histoplasmosis in Florida: I. Report of a case and epidemiologic studies. *Am. Rev. Respir. Dis.* 101:299–305, 1970.

Kaplan, W. Epidemiology of the principal systemic mycoses of man and lower animals and the ecology of their etiologic agents. *J. Am. Vet. Med. Assoc.* 163:1043–1047, 1973.

Kaufman, L. Serology of systemic fungus diseases. *Public Health Rep.* 81:177–185, 1966.

Kirk, R. W., ed. *Current veterinary therapy*, vol. 6: *Small animal practice*. Philadelphia: Saunders, 1977.

Klite, P. D., and Diercks, F. H. *Histoplasma capsulatum* in fecal contents and organs of bats in the Canal Zone. *Am. J. Trop. Med. Hyg.* 14:433–439, 1965.

Kreske, R. D., and Swieconek, R. A. *Histoplasmosis* (*Histoplasma capsulatum, Histoplasma duboisii*): *A comprehensive bibliography*. Transactions of the Miami Geographical Society. Coral Gables: University of Miami, 1971.

Lainson, R., and Shaw, J. J. Pneumocystis and histoplasma infections in wild animals from the Amazon region of Brazil. *Trans. R. Soc. Trop. Med. Hyg.* 69:505–508, 1975.

Levine, N. D., Dunlap, G. L., and Graham, R. An intracellular parasite encountered in a ferret. *Cornell Vet.* 28:249–251, 1938.

Mariat, E., and Segretain, G. Etude mycologique d'une histoplasmose spontanee du singe africain (*Cynocephalus babuin*) [Mycological study of spontaneous histoplasmosis of the African monkey (*Cynocephalus babuin*)]. *Ann. Inst. Pasteur* 91:874–891, 1956.

Marinkelle, C. J., and Grose, E. *Histoplasma capsulatum* from the liver of a bat in Colombia. *Science* 147:1039–1040, 1965.

Menges, R. W. Histoplasmin sensitivity among animals in central Missouri. *CDC Bull.* pp. 8–11. Atlanta: Federal Security Agency, Public Health Service, Communicable Disease Center, May 1951.

Menges, R. W., Furcolow, M. L., Habermann, R. T., and Weeks, R. J. Epidemiologic studies on histoplasmosis in wildlife. *Environ. Res.* 1:129–144, 1967.

Menges, R. W., Furcolow, M. L., and Hinton, A. The role of animals in the epidemiology of histoplasmosis. *Am. J. Hyg.* 59:113–118, 1954.

Menges, R. W., Habermann, R. T., Selby, L. A., Ellis, H. R., Behlow, R. F., and Smith, C. D. A review and recent findings on histoplasmosis in animals. *Vet. Med.* 58:331–338, 366, 1963.

Menges, R. W., and Kintner, L. D. Bovine histoplasmosis. *North Am. Vet.* 32:692–695, 1951.

Murdock, W. T., Travis, R. E., Sutliff, W. D., and Ajello, L. Acute pulmonary histoplasmosis after exposure to soil contaminated by starling excreta. *J. Am. Med. Assoc.* 179:73–75, 1962.

Negroni, P. *Histoplasmosis: Diagnosis and treatment*, p. 44, trans. Shirley McMillen. Springfield: Thomas, 1965.

Oels, H. C., Branum, E. L., Zollman, P. E., and Markowitz, H. Antibodies to *Histoplasma capsulatum* in human and animal populations of southeastern Minnesota. *Am. Rev. Respir. Dis.* 99:443–446, 1969.

Olson, B. J., Bell, J. A., and Emmons, C. W. Studies on histoplasmosis in a rural community. *Am. J. Public Health* 37:441–449, 1947.

Richman, H. Histoplasmosis in a colt. *North Am. Vet.* 29:710, 1948.

Schwarz, J., Baum, G. L., Wang, C. J. K., Bingham, E. L., and Rubel, H. Successful infection of pigeons and chickens with *Histoplasma capsulatum*. *Mycopathol. Mycol. Appl.* 8:189–193, 1957.

Schwarz, J., and Kauffman, C. A. Occupational hazards from deep mycoses. *Arch. Dermatol.* 113:1270–1275, 1977.

Schwarz, J., and Sethi, K. K. Recognition of changing sources in histoplasmosis infection. *Mycopathol. Mycol. Appl.* 37:77–80, 1969.

Shacklette, M. H., Diercks, F. H., and Gale, N. B. *Histoplasma capsulatum* recovered from bat tissues. *Science* 135:1135, 1962.

Smith, H. A., Jones, T. C., and Hunt, R. D. *Veterinary pathology*, 4th ed. Philadelphia: Lea and Febiger, 1972.

Taylor, R. L., and Shacklette, M. H. Naturally acquired histoplasmosis in the mammals of the Panama Canal Zone. *Am. J. Trop. Med. Hyg.* 11:796–799, 1962.

Tesch, R. B., and Schneidau, J. D. Naturally occurring histoplasmosis among bat colonies in southeastern United States. *Am. J. Epidemiol.* 86:545–551, 1967.

Velasco-Castrejon, O., and Gonzalez-Ochoa, A. Primary pulmonary epidemic of histoplasmosis in an abandoned mine. *Mykosen* 20:393–399, 1977.

Walker, J., and Spooner, E. T. C. Natural infection of the African baboon *Papio papio* with the large-cell form of *Histoplasma*. *J. Pathol. Bacteriol.* 80:436–438, 1960.

Zeidberg, L. D., Ajello, L., Dillon, A., and Runyon, L. C. Isolation of *Histoplasma capsulatum* from soil. *Am. J. Public Health* 42:930–935, 1952.

36 *Coccidioidomycosis*

JOHN W. DAVIS

Synonyms: **San Joaquin fever, coccidioidal granuloma, desert rheumatism, valley fever, Posada-Wernick's disease.**

Coccidioidomycosis is a primary respiratory infection caused by the fungus *Coccidioides immitis*. It infects a wide variety of wildlife species as well as man. Most infections are localized and often asymptomatic. It is the most infectious disease of the systemic mycoses.

HISTORY. The first documented case of coccidioidomycosis in a wild animal was reported in 1936 in a tropical monkey (*Cebus hypolecucus*) at the San Diego Zoo (McKenney et al. 1944). Wild animals reported to have had natural infections were a captive gorilla (McKenney et al. 1944), wild deer (Smith et al. 1972), baboon (Rapley and Long 1974), sea lion (*Zalophus californianus*) (Reed et al. 1976), giant red kangaroo (*Macropus rufus*) (Hutchinson et al. 1973), chimpanzees (Ingram 1975), monkey (*Cercocebus atys*) (Pappagianis et al. 1973), rhesus monkey (Breznock et al. 1975), and a wallaroo, South American tapir, aardvark, and Bengal tiger (Pappagianis, personal communication, 1978). *Coccidioides immitis* was found by direct examinaton or culture in the deer mouse (*Peromyscus eremicus*), pocket mice (*Perognathus baileyi, P. penicillatus, P. intermedius*), the kangaroo rat (*Dipodomys merriami*), and the ground squirrel (*Citellus harrisii*). Species of the genus *Perognathus* seem to be especially important hosts for the fungus. Emmons and Ashburn (1942) isolated *C. immitis* from a grasshopper mouse (*Onychomys torridus*), 15% of 124 pocket mice, and 17% of 29 kangaroo rats.

DISTRIBUTION. The geographic distribution of coccidioidomycosis is generally considered to be worldwide (Fiese 1958). It is very prevalent in the southwestern desert area of the United States (Emmons 1942); it appears to be rare in South America (Fiese 1958).

ETIOLOGY. Coccidioidomycosis is caused by *C. immitis*. The organism grows rapidly on Sabouraud medium or selective media containing cyclohexamide and chloramphenicol (Ajello et al. 1963; Merchant and Packer 1967). In body fluids or tissues, *C. immitis* exists in the form of spherical bodies which are commonly called spherules and range in size from 5 to 200 μ in diameter. When mature, the spherules possess a wall which is as much as 2 μ thick. The spherules are filled with a large number of globular or ellipsoidal spores called endospores, which range in size from 2 to 5 μ in diameter at maturity; a spherule may contain few or hundreds of endospores which are released at maturity, and each endosphore has the potential of becoming a spherule (Ajello et al. 1963; Conant et al. 1971).

On Sabouraud glucose agar *C. immitis* appears as a typical mold by the 3rd to 4th day after inoculation, and its colonies are moist, flat, and gray. The fungus quickly develops a cottony aerial mycelium which has barrel-shaped spores 25 × 3 × 3–4 μ in diameter and are called "arthrospores." These arthospores are highly infectious and readily airborne. The handling of cultures containing arthrospores presents a human health hazard in the laboratory (Ajello et al. 1963: Conant et al. 1971).

TRANSMISSION. Inhalation of *C. immitis* spores in dust or soil is the principal method of infection in animals and man (Cronkite and Lack 1940; Fiese 1958). Direct transmission from animal to animal is rare (Castleberry et al. 1963). Certain rodents such as deer mice and pocket mice apparently are important as reservoir hosts of *C. immitis* (Emmons 1942).

SIGNS. The clinical signs of coccidioidomycosis vary greatly; it can range from a benign upper respiratory infection to a disseminated fatal disease. In a captive mountain gorilla, the initial stage of acute coccidioidomycosis was characterized by apathy and anorexia. The axillary temperature was 39°C after 32 days. At 33 days a slight cough and pungent exudate occurred at the medial canthus of the eyes. The animal lost weight and strength and had a rough hair coat. Dyspnea and stertorous breathing developed on the 41st day. There was intermittent hemorrhage from the right nares, and the respiration rate increased to 43 times per minute. The animal died on the 45th day (McKenney et al. 1944).

A baboon had clinical signs that included nasal discharge, extensive coughing, and respiratory distress (Rapley and Long 1974). A sea lion exhibited anorexia for several days, edema without gas, and hemorrhagic myositis (Reed et al. 1976).

A rhesus monkey with radiographic evidence of coccidioidomycosis was asymptomatic (Breznock et al. 1975). Pappagianis et al. (1973) noted progressive weight loss, a wheezing, and swelling of the right knee in a monkey. Ingram (1975) observed weight loss and pale mucous membranes in a 10-year-old male laboratory-raised chimpanzee. This was followed by edema of the scrotal area and feet: 1 week later the animal became anorexic. Signs in a great red kangaroo included loss of appetite, progressive weight loss, debilitation, jaundice, and lethargy which resulted in euthanasia (Hutchinson et al. 1973).

PATHOLOGY. The gross lesions of coccidioidomycosis resemble those of tuberculosis in that they appear as distinct or confluent granulomas with or without calcification or suppuration; however, calcification is unusual. The lungs are most often affected and the great majority of these infections are benign. In a small percentage of cases, the infection is disseminated from the lungs, and secondary lesions may occur anywhere in the body. Where the disseminated form of the disease is encountered, nodules of varying size, shape, and consistency may be found in the liver, spleen, lungs, lymph nodes, meninges, or bone marrow. Granulomatous lesions usually heal by fibrosis.

The microscopic lesions are characteristic but somewhat variable, since the cellular reaction of the host is determined by the phase of the *Coccidioides* organism against which it is directed. The larger spherules are often surrounded by a wide zone of epithelioid cells mixed with a few giant cells, neutrophils, and lymphocytes. If a large spherule has ruptured and released its endospores, many neutrophils and lymphocytes, but few epithelioid cells, will be found associated with the tissue reaction. Organisms in different stages of growth are usually present; therefore, microscopically one sees a mixture of exudative and proliferative reactions. Lesions in the lungs, spleen, and liver are usually spherical and sharply circumscribed, whereas those in lymph nodes and bone marrow are more diffuse.

Ashburn and Emmons (1942) found gran-

ulomata in pocket mice and a kangaroo rat. These lesions were approximately 0.1 mm in diameter and occurred primarily in the lower lobes of the lungs. Diffuse masses of fusiform epithelioid cells occurred in the center of some nodules. Central zones of caseous necrosis varying from 300 to 800 μ in diameter were found in some of the granulomata. Fungus cells of varying sizes were present in all granulomata and were also scattered throughout the lungs. A second series of infected rodents had nodular lung lesions composed of fusiform epithelioid cells (Emmons and Ashburn 1942). The nodules were circumscribed, often had a peripheral zone of compactly arranged lymphocytes, and caseous necrosis occurred in approximately 90% of them. Two-thirds of the lesions had fibrosis.

Gross pathologic lesions in a captive gorilla that had died of coccidioidomycosis included enlargement and caseation of the peribronchial lymph glands and a soft and pulpy spleen that contained numerous tubercles scattered over the pleural surface (McKenney et al. 1944). Histologically, there were irregular areas of necrosis resembling tubercles in the spleen; the liver had more definitely formed tubercles with giant cells, and the lungs had well-defined tubercles which contained fewer neutrophils than the spleen.

Three of five coyotes caught in traps in the vicinity of Tucson, Arizona, had small single foci of coccidioidomycosis in the lungs. These foci were 2 mm in diameter, were located subpleurally in the right apical lobe or the right diphragmatic lobe, and were well-circumscribed, small, pneumonic consolidations containing lymphocytes, plasma cells, polymorphonuclear leukocytes, and histocytes. The elastic tissue from the alveolar walls had largely disappeared; one lesion had a slightly necrotic center and another an extensive caseation (Straub et al. 1961).

Rapley and Long (1974) described a baboon as having gross pathologic lesions that consisted of numerous firm white lesions randomly distributed in all lobes. The peribronchial lymph nodes were enlarged and contained purulent exudate. There were grayish white foci lesions 1–3 mm in diameter located in the subcapsular areas on one kidney. On histologic examination the bronchi and bronchioles were filled with necrotic debris that contained inflammatory cells. A few multinucleated giant cells and various sized spherules containing endospores were observed in the exudate. Obliterative bronchiolitis was observed, and complete destruction of the epithelial lining in other bronchioles was found. The lamina propria contained mononuclear cells. There were inflammatory changes that varied from a purulent exudate consisting chiefly of neutrophils to extensive accumulations of mononuclear cells. There was interstitial edema. The pleura was thickened and the pleura papilliform projections were highly vascular connective tissue. The lung parenchyma contained extensive fibrosis and granular formation. The mediastinal lymph nodes were actively involved with extensive purulent exudate, but granulomatous lesions were predominant. A small granulomatous lesion was found in the renal cortex.

Reed et al. (1976) described the gross pathology in a sea lion. The lungs had patchy areas of consolidation, and there were multiple white foci in the pale liver, spleen, and kidney. Histologic examination revealed suppurative granulomas in the liver and spleen. Large thick-walled spherules 20–30 μ in diameter were seen in the granulomas. A mild pneumonitis was recorded, and the kidney had a mild chronic inflammation.

Some of the pathology described by Breznock et al. (1975) in a rhesus monkey that had clinically appeared normal but was found to have diffuse pulmonary disease after radiographic findings was as follows: gross lesions were confined to the thoracic viscera; the right cranial, middle, and caudal lobes adhered to one another near their hiatus and to the pericardial sac. The left caudal lobe was partially collapsed, small in size, and purplish red and had a wrinkled pleural surface. The larger nodules were cavitated and often connected with a large air passage. The right caudal and left cranial lobes contained large cavitated lesions. Histologically there were two forms of reaction: (1) primarily neutrophilic and (2) granulomatous. Also noted was extensive destruction of airway walls and adjacent parenchyma.

Blundell et al. (1961) exposed a *Macaca mulatta* monkey to arthrospores of *C. immitis* by aerosol infection, and microscopic lesions were observed in the lungs on the 5th day after inoculation and were filled with endospores. On the 7th day, necrotic centers were observed in these lung lesions. Similar lesions appeared in the other body organs 15 days after inoculation. Dissemination of the disease from the lung occurred on the 30th day after inoculation.

Gross pathologic findings described in *Cercocebus atys* by Pappagianis et al. (1973) included gelatinous degeneration of the muscle sheath of the right knee along with a protrusion of the muscle fibers and abscess in the left lung and upper mediastinum. The spleen was slightly enlarged and lytic lesions were noted in the tibia, femur, and vertebrae.

Ingram (1975) observed the following pathology in a laboratory-raised male chimpanzee: radiographs showed a diffuse interstitial pattern for both lungs. There was fluid in the abdomen with possible adhesions. Disseminated lesions of coccidioidomycosis were found throughout the abdomen and thorax. There was complete adhesion of the dorsal and lateral chest wall. White foci were noted throughout the dark edematous parenchyma. Whitish foci were seen on the surface of the diaphragm and left abdominal wall. There were adhesions throughout the abdomen, and the spleen was enlarged. There were white foci in the swollen liver and multiple foci were found in the pale kidney. Microscopic lesions of dense subpleural scarring and multiple parenchymal granulomas as well as spherules of *C. immitis* were found in the lungs. Edema was found in many of the alveoli. The pleural surface of the diaphragm contained spherules and was covered with granulomas. Granulomas were found in the liver, pancreas, and spleen. Granulomatous abscesses were noted in the liver. Active granulomas were found in the thyroid gland and adrenal cortex.

Necropsy examination of a giant red kangaroo showed a fibrocalcified granuloma in the superior segment of the lower left lung lobe; its contents consisted of a yellowish tan thick material (Hutchinson et al. 1973). On histologic examination, gross findings of the necrotic contents were found within a fibrinous walled lesion. Spherules and endospores were also noted.

DIAGNOSIS. One can usually diagnose coccidioidomycosis by microscopic demonstration of typical *C. immitis* in a characteristic lesion. Wet, unstained, microscopic preparations of clinical materials should be examined for spherules. Mature spherules have thick refractile walls and contain endospores. If young spherules having thinner walls are found, the coverglass should be sealed with petrolatum and allowed to stand several hours. Spherules that are present will have mycelial filaments develop from the endospores (Ajello et al. 1963). If a diagnosis of coccidioidomycosis cannot be made by microscopic demonstration of *C. immitis* in characteristic lesions, infected clinical material should be inoculated into a selective medium such as Sabouraud glucose agar slant plus or minus antibiotics and incubated at room temperature (Conant et al. 1971). Cotton plugged tubes, not screw-capped tubes, should be used, since semianaerobic conditions inhibit the formation of spores in some strains of *C. immitis* (Hampson 1954). After 10–14 days of incubation, the aerial mycelium may be examined for diagnostic arthrospores (Ajello et al. 1963). The tubes containing aerial mycelium should be flooded with sterile physiologic saline before the culture is examined. If structures are found suggestive of *C. immitis*, their identification must be confirmed by animal inoculation; coupled with signs and lesions, this is sufficient to make a diagnosis. This disease must be differentiated from adiaspiromycosis (Emmons and Jellison 1960) and rhinosporidiosis (Conant et al. 1971).

Extreme care should be exercised when working with this organism in the laboratory since man can easily become infected by arthrospore inhalation. Double electroimmunodiffusion (EID) was adapted for detection of antibodies to *C. immitis*. In a limited experiment with canine serum the test was found to be qualitatively as sensitive as the complement fixation test. Advantages of EID include shorter time period (30 minutes) and the need for a small amount of antigen and antibody (10 µl) (Shifrine et al. 1975).

IMMUNITY. *Coccidioides immitis* infection results in a rapid and ordinarily effective immunologic response on the part of the host and the immunity conferred is lifelong and complete.

Little is known concerning immunity in wild animals exposed under natural conditions, but the precipitin and complement fixation tests may be useful for determining the extent of exposure of such animals to *C. immitis*. Skin tests and X rays have been used in confined wild animals.

Converse et al. (1963) vaccinated monkeys (*M. mulatta*) subcutaneously with 10^7 to 10^8 viable *C. immitis* arthrospores; 6 months after inoculation they were protected against a respiratory challenge of approximately 7,000 viable arthrospores, whereas unvaccinated monkeys receiving a similar challenge developed a severe disease. After 20 days the vaccinated monkeys had very minor pulmonary changes and 80% had negative lung cultures.

TREATMENT AND CONTROL. K. A. Ingram (personal communication, 1978) has had good results treating dogs with amphotericin B when

given intravenously 2–3 times per week until a total dose of 5 mg/0.454 kg has been given. However, Wertlake et al. (1963) reported tubular damage and calcium deposition in the kidneys following amphotericin B therapy in man and dogs.

Lawrence and Hoeprich (1976) compared the methyl ester of amphotericin B with the parent compound in terms of therapeutic efficacy and toxicity in experimental murine coccidioidomycosis. At low doses the methyl ester was less effective therapeutically than amphotericin B; however, at higher doses amphotericin B was directly lethal or nephrotic, whereas the methyl ester was therapeutically effective and nontoxic. In contrast to amphotericin B, the methyl ester did not cause either azotemia or histopathologic changes in the kidney.

REFERENCES

Ajello, L., Georg, L. K., Kaplan, W., and Kaufman, L. Laboratory manual for medical mycology. U.S. Department of Health, Education and Welfare, Public Health Serv. *CDC Bull.*, pp. 631–638, 1963.

Ashburn, L. L., and Emmons, C. W. The pathology of spontaneous coccidioidal granuloma in the lungs of wild rodents. *Am. J. Pathol.* 18:753–755, 1942.

Blundell, G. P., Castleberry, M. W., Lowe, E. P., and Converse, J. L. The pathology of *Coccidioides immitis* in the *Macaca mulatta*. *Am. J. Pathol.* 39:613–630, 1961.

Breznock, A. W., Henrickson, R. V. Silverman, S., and Swartz, L. W. Coccidioidomycosis in a rhesus monkey. *J. Am. Vet. Med. Assoc.* 167:657–661, 1975.

Castleberry, M. W., Converse, J. L., and del Favero, J. E. Coccidioidomycosis transmission to an infant monkey from its mother. *Arch. Pathol.* 75:459–461, 1963.

Conant, N. E., Smith, D. T., Baker, R. D., and Callaway, J. L. *Manual of clinical mycology*, 4th ed., pp. 192–195. Philadelphia: Saunders, 1971.

Converse, J. L., Castleberry, M. W., and Snyder, E. M. Experimental viable vaccine against pulmonary coccidioidomycosis in monkeys. *J. Bacteriol.* 86:1041–1051, 1963.

Cronkite, A. E., and Lack, A. R. Primary pulmonary coccidiodomycosis experimental infection with *Coccidiodes immitis*. *J. Exp. Med.* 72:167–174, 1940.

Emmons, C. W. Isolation of *Coccidioides* from soil and rodents. *Public Health Rep.* 57:109–111, 1942.

Emmons, C. W., and Ashburn, L. L. The isolation of *Haplosporangium parvum* n. sp. and *Coccidioides immitis* from wild rodents. *Public Health Rep.* 57:1715–1727, 1942.

Emmons, C. W., and Jellison, W. L. *Emmonsia cres-*

cens sp. n. and adiaspiromycosis (haplomycosis) in mammals. *Ann. N.Y. Acad. Sci.* 89:91–101, 1960.

Fiese, M. J. *Coccidioidomycosis.* Springfield, Ill.: Thomas, 1958.

Hampson, C. R. Sporulation capacity of *Coccidioides immitis* affected by cultural conditions. *J. Bacteriol.* 67:739–740, 1954.

Hutchinson, L. R., Duran, F., Lane, D. D., Robertstad, G. W., and Portillo, M. Coccidioidomycosis in a giant red kangaroo (*Macropus rufus*). *J. Zoo Anim. Med.* 4:22–24, 1973.

Ingram, K. A. Coccidioidomycosis in a colony of chimpanzees. *Amer. Assoc. of Zoo Vets. Ann. Proc.*, pp. 127–132, 1975.

Lawrence, R. M., and Hoeprich, P. D. Comparison of amphotericin B and toxicity. *J. Infect. Dis.* 133:168–174, 1976.

McKenney, F. D., Traum. J., and Bomestall, A. E. Acute coccidioidomycosis in mountain gorilla (*Gorilla beringeri*) with anatomical notes. *J. Am. Vet. Med. Assoc.* 104:136–140, 1944.

Merchant, I. A., and Packer, R. A. *Veterinary bacteriology and virology*, 7th ed. Ames: Iowa State University Press, 1967.

Pappagianis, D., Vanderlip, J., and May, B. Coccidioidomycosis naturally acquired by a monkey, *Cercocebus atys*, in Davis, California. *Sabouraudia* 2 (pt. 1):52–55, 1973.

Rapley, W. A., and Long, J. R. Coccidioidomycosis in a baboon recently imported from California. *Can. Vet. J.* 15:39–41, 1974.

Reed, R. E., Migaki, G., and Cummings, J. A. Coccidioidomycosis in a California sea lion (*Zalophus californianus*) *J. Wild. Dis.* 12:372–375, 1976.

Shifrine, M., Pappagianis, D., and Neves, J. Double electroimmunodiffusion: A rapid diagnostic test for canine coccidioidomycosis. *Am. J. Vet. Res.* 36:819–820, 1975.

Smith, H. A., Jones, T. C., and Hunt, R. I. *Veterinary pathology*, 4th ed. Philadelphia: Lea and Febiger, 1972.

Straub, M., Troutman, R. J., and Greene, J. W. Coccidioidomycosis in 3 coyotes. *Am. J. Vet. Res.* 89:811–812, 1961.

Wertlake, P. J., Butler, W. T., Hill, G. J., and Utz, J. P. Nephrotoxic tubular damage and calcium deposition following amphotericin B. *Am. J. Pathol.* 43:449–458, 1963.

37 *Adiaspiromycosis*

WILLIAM L. JELLISON

Synonyms: **Adiaspiromycosis is a name proposed by Emmons and Jellison (1960) for an infection of mammals formerly called haplomycosis.**

Adiaspiromycosis is a mycotic infection of many small mammals caused by very unusual fungi of the genus *Emmonsia*. Two species are well recognized, *Emmonsia parva* and *E. crescens*. Other species names have been proposed. *Emmonsia* organisms, especially *E. crescens*, are unusual in that they produce the largest yeast cell stage or tissue spherule of any pathogenic fungus known, 400–700 μ in diameter. There is no multiplication in the tissue phase, yet massive infections have been observed in small mammals in nature. Infection in nature is limited to the lungs. Experimental infection can be induced in any organ or location in mammals. *Emmonsia crescens* certainly has the widest host range and widest geographic distribution of any mycotic pathogen.

A few human cases have been reported in patients with clinical illness and pulmonary symptoms diagnosed by biopsy. Other human cases have been diagnosed by examination of preserved pathologic specimens.

HISTORY AND DISTRIBUTION. With the known presence of *E. crescens* in considerable abundance in Korea to the east and the Scandinavian countries to the west, it was certain that it would be found in the USSR (Jellison 1969). The first report was by Sharapov (1969). He examined 5,647 mammals of more than 45 species and found 407 infected. These included Carnivora, Rodentia, and Insectivora. Prominent in the examination were the vole rat (*Arvicola terrestris*), and the American muskrat (*Ondatra zibethica*), which is widely dispersed in the USSR. Among the carnivores the stout (*Mustela eversmanni*) and the sable (*Mustela zibellina*) showed a high proportion of infection, 16 of 22 and 52 of 80, respectively.

The most severe infection the author has observed was in a vole from Switzerland (Fig. 37.1). Each spherule in the figure represents a separate infection as multiplication does not occur in the animal host.

Sharapov (1972) stated that the agents of adiaspiromycosis in small wild animals in a mycelium form are components of rhizosphere-root mycoflora of some plants; this has been confirmed by experiments and field observations. This observation seems very unusual, and it is possible that spores of the fungus genus *Endogone* were mistaken for *Emmonsia*. These spores are frequently found in the stomach contents of small rodents. Sharapov also stated that the fungus has been isolated from the rhizosphere of rhizome *Scolochloa festucacea* Link and from two species of the field vole (*Microtus socialis* Pall., *M. arvalis* Pall.). In personal correspondence Sharapov (1974) stated that adiaspiromycosis has been found on the floodplain of the Amur River.

The discovery and report of a severe human case in Czechoslovakia based on biopsy has been a stimulus in a search for other human cases and surveys for the organisms in other animals (Kodousek et al. 1971).

Two excellent symposiums held in Czechoslovakia (Dvorak and Otcenasek 1970) reported human infection as well as a clinical pattern and therapy based on one case. Antigenic activity, life cycle and experimental infection in mice, histochemistry, ultrastructure, enzyme-cytochemistry, and electron microscopy are also discussed, 175 references are listed. A later publication by Kodousek (1974) lists 216 references.

A human case in Honduras was reported by Cueva and Little (1971). Diagnosis was based on examination of a lung biopsy specimen. One from Guatemala, also based on lung biopsy, was studied by Watts et al. (1975).

The monograph on adiaspiromycosis by Dvorak et al. (1973) contains an 11-page table listing animals that have been examined, those found infected, and their geographic locality and reporting author.

The first valid report of natural infection in a domestic animal, a dog, was reported from Klamath Falls, Oregon, by Koller et al. (1976), although the geographic source of the dog was not given. This diagnosis was confirmed by several others, including W. J. Hadlow and me.

TAXONOMY AND ETIOLOGY. In regard to the

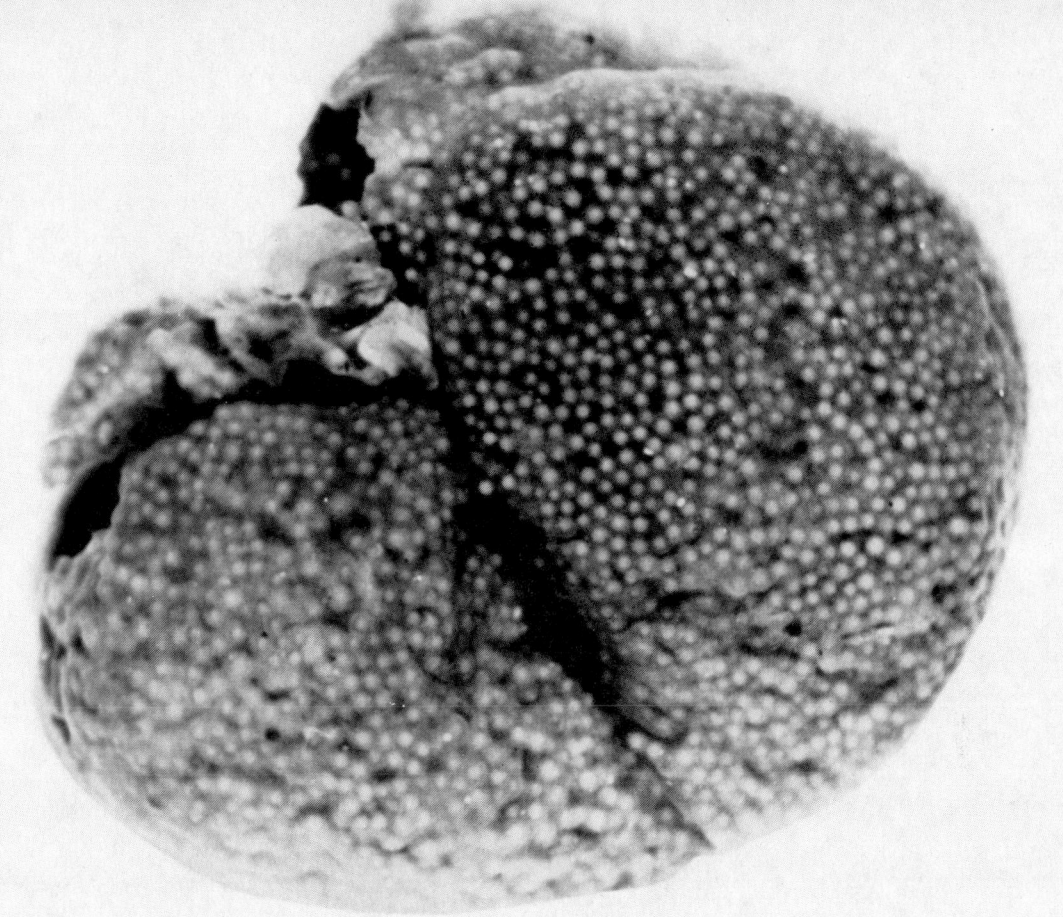

FIG. 37.1 Natural infection of *Emmonsia crescens* in the lungs of a vole (*Arvicola* sp.) from Switzerland. (Dr. B. Horning, collector; Rocky Mountain Laboratory 37778, photo by N. J. Kramis).

taxonomy of these fungi, it was recognized that the organism described as *E. crescens* in 1960 was probably the same as that described earlier as *Rhinosporidium pulmonale* by Kirschenblatt (1939). Thus his name would have had priority, if he had given a Latin description. Because he did not, the name is not valid by the rules of botanical nomenclature.

An even earlier publication and figure by Splendore (1920) of bodies found in *Pitymys savii* in the Province of Capitanata, Italy, are almost certainly *E. crescens*. The organisms were identified as the eggs of a worm "vermi sconoscutti."

Two other cultures were described as new species of *Emmonsia*. These were *E. brasiliensis* Batista, Lima, Pessoa, and Shome, 1963, and *E. ciferrina* Thirumalachuar, Padhye, and Srinivasan, 1965, from India. Padhye and Carmichael (1968) consider both these names to be synonyms of *Chrysosporium pruinosum* (Gilman and Abbott 1927).

In a survey for mycotic agents in Utah at Dugway Proving Grounds, 21 cultures of *Em-* *monsia* were isolated by culture of small bits of lung tissue (Jellison and Emmons 1955). All cultures were tested by inoculation into white mice, and some were retested. Although these cultures appeared to be typical of *Emmonsia*, none produced an infection, contrary to all previous experience with *Emmonsia*.

In several earlier publications, including the book *Korean Hemorrhagic Fever and Related Diseases: A Critical Review and a Hypothesis* (Jellison 1971), the theory is advanced that *Emmonsia crescens* could be the etiologic agent of hemorrhagic fever. After 25 years of both intensive and sporadic research by many investigators, the causative agent of Korean hemorrhagic fever remains unknown. Confidence in this theory prompted the author to search for and find *E. crescens* in Norway, Sweden, Finland, France, Yugoslavia, and Argentina where hemorrhagic feverlike diseases have been recognized.

Although the agent is not named, Lee et al. (1978) presume the Causative Agent of Korean hemorrhagic fever to be a virus.

LITERATURE. A section on adiaspiromycosis is included in Emmons et al. 1971. This account features the medical aspects. It is included in a section entitled "Miscellaneous or Rare Mycoses," which does not seem appropriate for a mycotic agent that probably has such a wide geographic and host range and an incidence from 10 to over 50% in some localized mammal populations.

In the course of the author's studies on adiaspiromycosis, first known as haplomycosis, and of the causative agents, *Emmonsia parva* and *Emmonsia crescens*, a considerable volume of literature and correspondence has been accumulated. Much of the accumulated information on this infection is reviewed in *Adiaspiromycosis* (Jellison 1969), which is still available from the Mountain Press, Missoula, Montana.

This literature could be made available to any serious student on the subject.

REFERENCES

Adiaspiromykosa. Stud. Pneumol. Phtiseol. Czech. 30:293–336, From Avicenum-Zdravotnicke Nakladatelstvi. N. P. Praha, 1970. Four articles by various authors. [This apparently constitutes the first symposium on adiaspiromycosis.]

Adiaspiromycosis. Acta. Univ. Palackianae. Proceedings of the Second Symposium on Adiaspiromycosis. Sumperk, Czechoslovakia, June 25. *Olomucensis* 63:7–112, 1972. (Available from Dr. R. Kodousek, University of Palackeho, Olomouc 5, Czechoslovakia.)

Al-Doory, Y, Vice, T. E. and Mainster, M. E. Adiaspiromycosis in a dog. *J. Am. Vet. Med. Assoc.* 159:87–90, 1971.

Batista, A. C., Lima, J. A. de, Pessoa, F. P., and Shome, S. K. *Emmonsia brasiliensis* s. sp.: Um hifomiceto de interessa para micopatologia humana. *Rev. Fac. Med. Univ. Ceara* 3:45–53, 1963.

Cueva, J. A., and Little, M. D., *Emmonsia crescens* infection (adiaspiromycosis) in man in Honduras. *Am. J. Trop. Med.* 20:282–287, 1971.

Dvorak, J., and Otcenasek, M. I symposium o adiaspiromykoze. *Hradec Kralov* 28:1, 1970.

Dvorak, J., Otcenasek, M., and Rosicky, B. Adiaspiromycosis caused by *Emmonsia crescens*, Emmons and Jellison, 1960. Studies of Czechoslovak Academy of Sciences No. 14. Prague: Academia, 1973.

Emmons, C. W., Binford, C. H. and Utz, J. P. Adiaspiromycosis. In *Medical mycology*, pp. 442–451. Philadelphia: Lea and Febiger, 1971.

Emmons, C. W., and Jellison, W. L. *Emmonsia crescens* sp. n. and adiaspiromycosis (haplomycosis) in mammals. *Ann. N.Y. Acad. Sci.* 89:91–101, 1960.

Gilman, J. C., and Abbot, E. V. A summary of soil fungi. *J. of Science, Iowa State College* 1:225–343, 1927.

Jellison, W. L. The presence of a pulmonary fungus in Korean rodents. Public Health Rep. 69:996–997, 1954.

———. *Adiaspiromycosis (= haplomycosis)*. Missoula, Mont.: Mountain Press, 1969.

———. Adiaspiromycosis. *Infectious diseases of wild mammals*. Ames, Iowa: The Iowa State University Press, pp. 321–323, 1970.

———. *Korean hemorrhagic fever: A critical review and a hypothesis*. Missoula, Mont. Mountain Press, 1971.

Jellison, W. L., and Emmons, C. W. Informal remarks. In *Symposium on Ecology of Disease Transmission in Native Animals*. Dugway Proving Grounds, Dugway, Utah, p. 112. Sponsored by and publication by Ecological Research, University of Utah, Salt Lake City, Utah, 1955.

Jellison, W. L., and Vinson, J. W. The distribution of *Emmonsia crescens* in Europe. *Mycologia* 53:524–535, 1961.

Kirschenblatt, J. D. A new parasite in the lungs of rodents. *C. R. Acad. Sci.* 23:406–408, 1939.

Kodousek, R. Adiaspiromycosis. *Acta Univ. Palackianae Olomucensis* 70:4–68, 1974.

Kodousek, R., Vortel, V., Fingerland, A., Vojtek, V., Sery, Z., Hajeck, V., and Kucera, K. Pulmonary adiaspiromycosis in man caused by *Emmonsia crescens*: Report of a unique case. *Am. J. Clin. Pathol.* 56:394–399, 1971.

Koller, L. D., Patton, N. M., and Whitsett, D. K. Adiaspiromycosis in the lungs of a dog. *J. Am. Vet. Med. Assoc.* 169:1316–1317, 1976.

Lee, H. W., Lee, P.W., and Johnson, K. M. Isolation of the etiologic agent of Korean hemorrhagic fever. *J. Infect. Dis.* 137:298–308, 1978.

Padhye, A. A., and Carmichael, J. W. *Emmonsia brasiliensis* and *Emmonsia ciferrina* are *Chrysosporium pruinosum*. *Mycologia* 60:445–447, 1968.

Sharapov, V. M. Adiaspiromycosis in USSR. (Translation). *Izv. Sibirsk. Otdel Acad. SSR.* 1:86–95, 1969.

———. Adiaspiromycosis in Mustelidae. *Trans. 9th Int. Cong. Game Biol.* (Moscow), pp. 662–665, 1970.

———. On the natural focality of adiaspiromycosis. (Russian article with English summary.) 50–51, 1972.

Splendore, D. A. Sui parassiti delle arvicole. *Ann. Igiene* 30(8):445–468, 1920.

Thirumalachar, M. J., Padhye, A. A., and Srinivasan, M. C. *Emmonsia ciferrina*, a new species from India. *Mycopathol. Mycol. Appl.* 26:323–332, 1965.

Watts, J. C., Callaway, C. S., Chandler, F. W., and Kaplan, W. Human pulmonary adiaspiromycosis. *Arch. Pathol.* 99:11–15, 1975.

38 *Rocky Mountain Spotted Fever*

J. FREDERICK BELL

Synonyms: **The synonyms "spotted fever" and "black measles," are misleading because they are also synonyms for other maladies. Very similar diseases caused by closely related rickettsias are: Sao Paulo exanthematic typhus, tobia fever (South America), boutonneuse fever (Mediterranean area), North Queensland tick typhus, Siberian tick typhus, Kenya tick typhus.**

Rocky Mountain spotted fever (RMSF) is one of a group of acute, severe rickettsial zoonoses. In man it is characterized by a macular rash that appears first on the wrists and ankles.

HISTORY. RMSF was recognized as a distinct danger by the Indians who frequented the Bitterroot Mountains of western Montana. Illness was most severe in this area, although a description of the disease in southern Idaho was the first to be published. The history of RMSF has been described by Price (1948) and by Aikawa (1966).

DISTRIBUTION AND ECOLOGY. Although Aikawa (1966) describes RMSF as uniquely American, this is true of the name only; the degree of separation from some other diseases reflects preferences in nomenclature as much as biological differences.

The common name itself is misleading; the characteristic disease is found in nearly all the contiguous states and is now most frequently recognized outside the Rocky Mountain area, especially along the East Coast where there was a marked increase in numbers of cases in the period 1970–1977 (Morbidity and Mortality Weekly Report 1979). About 25% of the reported cases in the United States occur in Virginia.

The ecology of *Rickettsia rickettsii* is essentially the ecology of its tick hosts and vectors. Although the organism is specifically adapted to ixodid ticks, the adaptation does not limit it to a particular species or genus; many are known to be infected. Since the various species of tick hosts are adapted to habitats ranging from human domiciles to forests, mountains and plains, and from humid or arid climates, the complexity of the ecology of the rickettsia is correspondingly great.

ETIOLOGY

Etiologic agent: *Rickettsia rickettsii* (also *R. rickettsi* or *Dermacentroxenus rickettsii*)
Classification: (Moulder 1974)

Class III.	Microtatobiotes Philip
Order I.	Rickettsiales Gieszczkiewicz 1939
Family I.	Rickettsiaceae Pinkerton 1936
Genus I.	*Rickettsia*
Species.	*rickettsii* (type species of the genus)

The organism cannot be cultivated in the absence of living cells. It propagates readily in yolk sacs of chick embryos, several kinds of tissue culture, susceptible laboratory animals (especially guinea pigs), and arthropods (especially ixodid ticks). Optimum temperature for propagation is 32°C in tissue culture and 35°C in chick embryos. The rickettsia is killed by temperature of 50°C for 10 minutes, 0.5% phenol, 0.1% formalin, and ordinary desiccation.

For proper definition of *R. rickettsii* it must be compared with other organisms that comprise the RMSF group. Lackman et al. (1965) used a mouse toxin neutralization test, the complement fixation (CF) test, and the older standard tests. Philip et al. (1978) used a microimmunofluorescence (micro-IF) technique to determine relationships of rickettsiae from various host and geographic sources and found general agreement with the results of other serologic procedures. Closeness of relationship of established species, and of some new ones proposed for species status within the genus, is defined.

Rickettsia rickettsii is gram-negative. Generally useful stains are Machiavello and Giemsa for smears and imprints (Gradwohl 1956) and the Wright-buffer sequence for formalin-fixed sections (Wolf and Cole 1966). The first procedure stains the organisms bright red, whereas they are bluish purple with Giemsa stain. Shape, size, and arrangement of the organism vary with the location and conditions of growth. Characteristically, *R. rickettsii* occurs within the nucleus as well as in the cytoplasm of cells.

TRANSMISSION AND HOSTS. In spite of long continuous efforts, relatively little is known of the intimate relationships of this organism of its vertebrate and invertebrate hosts. Several basic facts have been documented such as the transmission of infection from female tick to their offspring as discovered by Ricketts (1909). He reported that transovarial passage in *Dermacentor andersoni* is irregular, and Price (1954a) confirmed those observations. However, Burgdorfer (1963), in his studies of ticks experimentally infected with a highly virulent strain, demonstrated uniform transmission and also infection of the F² generation.

In North America the following species of ticks have been found naturally infected with *R. rickettsii* or closely related organisms (Burgdorfer et al. 1975; Hughes et al. 1976; Loving et al. 1978): *Dermacentor andersoni, D. variabilis, D. occidentalis, D. parumapertus, Amblyomma americanum, A. maculatum, A. cajennense, Rhipicephalus sanguineus, Haemaphysalis leporispalustris, Otobius lagophilus, Ixodes dentatus, I. scapularis,* and *I. pacificus.* Several of these are known vectors, and others are presumed. *Haemaphysalis* does not ordinarily feed on man but is undoubtedly important because of its wide distribution and host range and the tremendous numbers that occur under certain conditions. More than 17,000 ticks of this species have been found on a snowshoe hare, and 12,000 on a ruffed grouse in Minnesota.

Ectoparasites other than ticks are not known to be involved in the epizoology of RMSF.

Sufficient emphasis has not been placed on the limitations of spread of *R. rickettsii.* Theoretically, an infection that may be acquired by large numbers of ticks on an infected host and that is capable of being transmitted to 100% of the progeny should eventually infect the entire tick population. Since the incidence of infection of ticks varies from year to year, it is axiomatic that inhibitory factors occur. One possible inhibitory factor, feeding infected ticks on immune hosts, was not effective in freeing *H. asiaticum* of infection by *R. siberica,* and complete engorgement on such hosts did not prevent transovarial passage (Grokhovskaya et al. 1964). Other possible factors should be investigated for better understanding of limiting effects.

Although great effort has been expended on the study of wild vertebrate hosts of *R. rickettsii,* very little is known about their role in perpetuation of this rickettsia. In the eastern United States the organism has been isolated from opossum (*Didelphis*), cottontail rabbit

(*Sylvilagus*), white-footed mouse (*Peromyscus*), cotton rat (*Sigmodon*), meadow vole (*Microtus*), and pine vole (*Pitymys*) (Fuller 1963). Burgdorfer et al. (1962) obtained isolates from a snowshoe hare (*Lepus*), a golden-mantled ground squirrel (*Citellus*), and five chipmunks (*Eutamias*) in the Bitterroot Valley of Montana.

Much more evidence of infection of wild animals has been inferred from serologic surveys. Complement fixation titers of 24 or higher were found in a large proportion of the above species and also in the Columbian ground squirrel (*Citellus*) in western Montana. Fuller (1963) reported CF antibodies in red and gray foxes (*Vulpes* and *Urocyon*), raccoons (*Procyon*), striped skunks (*Mephitis*), and white-tailed deer (*Odocoileus*), and well as in rodents and lagomorphs. Burgdorfer et al. (1962) found concomitant presence of rickettsias and homologous antibodies in two rodent species and conversion from negative to strongly positive CF in retrapped animals within a period of 2 weeks in midsummer. Bozeman et al. (1967) isolated *R. rickettsii* from 6 species of native wild mammals in Virginia. In addition they found serologic evidence of infection in sera of 15 species of mammals of 5 orders and in 18 species of birds of 3 orders.

Stoenner et al. (1959) and Vest et al. (1965) conducted serologic surveys among the indigenous fauna of Utah and found that many individuals of a wide range of species had CF of agglutinating antibodies. Only 2 of 326 birds tested had significant CF titers. *R. rickettsii* was isolated readily from many of the ticks infesting the animals, but no isolates were obtained from the tissues of several thousand animals examined. Pagan et al. (1961) found significant titers of RMSF antibodies in the sera of 26 black-tailed jackrabbits (*Lepus*) in Kansas.

An excellent study of the prevalence of *R. rickettsii* in a complex ecosystem is reported in detail by the University of Utah Ecology and Epizoology Series (1964–1969) and, later, in the annual reports of Ecodynamics, (1970–1976). Data collected from year to year show wide fluctuations (cycles?) in the prevalence of *R. rickettsii* in animal populations on the Utah test site.

In spite of the paucity of data on demonstrable infection with rickettsemia in wild animals, there is a general inference that these hosts perform a significant role in the maintenance of *R. rickettsii* in addition to supporting the tick populations. This inference is based primarily on the fact that animals infected in the laboratory will infect ticks fed upon them.

Enough is known about the ecology of *R.*

rickettsii to afford an understanding of its epidemiology. The disease occurs most frequently in persons exposed to tick bite and especially among those whose facilities for grooming are limited. Thus, hikers, campers, sheepherders, surveyors, explorers, soldiers on maneuvers, and forest workers are at risk from infected *D. andersoni, D. variabilis,* and *A. americanum,* and owners of dogs may become infected, even in urban areas, where *Rhipicephalus* or *D. variabilis* are abundant. Infection may be contracted from ticks by crushing them, and the possibility of inhalation infection exists. Seasonal distribution of RMSF corresponds to the time of abundance of local vector ticks, and ordinarily cases are sporadic, but grouping may occur, for example, in summer recreation camps. Cases may occur rarely as a result of contact with an aberrant tick or from laboratory contact.

EXPERIMENTAL INFECTION OF WILD ANIMALS.

In spite of the difficulties of studying experimental infection in captive wild animals, innate resistance or susceptibility may be dominant over the conditions imposed, and antibody response or lack of it may be demonstrated. Because naturally infected wild animals are found so rarely, the nature of the disease in them is not known; but occurrence of a high incidence of serologically positive animals presumably implies frequent recovery from infection.

Burgdorfer et al. (1966) studied the susceptibility of small mammals inoculated via feeding ticks to a strain of rickettsia that produced fever of 39.8–41.5°C for 5–12 days in cavies. Concentration of rickettsias in the blood was determined and was correlated with the infectivity for normal ticks fed upon the animals at various stages. Columbian ground squirrels, golden-mantled ground squirrels, chipmunks, and voles responded to infection with rickettsemia that was infectious for immature *D. andersoni.* The minimal concentration of organisms necessary to infect 50% of the ticks ranged from 20–200 cavy infectious doses/ml; incidence of infection was highest in ticks that fed during periods of highest rickettsemia. *Rickettsia rickettsii* was detected in the blood of snowshoe hares for as long as 9 days, but in this species titers were lower. The bushy-tailed wood rat (*Neotoma*) was not infected under the conditions of the test. Jellison (1934) reported both deaths and severe scrotal reactions in voles (*Microtus*), but in this study voles were not severely affected and slight scrotal involvement occurred only rarely.

Rabbits (*Oryctolagus*) and rats (*Rattus*) develop less severe reactions to the organism than do cavies, but in the rabbit, at least, fever and Weil-Felix antibodies develop.

Lundgren et al. (1966) inoculated birds of several species and found rickettsemia comparable to that in rodents and lagomorphs in pigeons (*Columba*) chickens (*Gallus*), and pheasants (*Phasianus*). Minimal rickettsemia or none was found in three hawks (*Falco, Buteo,* and *Circus*), ravens (*Corvus*), and magpies (*Pica*). Pigeons, a marsh hawk, and a red-tailed hawk were the only birds that developed CF antibody. Lundgren and coworkers concluded that some birds may be involved in the cycle of RMSF in nature.

Carnivores are exposed to *R. rickettsii* in nature by feeding on infected rodents and as hosts to infected ticks. Lundgren et al. (1963) tested the susceptibility of young coyotes by oral and parenteral routes. Subcutaneous injection of 10^5 egg LD_{50} did not result in overt illness; but rickettsemia occurred for as long as 8 days, and CF antibodies developed. A much smaller inoculum resulted in antibody formation without rickettsemia; this was also true of orally infected animals which were subsequently immune to challenge by large subcutaneous doses. Miller (1950) inoculated foxes (*Vulpes?*) and raccoons which developed CF antibodies but not patent illness. He did not test the blood for presence of rickettsias. Badger (1933) tested the susceptibility of dogs by injection and by tick feeding; the reactions were similar to those of coyotes. Rickettsemia without patent illness occurred in mature animals, and a puppy had fever and cough as well as rickettsemia. Keenan et al. (1977) observed clinical syndromes ranging from mild febrile exanthema to death within 6 days after inoculation in dogs.

Susceptibility of monkeys to this disease was demonstrated by Howard Taylor Ricketts in the early 1900s, and the infection produced in rhesus and cynomolgous monkeys by aerosols has been studied by Saslaw et al. (1966). In spite of the unusual route of inoculation, the resulting picture was quite similar to the syndrome in man; there was no evidence of primary rickettsial pneumonia. Mortality was high in both species, and peripheral gangrene was a common sequel. Diagnostic CF titers reached a peak between 14 and 35 days, but only 10 of 14 animals showed significant increases in OX-19 agglutinins.

Only limited studies of susceptibility have been done in the ungulates. Badger (1933) found that an inoculated lamb (*Ovis*) responded to inoculation with rickettsemia that persisted for 7 days and production of OX-19 antibody to a titer of 1:640.

PATHOGENESIS. In all susceptible species, including man, the disease is primarily an infection of the blood vessels. Invasion and proliferation of rickettsia take place not only in endothelial cells but also in the smooth muscle of peripheral vessels; and the consequent destruction leads to thromboses, inflammation, and necrosis. Secondary effects of severe infection are generalized edema, shock, hypoproteinemia, thrombocytopenia, hypofibrinogenemia, azotemia, hepatitis, cardiac failure, and signs referable to central nervous system damage.

Virulence. In the evaluation of virulence, the age, species, and even sex of test animals, as well as the route of inoculation, dose of organisms, and other factors are important. Because of common use of antibiotics, mortality is now very low, and variations in virulence for man cannot be determined. In animals, too, the disease can vary from an imperceptible but immunogenic infection to a malignant and fatal illness. Production of scrotal swelling and necrosis of varying degrees in cavies is considered a criterion of virulence, but virulence for man does not parallel virulence for cavies. Undoubtedly, some of the differences in severity can be attributed to different doses (Saslaw et al. 1966), which also affects the length of incubation period.

An effect on virulence of the species of source animal has been postulated, and reduction of virulence for cavies by passage through Brazilian opposums has been reported (Miller 1950). Ricketts believed that the tick host species affected virulence, and for a long time it was thought that *R. rickettsii* resident in rabbit ticks (*H. leporispalustris*) had characteristically low virulence; but Parker et al. (1952) obtained several cavy-virulent isolates from ticks of this species collected on the East Coast of the United States. A remarkable but well-established feature affecting virulence is the enhancement by a blood meal, apparently without relation to numbers of organisms—the "reactivation" phenomenon. This effect of a blood meal is noted only in strains of organisms that are inherently virulent (Price 1953). Reactivation also occurs when infected ticks are merely kept at 37°C for 24 hours. Price concluded that passage of the organism through natural hosts

(mammals) decreases virulence, but arthropod passage causes enhancement (Price 1954a).

Bell and Pickens (1953) discovered that a specific toxin is elaborated by living *R. rickettsii*. Several variables affect the amount of toxin produced, but the amount is not proportional to virulence for cavies.

The Disease in Humans. The usual incubation period in humans is from 3 to 7 days after an infective tick bite. More severe cases are correlated with shorter incubation periods. Distressing prodromal signs and symptoms—headache, generalized aching, malaise, and severe chills—often precede the definitive syndrome. Fever as high as 40°C or more develops rapidly and is accompanied by severe headache, weakness, and painful tender extremities. The patient is weak, listless, and irritable; a dry cough is common. After a few days of illness there may be generalized edema, and a macular rash appears on the wrists and ankles and spreads rapidly to other areas of the body. In the early stages the rash fades on pressure; later it becomes maculopapular. In severe cases it may become purpuric and coalescent. Illness may be severe for 2 weeks, and convalescence is slow. Exceptionally, complications caused by involvement of the central nervous system or the cardiovascular or genitourinary systems occur. As a result of the vascular and perivascular inflammation from rickettsial invasion, peripheral gangrene occurs in some cases.

DIAGNOSIS. Laboratory confirmation of diagnosis may be obtained by isolation of the rickettsia, if appropriate laboratory facilities are available. Blood is taken from the patient in the febrile stage and injected by the intraperitoneal route into male cavies. Fever followed by scrotal inflammation typically occurs within a few days, but inapparent infection may occur and result in immunity to subsequent challenge. The agent may be identified by stains of scrotal smears and by cross-protection tests with immunized animals. The yolk sacs of embryonated hen eggs may also be inoculated with blood from the patient or cavy or with spleen or testicular washings of the latter. By this enrichment procedure, antigens may be prepared for use in serologic tests or for use as vaccines.

A neutralization test is performed by mixing patient's serum with graded infectious doses of the blood of a febrile cavy. After incubation the mixture is injected into male cavies. Serum of a convalescent RMSF patient will protect the animals.

Several in vitro serologic tests are available. Ricketts performed agglutination tests with suspensions of the organism, but the procedure did not become practical until Cox developed the yolk sac propagation of rickettsias. The great advantage of this test is that it is positive earlier than *Proteus* (Weil-Felix) agglutination. The latter reaction depends on the presence of a common antigen in certain strains of *Proteus* and in *R. rickettsii*. Agglutination occurs with OX-19 but not with OX-K strains.

The CF test is useful in this disease as in so many others, and CF antigen is now commonly prepared from infected yolk sacs (Cox 1979).

Other tests based on toxin neutralization and precipitin reactions are used for special purposes (Cox 1979; Lennette and Schmidt 1964). The direct fluorescent antibody (FA) reaction is useful for identifying the organism in tissues (Coons and Kaplan 1950) and has been used to demonstrate infection in the viscera of ticks (Burgdorfer and Lackman 1960). The rickettsia can be found also in tick hemolymph which is easily obtained by severing a leg (Burgdorfer 1970; Rehacek et al. 1971). The technique can be used successfully even on ticks that have been dead as long as 18 hours (Kurz and Burgdorfer 1978). The indirect FA test can be used for antibody titration. Philip et al. (1977) have compared the various serologic methods for diagnosis of RMSF.

PROGNOSIS. Prior to the use of antibiotics it was found that prognosis was best in vaccinated persons and young patients. Early antibiotic treatment greatly improves prognosis at all ages.

TREATMENT AND CONTROL. RMSF can be treated effectively with chloramphenicol and the tetracyclines; therefore, it is important to differentiate this disease from others not susceptible to this therapy. A history of tick bite or the finding of an engorged tick or a tick bite lesion is very helpful in diagnosis. The hemolymph test makes it possible to determine probable exposure, even before onset of signs, if the biting tick is available for test (Burgdorfer 1970; Rehacek et al. 1971). Necessity for earliest possible diagnosis and early treatment renders the later serologic tests of less importance.

RMSF retains little of the fearsome aspect it presented prior to the discovery of antibiotics. In addition to the effectiveness of treatment, there has been a decline in the number of cases in areas of former high endemicity beyond the

expected reduction as a result of limited use of vaccine. Some of this reduction is undoubtedly attributable to the use of antibiotics and abortion of the illness in early stages. However, reported incidence has increased markedly in some East Coast states in the past several years.

Until very recently, vaccine available commercially was prepared from infected hen egg yolk sac, but because of low potency and frequent side effects, it was withdrawn from the market. A new vaccine prepared from infected duck embryo monolayers has been found to obviate those faults and should be available soon (Ascher et al. 1978; Maugh 1978).

Vaccination should be limited to those who are especially exposed by reason of occupation or residence in tick-infested premises in a known endemic area. Even among those who are occupationally exposed to ticks, vaccination is not essential if adequate opportunity for twice-daily examination of the body for ticks exists and if medical facilities are accessible. In case of illness a recent history of tick bite should be told to the physician. Mere presence of a tick on the body or clothing does not necessarily constitute exposure, and a period of feeding of several hours is necessary for reactivation of infection in a tick.

Measures to prevent or minimize exposure to ticks are of great importance. Clothing that will reduce the risk of tick bite should be worn, and use of repellents is recommended in tick-infested areas. Infested dogs should be treated with acaricides at regular intervals, and dog quarters should be separate from the house and treated regularly where ticks are abundant. Ticks should not be picked with the bare hands, and they should be removed carefully to avoid leaving the hypostome in the skin.

Reduction of rodent populations in limited areas is considered effective because of the resulting decrease in ticks. Grazing by sheep and weed and brush removal by burning or chemicals have been used to decrease rodent habitat; these methods probably have more durable results than shooting, trapping, or poisoning the rodents. Poisoning of predators has had the unfortunate effect of causing great increases of rodents and commensurate increase of disease.

Direct application of acaricides probably has only temporary effect. They have been applied in limited areas to walks and pathways because of a peculiar propensity of ticks to concentrate in those locations rather than to be diffusely and homogeneously distributed.

A good source of information on control of

ticks is the Atlanta Communicable Disease Center's *Training Guide 772.*

ADDENDUM. *Rickettsia prowazekii,* the etiologic agent of epidemic typhus, has long been thought to infect only man among the vertebrates and to be transmitted only by *Pediculus* spp. However, the organism has recently been isolated from flying squirrels. (*Glaucomys volans*) in Florida and Virginia (Bozeman et al. 1975).

REFERENCES

Aikawa, J. K. *Rocky Mountain spotted fever.* Springfield, Ill.: Thomas, 1966.

Ascher, M. S., Oster, C. N., Harber, P. I., Kenyon, R. H., and Pedersen, C. E., Jr. Initial clinical evaluation of a new Rocky Mountain spotted fever vaccine of tissue culture origin. *J. Infect. Dis.* 138:217–221, 1978.

Badger, L. F. Rocky Mountain spotted fever: Susceptibility of the dog and sheep to the virus. *Public Health Rep.* 48:791–795, 1933.

Bell, E. J., and Pickens, E. G. A toxic substance associated with the rickettsias of the spotted fever group. *J. Immunol.* 70:461–472, 1953.

Bozeman, F. M., Masiello, S. A., Williams, M. S., and Elisberg, B. L. Epidemic typhus rickettsiae isolated from flying squirrels. *Nature* 225:545–547, 1975.

Bozeman, F. M., Shirai, A., Humphries, J. W., and Fuller, H. S. Ecology of Rocky Mountain spotted fever: II. Natural infection of wild mammals and birds in Virginia and Maryland. *Am. J. Trop. Med. Hyg.* 16:48–59, 1967.

Burgdorfer, W. Investigation of "transovarial transmission" of *Rickettsia rickettsii* in the wood tick, *Dermacentor andersoni. Exp. Parasitol.* 14: 152–159, 1963.

———. Hemolymph test: A technique for detection of rickettsiae in ticks. *Am. J. Trop. Med. Hyg.* 19:1010–1014, 1970.

Burgdorfer, W., Friedhoff, K. T., and Lancaster, J. L. Natural history of tick-borne spotted fever in the USA: II. Susceptibility of small mammals to virulent *Rickettsia rickettsii. Bull. WHO* 35:149–153, 1966.

Burgdorfer, W., and Lackman, D. Identification of *Rickettsia rickettsii* in the wood tick, *Dermacentor andersoni,* by means of fluorescent antibody. *J. Infect. Dis.* 107:241–244, 1960.

Burgdorfer, W., Newhouse, V. F., Pickens, E. G., and Lackman, D. B. Ecology of Rocky Mountain spotted fever in western Montana: I. Isolation of *Rickettsia rickettsii* from wild mammals. *Am. J. Hyg.* 76:293–301, 1962.

Burgdorfer, W., Sexton, D. J., Gerloff, R. K., Anacker, R. L., Philip, R. N., and Thomas, L. A. *Rhipicephalus sanguineus:* Vector of a new spotted fever group *Rickettsia* in the United States. *Infect. Immunol.* 12:205–210, 1975.

Coons, A. H., and Kaplan, M. H. Localization of antigen in tissue cells: IV. Antigens of rickettsiae and mumps virus. *J. Exp. Med.* 91:31–38, 1950.

Cox, H. R. Rickettsia. In F. Milgrom, C. J. Abeyounis, K. Kano, eds. *Principles of immunological diagnosis in medicine.* Philadelphia: Lea and Febiger, 1981.

Ecodynamics. *Ecology studies in western Utah,* series (1970–1976). Salt Lake City: Ecodynamics.

Fuller, H. S. Epidemiologie des rickettsioses: Donnees recentes sur l'ecologie de la fievre americaine par piqures de tiques. *Bull. Soc. Pathol. Exot.* 56:568–570, 1963.

Gradwohl, R. B. H. *Clinical laboratory methods and diagnosis,* 5th ed. St. Louis: C. V. Mosby, 1956.

Grokhovskaya, I. M., Sidorov, V. E., and Korshunova, O. S. Does feeding of ticks on immune animals influence *Rickettsia sibirica? Med. Parazitol.* (Mosk.) 33:178–181, 1964. Abstr. *Trop. Dis. Bull.* 61:778, 1964.

Hattwick, M. A., O'Brien, R. J., and Hanson, B. F. Rocky Mountain spotted fever: Epidemiology of an increasing problem. *Ann. Intern. Med.* 84:732–739, 1976.

Hughes, L. E., Clifford, C. M., Gresbrink, R., Thomas, L. A., and Keirans, J. E. Isolation of a spotted fever group *Rickettsia* from the Pacific Coast tick, *Ixodes pacificus,* in Oregon. *Am. J. Trop. Med. Hyg.* 25:513–516, 1976.

Jellison, W. L. Rocky Mountain spotted fever: The susceptibility of mice. *Public Health Rep.* 49(1):363–367, 1934.

Keenan, K. P., Buhles, W. C., Huxsoll, D. L., Williams, R. G., Hildebrandt, P. K., Campbell, J. M., and Stephenson, E. H. Pathogenesis of infection with *Rickettsia rickettsii* in the dog: A disease model for Rocky Mountain spotted fever. *J. Infect. Dis.* 135:911–917, 1977.

Kurz, J., and Burgdorfer, W. Detection of the Rocky Mountain spotted fever agent, *Rickettsia rickettsii,* in dead ticks, *Dermacentor andersoni. Infect. Immun.* 20:584–586, 1978.

Lackman, D. B., Bell, E. J., Stoenner, H. G., and Pickens, E. G. The Rocky Mountain spotted fever groups of rickettsias. *Health Lab Sci.* 2:135–141, 1965.

Lennette, E. H., and Schmidt, N. J. *Diagnostic procedures for viral and rickettsial diseases,* 3d ed., pp. 743–772. New York: American Public Health Association, 1964.

Loving, S. M., Smith, A. B., DiSalvo, A. F., and Burgdorfer, W. Distribution and prevalence of spotted fever group Rickettsiae in ticks from South Carolina, with an epidemiological survey of persons bitten by infected ticks. *Am. J. Trop. Med. Hyg.* 27:1255–1260, 1978.

Lundgren, D. L., Thorpe, B. D., and Haskell, C. D. Infectious diseases in wild animals in Utah: VI. Experimental infection of birds with *Rickettsia rickettsii. J. Bacteriol.* 91:963–966, 1966.

Lundgren, D. L., Ushijima, N., and Sidwell, R. W. Studies on infectious diseases in wild animals in Utah: V. Experimental Rocky Mountain spotted fever in the coyote, *Canis latrans lestes* Merriam. *Zoonoses Res.* 21:125–134, 1963.

Maugh, T. H., II. Rickettsiae: A new vaccine for Rocky Mountain spotted fever. *Science* 201:604, 1978.

Merrell, C. L., and Wright, D. N. A serological survey of mule deer and elk in Utah. *J. Wildl. Dis.* 14:471–478, 1978.

Miller, J. K. Rocky Mountain spotted fever on Long Island. *Ann. Intern. Med.* 33:1398–1406, 1950.

Moulder, J. W. The rickettsias. In R. E. Buchanan and N. E. Gibbons, eds., *Bergey's manual of determinative bacteriology*, p. 18, pp. 882–897. Baltimore: Williams and Wilkins, 1974.

Morbidity and Mortality Weekly Report, April 27, 1979. Surveillance summary: Rocky Mountain spotted fever, United States. *MMWR* 28:181–182, 1978.

Pagan, E. F., McMahon, K. J., and Bowen, R. E. Complement-fixing antibodies for *R. rickettsii* in serums of black-tailed jackrabbits. *Public Health Rep.* 76:1120–1122, 1961.

Parker, R. R., Bell, J. F., Chalgren, W. S., Thrailkill, F. B., and McKee, M. T. The recovery of strains of Rocky Mountain spotted fever and tularemia from ticks of the eastern United States. *J. Infect. Dis.* 91:231–237, 1952.

Philip, R. N., Casper, E. A., Burgdorfer, W., Gerloff, R. K., Hughes, L. E., and Bell, E. J. Serologic typing of rickettsiae of the spotted fever group by microimmunofluorescence. *J. Immunol.* 121:1961–1968, 1978.

Philip, R. N., Casper, E. A., MacCormack, V. N., Sexton, D. J., Thomas, L. A. Anacker, R. L., Burgdorfer, W., and Vick, S. A comparison of serologic methods for diagnosis of Rocky Mountain spotted fever. *Am. J. Epidemiol.* 105:56–67, 1977,

Price, E. G. *Fighting spotted fever in the Rockies.* Helena, Mont.: Naegele Printing Co., 1948.

Price, W. H. A quantitative analysis of the factors involved in the variations in virulence of rickettsiae. *Science* 118:49–52, 1953.

———. The epidemiology of Rocky Mountain spotted fever: II. Studies on the biological survival mechanism of *Rickettsia rickettsii*. *Am. J. Hyg.* 60:292–319, 1954a.

———. Variation in virulence of *Rickettsia rickettsii* under natural and experimental conditions. In E. W. Hartman, F. L. Horsfall, and J. G. Kidd, eds., *The dynamics of viral and rickettsial infections.* Garden City, N.Y.: Country Life Press, 1954b.

Rehacek, J., Brezina, R., Zupancicova, M., and Kovacova, E. Demonstrations of rickettsiae in tick haemocytes. *J. Hyg. Epidemiol. Microbiol. Immunol.* 15:424–435, 1971.

Ricketts, H. T. Some aspects of Rocky Mountain spotted fever as shown by recent investigations. *Med. Rec.* 76:843–855, 1909.

Saslaw, S., Carlisle, H. N., Wolf, G. L., and Cole, C. R. Rocky Mountain spotted fever: Clinical and laboratory observations of monkeys after respiratory exposure. *J. Infect. Dis.* 116:243–255, 1966.

Stoenner, H. G., Holdenried, R., Lackman, D., and Osburn, J. S. The occurrence of *Coxiella burnetii, Brucella,* and other pathogens among fauna of the Great Salt Lake Desert in Utah. *J. Trop. Med. Hyg.* 8:590–596, 1959.

University of Utah. A study of the ecology and epizoology of the native fauna of the Great Salt Lake Desert. *Ecology and Epizoology Series* (1964–1969). Salt Lake City: University of Utah.

Vest, E. D., Lundgren, D. L., Parker, D. D., Johnson, D. E., Morse, E. L., Bushman, J. B., Sidwell, R. W., and Thorpe, B. D. Results of a five-year survey for certain enzootic diseases in the fauna of western Utah. *J. Trop. Med. Hyg.* 14:124–135, 1965.

Wolf, G. L., and Cole, C. R. Staining rickettsiae in sections of formalin-fixed tissue: A 12-minute Wright-buffer sequence. *Stain Technol.* 41:185–188, 1966.

39 *Salmon Poisoning Disease*

STUART E. KNAPP   RAYMOND E. MILLEMANN

Synonyms: **Salmon disease, salmon poisoning.**

Salmon poisoning disease (SPD), which is enzootic in the Pacific Northwest, is a helminth-borne, almost always fatal disease of dogs, foxes, and coyotes. The name is a misnomer because the salmon are not poisoned nor do they poison the canid; however, the designation is retained because of long use. The vector of the disease is the digenetic trematode *Nanophyetus salmincola* (Chapin); and a rickettsialike organism, *Neorickettsia helminthoeca*, is the etiologic agent.

HISTORY. SPD was first reported from northwestern Oregon by Jesse Quinn Thornton (1849) who stated that dogs are very fond of raw fresh salmon; but it is usually fatal to them. Cooper and Suckley (1859) also reported the disease in Oregon and stated, "The native dogs of Oregon subsist well upon fish, which they even do not hesitate to eat *raw.* Salmon ... will make any blooded dog from the States very ill; scarcely one dog out of ten recovers. They concluded, however, that the disease "salmon sickness" was distemper. Pernot (1911) reported that minute cysts he observed in salmonids caused the disease and concluded that the cysts were amoebas. He infected two dogs by feeding them salmon kidneys. This was the first report of experimentally produced infections. Donham (1925) reported that the amoebalike cysts in salmon and trout were trematodes. Donham et al. (1926) showed that SPD was caused by a trematode maturing in intestines of infected animals and that animals recovering from the disease were immune to further infection.

The trematodes were described as *Nanophyes salmincola* by Chapin in 1926, but he changed the name to *Nanophyetus salmincola*

in 1928. The genus *Nanophyetus* was shifted to *Troglotrema* by Witenberg (1932), but Wallace (1935) insisted the name *Nanophyetus* was valid.

Simms et al. (1931b) confirmed Donham's finding that an intestinal trematode was involved with the disease and reported that the disease could be produced by intraperitoneal injection of mature trematodes into dogs. They were not certain of the specific cause of salmon poisoning but knew the disease had a characteristic incubation period followed by typical acute symptoms. Pathologic lesions limited to the "digestive tube" were also described.

Simms et al. (1931b) stated that the snail *Goniobasis plicifera* var. *silicula* was the molluscan intermediate host for the trematode. According to Henderson (1936) and Morrison (1954) the correct name of the snail is *Oxytrema silicula*. Simms et al. (1931b), Bennington and Pratt (1960), Schlegel et al. (1968), Law (1969), and Carter (1973) also reported details of the life cycle of the trematode, including naturally and experimentally infected definitive hosts.

Simms et al. (1931b) reported that metacercarial stages of the trematode were found in young salmon before they left fresh water, in mature salmon after they returned to fresh water, but not in salmon returning from the ocean. They therefore concluded that "cleansing" of the fish must occur during the years the salmon are in salt water. Thornton (1849) had indicated that this was popularly believed by local inhabitants in 1848.

Simms and Muth (1934) described many of the characteristics of the disease agent and provided conclusive evidence that the trematode acts as a vector for transmission of the disease. They postulated that the cause of the disease was a rickettsia or a hemosporidian.

Cordy and Gorham (1950) were the first to discover the disease agent and to report detailed descriptions on the pathogenesis of SPD in dogs and foxes. Their report provided a comprehensive account of the course of the disease in canids excluding lesions of the central nervous system. Descriptions of central nervous system and lymphoreticular lesions of SPD were reported by Hadlow (1957) and Frank et al. (1974b), respectively.

The work of the authors reported here was supported by Public Health Service Research Grant 5 ROI AI 06599 from the National Institute of Allergy and Infectious Diseases. Publication No. 1314, Environmental Sciences Division, Oak Ridge National Laboratory (operated by Union Carbide Corporation under contract W-7405-eng-26 with the U.S. Department of Energy).

Cordy and Gorham (1950) suggested that the agent belonged in the order Rickettsiales, and Philip et al. (1953) proposed the name *Neorickettsia helminthoeca*. Evidence that the agent is a rickettsia is provided by the results of the study by Brown et al. (1972) who first propagated the agent in vitro. It was subsequently cultivated by Noonan (1973) and Frank et al. (1974a).

The SPD literature was reviewed by Philip (1955), and more recently by Millemann and Knapp (1970) with emphasis on the biology of the trematode vector.

Skrjabin and Podjapolskaja (1931) described a new species of *Nanophyetus* (*N. schikhobalowi*) from far eastern Siberian people. Filimonova (1963, 1965, 1966) reported on the life cycle of this species. The first intermediate hosts are snails (*Semisulcospira laevigata* and *S. cancellata*); the second intermediate hosts are salmonid and some nonsalmonid fishes; and the adult trematode occurs naturally in man, dog, cat, red fox (*Vulpes vulpes*), gray wolf, Alaskan brown bear, Asiatic black bear, raccoon dog, American mink, yellow-throated Asiatic marten, Old World badger, wolverine, sea otter, Norway rat, and weasel (*Mustela sibirica*). There is no mention in the Russian literature that *N. schikhobalowi* either carries a rickettsia or causes SPD in dogs or humans. Witenberg (1932), Gebhardt et al. (1966), and Filimonova (1966, 1968) believed that *N. schikhobalowi* is conspecific with *N. salmincola*.

DISTRIBUTION. Simms et al. (1931a,b) stated that the geographic distribution of the snail intermediate host of the trematode vector determined the enzootic area of the disease. The snail occurs along the U.S. Pacific Coast from the Sacramento River north to the southern portion of the Olympic Peninsula in Washington and inland only as far as the western slope of the Cascade Mountains.

ETIOLOGY. *Neorickettsia helminthoeca*, a rickettsialike organism, is the etiologic agent of the disease (Fig. 39.1). The organisms, approximately 0.3 μm in size, are coccoid or coccobacillary in shape and occur singly, in multiple colonies, or in morulalike clumps in infected canid cells. Pleomorphic forms that appear as rods of varying lengths up to 2 μm and are sometimes crescent or ring shaped have been observed (Philip 1955). The organisms stain purple with Giemsa stain, blue or red with Macchiavello stain, and are gram-negative.

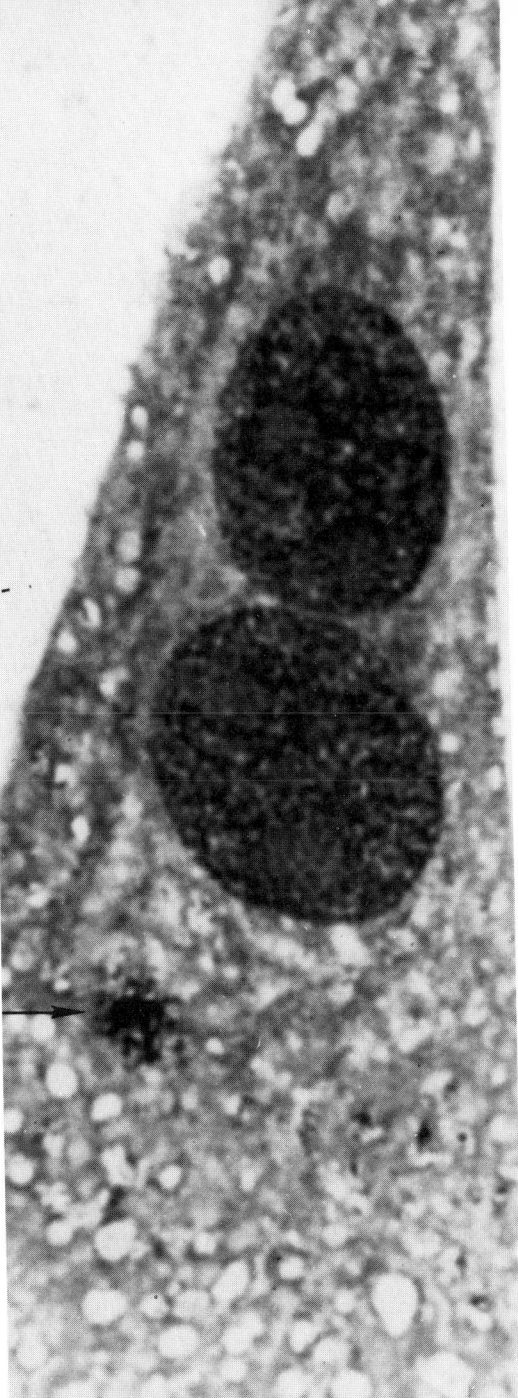

FIG. 39.1 Canine macrophage infected with *Neorickettsia helminthoeca*. An isolated colony (arrow) and individual minute coccoid organisms are present. Cells were from a homogenate of a lymph node taken from a dog with acute SPD and were cultured in Eagle's minimal essential medium supplemented with calf serum (×2,000, approx.). (Courtesy of G. L. Zimmerman and D. R. Stevens, Oregon State University.)

Initial attempts to grow the organisms on bacteriologic media in embryonated chicken eggs and in chick embryo tissue culture were unsuccessful (Philip 1955). Brown et al. (1972) cultivated the SPD agent in primary canine monocyte cell cultures and fulfilled Koch-Rivers's postulates. They also showed by specific immunofluorescence that antigen cross-reactivity did not exist between the SPD agent and *Ehrlichia canis*, the causative agent of a tick-borne canine rickettsiosis (Philip 1959). Noonan (1973) reported successful cultivation of the SPD agent in canine leukocytes and sarcoma cells and in mouse lymphoblasts; Frank et al. (1974a) cultivated the agent in canine monocytes. The agent can be preserved for up to 3 months by freezing infected cell cultures at −80°C (Brown et al. 1972).

Farrell (1966) and Farrell et al. (1973a) reported the existence of a second rickettsialike disease of dogs, which they named Elokomin fluke fever (EFF), that is also transmitted by *N. salmincola*. This disease has a high morbidity and low mortality for dogs; raccoons (*Procyon lotor*) and black bears (*Ursus americanus*), which are refractory to SPD, are susceptible to EFF; and EFF and SPD are immunologically and serologically distinct (Frank et al. 1974a,b; Kitao et al. 1973; Sakawa et al. 1973). The two agents are also antigenically distinguishable by fluorescent antibody studies from the human disease agent *Rickettsia sennetsu* (Sakawa et al. 1973). The last organism is morphologically similar to the SPD and EFF agents and may also be transmitted (not yet proven) by endoparasites. Whether the SPD and EFF agents are distinct entities or represent different antigenic types is not clear. The results of studies by Frank et al. (1974a,b) support the latter view. They found no differences between the two agents when grown in tissue culture; their ultrastructures and intracellular growth patterns are similar; macrophage response to infection with the agents is comparable; and the histopathology of the infections in dogs is similar but less severe in EFF.

TRANSMISSION

Natural. The digenetic trematode *N. salmincola* is the vector for the SPD agent. The infective agent has been demonstrated in all the trematode stages. Its presence in adult trematodes was shown by Nyberg et al. (1967), Philip et al. (1954b), Simms and Muth (1934), and Simms et al. (1931a,b); in metacercariae by Philip et al. (1954a) and Simms et al. (1932); in helminth-infected snail livers by Philip et al. (1954b); and in helminth eggs by Nyberg et al. (1967).

The trematode requires three hosts for completion of its life cycle (Fig. 39.2). The first intermediate host is *Oxytrema* (= *Goniobasis*) *silicula*, a pleurocerid stream snail found in northwestern California, in Oregon west of the Cascade Mountains, and in the Olympic Peninsula in Washington. The parasite can develop only in this snail, and thus the geographic distribution of the snail limits the enzootic area in which canine infection occurs (Simms et al. 1931a,b). The sporocyst stage of the parasite in the snail was unknown until it was recently described by Carter (1973) who was also the first to report successful in vitro development and hatching of the eggs. The parasites as cercariae emerge from the snail host through the ctenidial leaflets (Law 1969). They then enter and encyst in the second intermediate hosts, which are various salmonid and some nonsalmonid fishes and also the Pacific giant salamander (Table 39.1). Anadromous fish, which acquire the infection during their residence in fresh water, retain both the trematode and the rickettsiae during their residence in the ocean for periods of up to 3 years, and dogs fed such fish develop SPD (Farrell et al. 1964; Millemann et al. 1964; Weiseth et al. 1974). The definitive hosts are fish-eating mammals and birds (Table 39.2) that acquire the trematodes by eating raw infected fish. However, Farrell et al. (1968, 1974) reported trematode infection and SPD in two dogs that reportedly had eaten only kippered salmon. The fish had been soaked in brine and then smoked at 82°C for 10–16 hours.

Animals that have been examined but not found to be naturally infected are: squirrel, crow, robin, turkey vulture, ring-billed gull, American merganser, Bonaparte's gull, red-tailed hawk, white-winged scoter, water snake, meadow mouse, shrew-mole, belted kingfisher, Trobridge shrew, nutria, black bear, muskrat, bushy-tailed wood rat, opossum, striped skunk, and cougar (Donham et al. 1926; Schlegel et al. 1968). However, for many of these species only a few individuals were examined.

Only canids are susceptible to SPD. However, parasites from noncanid hosts harbor the agent. Philip (1955) produced disease in a dog by intraperitoneal injection of 500 adult trematodes (but not of lymph nodes) recovered from a symptomless infected raccoon.

Experimental. The second intermediate hosts and the definitive hosts that have been experi-

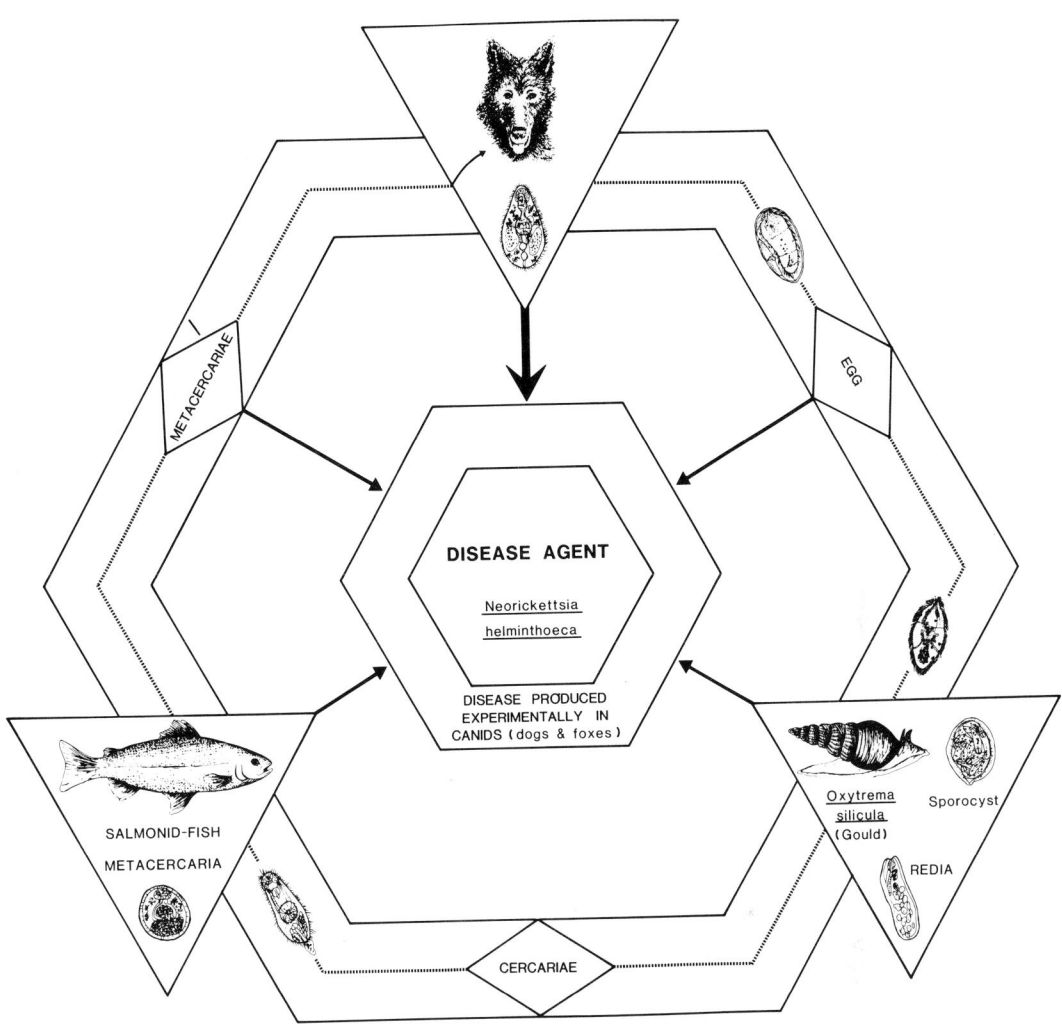

FIG. 39.2   Life cycle of *Nanophyetus salmincola* showing that the disease
agent (*Neorickettsia helminthoeca*) in an infectious state for canids is present
in all stages of the trematode vector. (Original—Knapp.)

mentally infected with the trematode are listed
in Tables 39.1 and 39.2, respectively.

SPD has been transmitted to canids by
feeding them infected fish (many authors), and
by injection of infected blood, spleen, and lymph
node suspensions (Cordy and Gorham 1950;
Philip et al. 1954a; Simms et al. 1932), adult
flukes (Nyberg et al. 1967; Simms and Muth
1934; Simms et al. 1931b), metacercariae
(Simms et al. 1932), helminth-infected snail
livers (Philip et al. 1954b), and helminth eggs
(Nyberg et al. 1967). Philip (1955) reported
partial success in transmitting SPD to dogs by

allowing ticks (*Haemaphysalis leachi* and *Rhipicephalus sanguineus*) to feed on the animals
or by injection of suspensions of *R. sanguineus*
ticks. Bosman et al. (1970) transmitted SPD to
dogs by aerosols and rectal administration of
infectious dog lymph node suspensions and rectal mucosa homogenates.

Simms et al. (1931b, 1932) failed to produce
SPD in 2 bobcats and 1 bear by feeding infected
fish, and in 1 guinea pig, 1 white rat, and 1
rabbit by intraperitoneal injection of blood from
a sick dog. Cordy and Gorham (1950) failed to
produce disease in mink, cats, guinea pigs,

hamsters, and white mice. Philip et al. (1954a) were unable to adapt the agent to guinea pigs, hamsters, and white mice. Monkeys are susceptible to infection with the trematode but are apparently refractory to the disease (Farrel et al., unpublished, cited in Farrell et al. 1974; Karr and Wong 1974). Philip (1958) intentionally infected himself by eating raw infected trout, samples of which produced a fatal infection when fed to a dog. He suffered no ill effects,

TABLE 39.1   Second Intermediate Hosts for *Nanophyetus salmincola*.

Scientific Name	Common Name	Observed Infection[a]		Reference
		N	E	
Ambystomidae				
Dicamptodon ensatus	Pacific giant salamander	+	0	Gebhardt et al. 1966
Hylidae				
Hyla regilla	Pacific tree frog	0	+	Winward and Lattig 1970
Catostomidae				
Catostomus macrocheilus	largescale sucker	0	+	Gebhardt et al. 1966
Centrarchidae				
Lepomis macrochirus	bluegill	0	+	Gebhardt et al. 1966
Cottidae				
Cottus perplexus	reticulate sculpin	+	+	Bennington and Pratt 1960; Gebhardt et al. 1966
Cyprinidae				
Carassius auratus	goldfish	0	+	Bennington and Pratt 1960; Gebhardt et al. 1966
Rhinichthys osculus	speckled dace	0	+	Bennington and Pratt 1960
Richardsonius balteatus	redside shiner	+	+	Gebhardt et al. 1966
Gasterosteidae				
Gasterosteus a. aculeatus	threespine stickleback	0	+	Gebhardt et al. 1966
G. a. microcephalus	threespine stickleback	0	+	Gebhardt et al. 1966
Petromyzontidae				
Lampetra richardsoni	Western brook lamprey	+	+	Gebhardt et al. 1966
L. tridentata	Pacific lamprey	+	0	Gebhardt et al. 1966
Poeciliidae				
Gambusia affinis	mosquito fish	0	+	Gebhardt et al. 1966
Salmonidae				
Oncorhynchus tshawytscha	chinook salmon	+	+	Donham et al. 1926; Bennington and Pratt 1960
O. kisutch	coho salmon	+	+	Donham et al. 1926; Baldwin et al. 1967
O. keta	chum salmon	+	0	Simms et al. 1931b
O. nerka	kokanee	0	+	Baldwin et al. 1967
O. gorbuscha	pink salmon	−	0	Weiseth et al. 1974
Salmo gairdneri	rainbow trout	+	+	Simms et al. 1931b; Baldwin et al. 1967
S. clarki clarki	cutthroat trout	+	+	Donham et al. 1926; Baldwin et al. 1967
S. clarki lewisi	Montana black-spotted cutthroat trout	0	+	Baldwin et al. 1967
S. clarki henshawi	Lahontan cutthroat trout	0	+	Baldwin et al. 1967
S. salar	Atlantic salmon	0	+	Gebhardt et al. 1966
S. trutta	brown trout	0	+	Gebhardt et al. 1966
Salvelinus fontinalis	brook trout	+	+	Simms et al. 1931b; Gebhardt et al. 1966
S. namaycush	lake trout	0	+	Gebhardt et al. 1966

Note: Hosts for *N. schikhobalowi* not listed.

[a]N = natural and E = experimental. 0 = no information available.

but some parasites did attain maturity as evidenced by the appearance of a few eggs in the stools 10 days after ingestion of the fish. Although *N. schikhobalowi* occurs in man in far eastern Siberia (Filimonova, 1963, 1965, 1966; Skrjabin and Podjapolskaja 1931), natural human infections with the New World species of *Nanophyetus* have not been reported until recently. J. R. Berry, R. Eastburn, and T. P. Kistner (personal communication, 1979) found eggs of *N. salmincola* in the stools of two young men who had histories of eating raw salmon in

TABLE 39.2 Definitive Hosts of *Nanophyetus salmincola.*

Scientific Name	Common Name	N	E	Reference
Homo sapiens	man	0	+	Philip 1958
Cercocebus atys	sooty mangabey	0	+	Karr and Wong 1974
Macaca mulatta	rhesus monkey	0	+	Karr and Wong 1974; Farrell et al. 1974
M. nemestrina	pig-tailed macaque	0	+	Farrell et al. 1974
Ardea herodias	great blue heron	+	0	Schlegel et al. 1968
Lophodytes cucullatus	hooded merganser	+	0	Schlegel et al. 1968
Megaceryle alcoyon	belted kingfisher	+	0	Donham 1928
Alopex lagopus	Arctic fox	+	+	Simms et al. 1931a,b
Canis familaris	domestic dog	+	+	Many authors
C. latrans	coyote	+	+	Cram 1926; Donham and Simms 1927; Schlegel et al. 1968
Cavia porcellus	guinea pig	0	+	Simms et al. 1931b
Didelphis virgiana	opossum	0	+	Schlegel et al. 1968
Felis domestica	domestic cat	+	+	Simms et al. 1931b; Schlegel et al. 1968
Lutra canadensis	river otter	+	0	Schlegel et al. 1968
Lynx rufus	bobcat	+	+	Cram 1926; Simms et al. 1931b; Schlegel et al. 1968
Meriones unguiculatus	jird	0	+	Nyberg and Knapp (unpublished)
Mesocricetus auratus	golden hamster	0	+	Philip 1959; Bennington and Pratt 1960
Mus musculus	white mouse	0	+	Philip 1959
Mustela erminea	short-tail weasel	+	0	Schlegel et al. 1968
M. vison	mink	+	0	Donham et al. 1926; Simms et al. 1931b; Baker 1950; Schlegel et al. 1968
Neotoma spp.	woodrat	0	+	Bennington and Pratt 1960
Procyon lotor	raccoon	+	+	Cram 1926; Simms et al. 1931b; Bennington and Pratt 1960; Schlegel et al. 1968
Rattus norvegicus	Norway rat	+	+	Simms et al. 1931b; Schlegel et al. 1968
Spilogale putorius	spotted skunk	+	0	Schlegel et al. 1968
Ursus americanus	black bear	0	+	Simms et al. 1931b; Farrel et al. 1973a
Vulpes fulva	red fox	+	+	Donham et al. 1926; Simms et al. 1931b; Cordy and Gorham 1950; Schlegel et al. 1968

Note: Hosts for *N. schikhobalowi* not listed.
[a]N= natural and E = experimental. 0 = no information available.

Oregon. One man was symptomless, but the other had abdominal discomfort, nausea, weight loss, and gastric tenderness of several weeks duration when examined. After drug treatment, his symptoms disappeared and the stools of both men were negative for helminth eggs. Whether the illness of the one individual was caused by the trematode or the rickettsiae is not known. However, gastrointestinal symptoms occur in humans in Siberia with *N. schikhobalowi* infections (Sinovich 1959), and this trematode apparently does not carry rickettsiae.

Philip (1955) reported that raccoons develop a mild temperature rise after eating infected fish or after injection with proved infectious lymph nodes but otherwise remain symptomless. Farrell et al. (1973a) observed the same reaction, together with other mild signs, in black bears and dogs. They named this disease Elokomin fluke fever to distinguish it from the more severe SPD, which develops only canids.

SIGNS. Signs of infection in dogs and foxes are similar (Cordy and Gorham 1950). The incubation period averages 5–7 days, although some dogs have long incubation periods of 19–33 days (Philip 1955), after which there is a sudden onset of fever and anorexia, sometimes accompanied by vomiting and diarrhea or dysentery. The fever with a temperature peak of 40–42.8°C lasts from 4–7 days and is followed by a period of defervescence during which the temperature returns to normal or falls below. Constant inappetence results in marked dehydration and weight loss. The animal will occasionally drink excessive amounts of water. Remensynder (1974) reported the presence of a rancid odor of the breath in the majority of the dogs he treated for SPD. A serous nasal discharge may occur early in the febrile period. A conjunctival exudate may be present at the inner canthus. The somatic lymph nodes become enlarged, as well as the mesenteric lymph nodes in later stages of the disease. Death usually occurs within 10 days to 2 weeks after onset of signs. Figure 39.3 shows the course of a typical infection.

Some dogs that succumb to the disease may be afebrile or show a slight temperature rise or a shortened febrile period (Philip 1955).

PATHOGENESIS AND PATHOLOGY. SPD is acquired by the ingestion of raw infected salmonid fish. But, as noted above, Farrell et al. (1968) reported that two dogs developed SPD after they had supposedly eaten only kippered salmon. The way that the etiologic agent leaves the trematode vector and gains access to the host tissues is not known. The organisms are present in reticuloendothelial cells of lymph nodes, tonsils, spleen, and intestinal lymph follicles of dogs and foxes, and occasionally in macrophages of the liver, lungs, and blood (Cordy and Gorham 1950).

The principal gross lesions include variable enlargement of the ileocecal, mesenteric, portal, and internal iliac lymph nodes (Fig. 39.4). The thymus may be enlarged and edematous in young animals. The spleen and tonsils may also

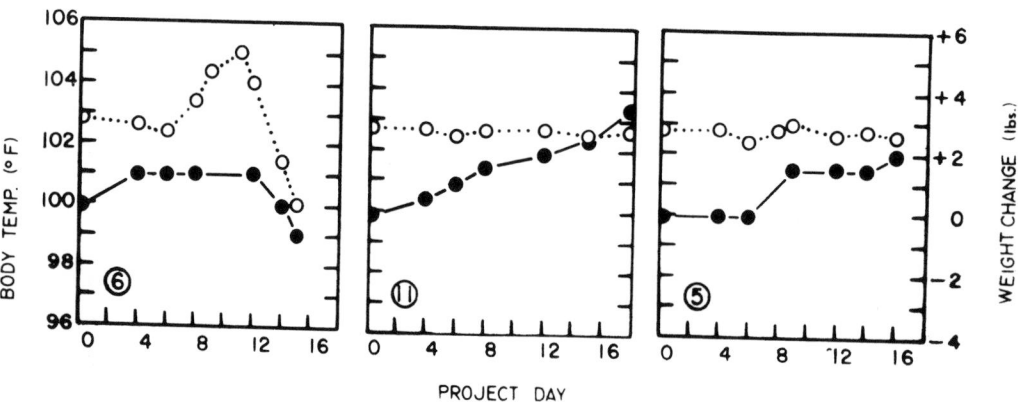

FIG. 39.3 Body temperatures (broken lines) and weight changes (unbroken lines) for a dog (6) with salmon poisoning disease, a noninfected control dog (11), and an immune dog (5) challenged with *Nanophyetus salmincola* metacercariae. Dog 6 was injected intraperitoneally with 100,000 ground *N. salmincola* eggs. (Original—Nyberg, Knapp, and Millemann.)

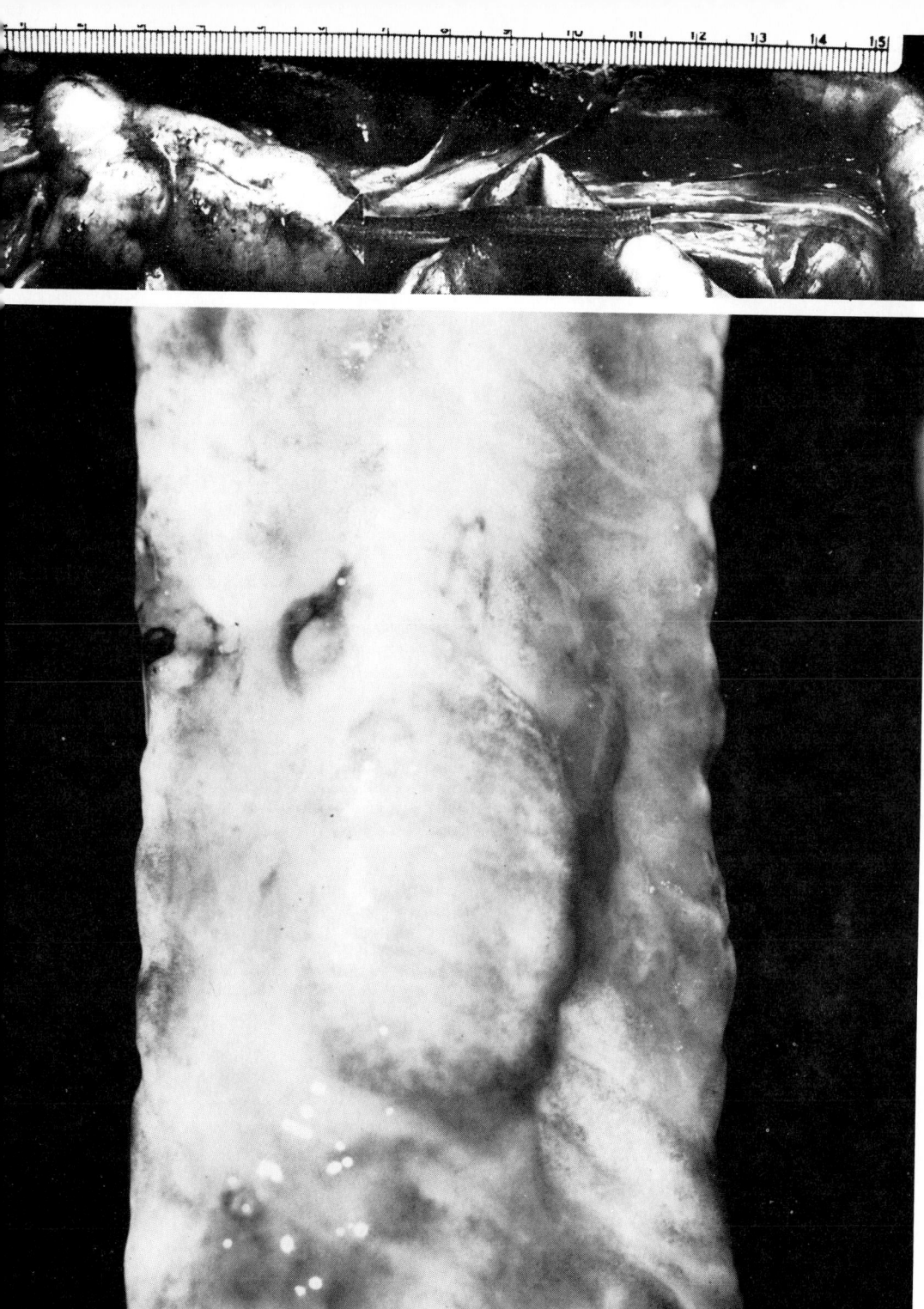

FIG. 39.4. (*Above*) Characteristically enlarged ileocecal lymph node (at end of arrow) from a dog that died of salmon poisoning disease. (Original—Nyberg, Knapp, and Millemann.) (*Below*) Higher magnification. (Courtesy of G. L. Zimmerman and D. R. Stevens, Oregon State University.)

show enlargement, hemorrhage, and hyperplasia. Occasional enlargement of other lymphatic tissues may occur. Necrosis and hyperplasia of intestinal lymph follicles can lead to ulceration and severe hemorrhage (Cordy and Gorham 1950).

Microscopic necrotic foci appear in the lymph follicles and also may occur in other tissues. Leukocytic infiltration is a common occurrence. Other changes include a severe depletion of small lymphocytes from the lymph node cortex with loss of germinal centers and marked infiltration of macrophages (Frank et al. 1974b). Splenic follicular necrosis and loss of thymic architecture from macrophage infiltration can also occur. The presence of these lesions distinguishes SPD from EFF in dogs (Frank et al. 1974b). Neuropathologic changes in SPD are characterized by a nonsuppurative meningitis or meningoencephalitis (Hadlow 1957).

The trematodes embedded in intestinal tissue account for slight tissue damage and are found predominantly in the duodenum. The enteric ulceration and hemorrhage resulting from lymph follicle necrosis are frequently confined to areas of the alimentary tract adjacent to the ileocecal valve.

Cordy and Gorham (1950) have compared pathologic lesions of SPD in dogs and foxes. Macroscopic lesions were more extensive in foxes, and apparently the foxes are more susceptible to the disease. In most of the dogs examined, the livers appeared to be normal, but in most of the foxes they were soft and friable. Hemoperitoneum and hemorrhage of the gall bladder wall, kidney necrosis, and heart lesions were observed only in foxes.

The mechanism by which the organisms cause disease in canids is not known.

DIAGNOSIS. A history of the animal's eating raw fish and appearance of the signs provide a presumptive diagnosis for SPD.

Trematode eggs first appear in the feces of dogs 5–8 days after the animals have eaten infected fish and disappear by the 250th day of infection (Simms et al. 1931b). The eggs are 87–97 μm by 38–55 μm in size (Bennington and Pratt 1960). They are light brown with an indistinct operculum at one end and a small blunt point at the other (Fig. 39.5). Eggs can be detected by a direct smear of the feces in heavy infections. A more reliable method is the technique of Dennis et al. (1954). Farrell et al. (1955) stated that this technique is applicable to recovery of *N. salmincola* eggs; they described the technique as follows:

It consists of a washing-sedimentation technique, using a mixture of 5 cc. of a household liquid detergent and 995 cc. of tap water to which a few drops of 1 per cent alum (aluminum potassium sulfate, U.S.P.) have been added. This fluid becomes somewhat gelatinous on standing; therefore, it is prepared at frequent intervals. A 1- to 3-Gm. fecal sample is thoroughly mixed with about 15 cc. of the detergent solution in a large test tube or other container and the mixture is strained into a 50-cc. centrifuge tube. The material on the strainer is washed with more detergent solution until the centrifuge tube is filled to the 50-cc. mark. The suspension is allowed to stand for five to ten minutes and then the supernatant fluid is carefully decanted or siphoned off, allowing 2 or 3 cc.

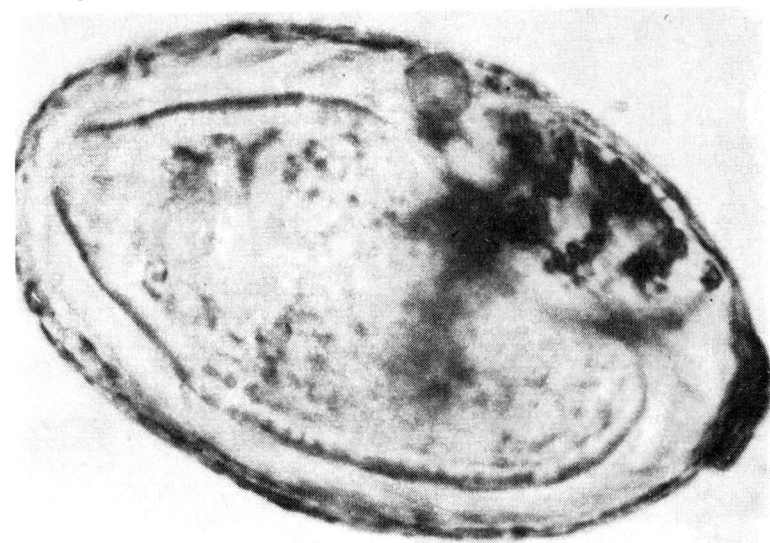

FIG. 39.5 *Nanophyetus salmincola* egg showing characteristic shape, indistinct operculum, and abopercular knob. Eggs passed in the feces of definitive hosts do not contain a developed miracidium as this one does (×1440). (Original—Nyberg, Knapp, and Millemann.)

of the liquid and debris to remain in the centrifuge tube. The sediment is again washed by refilling the centrifuge tube to the 50-cc. mark with the detergent solution and allowing it to stand for another five to ten minutes. The supernatant fluid is then separated as before. (The ova will settle quickly in water, but the detergent solution floats off more debris.) A small amount of the sediment is transferred to a slide and examined for fluke ova (pp. 241–242).

The finding of trematode eggs in the feces does not establish the diagnosis, because dogs that have recovered from the disease can be reinfected with the trematode, and the eggs of other canine parasites can be confused with those of *N. salmincola*.

A successful skin test has not been developed (Farrell et al. 1955).

Farrell et al. (1955) described another technique for diagnosis of SPD. The mandibular lymph nodes, medial and ventral to the mandible of the dog, are palpated, then one of the nodes is pulled ventrally and a curved intestinal clamp placed behind it, fixing the node in position. A few drops of fluid can be aspirated from the node, using a 20-gauge needle attached to a syringe. The plunger is withdrawn and the node compressed at the same time. The aspirated fluid, which usually remains in the needle, is expressed onto a clean microscope slide. The drop is smeared, air-dried, fixed, and defatted for 1 minute with a mixture of equal parts of ether and alcohol. The smear is stained by either Giemsa's or Macchiavello's technique. In addition to the usual Giemsa technique, which is used if there is any doubt as to the presence of rickettsiae, Farrell et al. (1955) described a rapid Giemsa method. This involves staining the smears for 2 minutes with a 1:1 dilution of stock Giemsa and buffered water at pH 7.2, followed by washing of the slides. The cells in the smears are examined for the typical intracytoplasmic rickettsial bodies. Extracellular organisms cannot be reliably distinguished from debris.

PROGNOSIS. SPD is an almost uniformly fatal disease for dogs. About 90% of naturally infected animals die (Philips 1955). Simms et al. (1931a) reported that only 4 of 102 dogs with SPD recovered naturally. The disease is equally fatal for foxes (Cordy and Gorham 1950) and coyotes (Donham and Simms 1927).

IMMUNITY. Canines that recover from the disease either spontaneously or after drug treatment develop a lasting and solid immunity to the disease agent, but not to the fluke (Philip

1950; Shaw and Howarth 1939; Simms et al. 1931a). Simms et al. (1931a) reported that dogs from an immune female were susceptible to SPD. There is no cross-protection between SPD and EFF (Farrell et al. 1973a).

TREATMENT. Various sulfonamides given orally or parenterally have been successful in treatment (Coon et al. 1938; Cordy and Gorham 1951; Philip 1955). Dosage at therapeutic blood levels should be maintained for at least 3 days. Effective results also have been obtained with penicillin, chlortetracycline, chloramphenicol, and oxytetracycline but not with streptomycin (Farrell 1971). The best results follow administration of large divided doses. If the animal is dehydrated, intravenous fluid therapy is essential to avoid nephrotoxic effects. Treatment in the late stages of the disease may not be successful. General supportive treatment, aimed at correcting and maintaining fluid and electrolyte balance, providing nutritional requirements, and controlling diarrhea, often is essential unless there is a prompt favorable response.

CONTROL. No vaccine or other prophylatic is currently available. However, now that the SPD agent can be grown in tissue culture, development of a vaccine should be possible.

Shaw and Howarth (1939) suggested that dog owners feed their animals infected fish and institute early sulfonamide therapy to produce solid immunity.

Preventive measures include: avoiding the feeding of raw trout or salmon to dogs; freezing (−20°C for 24 hours) or thoroughly cooking infected fish, both of which inactivate the rickettsiae and the trematode (Farrell et al. 1974); and keeping the dogs away from streams during the peak period of salmon migration. Additional possible preventive measures include: the avoidance of feeding kippered fish to dogs; isolation of dogs with SPD; and appropriate sterilization of instruments, feed pans, and other hospital or kennel equipment.

Control of the infection by eradication of the snail host by use of molluscicides is not practical.

Infection of hatchery fish could be prevented by destruction of the free-living cercariae in the incoming water. This has been achieved experimentally by passing water containing cercariae through an electrically charged grid (Combs 1968) or past an ultrasonic generator (Farrell et al. 1973b), but large-scale sustained efforts routinely using these methods have not been made.

REFERENCES

Baker, G. A. *Troglotrema salmincola* in mink. *J. Parasitol.* 36:503, 1950.

Baldwin, N. L., Millemann, R. E., and Knapp, S. E. "Salmon poisoning" disease: III. Effect of experimental *Nanophyetus salmincola* infection on the fish host. *J. Parasitol.* 53:556–564, 1967 .

Bennington, E., and Pratt, I. The life history of the salmon-poisoning fluke, *Nanophyetus salmincola* (Chapin). *J. Parasitol.* 46:91–100, 1960.

Bosman, D. D., Farrell, R. K., and Gorham, J. R. Non-endoparasite transmission of salmon poisoning disease of dogs. *J. Am. Vet. Med. Assoc.* 156:1907–1910, 1970.

Brown, J. L., Huxsoll, D. L., Ristic, M., and Hildebrandt, P. K. *In vitro* cultivation of *Neorickettsia helminthoeca*, the causative agent of salmon poisoning disease. *Am. J. Vet. Res.* 33:1695–1700, 1972.

Carter, R. T. Development of the egg of *Nanophyetus salmincola* (Chapin) and infection of the first intermediate host. Ph.D. thesis. Oregon State University, 1973. Abstr. *Diss. Abstr.* 33:4582, 1973.

Chapin, E. A. A new genus and species of trematode, the probable cause of salmon-poisoning in dogs. *North Am. Vet.* 7:36–37, 1926.

——. Note. *J. Parasitol.* 14:60, 1928.

Combs, B. D. An electrical grid for controlling trematode cercariae in hatchery water supplies. *Prog. Fish-Cult.* 30:67–75, 1968.

Coon, E. W., Myers, F. C., Phelps, T. R., Ruehle, O. J., Snodgrass, W. B., Shaw, J. N., Simms, B. T., and Bolin, F. M. Sulphanilamide as a treatment for salmon poisoning in dogs. *North Am. Vet.* 19:57–59, 1938.

Cooper, J. G., and Suckley, G. *The natural history of Washington Territory with much relating to Minnesota, Nebraska, Kansas, Oregon, and California, between the thirty-sixth and forty-ninth parallels of latitude, being those parts of the final reports on the survey of the Northern Pacific Railroad route, containing the climate and physical geography, with full catalogues and descriptions of the plants and animals collected from 1853 to 1857,* pt. 3. Zoological report, p. 112. New York: Bailliere Bros., 1859.

Cordy, D. R., and Gorham, J. R. The pathology and etiology of salmon disease in the dog and fox. *Am. J. Pathol.* 26:617–637, 1950.

——. Certain sulfonamides and antibiotics in the treatment of experimental "salmon poisoning" in dogs. *J. Am. Vet. Med. Assoc.* 118:305, 1951.

Cram, E. G. Wild carnivores as hosts for the trematode previously found in dogs as the result of salmon poisoning. *North Am. Vet.* 7:42–43, 1926.

Dennis, W. R., Stone, W. M., and Swanson, L. E. A new laboratory and field diagnostic test for fluke ova in feces. *J. Am. Vet. Med. Assoc.* 124:47–50, 1954.

Donham, C. R. So-called salmon poisoning of dogs. *Science* 61:341, 1925.

——. Salmon poisoning in dogs. M.S. thesis, Oregon State University, 1928.

Donham, C. R., and Simms, B. T. Coyote susceptible to salmon poisoning. *J. Am. Vet. Med. Assoc.* 71:215–217, 1927.

Donham, C. R., Simms, B. T., and Miller, F. W. So-called salmon poisoning in dogs (progress report). *J. Am. Vet. Med. Assoc.* 68:701–715, 1926.

Farrell, R. K. Transmission of two rickettsia-like disease agents of dogs by endoparasites in northwestern U.S.A. *1964 Proc. 1st Int. Congr. Parasitol. (Rome)* 1:438, 1966.

——. Canine rickettsiosis. In *Current veterinary therapy*, vol. 4. R. W. Kirk, ed., Philadelphia: Saunders, 1971.

Farrell, R. K., Dee, J. F., and Ott, R. L. Salmon poisoning in a dog fed kippered salmon. *J. Am. Vet. Med. Assoc.* 152:370–371, 1968.

Farrell, R. K., Leader, R. W., and Johnston, S. D. Differentiation of salmon poisoning disease and Elokomin fluke fever: Studies with the black bear (*Ursus americanus*). *Am. J. Vet. Res.* 34:919–922, 1973a.

Farrell, R. K., Lloyd, M. A., and Earp, B. Persistence of *Neorickettsia helminthoeca* in an endoparasite of the Pacific salmon. *Science* 145:162–163, 1964.

Farrell, R. K., Ott, R. L., and Gorham, J. R. The clinical laboratory diagnosis of salmon poisoning. *J. Am. Vet. Med. Assoc.* 127:241–244, 1955.

Farrell, R. K., Soave, O. A., and Johnston, S. D. *Nanophyetus salmincola* infections in kippered salmon. *Am. J. Public Health* 64:808–809, 1974.

Farrell, R. K., Watson, R. E., and Lloyd, M. Effect of ultrasound on trematode cercariae. *J. Parasitol.* 59:747–748, 1973b.

Filimonova, L. V. The biological cycle of the trematode *Nanophyetus schikhobalowi*. *Trans. Helminthol. Lab. Acad. Sci. USSR* 13:347–357, 1963.

——. An experimental investigation of the biology of *Nanophyetus schikhobalowi* Skrjabin and Podjapolskaja, 1931 (Trematoda, Nanophyetidae). *Trans. Helminthol. Lab. Acad. Sci. USSR* 15:172–184, 1965.

——. Distribution of nanophyetosis in the territory of the Soviet Far East. *Trans. Helminthol. Lab. Acad. Sci. USSR* 17:240–244, 1966.

——. On changing the taxonomic status of *Nanophyetus schikhobalowi* Skrjabin and Podjapolskaja, 1931 (Trematoda: Nanophyetidae). In *Helminths of man, animals and plants and means of combating them*, pp. 321–329. Moscow: Akad. Nauk SSSR Vses. Obsch Gelmintol., 1968.

Frank, D. W., McGuire, T. C. Gorham, J. R., and Davis, W. C. Cultivation of two species of *Neorickettsia* in canine monocytes. *J. Infect. Dis.* 129:257–262, 1974a.

Frank, D. W., McGuire, T. C., Gorham, J. R., and Farrell, R. K. Lymphoreticular lesions of canine neorickettsiosis. *J. Infect. Dis.* 129:163–171, 1974b.

Gebhardt, G. A., Millemann, R. E., Knapp, S. E., and Nyberg, P. A. "Salmon poisoning" disease: II.

Second intermediate host susceptibility studies. *J. Parasitol.* 52:54–59, 1966.

Hadlow, W. J. Neuropathology of experimental salmon poisoning of dogs. *Am. J. Vet. Res.* 18:898–908, 1957.

Henderson, J. The non-marine mollusca of Oregon and Washington, supplement. *Univ. Colo. Stud.* 23:251–278, 1936.

Karr, S. L., Jr., and Wong, M. M. Experimental infection of monkeys with *Nanophyetus salmincola. J. Parasitol.* 60:358, 1974.

Kitao, T., Farrell, R. K., and Fukuda, T. Differentiation of salmon poisoning disease and Elokomin fluke fever: Fluorescent antibody studies with *Rickettsia sennetsu. Am. J. Vet. Res.* 34: 927–928, 1973.

Law, D. T. The biology of *Nanophyetus salmincola* (Chapin) in its snail intermediate host, *Oxytrema silicula.* M.S. thesis, Oregon State University, 1969.

Millemann, R. E., Gebhardt, G. A., and Knapp, S. E. "Salmon poisoning" disease: I. Infection in a dog from marine salmonids. *J. Parasitol.* 50: 588–589, 1964.

Millemann, R. E., and Knapp, S. E. Biology of *Nanophyetus salmincola* and "salmon poisoning" disease. *Adv. Parasitol.* 8:1–41, 1970.

Morrison, J. P. E. The relationships of Old and New World melanians. *Proc. U.S. Nat. Mus.* 103: 357–394, 1954.

Noonan, W. E., *Neorickettsia helminthoeca* in cell culture. Ph.D. thesis, Oregon State University, 1973. Abstr. *Diss. Abstr.* 33:4046, 1973.

Nyberg, P. A., Knapp, S. E., and Millemann, R. E. "Salmon poisoning" disease: IV. Transmission of the disease to dogs by *Nanophyetus salmincola* eggs. *J. Parasitol.* 53:694–699, 1967.

Pernot, E. F. "Salmoning" of dogs. *Oreg. State Bd. Health Bull.* 5:1, 1911.

Philip, C. B. There's always something new under the "parasitological sun" (the unique story of helminth-borne salmon poisoning disease). *J. Parasitol.* 41:125–148, 1955.

———. A helminth replaces the usual arthropod as a vector of a rickettsialike disease. *1956 Proc. 10th Int. Congr. Entomol.* 3:651–653, 1958.

———. Canine rickettsiosis in western United States and comparison with a similar disease in the Old World. *Arch. Inst. Pasteur Tunis* 36:595–603, 1959.

Philip, C. B., Hadlow, W. J., and Hughes, L. E. *Neorickettsia helmintheca,* a new rickettsia-like disease agent of dogs in western United States transmitted by a helminth. *Int. Congr. Microbiol. Rep. Proc. 6th Congr.,* Rome 4:70–82, 1953.

———. Studies on salmon poisoning disease of canines. I. The rickettsial relationships and pathogenicity of *Neorickettsia helminthoeca. Exp.*

Parasitol. 3:336–350, 1954a.

Philip, C. B., Hughes, L. E., Locker, B., and Hadlow, W. J. Salmon poisoning disease of canines: II. Further observations on etiologic agent. *Proc. Exp. Biol. Med.* 87:397–400, 1954b.

Remensynder, R. J. Salmon poisoning in a dog in Oregon. *Vet. Med. Small Anim. Clin.* 69:562, 1974.

Sakawa, H., Farrell, R. K., and Mori, M. Differentiation of salmon poisoning disease and Elokomin fluke fever: Complement fixation. *Am. J. Vet. Res.* 34:923–925, 1973.

Schlegel, M. W., Knapp, S. E., and Millemann, R. E. "Salmon poisoning" disease: V. Definitive hosts of the trematode vector, *Nanophyetus salmincola. J. Parasitol.* 54:770–774, 1968.

Shaw, J. N., and Howarth, C. R. Immunity to salmon poisoning follows treatment of affected dogs with sulfanilamide. *North Am. Vet.* 20:67–68, 1939.

Simms, B. T., Donham, C. R., and Shaw, J. N. Salmon poisoning. *Am. J. Hyg.* 13:363–391, 1931a.

Simms, B. T., Donham, C. R., Shaw, J. N., and McCapes, A. M. Salmon poisoning. *J. Am. Vet. Med. Assoc.* 78:181–195, 1931b.

Simms, B. T., McCapes, A. M., and Muth, O. H. Salmon poisoning: Transmission and immunization experiments. *J. Am. Vet. Med. Assoc.* 81: 26–36, 1932.

Simms, B. T., and Muth, O. H. Salmon poisoning: Transmission and immunization studies. *Proc. 5th Pacific Sci. Congr. Can. (1933)* 4:2949–2960, 1934.

Sinovich, L. I. Nanophyetosis in the Soviet Far East. *10th Conference on Parasitological Problems and Diseases with Natural Reservoirs,* vol. 2. Moscow and Leningrad: Acad. Sci. USSR, 410–411, 1959.

Skrjabin, K. J., and Podjapolskaja, W. P. *Nanophyetus schikhobalowi* n. sp. ein neuer Trematode aus dem Darm des Menschen. *Zentralbla. Bakteriol.* [*Orig. A*] 119:294–297, 1931.

Thornton, J. Q. *Oregon and California in 1848,* vol. 1. New York: Harper and Bros., 1849.

Wallace, F. G. A morphological and biological study of the trematode. *Sellacotyle mustelae* n.g., n.sp. *J. Parasitol.* 21:143–164, 1935.

Weiseth, P. R., Farrell, R. K., and Johnston, S. D. Prevalence of *Nanophyetus salmincola* in ocean-caught salmon. *J. Am. Vet. Med. Assoc.* 165: 849–850, 1974.

Winward, L. D., and Lattig, G. M. A new experimental second intermediate host of *Nanophyetus salminocola* with evidence of transmission of *Neorickettsia helminthoeca. J. Parasitol.* 56:621–622, 1970.

Witenberg, G. On the anatomy and systematic position of the causative agent of so-called salmon poisoning. *J. Parasitol.* 18:258–263, 1932.

40 *Q Fever*

J. FREDERICK BELL

Synonyms: **Abattoir fever, Nine-Mile fever, Balkan grippe, coxiellosis.**

Q fever is a generalized rickettsial infection characterized by absence of rash and usually by pneumonitis. Ordinarily the disease is acute, self-limited, and nonfatal; but cases with insidious onset and chronic course occur.

HISTORY AND DISTRIBUTION. In studies in Montana, Davis and Cox (1938) found the organism causing Q fever, before the disease was recognized in the United States, by feeding ticks on guinea pigs. In 1938 Rolla Dyer, who contracted Nine-Mile fever while working in Cox's laboratory, proved the identity of that disease with the Q fever of Australia.

Q fever is absent from large areas such as Scandinavia and is sporadic in others (Liebisch 1979). All of 6 cases reported in Finland were attributed to exotic sources (Palosuo et al. 1974). The illness is sometimes disabling in man and may occur in extensive epidemics, but its importance has been considered minor when compared to more severe zoonoses, such as rabies, brucellosis, and tuberculosis, that rage unchecked in the livestock of many countries. Under such circumstances, Q fever is likely to be overlooked or neglected, and there is increasing evidence that it is often undiagnosed (D'Angelo et al. 1979).

ETIOLOGY. The etiologic agent of this disease is a rickettsia that differs in several important respects from other members of the order.

Classification of the organism according to *Bergey's Manual of Determinative Bacteriology* (Weiss and Moulder 1974) is as follows:

Class II.	Microtatobiotes
Order I.	Rickettsiales
Family I.	Rickettsiaceae
Tribe I.	Rickettsieae
Genus II.	*Coxiella*
Species.	*burnetii* (= *C. burneti, Rickettsia diaporica, R. burneti*)

The genus *Coxiella* is differentiated from the genus *Rickettsia* because the former organism is filterable (through Berkefeld N and W and the Seitz EK filter), does not cause rash, and does not elicit Weil-Felix agglutinins in man. It is further characterized as rod shaped or coccoid, and it occurs in the cytoplasm of infected cells. The organism stains lightly with aniline dyes. It is gram-positive. It has not yet been cultivated in cell-free media. Resistance to chemical and physical agents is exceptional; it resists 60°C for 1 hour, and 0.5% formalin and 1% phenol for 24 hours. The organism remains viable for several years in dried tick feces and survives without loss of titer in cell-free media for at least 109 days. Undoubtedly, the latter attributes are important in the epidemiology of Q fever.

The genus *Coxiella* is monotypic, and its major antigenic composition does not overlap that of other rickettsias, with the possible exception of *R. akari* (Marchette 1965). There are two mutable antigenic phases. The naturally occurring organism appears always to be an antigenic phase I, whether isolated from sheep placentas, cows' milk, or ticks. However, when propagated in the yolk sacs of embryonated hen eggs, the organism gradually changes to phase II (Stoker and Fiset 1956). Ascendancy of the phase I form is rapid when the egg-adapted rickettsias are inoculated into laboratory animals.

TRANSMISSION AND HOSTS

Occurrence in Humans. The occurrence of Q fever as sporadic infections in the general population, even in remote areas, has been established by means of skin tests and serologic reactions. Presumably some infections are asymptomatic, many cause pyrexia without localizing signs, and others may be confused with influenza or other illness at the time of occurrence. The disease occurs in epidemic proportions in some industries and under certain conditions. The first recognized association of industry with illness was in slaughterhouse workers in Australia, and this association has been confirmed in other countries. Another relationship is with sheep and cattle husbandry, but as many as 85% of patients have no history of exposure. The placentas of animals pose great danger to workers, and infection occurs even in people who merely reside near infected premises. There is much serologic evidence of asymptomatic infection in residents of dairy premises (Luoto et al. 1965) and among groups who drink unpasteurized milk from infected herds (Benson et al. 1963). The oral route is a relatively inefficient one for production of overt infection of man. It is possible that the high titers of antibody associated with the organism in milk may also alter its infectivity.

Spectacular epidemics have occurred in armed forces billeted in farm buildings, and among people exposed to migrating herds.

Multiple cases have occurred within a household (Kaplan and Hulse 1961) but, in spite of the danger of infection from experimental animals and frequent involvement of the lungs in man, transfer from person to person is uncommon.

In areas where cycles of Q fever occur in both domestic and wild animals, the source of occasional human infections is difficult to ascertain, but circumstantial evidence implicates the cycle in wild animals in some cases (Marchette 1965).

Domestic and Domiciliated Animals. All common domestic mammals except the cat have frequently been reported to be seropositive, but there are wide variations of incidence in different parts of the world.

Coxiella burnetii, or antibodies to it, have been found in cattle, sheep, goats, pigs, horses, buffalo, camels, and dogs. Whether the disease is self-perpetuating in all these species is unknown. It appears that among ruminants, at least, an activation of cryptic infection occurs during gestation, and contagion occurs from the placenta, secretions, and excretions of the dam. Activation may recur in successive pregnancies. Shepard (1959) believes that the high incidence of Q fever in dairy cattle breeders is attributable to the crowded conditions under which these cattle are kept. Presumably other factors such as dryness, exposure to wind, and kind of bedding may also be involved. The infection may be maintained at a low level in herds in some areas and then increase following importation of herds from remote sources. In view of the great infectivity of this agent and the relatively great homogeneity of dairy herds, it is astonishing that infection is often present in only a small fraction of a herd. However, many factors may be involved in the host-parasite relationship (Evans 1978).

In spite of an apparent self-perpetuating cycle in ungulates, some question remains as to whether infection in domestic species may be renewed or reinforced from the cycle in wild animals. Several species of ticks parasitic on domestic animals have been found to be infected with the rickettsia, and some of them, such as *Dermacentor, Ixodes, Amblyomma,* and *Haemaphysalis* spp., are multihost ticks and could transmit the disease from wild to domestic animals or the reverse. Infection of livestock and house rats is infrequent in Malaya but common in wild rodents, and Marchette (1965) believed that domestic species and man become infected through frequent exposures in the wild habitat.

It has been postulated on epidemiologic grounds that coxiellosis is essentially an infection of a savannah habitat, and this may be true of the domestic cycle in which both concentration of herds and dust formation are important; but as Marchette has pointed out, infection may also be found in forest-dwelling wild species.

Infections have been demonstrated in *Rattus rattus, R. norvegicus,* and *Mus musculus.* It seems obvious but is unproved that these animals may be infected from both barnyard and sylvatic sources.

Wild Animals. The range of species of mammals reported to be naturally or experimentally infected is so vast that a comprehensive review is not feasible here. There is no large taxonomic group of mammals known to be refractory to the infection, but there are wide variations in reactions to infection and in incidence of antibody-containing serums. Despite the great amount of general information regarding presence of the organisms in populations of domestic mammals, surprisingly little is known about the details of epizoology of Q fever in wild animals.

Because *C. burnetii* is so easily spread within laboratory animal colonies, some reported isolations must be considered of dubious validity. Investigators should not only take extreme precautions to prevent cross-contamination of animals but, when results are published, they should also describe the measures taken. Also, adequate controls must be included in all serologic studies because, as mentioned by Marchette, cross-reaction with another antigen may occur.

The best known and one of the most thorough studies of the ecology of *C. burnetii* in wild animals was that of Derrick and Smith (1940) on the bandicoots of Moreton Island, Australia. These animals supported heavy infestations of *Haemaphysalis humerosa,* and the rickettsia was exchanged reciprocally between host and parasite. Another ixodid parasite of bandicoots (*Ixodes holocyclus*) also fed on cattle and transmitted infection to them. Rodents occupying the bandicoot habitat had serologic evidence of infection (Freeman et al. 1940), but their part in the cycle is not clear. Evidence of a cycle of infection involving the kangaroos, *Megaleia rufa* (red) and *Macropus major* (gray), and the tick, *Amblyomma triguttatum* in western Queensland was adduced by Pope et al. (1960) Sheep and goats were also infected by the tick.

In the United States *Coxiella* was first isolated from wild animals by Stoenner et al. (1959) in Utah. Isolates were obtained from tissues of *Dipodomys microps* and *D. ordii* and from the tick *Dermacentor parumapertus*. Additional evidence of infection in rodents, lagomorphs, and other animals was obtained by serology. All these species were hosts of *D. parumapertus*, and a cycle involving the ectoparasite was inferred. It was especially noteworthy that the disease was undetected in extensive studies between December 1955 and March 1957 when major epizootics in three areas began. However, prior to December 1955 their studies had revealed diagnostic titers of antibody in indigenous animals. In subsequent studies in the same area, Vest et al. (1965)

found much additional evidence of infection; a peak incidence of epizootic proportions was reached in 1960. Ninety-one isolations of *Coxiella* were made by these workers, and 1,367 specimens from 19 species were seropositive. Several genera were added to the list as a result of surveys by Enright et al. (1971), Riehmann et al. (1978, 1979), and Randhawa et al. (1977). A composite table listing some of the known infected mammalian genera in North America has been prepared from the results obtained by several authors (Table 40.1). *Coxiella*-infected ticks (*Dermacentor andersoni*) have been collected from a Rocky Mountain goat (*Oreamnos*) (Eklund et al. 1947).

In some of the listed genera several species were involved, and repeated isolations were obtained from some of them. Because *Dipodomys microps* maintained the rickettsia in its tissues for several months after experimental infection, it was considered a probable reservoir species; *Lepus californicus* was thought to have a role in "amplification" of the infection in nature (University of Utah 1969). Evidence of infection has been found in a wide range of species in other lands. Presence of infection in bats (*Eptesicus*), bandicoots (*Isoodon*), tree shrews (*Tupaia*), hamsters (*Cricetulus*), merions

TABLE 40.1 Genera Affected by *Coxiella*.

Genus	Common Name	Isolation	Serology
Ammospermophilus	antelope ground squirrel	−	+
Antilocapra	pronghorn	−	+
Canis	coyote	+	+
Citellus	ground squirrel	+	+
Didelphis	opossum	−	+
Dipodomys	kangaroo rat	+	+
Erethizon	porcupine	−	+
Eutamias	chipmunk	+	+
Lepus	jackrabbit	+	+
Mephitis	striped skunk	+	−
Mus	house mouse	−	+
Neotoma	wood rat	+	+
Odocoileus	deer	+	+
Onychomys	grasshopper mouse	−	+
Perognathus	pocket mouse	+	+
Peromyscus	deer mouse	+	+
Procyon	raccoon	−	+
Rattus	Norway rat	+	−
Reithrodontomys	harvest mouse	+	+
Spilogale	spotted skunk	+	−
Sus	hog (feral)	−	+
Sylvilagus	cottontail rabbit	+	+
Taxidea	badger	−	+
Thomomys	pocket gopher	+	+
Urocyon	gray fox	+	−
Vulpes	kit fox	−	+

(*Meriones*), shrews (*Sorex*), voles (*Clethrion-omys*), weasels (*Mustela*), and hedgehogs (*Hemiechinus*) demonstrates the wide range of species that *Coxiella* can infect in nature. Antibodies to *Coxiella* were found in many species of African animals by Heisch et al. (1962).

Arthropod Vectors. The range of kinds of infected ectoparasites is also very large. Flies, fleas, chiggers, and other mites; lice; and many species of ticks have been found infected or have been infected experimentally. Some of the tick genera involved are *Haemaphysalis, Amblyomma, Ixodes, Dermacentor, Ornithodoros,* and *Otobius*; but no group or species should be considered above suspicion. *Coxiella burnetii* not only infects many species of arthropods but also invades many of their tissues and the lumen of the gut and propagates there. In some species it is believed to exist only in the gut, but since feces can infect the host or other animals by inhalation or via broken or unbroken skin, limited invasiveness in the arthropod may not be important.

Whether ectoparasites are essential for propagation of *Coxiella* in wild animals is unknown, although frequent infection of arthropods and proved vector potential seem to imply that role (Sidwell et al. 1964a). Liebisch (1979) concluded, as a result of extensive studies of various ecosystems in Europe, that "complete" natural foci of Q fever involve the rickettsiae, the tick vector (*D. marginatus* in Germany), reservoir hosts of wild animals (for example, mice and deer), and susceptible farm animals. Since some species of rodents and ungulates remain infective and excrete the organisms for long periods, the airborne route may also be involved. Predation and cannibalism are possible mechanisms of exchange of infection, even among the rodents. Infective contact with domestic sources is likely in certain areas, but Burgdorfer et al. (1963) isolated the etiologic agent from rodents in the mountains of Montana in an area inaccessible to livestock. In wild ungulates (Enright et al. 1971) the presence of *C. burnetii* has been established in deer, and it seems reasonable to assume that the disease is common at times among ungulates that congregate in large herds in enzootic areas. However, evidence of such occurrence is lacking.

SIGNS, SYMPTOMS, AND PATHOLOGY

Humans. A complete spectrum of severity of illness ranging from inapparent infection to fatal disease occurs in humans. Death, however, is rare, and the preponderance of cases are mild. Incubation periods are variable and, as shown by experimental infection by aerosol, the length of this period is inversely related to dose: as doses are increased from minimal to large, symptoms occur at shorter intervals (from 10 to 17 days) (Tigertt 1959). The dose of inoculum is known to affect severity of the disease. Individual susceptibility, virulence of the inoculum, and route of infection may also be important. Headache, backache, anorexia, and fever are common at onset, but chills are uncommon. Pneumonia is common. Duration of illness and convalescence is variable, and there may be relapses. Intractable rickettsial endocarditis as a sequel is being found with increasing frequency (Morbidity and Mortality Weekly Report 1979). Differential diagnosis is aided by the absence of rash, the occurrence of other cases, and sometimes by occupation or location of the patient, but pyrexia without localizing signs and failure of anamnesis are common. Tetracyclines and chloramphenicol are usually effective antibiotics and to prevent relapse should be continued several days after the temperature reaches normal. Endocarditis often persists in spite of rigorous antibiotic therapy.

Livestock. The striking feature of coxiellosis in livestock is its mildness. In fact, the term *disease* is inappropriate here because ordinarily there is no detectable clinical symptomatology. Normal calves and lambs are born to dams with heavily infected placentas, and they are reared without difficulty on heavily infected milk. This heavy infestation of placenta and milk persists in the presence of high antibody titers in serum and milk, thus differing from the phenomenon of tolerance, as exemplified by congenital lymphocytic choriomeningitis infection in rodents. Goats have been reported to suffer abortions as a result of infection.

From a public health standpoint, it is unfortunate that control of Q fever lacks the reinforcement that is afforded by economic considerations in the diseases of livestock of veterinary importance.

Laboratory Animals. All common laboratory animals are susceptible to Q fever to such an extent that they will usually support propagation of the organisms and often will react with fever, splenomegaly, and antibody formation. Death is unusual in all species. Cavies and hamsters are the animals favored for isolation, but mice, rabbits, and rats can be used. Variations in susceptibility reported by different investigators are usually attributed to variations in virulence of the isolate, but again it is probable that individual and strain differences of the test animals and abundance of organisms in the original specimen are also involved. There are many reports of fresh isolates that fail to cause febrile reaction in cavies and of isolates that are difficult to propagate in cavies and mice. When fever results from parenteral injection, it occurs on the 4th day or later, reaches 40°C or more, and may persist for more than a week. The gross lesions are splenomegaly and peritoneal exudate, but these are common in other diseases. Absence of orchitis aids in differentiation from virulent Rocky Mountain spotted fever. Rash has been reported in infected rabbits.

Perrin and Bengtson (1942) have described the microscopic lesions in experimentally infected mice. After inoculation by intranasal or intraperitoneal routes, nodular lesions composed chiefly of large mononuclear cells were found in spleen, liver, kidney, lymph nodes, and adrenals. Patchy areas of aplasia and degeneration were found in the bone marrow. Lesions in spleen and liver were the first to appear. Proliferative pneumonic changes with a predominance of mononuclear cells in the exudate were seen only in mice inoculated intranasally. *Coxiella* is widely distributed in the organs and tissues and can be found in the urine of laboratory animals.

Virulence. The manifestations of virulence of an organism ordinarily occur in inverse proportion to the resistance of the host, and resistance varies among individuals as well as among species or strains of animals. Dose and route of inoculation affect the results of injection, and adaptation to a host also is a determinant of reaction; thus, a strain that may cause severe illness in cavies or man does not produce death of chick embryos on first passage. Stoenner and Lackman (1960) and Enright et al. (1971) used the criteria of febrile response, splenomegaly, numbers of organisms in tissue, lesions at the site of injection, and mortality in cavies to compare the virulences of isolates from diverse host and geographic sources and found wide variations in several respects. They also found that hamsters were much more susceptible than cavies to isolates from rodents in Utah, whereas this was not true of other isolates tested in the same laboratory.

If ability to produce infection in very small doses were the sole criterion of virulence, *C. burnetii* would rank high, inasmuch as one or-

ganism of certain strains will induce progressive infection when injected into a cavy or inhaled by a man (Tigertt et al. 1960). On the other hand, death from the disease is exceptional in man and in naturally and experimentally infected animals.

Several of the rickettsias possess specific toxins that may be demonstrated by intravenous injection of the living organisms into mice (Bell and Pickens 1953). A toxic effect of killed phase I, but not phase II, organisms was demonstrated when they were injected intraperitoneally into cavies (Fiset 1959). However, this toxicity was neutralized by normal rabbit serum. Fatal infection is not known to occur in wild animals.

Experimental Infection in Wild Mammals. Marchette et al. (1962) have conducted carefully controlled studies on infections in rodents (*Citellus, Perognathus, Dipodomys, Reithrodontomys, Peromyscus, Neotoma,* and *Microtus*) and in lagomorphs indigenous to an enzootic area in Utah. All species were uniformly susceptible to subcutaneous injection, but death was exceptional. Antibody was present in significant titer in rodent serums in the 2nd week, but *Coxiella* could be isolated from the blood in the 4th week, from the brain and liver up to 49 days, from the lung to 34 days, and from the spleen and kidney up to 252 days. In *Sylvilagus,* rickettsemia occurred from the 3rd to the 20th days. Blood samples from infected *Peromyscus* were tested for complement fixation (CF) antibodies; a significant titer was demonstrated in the 2nd week and persisted for 48 weeks. Coyotes (*Canis*) were inoculated by the subcutaneous and oral routes. Rickettsias were found in blood and tissues in both cases for as long as 3 weeks in subcutaneously infected animals. Significant CF antibody titers were detected in all coyotes; one had a high titer before inoculation. Two bobcats (*Lynx*) were exposed to infection by feeding. One had circulating *Coxiella* and developed CF antibodies, but the other was not detectably infected.

Because nearly all animals survived infection and were kept for serology, lesions were not described.

Sidwell and Gebhardt (1962) conducted a similar study on several rodent species (*Peromyscus, Microtus, Neotoma, Dipodomys*) inoculated by the intraperitoneal route. Phase II CF antibody was produced at 1–2 weeks in all species and reached a peak in 3–5 weeks. Phase I CF and agglutinating antibodies were demonstrable at 3–5 weeks and increased slowly, in some cases to the 36th week, but the wild-caught *Dipodomys* possessed little of the latter kind of antibody.

Natural Infection in Wild Mammals. Almost nothing is known about naturally acquired Q fever in wild animals. The frequent occurrence of antibodies in many wild species suggests that recovery is common, and many isolations from tissues and blood may indicate that the course of natural infection is similar to the experimental infection in laboratory animals and in wild species. *Coxiella* infection in domestic animals is known to be activated by the stress of pregnancy and also by cortisone injection (Sidwell et al. 1964b); other pathogens (such as *Francisella tularensis* in snowshoe hares) are known to be activated by the stress of crowding in nature. Whether there is a similar relationship of *coxiellosis* in wild animals has not been discovered.

DIAGNOSIS

Serologic Tests. Several useful serologic tests for Q fever antibodies have been developed. The multiplicity of tests reflects the fact that no one is generally most useful; each has advantages for special purposes, and selection of a test may depend on preference or prior experience. All tests depend upon rise of specific antibodies during infection, and sera taken early and late in the disease should be compared for diagnostic purposes. Serologic diagnosis by the methods now available has been reviewed by Cox (1981). Techniques that have been used frequently or are coming into use are: (1) complement fixation, (2) capillary agglutination test, (3) standard rickettsial agglutination, (4) microscopic slide agglutination, (5) agglutination resuspension, (6) radioisotope precipitation test (RIP), (7) opsonin test, (8) serum neutralization (3 variations), (9) serum protection, (10) fluorescent antibody (FA), direct and indirect, (11) passive cutaneous anaphylaxis, and (12) enzyme-linked immunoassay. Results obtained by the various tests are not necessarily transposable; even the results obtained with phase I and phase II antigens in the CF test may be very different.

The Weil-Felix test (agglutination of bacteria of the genus *Proteus*), useful in diagnosis of several of the rickettsial diseases, is not applicable in Q fever; this is also true for cold agglutinins which are not produced.

A skin test (ST) may also be used to diagnose Q fever. A relatively small proportion of the general population develops severe reactions at the site of vaccination when given Q fever vaccine. Some persons who do not react to the first injection develop lesions after subsequent vaccination. The test would appear to be applicable to wild animal populations only in very special cases and after preliminary experimentation with the species tested.

Isolaton of C. burnettii. The common materials tested for the presence of *C. burnetii* are milk, blood, parasitic arthropods, and tissues such as rodent spleen or ruminant placenta. In special studies sputum, urine, feces, dust, or air samples may be examined. Unlike many other pathogens, this species is remarkably tolerant of abuse or neglect and can be isolated from contaminated and poorly preserved menstrua. Nevertheless, the chances of successful isolation are greatly improved by proper care in collecting and transporting specimens. When field studies are to be correlated with laboratory studies, prior consultation between the parties concerned will ensure coordination and use of the most efficient techniques. The general principles of preservation, transport, and processing of specimens have been published (Lennette and Schmidt 1964). Aseptic techniques should be used in collecting specimens whenever possible not only to reduce contamination by extraneous organisms but also to avoid specific contamination among specimens.

When blood is taken, serum should be separated from the clot in order to prevent hemolysis, which interferes with some serologic techniques. The serum can be used for serology and the clot for isolation of the organism. After separation, both portions can be frozen. Tissues may also be frozen and shipped, but the freezing and thawing processes preclude histologic examination; therefore, other portions of the same tissues should be fixed in 10% formalin if microscopic pathology is desired.

Milk, whey, sputum, or urine may also be shipped frozen; and formalin (approximately 0.5% final concentration) may be added to milk or whey as a preservative if they are to be tested for antibody (except neutralizing antibody) titer only, but not, of course, if isolation procedures are to be applied. Penicillin (1,000 units per milliliter) and streptomycin (250 units per milliliter) may be added when freezing is not feasible or when contamination by bacteria has been unavoidable. Several of the other common antibiotics are rickettsiostatic.

Arthropods may also be transported in the frozen state, but it is usually desirable to send them alive. Several rules should be followed when collecting and testing parasites:

1. In labeling as to place of collection, host species, date, and so on, for epidemiologic purposes, each group should be as homogeneous as possible in all respects.
2. Identification and separation of genus, species, and instar may be done by sender or receiver.
3. Suitable containers must be used. In general, both adequate humidity and adequate ventilation are required, and these requirements preclude the use of sealed or tightly stoppered containers. Cloth-covered or screened containers are suitable, and there should be damp absorbent cotton, sponge, or plaster of paris present, preferably not in contact with the arthropods. It is important to ensure that the parasites cannot escape from either the inner or outer container. Some species will not survive unless fed daily, and these present a special problem.
4. The recipient should be informed before shipment. Time in passage should be as short as possible, and shipment should be scheduled to arrive on a regular working day unless another time has been agreed on. For shipments between countries, entry permits are often required. In the United States, these can be obtained from: Chief Staff Veterinarian, Organisms and Vectors, Veterinary Services, Animal and Plant Health Inspection Service, Federal Center Building, U.S.D.A., Hyattsville, Md. 20781. The permit must be attached to the container or, if enclosed, the shipping label should state this.

Ectoparasites in many parts of the world are infected with pathogens of several kinds. For example, in western Montana ticks may be infected with *F. tularensis*, Colorado tick fever, California virus, *R. rickettsii*, and other related rickettsias. Sometimes an agent such as *F. tularensis* may be so prevalent in ticks that it will interfere with demonstration of the organism sought. There is no substantial evidence that presence of one kind of pathogen in an arthropod will preclude the presence of another kind; moreover, in a pool of ectoparasites one individual could have one kind of organism, while another could have a different one.

Several methods are available for identification of the specific organism in the presence of dual infections:

1. Arthropods may be washed in aqueous merthiolate solution (1:10,000) and rinsed thoroughly prior to trituration. This procedure frees the ectoparasites of external contamination by *Staphylococcus*, *Pseudomonas*, and so on.
2. Selection of antibiotics may permit proliferation of one organism while hindering others.
3. Test animals may be immunized to the undesired contaminating organism.
4. Selection of appropriate species, age, or sex of animals may favor some organisms over others.
5. Select the route of inoculation most appropriate to demonstration of the organism.
6. Filtration through bacterial filters of appropriate size for example, Seitz EK, will permit passage of *C. burnetii*.
7. The hemolymph test can be used (Liebisch 1979).

Animal Inoculation. An inoculum is prepared by triturating the specimen in saline solution, broth, or other liquid. Homogenization of tough materials, such as ticks, is facilitated by the use of sterile sand or granular Alundum with a mortar and pestle. Ordinarily, sufficient diluent is used to prepare a 10% suspension, and 1 or 2 ml are injected intraperitoneally into each of two young adult male prebled guinea pigs. Temperatures of the inoculated animals should be recorded daily for 2 weeks. In event of infection by *C. burnetii* a fever of 40°C or more will be noted after an incubation period of 5–12 days. After 2 or 3 days of fever one of the animals may be killed for demonstration of the organism and for passage of spleen suspension to other animals or to chick embryos. Signs of inflammation, such as peritoneal exudate or splenomegaly, suggest the presence of rickettsias; and impression smears or slides from a cut spleen surface should be stained for microscopic examination. Samples should be cultured at this time to detect bacterial contaminants or pathogens.

Alternatively, blood may be taken from febrile animals for bacterial culture, passaged to other animals, and inoculated into yolk sacs of embryonated hen eggs. If animals previously immunized to Q fever are available, they can be inoculated at the same time as the normal animals, and comparison of reactions in the two groups is helpful in identification. The animals should be bled again 28 days after injection, and the early and late serums should be tested for CF antibodies. For isolation in chick embryos, fertile eggs at the 5th–7th day of incubation are used. Test material is injected into the yolk sac, and the eggs are candled daily. Stained smears are prepared from the yolk sacs of embryos that die after the 3rd day. If no deaths occur by the 8th day, blind passage to other embryonated eggs is made. Preliminary identification of isolates may be done on smears stained by Giemsa, Machiavello, and FA techniques; confirmatory evidence is obtained by development of specific antibodies in inoculated animals or by use of embryo-grown organisms as CF antigens.

Hamsters may be used instead of cavies. Mice are susceptible to Q fever but less so than hamsters or cavies and should not be used as a substitute for cavies. *Coxiella burnetii* may also be grown in tissue culture, but this technique is not used for isolation (Pickens and Gaon 1961; Roberts and Downs 1959).

A cautionary note on the interpretation of results of inoculation of laboratory animals is in order. In any laboratory actively engaged in the study of living *C. burnetii*, escape of organisms and infection of laboratory animals as well as man should be regarded as inevitable. Publication of extensive new data on isolations of the organism has been withheld by the Rocky Mountain Laboratory because of the occurrence of specific antibodies in uninoculated laboratory animals, even among those just received from a local supplier. It follows that only pretested animals should be used for primary isolation and that sentinel animals should be distributed in the animal quarters and tested at regular intervals. Reisolation from a portion of the original material held in the frozen state affords additional confidence in isolation results.

Stains. Besides the FA technique, two general stains are commonly used for demonstrating the organism on slides. Smears are prepared by touching a slide to a cut surface of spleen or by spreading a loopful of yolk sac contents thinly on the slide. Known uninfected smears are useful as controls until confidence in use of the techniques is established.

1. With Giemsa stain the smear is fixed with methanol before staining. The rickettsias may be either intracellular or extracellular, single, or in small groups; they stain violet red. In smears of guinea pig spleens, the normal lymphocytic inclusions may be confused with rickettsias. Wolbach's modification of Giemsa stain may be used for histopathology and for staining the organism in

alcohol-fixed tissues (Mallory 1938).
2. Machiavello stain is most frequently used in the Rocky Mountain Laboratory. The smear is fixed by gentle heat, stained with basic fuchsin, and counterstained with methylene blue (Lennette and Schmidt 1964). The organisms stain bright red.

Gram stain has also been used on rickettsias. *Coxiella burnetii* is gram-positive (Gimenez 1965), whereas other rickettsias and the psittacosis-lymphogranuloma agents are gram-negative.

CONTROL. The known epidemiology and epizoology of Q fever afford clues to sources of exposure of man. However, prolonged and intensive exposure to large numbers of viable organisms under certain circumstances (for example, milk from infected herds) does not ordinarily cause overt infection, whereas remote, and presumably minimal, exposure under other circumstances will frequently cause severe infection. The route of infection of man appears to be of predominant importance. Inhalation of aerosolized organisms, as in a laboratory or downwind from infected dairy premises, is a relatively grave risk; whereas ingestion of heavily infected milk seems to produce little clinical or subclinical disease. The occurrence of cases is, of course, unequivocal evidence of risk; but unless Q fever is suspected, sporadic cases, as in abattoirs, may be misdiagnosed as influenza or atypical pneumonia. Several states lack laboratory facilities for serodiagnosis of Q fever and therefore fail to identify the disease (D'Angelo et al. 1979).

For occupationally exposed persons, vaccine is recommended, but currently it is not available in the United States. Frequent moderately unpleasant reactions to the vaccine and occasional severe reactions have tended to discourage use of the vaccine to the desired extent. However, it has been recognized that occasional reactions to primary vaccination are not due to inherent toxicity of the vaccine but are manifestations of allergic status as a result of previous infection or vaccination (Bell et al. 1964). Recognition of the mechanism of the "toxicity" of Q fever vaccine has led to elimination of reactors by ST prior to vaccination.

At the Rocky Mountain Laboratory where Q fever has been studied continuously since its discovery, conscientious attempts have been made to prevent escape of the organism. Nevertheless, a long series of cases has occurred, some among even the most casual visitors and in those who have refused vaccination. On the other hand, there has been no Q fever in persons vaccinated 1 month or more prior to exposure.

Prospects for the eradication of Q fever are nil in the foreseeable future. Control of the disease in man rests upon avoidance, prophylaxis for persons necessarily exposed, and environmental sanitation. Sufficient information and techniques are available to identify the major occupational hazards. Unfortunately, vigilance is probably inadequate for detecting periodic increases in enzootic areas or invasion of new areas before cases occur. Persons intimately exposed to large numbers of wild animals or their ectoparasites in enzootic areas should probably be vaccinated.

Appropriate zoning laws that take cognizance of Q fever undoubtedly would prevent many of the cases that occur as a result of exposure to dust-laden wind from livestock herds. Vaccinating cattle, use of antibiotics, prevention of dust formation, and isolating herds at time of parturition are measures that have not been fully exploited.

REFERENCES

Babudieri, B. Laboratory techniques for diagnosis of Q fever. *WHO Monogr.* ser. 19, pp. 193–209, 1953.

Bell, E. J., and Pickens, E. G. A toxic substance associated with the rickettsias of the spotted fever group. *J. Immunol.* 70:461–472, 1953.

Bell, J. F., Meis, A., and Hadlow, W. J. Recurrent reaction at site of Q fever vaccination in a sensitized person. *Military Med.* 129(7):591–595, 1964.

Benson, W. W., Brock, D. W., and Mather, J. Serologic analysis of a penitentiary group using raw milk from a Q fever infected herd. *Public Health Rep.* 78:707–710, 1963.

Burgdorfer, W., Pickens, E. G., Newhouse, V. F., and Lackman, D. B. Isolation of *Coxiella burneti* from rodents in western Montana. *J. Infect. Dis.* 112:181–186, 1963.

Cox, H. R. Rickettsia. In F. Milgrom, C. J. Abeyounis, K. Kano, eds., *Principles of immunological diagnosis in medicine.* Philadelphia: Lea and Febiger. (In press.)

D'Angelo, L. J., Baker, E. F., and Schlosser, W. Q fever in the United States. *J. Infect. Dis.* 139:613–615, 1979.

Davis, G. E., and Cox, H. R. A filter-passing infectious agent isolated from ticks: I. Isolation from *Dermacentor andersoni*: Reactions in animals and filtration experiments. *Public Health Rep.* 53:2259–2267, 1938.

Derrick, E. H., and Smith, D. J. W. Studies in the epidemiology of Q fever: II. The isolation of three strains of *Rickettsia burneti* from the bandicoot

Isoodon torosus. Aust. J. Exp. Biol. Med. Sci. 18:99–102, 1940.

Ecodynamics. *Ecology studies in western Utah, 1972,* ser. 72-1. Annual report. Salt Lake City, Utah: Ecodynamics, April 3, 1973.

Eklund, C. M., Parker, R. R., and Lackman, D. B. A case of Q fever probably contracted by exposure to ticks in nature. *Public Health Rep.* 62:1413–1416, 1947.

Enright, J. B., Behymer, D. E., Franti, C. E., Dutson, V. J., Longhurst, W. M., Wright, M. E., and Goggin, J. E., The behavior of Q fever rickettsiae isolated from wild animals in Northern California. *J. Wildl. Dis.* 112:181–186, 1963.

Enright, J. B., Longhurst, W. M., Wright, M. E., Dutson, V. J., Franti, C. E., and Behymer, D. E. Q fever antibodies in birds. *J. Wildl. Dis.* 7:14–27, 1971.

Evans, A. S. Causation and disease: A chronological journey. *Am. J. Epidemiol.* 108:249–258, 1978.

Fiset, P. *Symposium on Q fever: Serological diagnosis, strain identification and antigenic variation.* Med. sci. publ. 6, Walter Reed Army Inst. Res. Washington, D.C.: U.S. Government Printing Office, 1959.

Freeman, M., Derrick, E. H., Brown, H. E., Smith, D. J. W., and Johnson, D. W. Studies in the epidemiology of Q fever: V. Surveys of human and animal sera for *Rickettsia burneti* agglutinins. *Aust. J. Exp. Biol. Med. Sci.* 18:193–200, 1940.

Gimenez, D. F. Gram staining of *Coxiella burneti. J. Bacteriol.* 90:834–837, 1965.

Heisch, R. B., Grainger, W. E., Harvey, A. E. C., and Lister, G. Feral aspects of rickettsial infections in Kenya. *Trans. R. Soc. Trop. Med. Hyg.* 56:272–282, 1962.

Horsfall, W. R., and Ferris, D. H. *Coxiella burneti,* causative agent of Q fever: A composite abstract of the literature to 1961. *Wildl. Dis.,* vol. 28 (microcard), 1962.

Kaplan, M. M., and Hulse, E. C. Prevalence of Q fever in Europe and survey methods for its detection. *WHO Monogr.* ser. Joint Seminar on Zoonoses FAO agr. ser. 25, 1961.

Lennette, E. H., and Schmidt, N. J. *Diagnostic procedures for viral and rickettsial diseases,* 3d ed. New York: American Public Health Association, 1964.

Liebisch, A. Ecology and distribution of Q fever rickettsiae in Europe, with special reference to Germany. In J. G. Rodriguez, ed., *Recent advances in acarology,* vol. 2, sect. 3, pp. 225–232. New York: Academic Press, 1979.

Luoto, L., Casey, M. L., and Pickens, E. G. Q fever studies in Montana: Detection of asymptomatic infection among residents of infected dairy premises. *Am. J. Epidemiol.* 81:356–369, 1965.

Mallory, F. B. *Pathological technique.* Philadelphia: Saunders, 1938.

Marchette, N. J. Rickettsioses (tick typhus, Q fever, urban typhus) in Malaya. *J. Med. Entomol.* 2:339–371, 1965.

Marchette, N. J., Sidwell, R. W., Nicholes, P. S., and

Bushman, J. B. Studies on infectious diseases in wild animals in Utah: III. Experimental Q fever in wild vertebrates. *Zoonoses Res.* 1:321–339, 1962.

Morbidity and Mortality Weekly Report. Q fever—United Kingdom. *MMWR* 28(May 25):230–231, 1979.

Palosuo, T., Leinikki, P., Petterson, T., Saikku, P. Jantti, V. Hazards of expanding tourism: Report of six cases of Q fever in Finland. *Scand. J. Infect. Dis.* 6:173–176, 1974.

Perrin, T. L., and Bengtson, I. A. The histopathology of experimental "Q" fever in mice. *Public Health Rep.* 57:790–798, 1942.

Pickens, E. G., and Gaon, J. A. Growth of *Coxiella burneti* on agar tissue culture. *Am. J. Trop. Med. Hyg.* 10:49–52, 1961.

Pope, J. H., Scott, W., and Dwyer, R. *Coxiella burneti* in kangaroos and kangaroo ticks in Western Queensland. *Aust. J. Exp. Biol.* 38:17–28, 1960.

Randhawa, A. S., Kelly, V. P., and Baker, E. F. Agglutinins to *Coxiella burneti* and *Brucella* spp., with particular reference to *Brucella canis*, in wild animals of Southern Texas. *J. Am. Vet. Med. Assoc.* 171:989–942, 1977.

Riemann, H. P., Behymer, D. E., Franti, C. E., Crabb, E., and Schwab, R. G. Survey of Q fever agglutinins in birds and small rodents in Northern California, 1975–76. *J. Wildl. Dis.* 15:515–23, 1979.

Roberts, A. N., and Downs, C. M. Study on the growth of *Coxiella burneti* in the L strain mouse fibroblast and the chick fibroblast. *J. Bacteriol.* 77:194–204, 1959.

Shepard, C. C. Symposium on Q fever. Med. sci. publ. 6, Walter Reed Army Inst. Res. Washington, D.C.: U.S. Government Printing Office, 1959.

Sidwell, R. W., and Gebhardt, L. P. Q fever antibody response for experimentally infected wild rodents and laboratory animals. *J. Immunol.* 89:318–322, 1962.

Sidwell, R. W., Lundgren, D. L., Buchman, J. B., and Thorpe, B. D. The occurrence of a possible epizootic of Q fever in fauna of the Great Salt Lake Desert of Utah. *Am. J. Trop. Med. Hyg.* 13:754–762, 1964a.

Sidwell, R. W., Thorpe, B. D., and Gebhardt, L. P. Studies of latent Q fever infections: II. Effects of multiple cortisone injections. *Am. J. Hyg.* 79:320–327, 1964b.

Stoenner, H. G., Holdenried, R., Lackman, D., and Osburn, J. S., Jr. The occurrence of *Coxiella burneti*, *Brucella* and other pathogens among fauna of the Great Salt Lake Desert in Utah. *Am. J. Trop. Med. Hyg.* 8:590–595, 1959.

Stoenner, H. G., and Lackman, D. B. The biologic properties of *Coxiella burneti* isolated from rodents collected in Utah. *Am. J. Hyg.* 71:45–51, 1960.

Stoker, M. G. P., and Fiset, P. Phase variation of the nine mile and other strains of *Rickettsia burnetii*. *Can J. Microbiol.* 2:310–321, 1956.

Tigertt, W. D. *Symposium on Q fever: Studies on Q fever in man.* Med. sci. publ. 6, pp. 28–36. Walter Reed Army Inst. Res. Washington, D.C.: U.S. Government Printing Office, 1959.

Tigertt, W. D., Benenson, A. S., and Gochenour, W. S. Conference on airborne infection. *Bacteriol. Rev.* 25:285–293, 1960.

University of Utah. A study of the ecology and epizoology of the native fauna of the Great Salt Lake Desert, 1969. *Ecology and Epizoology Series*, no. 145. Annual summary review, E and E Research Group, 342-S. Bioscience Research Building. Salt Lake City: University of Utah, May 15, 1969.

Vest, E. D., Lundgren, D. L., Parker, D. D., Johnson, D. E., Morse, E. L., Bushman, J. B., Sidwell, R. W., and Thorpe, B. D. Results of a five-year survey for certain enzootic diseases in the fauna of western Utah. *Am. J. Trop. Med. Hyg.* 14:124–135, 1965.

Weiss, E., and Moulder, J. W. Genus III, *Coxiella* (Philip). In R. E. Buchanan and N. E. Gibbons, eds. *Bergey's manual of determinative bacteriology*, pp. 891–893. Baltimore: Williams and Wilkins, 1974.

Yadav, M. P., Rarotra, J. R., and Sethi, M. S. The occurrence of coxiellosis among rodents and shrews in the Tarai area of Uttar Pradesh. *J. Wildl. Dis.* 15:11–14, 1979.

41 Tick-Borne Fever and Rickettsial Pox

J. FREDERICK BELL

Tick-Borne Fever

Synonyms: **Erlichiosis, pasture fever.**

Several febrile diseases of man and animals caused by viruses, bacteria, and rickettsias are transmitted by ticks and the term tick-borne fever is commonly used to designate them. However, present usage tends to restrict the appellation to a specific disease or complex of closely related diseases caused by rickettsia-like organisms of the tribe Ehrichiae, family Rickettsiaceae, which are found in the white blood cells.

DISTRIBUTION AND EPIZOOLOGY. Tick-borne fever has been reported in domestic animals over large areas of northern Europe where *Ixodes ricinus* is a common parasite; similar disease has been reported in India, Iran, and Africa. It has not been reported in North America. The disease has been reproduced by feeding *Ixodes* ticks from infected pastures on a susceptible cow (*Bos*). *Ehrlichia bovis* can also be transmitted by *Hyalomma* spp. and *E. ovina* and *Rhipicephalus bursa*. Primary clinical disease is restricted to the periods of tick activity; subclinical infection of livestock is thought to be common.

Both the numbers of ticks and the incidence of infection among them may vary from time to time and from place to place. Tuomi (1966) believed that nonsusceptible hosts such as hares may carry the ticks from infective to clean pastures.

ETIOLOGY. The etiologic agents of tick-borne fever and canine pancytopenia are classified within the order Rickettsiales (Moulder 1974) as follows:

Family: Rickettsiaceae
Tribe II. Ehrlichieae Philip
Genus IV. *Ehrlichia* Moshkovski 1945

The organisms are described as pleomorphic and coccoid. They occur within the cytoplasm of circulating leukocytes of mammals. At present the identified agents of tick-borne fever are *E. canis* of dogs, *E. equi* of horses, and *E. phagocytophila* of cattle, sheep, and deer. An apparently closely related organism is *Cytoecetes microti* which occurs as an infection of the neutrophils in *Microtus* (Foggie 1962). *C. ondiri* causes bovine petechial fever (BPF) in cattle and sheep (Ondiri disease), and *Rickettsia* (*Donatienella*) *delpyi* was isolated from the leukocytes of a splenectomized Iranian gerbil (Rousellott 1948).

Because the *Ehrlichiae* cannot be grown in artificial media, do not infect chick embryos, and are difficult to propagate in laboratory animals, the systematics of the group are not well defined. Accordingly, various authors include or exclude certain infectious entities when discussing the group, and some organisms given species rank in the past (such as the agents responsible for tick-borne fever in cattle and sheep) are now considered to be different strains of one species. Taxonomy within the genus must be regarded as especially unstable. *E. bovis*, *E. ovina*, and *E. kurlovi* are listed as species incertae sedis in *Bergey's Manual of Determinative Bacteriology* (Moulder 1974).

The organisms do not pass gradocol membranes of 1 μ average pore diameter; cannot be propagated on bacterial media or in chick embryos (exception, *E. kurlovi*); and stain dark blue with Leishman, and blue, purple, or lavender with Giemsa technique. Similar organisms infect monocytes and endothelial cells of pigs in North Africa and lymphocytes of pigeons in South Africa (Haig 1955).

HOSTS, SIGNS, AND PATHOLOGY. Although canine pancytopenia is not known to occur in wild animals, it has been produced experimentally in red (*Vulpes*) and gray (*Urocyon*) foxes (Amyx and Huxsoll 1973). It is discussed here because it was the first of the group to be described and because it has been the most thoroughly studied. It is widely distributed in Africa, the Mediterranean, and Southeast Asia. *Rhipicephalus sanguineus* is the vector of *E. canis*; there is some question as to whether it can be transmitted transovarially (Groves et al. 1975). The incubation period varies from 6 to 21 days. Ordinarily the disease is mild; intermittent fever on alternate days persists for 10–14 days. Besides the nonspecific signs of listlessness and inappetence, there may be shallow red erosions of the skin. Exceptionally, there is somnolence and mild paraplegia.

Ehrlichia infection in cattle, sheep, and wild animals is called pasture fever. According to Foggie (1962), the sheep strain can be transmitted serially in sheep and produces a severe reaction; whereas it is difficult to infect sheep (*Ovis*) with the bovine strain, and it cannot be propagated serially in sheep. It is difficult also to infect cattle with sheep strains. Foggie found that infection of sheep with an ovine strain protected against subsequent infection with the cattle strain but that sheep originally infected with the cattle strain were fully susceptible to the ovine strain.

In Great Britain attempts to isolate the organism from roe deer (*Capreolus*) in an infected area were unsuccessful, but Ehrlichiae indistinguishable from the sheep strain were found in red deer (*Cervus*). In Finland an elk (*Alces*) calf was tested for susceptibility to three different strains of Ehrlichiae without effect (Tuomi 1966). Tuomi also reported the case of a cow (*Bos*) that contracted the disease when it escaped to a forest where no domestic stock had grazed for years. Goats (*Capra*) are susceptible to the ovine strain, and McDiarmid (1965) has isolated an agent similar to the bovine strain from fallow (*Dama*) and roe deer.

The nature of the disease in wild animals is unknown and can be inferred only from data on infection in cattle, cows, and sheep. Severity of illness is variable, probably due in part to variations in virulence of the organism. Fever, reduced milk yield, and inappetence are common in cattle, though nonspecific. In approximately one-fourth of the cases, milk production is never fully reestablished. Late in the illness, coughing occurs in about 40% of cases. Late neutropenia is characteristic and is thought to decrease resistance to secondary bacterial infections. Recovery occurs in a few days with or without treatment, but tetracyclines and sulfonamides speed the lysis of fever.

The disease in sheep is similar, but coughing does not occur. Occasionally, abortion has been reported. Relapse may occur in both ovine and bovine disease. Immunity as a result of infection has been reported as short-lived in some cases and durable in others. There is some evidence that premunition may be responsible for immunity of long duration.

Ehrlichia ovina has been adapted to cavies and mice by serial transmission in splenecto-

mized animals. The cavy strain was subsequently adapted to normal, nonsplenectomized cavies by blind passage. The adapted strains did not lose virulence for sheep.

Ehrlichias are not known to be infectious for man, but nonhuman primates have been infected with *E. equi* experimentally (Lewis et al. 1975).

DIAGNOSIS. Microscopic identification of the agent in smears of tissue or blood is the only certain method of identification. The organisms can take the Giemsa stain; specific identification is aided by the use of fluorescent antibody (Ristic et al. 1972; Smith et al. 1976). Characteristically, the organisms are found as morular colonies in granulocytes and monocytes or lymphocytes at the height of febrile reaction (Gordon et al. 1962), but they have also been described in endothelial cells. Other tick-borne disease such as tick pyemia and piroplasmosis may occur in the same herd or the same individual. The Weil-Felix reaction is not positive in tick-borne fever, and inability to propagate the organism in the usual media has hindered use of other common serologic tests. The indirect fluorescent antibody test has been used by Ristic et al. (1972).

For the study of infection in ticks, the methods of Roshdy (1963) and of Smith et al. (1976) may be used.

CONTROL. The disease has not been controlled, but it has been noted that animals introduced from disease-free areas are most likely to contract the illness. Control or avoidance of vector ticks is the logical procedure, but these measures have not been practical on a large scale. No commercial vaccine is available.

Rickettsialpox

Synonyms: **Vesicular rickettsiosis, gamaso-rickettsiosis varicelliformis.**

Rickettsialpox is an acute, generalized, nonfatal infection characterized by a primary cutaneous lesion at the site of inoculation and a generalized papulovesicular eruption.

HISTORY. First recognition of this disease, in a suburb of New York City, is credited to two physicians, B. Shankman and L. N. Sussman

(Huebner et al. 1946b). The agent was isolated from a patient, from the mite vector (Huebner et al. 1946a), and from a mouse (Huebner et al. 1947). A few years later a similar or identical disease was detected in the USSR, where the agent is called *Dermacentroxenus murinus* and the disease is called vesicular rickettsiosis or gamaso-rickettsiosis varicelliformis (Zdrodovskii and Golinevich 1960). A feature of the history of this disease in man is that the great majority of cases were recognized within a period of a few years. Subsequently, the infection has been reported only occasionally (Zatulofsky et al. 1972), and similar low endemicity probably accounts for the failure to recognize it earlier (Paterson and Taylor 1966).

DISTRIBUTION AND EPIDEMIOLOGY. *Rickettsia akari*, or the disease it produces in man, has been identified in scattered areas of the United States, Korea, the USSR, and Africa. The vector mite parasitize rats and mice and has been found in widely scattered foci in the United States and Egypt. It is assumed that complete distribution of the disease has not been determined. Studies of Huebner et al. (1946a) and of Nichols et al. (1953) indicate that association of the mite, *Allodermanyssus sanguineus*, and *Mus* or *Rattus* is essential for perpetuation of the disease in urban environments. Whether other host-parasite associations are involved in sylvatic habitats is not known, although isolation of *R. akari* from a vole (*Microtus fortis pelliceus*) may imply other cycles (Jackson et al. 1957). The mite visits its hosts only for feeding, which may take an hour or two. When replete it retires to crevices for digestion of the blood meal and has been observed to survive for as long as 6 weeks without feeding. The life cycle of the species has been described by Baker et al. (1956). Infection with *R. akari* has not been demonstrated to be harmful to the mite, and transovarial passage of infection is likely.

Tropical rat mites, *Ornithonyssus* (*Liponyssus*) *bacoti*, (Philip and Hughes 1948) and lice (Weyer 1952) have been infected in the laboratory but are not known to be involved in the natural cycle.

ETIOLOGY. The agent of this disease is *Rickettsia akari* (=*Dermacentroxenus murinus*). Relationship of this organism to the Rocky Mountain spotted fever (RMSF) group has been noted by Zdrodovskii and Golinevich (1960) and also by Lackman et al. (1965). The organism is not distinguishable from other members of the group on the basis of morphology or staining,

and furthermore, it occurs within the nuclei of infected cells, as do others of this group. One feature that distinguishes it from other members of the group is its vector, the mite *A. sanguineus*. *Rickettsia akari* can be propagated in yolk sacs and on amniotic membranes of developing chick embryos, and test antigens are prepared in this way. It can be also be grown on embryonic tissue cultures.

SIGNS AND PATHOLOGY. Mice are susceptible to *R. akari*. After intranasal inoculation, fatal pneumonia occurs, with abundant occurrence of rickettsia in the affected cells. Intraperitoneal inoculation also produces severe illness; death may occur in 9–18 days on primary inoculation and earlier after injection of such passage materials as peritoneal exudate or organ emulsions. A few days before death the mice exhibit lassitude, inappetence, ruffled fur, and rapid breathing. At necropsy there is evidence of peritonitis marked by blood-tinged exudate, lymphadenitis, and greatly enlarged spleen. Some mice survive infection. Subcutaneous inoculation causes infection of about 1-month duration. Rickettsias are found in the spleen but not in urine or feces. Rats are similarly susceptible and develop periorchitis, with fever of several days duration. The infection is easily propagated in rats by intraperitoneal transfer of infected organ emulsions.

The response of cavies to infection is similar to that of rats. Rickettsias are abundant in the exudate on the tunica vaginalis.

Rickettsia akari has been isolated from domiciliated mice (*Mus*) and rats (*Rattus*) and from wild voles (*Microtus*), but the nature of the natural infection in these species is not known.

DIAGNOSIS. Rickettsialpox occurs so infrequently at present that awareness is a problem. The occurrence of other diagnosed cases and development of the characteristic syndrome facilitate diagnosis. Differentiation from chickenpox is aided by history, by the successive crops of vesicles that occur in that disease, and by the presence of a primary lesion with lymphadenitis in rickettsialpox. The Weil-Felix agglutination is not uniformly present, but complement fixation tests with early and late serum specimens show a significant rise in antibodies. Interpretation must take into consideration the cross-reactions that occur between various rickettsias of the spotted fever group (Cox 1979; Philip et al. 1978).

Rickettsia akari can be isolated from blood of febrile patients by animal inoculation. White mice are the animals of choice, and the organism can be identified in Machiavello-stained smears of the peritoneum or by subinoculation into embryonated eggs. The fluorescent antibody technique may be used for specific identification of organisms in smears.

Dolgopol (1948) has studied the histologic changes of the disease in man and recommends skin biopsy for early specific diagnosis in case of doubt. She noted the resemblance of the lesions to those of scrub typhus and their difference from those of typhus, RMSF, and boutonneuse fever in that there are incomplete thrombi and absence of arteritis and hemorrhages.

CONTROL. Control of rickettsialpox depends essentially upon control of mice, their parasites, or both, in human dwellings (see U. S. Department of Agriculture [1966] and various articles in the journal, *Pest Control*, published by Harvest Publishing, Cleveland).

REFERENCES

Amyx, H. L., and Huxsoll, D. L. Red and gray foxes: Potential reservoir hosts for *Ehrlichia canis*. *J. Wildl. Dis.* 9:47–50, 1973.

Baker, E. W., Evans, T. M., Gould, D. J., Hull, W. B., and Keegan, H. L. *A manual of parasitic mites of medical or economic importance*, pp. 18–20. New York: Technical Publ., National Pest Control Assoc., 1956.

Cox, H. R. Rickettsia. In F. Milgrom, C. J. Abeyounis, K. Kano, eds., *Principles of immunological diagnosis in medicine*. Philadelphia: Lea and Febiger. (In press.)

Dolgopol, B. B. Histologic changes in rickettsialpox. *Am. J. Pathol.* 24:119–133, 1948.

Foggie, A. Studies on tick pyaemia and tick-borne fever: Aspects of disease transmission by ticks. *Symp. Zool. Soc. Lond.* 6:51–57, 1962.

Gordon, W. S., Brownlee, A., Wilson, D. R., and MacLeod, J. The epizootiology of louping ill and tick-borne fever with observations on the control of these sheep diseases: Aspects of disease transmission by ticks. *Symp. Zool. Soc. Lond.* 6:1–27, 1962.

Groves, M. G., Dennis, G. L., Amyx, H. L., and Huxsoll, D. L. Transmission of *Ehrlichia canis* to dogs by ticks (*Rhipicephalus sanguineus*). *Am. J. Vet. Res.* 36:937–940, 1975.

Haig, D. A. Tickborne rickettsioses in South Africa. *Adv. Vet. Sci.* 2:318–322, 1955.

Huebner, R. J., Jellison, W. L., and Armstrong, A. Rickettsialpox: A newly recognized rickettsial disease: V. Recovery of *Rickettsia akari* from a house mouse (*Mus musculus*). *Public Health Rep.* 62:777–780, 1947.

Huebner, R. J., Jellison, W. L., and Pomerantz, D. Rickettsialpox: A newly recognized rickettsial disease: IV. Isolation of a rickettsia apparently identical with the causative agent of rickettsialpox from *Allodermanyssus sanguineus*, a rodent mite. *Public Health Rep.* 61:1677–1682, 1946a.

Huebner, R. J., Stamps, P., and Armstrong, A. Rickettsialpox: A newly recognized rickettsial disease: I. Isolation of the etiological agent. *Public Health Rep.* 61:1605–1614, 1946b.

Jackson, E. B., Danauskas, J. X., Coale, M. C., and Smadel, J. E. Recovery of *Rickettsia akari* from the Korean vole *Microtus fortis pelliceus*. *Am. J. Hyg.* 66:301–307, 1957.

Lackman, D. B. A review of information of rickettsialpox in the United States. *Clin. Ped.* 2:296–301, 1963.

Lackman, D. B., Bell, E. J., Stoenner, H. G., and Pickens, E. G. The Rocky Mountain spotted fever group of rickettsias. *Health Lab. Sci.* 2:135–141, 1965.

Lewis, G. E., Jr., Huxsoll, D. L. Ristic, M., Johnson, A. J. Experimentally induced infection of dogs, cats, and non-human primates with *Ehrlichia equi*, etiologic agent of equine ehrlichiosis. *Am. J. Vet. Res.* 36:85–88, 1975.

McDiarmid, A. Modern trends in animal health and husbandry: Some infectious disease of free-living wildlife. *B. Vet. J.* 121:245–257, 1965.

Moulder, J. W. The rickettsias. In R. E. Buchanan and N. E. Gibbons, eds., *Bergey's manual of determinative bacteriology*, p. 18, 8th ed. Baltimore: Williams and Wilkins, 1974.

Nichols, E., Rindze, M. E., and Russell, G. G. Relationship of habits of house mouse and mouse mite (*Allodermanyssus sanguineus*) to spread of rickettsialpox. *Ann. Inter. Med.* 39:92–102, 1953.

Paterson, P. Y., and Taylor, W. Rickettsialpox. *Bull. N.Y. Acad. Med.* 42:579–587, 1966.

Philip, R. N., Casper, E. A., Burgdorfer, W., Gerloff, R. K., Hughes, L. E., and Bell, E. J. Serologic typing of rickettsiae of the spotted fever group by microimmunofluorescence. *J. Immunol.* 121:1961–1968, 1978.

Philip, C. B., and Hughes, L. E. The tropical rat mite, *Liponyssus bacoti*, as an experimental vector of rickettsialpox. *Am. J. Trop. Med. Hyg.* 28:679–705, 1948.

Ristic, M., Huxsoll, D. L., Weisiger, R. M., Hildebrandt, P. K., and Nyindo, M. B. A. Serological diagnosis of tropical canine pancytopenia by indirect immunofluorescence. *Infect. Immun.* 6:226–231, 1972.

Roshdy, M. A. Feulgen-Schiffs technique for examination of the distribution of the intracellular rickettsia-like microorganisms in whole mounts of ticks or their tissues. *Nature* 199:827, 1963.

Rousselot, R. *Rickettsia* (*Donatiennella*) *delpyi*, n. sp. n. subgen. *Bull. Soc. Pathol. Exot.* 41:110–112, 1948.

Smith, R. D., Sells, D. M., Stephenson, E. H., Ristic, M., and Huxsoll, D. L. Development of *Ehrlichia canis,* causative agent of canine ehrlichiosis, in the tick *Rhipicephalus sanguineus* and its differentiation from symbiotic rickettsia. *Am. J. Vet. Res.* 37:119–126, 1976.

Tuomi, J. Studies in epidemiology of bovine tick-borne fever in Finland. *Ann. Med. Exp. Biol. Fenniae* 44 (suppl. 6):7–62, 1966.

U.S. Department of Agriculture. *Insecticide recommendations of the entomology research division.* Agr. Handbook 313, Supt. of Documents. Washington D.C.: U.S. Government Printing Office, 1966.

Weyer, F. Versuche zur Kunstlichen Infektion der Schweinelaus *Haematopinus* L. mit *Rickettsia prowazeki* und *R. quintana. Schweiz. Z. Allg. Path.* 15:203–216, 1952.

Zdrodovskii, P. F., and Golinevich, H. M. *The rickettsial diseases,* pp. 340–353. New York: Pergamon Press, 1960.

Zatulofsky, G. G., Shkolnik, L. Y., Anischenko, G. A., Mukhopad, V. A., and Fonberg, M. M. Concerning vesicular rickettsiosis in the Ukrainian SSR. *Zh. Mikrobiol. Epidemiol. Immunobiol.* 50: 124–128, 1972.

42 *Bovine Petechial Fever*

J. G. GROOTENHUIS

Synonyms: **None.**

Bovine petechial fever (BPF) is a hemorrhagic disease of cattle caused by the rickettsial agent *Cytoecetes ondiri* (Krauss et al. 1972). The disease is confined to high altitude areas of Kenya, and probably Tanzania, and occurs in a habitat with heavy shade from thick brush or dense understory cover (Walker et al. 1974).

ETIOLOGY, CLINICAL SIGNS, AND PATHOLOGY. *Cytoecetes ondiri* is found in the cytoplasm of neutrophilic granulocytes. The organism has also been demonstrated in some other tissues by inoculation of ground-up tissues into susceptible sheep; examples include lung, liver, heart, and vascular endothelial cells, apart from hematopoietic tissues, bone marrow, spleen, and lymph nodes. In experimental infections of cattle and sheep, the agent could most consistently be isolated from blood and the spleen, where multiplication probably occurs (Snodgrass 1975).

The morphology of *C. ondiri* varies from small spherical organisms (ca. 0.5 μm) and larger irregularly shaped bodies (1−2 μm), to aggregations of small bodies in a morula of 3−5 μm diameter (Fig. 42.1). In Giemsa-stained blood smears, the organisms are grayish blue and can easily be distinguished from cell debris and intracellular granules. Ultrastructural studies have demonstrated these rickettsial bodies in membrane-lined vacuoles within the cytoplasm of the neutrophils (Krauss et al. 1972).

The clinical signs are characterized by high body temperature (± 41°C) and hemorrhages in the mucous membranes, particularly in the oral and vaginal mucosae. Sometimes fever is the only clinical sign. Lactating cows will show a marked drop in milk yield. Pulmonary edema or heavy blood loss in feces indicate a grave prognosis (Danskin and Burdin 1963).

The lesions suggest an impairment of the blood clotting mechanisms, which correlates with thrombocytopenia (Danskin and Burdin 1963). Hemorrhages can be found on the mucosa and serosa of all internal organs, on the capsules of lymph nodes, on the perimysium, in intermuscular connective tissues, and in the subcutis. Other lesions described are lung edema, hydropericardium, degeneration of liver parenchyma, and hemorrhagic edema of the gall bladder (Plowright 1962).

TRANSMISSION. The mode of transmission is unknown. Attempts to transmit the disease experimentally with several tick species, trombiculid mites (Walker et al. 1974), and diptera of the *Stomoxys*, *Culex*, and *Anopheles* genera (Piercy 1953) have failed. Disease outbreaks regularly occur in cattle herds where intensive tick control is practiced.

EPIDEMIOLOGY AND WILDLIFE INVOLVEMENT. In Kenya BPF is confined to dense ground cover at altitudes of between 1,500 and 2,700 m. Outbreaks occur seasonally at the end of the rains and shortly thereafter (Plowright 1962). A possible explanation for seasonal occurrence is movement of cattle into wooded pastures at the end of a period of drought.

Cytoecetes ondiri can cause a serious disease in cattle, up to 50% morbidity and 10% mortality, and a symptomless persistent infection in bushbuck (*Tragelaphus scriptus*). A transient infection with mild clinical signs is produced in experimentally inoculated sheep

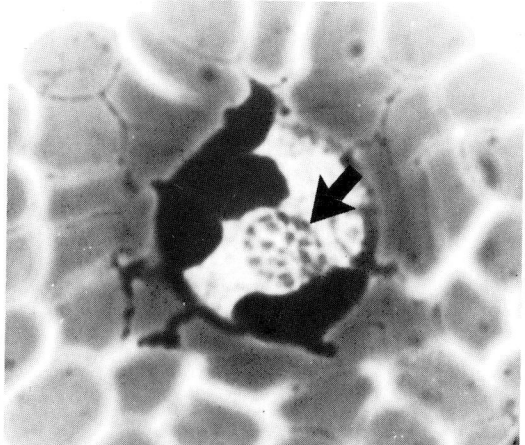

FIG. 42.1 Neutrophil with a morula of large irregular *Cytoecetes ondiri* bodies in its cytoplasm (arrow). Blood smear from sheep (Giemsa; ×2,000).

and goats. From nine wild ruminant species examined in an endemic BPF area, buffalo (*Syncerus caffer*), bushbuck, dikdik (*Rhynchotragus kirki*), duiker (*Sylvicapra grimmia*), impala (*Aepyceros melampus*), reedbuck (*Redunca fulvorufula*), steenbok (*Raphicerus campestris*), suni (*Nesotragus moschatus*), and waterbuck (*Kobus defassa*), only bushbuck were found to be carriers. The prevalence of *C. ondiri* in the blood of healthy bushbuck was 43% (L. Sileo, F. G. Davies, and L. Karstad, unpublished data, 1976). Transient infections of short duration were established in buffalo and wildebeest (*Connochaetes gnu*) after inoculation of infected blood.

DIAGNOSIS. Diagnosis is based on clinical signs and pathology but must be confirmed by demonstration of the agent in granulocytes in blood smears or by inoculation of blood into test sheep.

TREATMENT AND CONTROL. Cattle should be kept away from known endemic areas. Affected animals can be treated effectively with oxytetracyclines or dithiosemicarbazone, if treatment is administered early (Snodgrass 1976).

REFERENCES

Danskin, D., and Burdin, M. L. Bovine petechial fever. *Vet. Rec.* 75, 15:391–394, 1963.

FAO. Terminal report to the government of Kenya on wildlife disease research. AG: DP/K/N/68/013, 1978.

Krauss, H., Davies, F. G., Odegaard, O. A., and Cooper, J. E. The morphology of the causal agent of bovine petechial fever. *J. Comp. Pathol.* 82:241–251, 1972.

Piercy, S. E. Bovine infectious petechial fever. *E. Afr. Agr. J.* 18:65–68, 1953.

Plowright, W. Some notes on bovine petechial fever (Ondiri disease) at Muguga, Kenya. *Bull. Epizoot. Dis. Afr.* 10:499–505, 1962.

Snodgrass, D. R. Pathogenesis of bovine petechial fever. *J. Comp. Pathol.* 85:523–530, 1975.

———. Chemotherapy of experimental bovine petechial fever. *Res. Vet. Sci.* 20:108–109, 1976.

Snodgrass, D. R., Karstad, L. H., and Cooper, J. E. The role of wild ruminants in the epidemiology of bovine petechial fever. *J. Hyg. Camb.* 74:245–250, 1975.

Walker, A. R., Cooper, J. E., and Snodgrass, D. R. Investigations into the epidemiology of bovine petechial fever in Kenya and the potential of trombiculid mites as vectors. *Trop. Anim. Health Prod.* 6:193–198, 1974.

43 *Heartwater*

E. YOUNG

Synonyms: **None.**

Heartwater is a septicemic, rickettsial disease of ruminants, characterized by hyperthermia and nervous symptoms. The disease is restricted to tropical and subtropical regions such as Madagascar and parts of Africa and the infective agent, *Cowdria ruminantium*, is naturally transmitted by the "bont" tick (*Amblyomma* spp.) (Siegmund 1961). It may cause an inapparent, transient reaction in some wild animals and be responsible for clinical disease and mortalities in others.

ETIOLOGY AND TRANSMISSION. *Coudria ruminantium* is a parasite affecting the endothelial cells of the blood vessels, consequently causing a variety of pathologic lesions and signs. The characteristic rickettsial colonies are readily found in preparations made from the hippocampus, cerebral cortex, or the intima of large veins.

It has been experimentally proved that infected *Amblyomma herbraeum* can transmit heartwater to the blesbok (*Damaliscus dorcas*) and that clean ticks become infected when allowed to feed on an artificially infected blesbok. Similarly, other wild animals may also act as natural, asymptomatic hosts of heartwater (Neitz 1973). The infective agent can also be artificially transmitted by the inoculation of a susceptible animal with blood taken during the febrile stage.

SUSCEPTIBLE SPECIES. Springbok (*Antidorcas marsupialis*), eland (*Taurotragus oryx*), Indian nilgai (*Boselaphus tragocamelus*), Indian buffalo (*Bubalus bubalis*), fallow deer (*Dama dama*), Barbary sheep (*Ammotragus lervia*), Himalayan tahr (*Hemitragus jemlahicus*), blackbuck (*Antelope cervicapra*), and domestic cattle, sheep, and goats have been found to be clinically affected by heartwater (Hofmeyr

The author thanks the Onderstepoort Library and Andrew Hofmeyr and Lorraine Pienaar for assistance with the review of literature, and Dr. Durr Bezuidenhout, Onderstepoort, for valuable advice.

1956; Neitz 1944; Thirion and Bezuidenhout, personal communication, 1978; Young and Basson 1973). Fatal infection occurs in all these species. The black wildebeest (*Connochaetes gnu*) and blesbok can act as asymptomatic carriers (Neitz 1935), while preliminary experiments excluded impala (*Aepyceros melampus*), blue wildebeest (*Connochaetes taurinus*), African buffalo (*Syncerus caffer*), kudu (*Tragelaphus strepsiceros*), giraffe (*Giraffa camelopardalis*), and warthog (*Phacochoerus aethiopicus*) as susceptible species (Gradwell et al. 1976). A variable natural resistance, however, seems to be present in wild animals in enzootic areas, and more research is required to establish the natural host range of *C. ruminantium*.

INCUBATION PERIOD. Incubation periods are variable in domestic ruminants, and they are unknown for most wild animal species. Artificially infected springbok developed hyperthermia and noticeable signs after about 1–2 weeks, and Neitz (1944) found experimentally infected blesbok developed a parasitemia after 12 days. The period the blood remained infective could not be determined accurately. A splenectomized blesbok died from heartwater 21 days after inoculation with infected blood, and an artificially infected black wildebeest developed parasitemia about 13 days postinfection, lasting until about day 30 (Neitz 1944).

SIGNS AND PATHOLOGY. In peracute cases animals may die suddenly. The usual signs include hyperthermia, polypnea, tachycardia, hyperaesthesia, and circling with a stiff and unsteady, high-stepping gait followed by prostration, opisthotonus, muscle tremors and convulsions, blinking of the eyes, prolapse of the membrana nicitans, continuous grinding of the teeth, and the discharge of froth from the nostrils and mouth.

General congestion, isolated hemorrhages, hydrothorax, hydropericardium, ascites, pulmonary edema, and splenomegaly represent the most characteristic postmortem findings.

DIAGNOSIS. The described signs and lesions in possibly susceptible species in enzootic heart-

Gonzalez (1965) were unable to infect guinea pigs, mice, rats, and gerbils with *A. marginale*, despite attempts to increase their susceptibility by various methods. Gilruth et al. (1911) observed anaplasmalike bodies in small numbers in blood films from the dingo and several species of monotremes and marsupials in Australia but did not prove the identity of the structures and may have been observing erythrocytic nuclear fragments or parasites other than anaplasma. McMillan and Bancroft (1974) reported *Anaplasma* in blood films of the platypus in Australia.

DISTRIBUTION. Anaplasmosis is widely distributed throughout the tropical and subtropical regions of the world and occurs in certain portions of the temperate regions. Local incidence depends largely on the prevalence of potential arthropod vectors. Occurrence is usually greatest in spring, summer, and early fall—the time of year when the vectors are most active. The disease has been reported from most parts of Africa, southern Europe, the Soviet Union, Asia, Asia Minor, Australia, Taiwan, the Phillippines, the Antilles, South America, and the United States (Ristic 1960).

ETIOLOGY. Anaplasmosis is caused by *Anaplasma marginale*, an obligate intraerythrocytic parasite classified in the family Anaplasmataceae, order Rickettsiales (Buchanan and Gibbons 1974). It is gram-negative and non-acid-fast and, in Giemsa- or Wright-stained blood films, appears as dense, rounded dark blue structures 0.3−1.0μ in diameter lying at or near the periphery of red blood cells. The ovine form of the parasite (*A. ovis*) (Fig. 44.1) is morphologically identical with *A. marginale*. Cattle are refractory to *A. ovis* as sheep are to *A. marginale*. *Anaplasma centrale*, which occurs in the center of the erythrocyte instead of near the margin, is associated with a mild form of the disease in cattle.

Each marginal body is composed of one to eight subunits, or initial bodies (Fig. 44.2), formed from a single initial body by binary fission. On maturation the initial bodies separate from the erthrocyte in which they developed and enter a new erythrocyte by causing invagination of the cytoplasmic membrane, completing the reproductive cycle.

TRANSMISSION. Anaplasmosis may be transmitted mechanically by biting insects such as horseflies (*Tabanus*), stable flies (*Stomoxys*), and mosquitoes (*Psorophora*) and by surgical

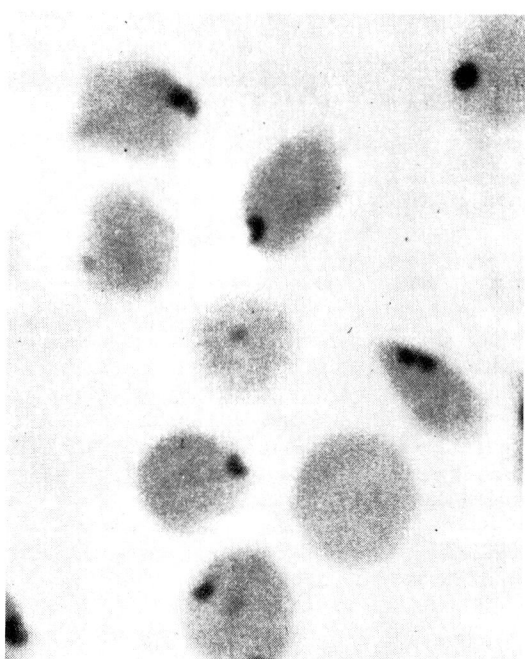

FIG. 44.1 *Anaplasma ovis* in deer (Giemsa stain; ×3,000). (Photomicrograph courtesy of J. P. Kreier.)

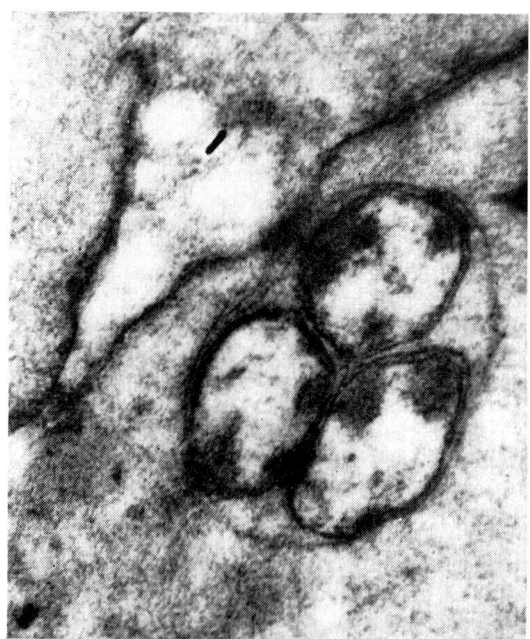

FIG. 44.2 *Anaplasma marginale*: marginal body with three initial bodies demonstrated by electron microscopy (×70,000). (Photomicrograph courtesy M. Ristic.)

instruments or hypodermic needles. Mechanical transmission must occur promptly; contact with the susceptible host must occur within a few minutes after the insect or instrument becomes contaminated with the infective blood in order to transfer anaplasma while they are still viable. According to Piercy (1956) the efficiency of transmission by prompt transfer of blood may exceed 50% when acute cases are involved, but with carrier animals transmission probably occurs less than 10% of the time.

Many species of ticks are known to act as biological vectors. One of the most efficient is *Dermacentor occidentalis*, a three-host tick considered by Osebold et al. (1962) and Christensen et al. (1962) to be the primary vector of anaplasmosis among deer and cattle in certain parts of the coastal range area of California. The tick is unique in that it occurs on ungulates in all stages of its life cycle and is capable of transovarian transmission of the anaplasma organism (Herms and Howell 1936). Other three-host ticks such as *D. andersoni* are found on ungulates only in the adult stage and have the opportunity of infecting only one definitive host.

Transovarian transmission of anaplasma has been demonstrated also in *D. andersoni* (Howell et al. 1941) and *Boophilus annulatus* (Kuttler 1971). This characteristic is essential for transmission by one-host ticks and three-host ticks such as *D. andersoni* which occur on susceptible or infected hosts only during the adult stage.

At least 18 species of ticks are potential anaplasmosis vectors, capable of harboring viable anaplasma for several weeks or months. Transstadial transfer of *A. marginale* has been demonstrated in *D. albipictus*, *D. variabilis*, *Ixodes scapularis*, *Rhipicephalus bursa*, *R. sanguineus* (Dikmans 1950), and *B. microplus* (Connell 1974). *Argas persicus* is another potential North American vector. In Australia and South America *A. marginale* is transmitted by *B. microplus*, and in north Caucasia by *B. calcaratus*. In Europe *Haemaphysalis cinnabarina* and *I. ricinus* are known vectors. In Africa the tick vectors of *A. marginale* are *B. decoloratus*, *Hyalomma excavatum*, *R. bursa*, and *R. simus*. *Anaplasma centrale* is transmitted by *B. decoloratus* in Africa and *H. cinnabarina* in Romania. *Anaplasma ovis* is transmitted by *D. silvarum* in the Ukraine and by *R. bursa* and *Ornithodoros lahorensis* in Russia (Neitz 1956).

Transplacental transmission of *A. marginale* can occur in cattle following acute infection during the third trimester of pregnancy (Swift and Paumer 1976). The significance of this occurrence remains to be seen, but since wild ruminants rarely experience acute anaplasmosis, it is doubtful that transplacental transmission is important in those species.

SIGNS. Anaplasmosis may occur as an acute, subacute, or chronic infection. The chronic form represents a premune state in a commensal host-parasite relationship. There are no documented reports of naturally occurring acute anaplasmosis in wild ruminants. Although this may be due to a lack of observation, it is more likely the result of natural immunity or host adaptation to the parasite over a long-time association. Evidence of this is derived from many observations of wildlife failing to develop clinical anaplasmosis from relatively large inoculums that have proven virulent for domestic animals.

Most members of the deer family (Cervidae) are susceptible to infection with *A. marginale*, but do not ordinarily show signs of disease unless they have undergone splenectomy. Clinical anaplasmosis in nonsplenectomized wild ruminants has been reported only in black-tailed deer infected with *A. marginale* (Christensen et al. 1958b) and in blesbuck infected with *A. ovis* (Neitz 1939).

The onset of clinical disease is signaled by a febrile reaction of several days duration which is accompanied by depression and inappetence. Destruction of infected erythrocytes occurs rapidly, and the severity of the resulting anemia depends on the proportion of the erythrocytes that have become infected with anaplasma. After the critical period the effects of the anemia will include pale mucous membranes, increased respiratory rate, rapid pulse, weakness, dehydration, thirst, and constipation; eventually, icterus and marked weight loss is evident in severe cases. Hemoglobinuria does not occur, but frequent passage of normal-colored urine may be observed.

Physical exertion during the period of anemia may easily cause death from hypoxia. Convalescence takes place over a period of several weeks or months, depending on the severity of the case, during which regeneration of red blood cells and restoration of body condition takes place.

Among infected wild ruminants the mortality is apparently insignificant, but it may reach 50% in mature cattle. Susceptibility within a species depends largely on age and physical condition, which will have considerable influence on the severity of infection and resulting mortality.

PATHOGENESIS. Introduction of anaplasma bodies into the bloodstream of a susceptible host is followed by an incubation period during which no outward signs of disease are evident. The length of incubation varies considerably, depending on the size and infectivity of the inoculum, but usually after 3–6 weeks anaplasma bodies begin to appear in the blood.

Ristic and Watrach (1963) proposed that the development of anaplasmosis occurs in four stages, the first of which is dominated by initial bodies, followed by an increase in marginal bodies, then a period of vigorous growth of marginal bodies and transfer of initial bodies to uninfected erythrocytes, and finally a massive multiplication stage during which the maximum parasitemia occurs. The four stages are roughly equal in duration, each lasting several days.

At the completion of the fourth stage the parasitized erythrocytes begin to disappear from the blood and are presumably removed by phagocytic action of the reticuloendothelial system. During this process the effects of the resulting anemia begin to be felt, and leukocytosis appears. Anaplasma bodies are observed on blood films in decreasing numbers during convalescence, which lasts for several weeks. Regeneration of erythrocytes is indicated by the appearance of anisocytosis, polychromatophilia, nucleated erythrocytes, and an increased number of Howell-Jolly bodies, which may be confused with the remaining anaplasma bodies.

In severe anemia the erythrocyte count, packed cell volume, and hemoglobin content may drop below 25% of normal. Death will usually occur if the blood values drop below this level, but death can also occur prior to this stage as a result of excessive physical exertion.

Abortion has been observed in cattle following experimental acute anaplasmosis (Fowler and Swift 1975). Fetal death was apparently due to hypoxia. Since wild ruminants rarely experience acute anaplasmosis, it is not likely that this sequela is important.

Recovered wild ruminants remain carriers of the anaplasma organism for a considerable length of time, possibly for life (Christensen et al. 1960; Howe et al. 1964), although infections may be lost in some instances (Howe and Hepworth 1965).

PATHOLOGY. Postmortem changes seen with anaplasmosis are related to the massive destruction of red blood cells and the resulting anemia. Typical gross lesions are pale mucous membranes, icterus, enlargement of the spleen up to 2.5 times normal, thin watery blood, distended gall bladder, and a slightly enlarged liver with a mottled mahogany-colored surface. Epicardial and endocardial hemorrhages may be seen in acute cases, signs of constipation may be evident, lymph nodes may be enlarged and edematous, and petechial hemorrhages may occur on the visceral and parietal pleura.

DIAGNOSIS. A diagnosis of anaplasmosis in wild ruminants depends on the demonstration of anaplasma bodies in the red blood cells of the subject or in the erythrocytes of a susceptible host inoculated with blood from the subject. Signs are seldom pronounced enough to be of diagnostic value in wild ruminants, but epizootiologic aspects such as the prevalence of vectors, time of year, and incidence of anaplasmosis in the various ruminant species in the area may be of value in anticipating the occurrence of the disease.

The complement fixation (CF) test and the capillary tube agglutination (CA) test were developed to detect anaplasmosis in cattle and are reliable diagnostic tools for that species. However, several authors have reported that these tests are unreliable when applied to sera of wild ruminants (Howarth et al. 1976). The CF test commonly gives both false negative and false positive results; the CA test gives many false negatives but very few false positives (Kuttler et al. 1968) and, therefore, might have limited value in a survey situation.

An indirect fluorescent antibody (IFA) test has been developed for use in cattle but has not been used extensively with wildlife sera. Lohr and Meyer (1973) and Lohr et al. (1974) reported results of IFA tests on numerous antelopes and other herbivora, but the accuracy of the test in wildlife was not established.

A rapid card agglutination test (Amerault and Roby 1968) developed for field use in cattle also proved to be unreliable when applied to deer sera (Howarth et al. 1969; Peterson et al. 1973). However, when the procedure was modified by the addition of bovine serum factor (Amerault et al. 1972), nonspecific reactions were reduced or eliminated and the modified card agglutination (MCA) test was used successfully to establish the anaplasmosis status of 35 Columbian black-tailed deer (Howarth et al. 1976). Although it is premature to state that the MCA test is the answer to anaplasmosis testing of wild ruminants, it is anticipated that it will improve our ability to detect infections in those species.

PROGNOSIS. In most wild ruminants, anaplasmosis occurs as a subclinical infection; therefore, the prognosis is favorable in the majority of cases. Older animals in poor physical condition, however, are more susceptible to infection and may suffer more severely from its effects.

IMMUNITY. Recovery of a susceptible host from anaplasmosis leaves the subject with a solid immunity that will persist as long as it remains host to the causative organism in a latent condition. This is known as a state of premunition. If premunition ceases as a result of therapeutic treatments or for any other reason, immunity will soon be lost and the subject will be susceptible to reinfection.

Cross-immunity occurs between A. marginale and A. centrale, so that an animal will gain immunity against infection with both forms after recovery from infection with either. Certain wild ruminants that are susceptible to infection with A. ovis as well as A. marginale would be expected to gain some cross-immunity from infections with these forms. Common antigenicity between A. ovis and A. marginale was demonstrated by Kreier and Ristic (1963) when they employed fluorescein-labeled anti-A. marginale globulin to demonstrate A. ovis in blood films of splenectomized white-tailed deer. Cross-antigenicity between A. ovis and A. marginale was also observed by Splitter et al. (1956) in carrying out complement fixation tests.

Some wild ruminants appear to be refractory to natural infection. For example, white-tailed deer may not contract anaplasmosis on exposure to infected ticks (Kuttler et al. 1971). Surveys of wild populations in areas where bovine anaplasmosis is enzootic have failed to demonstrate latent infections in pronghorn antelope (Howe and Hepworth 1965; Jacobson et al. 1977), elk (Vaughn et al. 1976), mule deer (Peterson et al. 1973), white-tailed deer (Beddell and Miller 1966), and bison (Peterson and Roby 1975).

Lohr and Meyer (1973) reported the failure of splenectomized calves to develop immunity against A. marginale after recovering from infection with Anaplasma obtained from naturally infected African antelopes. This suggests the possibility of more than one strain of A. marginale and could explain the apparent natural resistance of wild ruminants to infection with bovine strains of A. marginale and the failure

of transfer of infection between cattle and wildlife in some areas. In IFA tests the two Anaplasma were as antigenically similar as A. centrale and A. marginale, but the antelope Anaplasma appeared to be less virulent to calves than the bovine Anaplasma. The area of strain differences must be clarified before the significance of wildlife as reservoirs of bovine anaplasmosis can be established.

TREATMENT AND CONTROL. Treatment of anaplasmosis in wild ruminants will seldom be a consideration because of their apparent resistance to clinical infection. Furthermore, since a diagnosis of clinical disease will seldom be made before the effects of anemia are evident, treatment with chemotherapeutic agents is seldom of value even in domestic cattle. After the anemia is established, supportive treatment may be indicated. Blood transfusions and fluid therapy may be helpful in cases of severe anemia if such treatment can be administered without causing the subject undue excitement. The value of the treatment will be more than offset by the risk of immediate death from hypoxia in a highly excitable animal.

The carrier state of anaplasmosis in cattle can be eliminated by administering oxytetracycline or chlortetracycline as a feed additive in dosages of 7–11 mg/kg daily for periods of up to 60 days. Oxytetracycline is also useful in arresting the development of anaplasmosis during the incubation period by parenteral inoculation at the same dosage rate for 3–5 days.

A combination of dithiosemicarbazone given intravenously at 5 or 10 mg/kg along with oxytetracycline given intravenously at 11 mg/kg repeated twice at 24- or 48-hour intervals eliminated A. marginale from splenectomized calves (Kuttler 1972). Imidocarb dipropionate or dihydrochloride at the rate of 2–6 mg/kg subcutaneously or intramuscularly in single or multiple doses has given inconsistent results, and the drugs are extremely toxic when repeated at higher dosages (Adams and Todorovic 1974; McHardy and Simpson 1974; Roby and Mazzola 1972).

Effective control measures are based largely on herd management and control of potential parasite vectors. The removal or treatment of known carriers and reduction of external parasites will help considerably in reducing the incidence of anaplasmosis in infected herds. The management of disease in wildlife is difficult and may not be possible beyond periodic reductions of their numbers.

High morbidity is reported among deer in enzootic areas of California, while largely uninfected game herds are reported in other areas where anaplasmosis is common among cattle. One must consider the important modes of transmission and the possibility of more than one strain of *Anaplasma* in attempting to evaluate these seemingly contradictory situations. The tick *D. occidentalis* is a highly efficient vector in California, but in other areas less efficient vectors predominate. Various biting flies may serve to perpetuate the disease within cattle herds without involving wildlife reservoirs.

An inactivated *A. marginale* vaccine (Anaplaz, Fort Dodge Laboratories, Fort Dodge, Kans.) is effective in preventing acute infections in cattle. The product does not cause active infection, but natural infection can still be acquired after vaccination. Although response to infection is mild, a state of premunition develops in infected vaccinated animals, as it does in unvaccinated animals that have recovered from a clinical infection. Vaccination titers persist for about 6 months and cannot be serologically differentiated from disease titers (Amerault and Roby 1971). No reports are available on the use of vaccine in wildlife.

REFERENCES

Adams, L. G.., and Todorovic, R. A. The chemotherapeutic efficacy of imidocarb dihydrochloride on concurrent bovine anaplasmosis and babesiosis. *Trop. Anim. Health Prod.* 6:71–84, 1974.

Amerault, T. E., and Roby, T. O. A rapid card agglutination reaction in bovine anaplasmosis. *Proc. 5th Natl. Anaplasmosis Conf.* (U.S.A.), Stillwater, Okla., pp. 65–75, 1968.

———. Card agglutination and complement-fixation reactions after vaccination of cattle against anaplasmosis. *J. Am. Vet. Med. Assoc.* 159: 1749–1751, 1971.

Amerault, T. E., Rose, J. E., and Roby, T. O. Modified card agglutination test for bovine anaplasmosis: Evaluation with serum and plasma from experimental and natural cases of anaplasmosis. *Proc. 76th Ann. Meet. U. S. Anim. Health Assoc.*, pp. 736–744, 1972.

Beddell, D. M., and Miller, J. G. A report of the examination of 270 white-tailed deer, *Odocoileus virginianus*, from anaplasmosis enzootic areas of southeastern United States for evidence of anaplasmosis. Anim. Dis. Dept. Tifton: University of Georgia, 1966.

Boynton, W. H., and Woods, G. M. Deer as carriers of anaplasmosis. *Science* 78:559–560, 1933.

———. Anaplasmosis among deer in the natural state. *Science* 91:168, 1940.

Buchanan, R. E., and Gibbons, N. E. eds., *Bergey's manual of determinative bacteriology*, 8th ed. Baltimore: Williams and Wilkins, 1974.

Burridge, M. J. The role of wild mammals in the epidemiology of bovine theileriosis in East Africa. *J. Wildl. Dis.* 11:68–75, 1975.

Christensen, J. F., and McNeal, D. W. *Anaplasma marginale* infection in deer in the Sierra Nevada foothill area of California. *Am. J. Vet. Res.* 28:599–600, 1967.

Christensen, J. F., Osebold, J. W., and Douglas, J. R. Bovine anaplasmosis in the coastal range area of California. *J. Am. Vet. Med. Assoc.* 141: 952–957, 1962.

Christensen, J. F., Osebold, J. W., Harrold, J. B., and Rosen, M. N. Persistence of latent *Anaplasma marginale* infections in deer. *J. Am. Vet. Med. Assoc.* 136:426–427, 1960.

Christensen, J. F., Osebold, J. W., and Rosen, M. N. The incidence of latent *Anaplasma marginale* infection in wild deer in an area where anaplasmosis is enzootic in cattle. *Proc. 62nd Ann. Meet. U.S. Livestock Sanit. Assoc.*, Chicago, Ill., pp. 59–65, 1958a.

———. Infections and antibody response in deer experimentally infected with *Anaplasma marginale* from bovine carriers. *J. Am. Vet. Med. Assoc.* 132:289–292, 1958b.

Connell, M. L. Transmission of *Anaplasma marginale* by the cattle tick *Boophilus microplus*. Queensl. *J. Agr. Anim. Sci.* 31:185–194, 1974.

Darlington, P. B. Anaplasmosis in cattle (gallziekte) found to exist in Kansas. *North Am. Vet.* 7:39–41, 1926.

Dikmans, G. The transmission of anaplasmosis *Am. J. Vet. Res.* 11:5–16, 1950.

Dykstra, R. R., Lienhardt, H. F., Pyle, C. A., and Farley, H. Studies in anaplasmosis. *Kans. Agr. Exp. Sta. Rep.* 1:1–32, 1938.

Enigk, K. Die Empfanglichkeit der Elenantilope fur *Anaplasma ovis* und *Eperythrozoon ovis*. *Dtsch. Tropenmed. Z.* 46:48–52, 1942.

Fowler, D., and Swift, B. L. Abortion in cows inoculated with *Anaplasma marginale*. *Theriogenology* 4:59–67, 1975.

Gilruth, J. A., Sweet, G., and Dodd, S. Observations on the occurrence in the blood of various animals (chiefly monotremes and marsupials) of bodies apparently identical with *Anaplasma marginale*, Theiler, 1910. *Parasitology* 4:1–6, 1911.

Grobov, O. F. The susceptibility of the elk to anaplasmosis of cattle. *Veterinariya* 9:50, 1961.

Herms, W. B., and Howell, D. E. The western dog tick, *Dermacentor occidentalis* Neum., a vector of bovine anaplasmosis in California. *J. Parasitol.* 22:283–288, 1936.

Howarth, J. A., Hokama, Y., and Amerault, T. E. The modified card agglutination test: An accurate tool for detecting anaplasmosis in Columbian black-tailed deer. *J. Wildl. Dis.* 12:427–434, 1976.

Howarth, J. A., Roby, T. O., Amerault, T. E., and McNeal, D. W. Prevalence of *Anaplasma mar-*

ginale infection in California deer as measured by calf inoculation and serologic techniques. *Proc. U.S. Anim. Health Assoc.*, pp. 136–147, 1969.

Howe, D. L., and Hepworth, W. G. Anaplasmosis in big game animals: Tests on wild populations in Wyoming. *Am. J. Vet. Res.* 26:1114–1120, 1965.

Howe, D. L., Hepworth, W. G., Blunt, F., and Thomas, G. M. Anaplasmosis in big game animals: Experimental transmission and evaluation of serologic tests. *Am. J. Vet. Res.* 25:1271–1275, 1964.

Howell, D. E., Stiles, G. W., and Moe, L. H. The hereditary transmission of anaplasmosis by *Dermacentor andersoni* Stiles. *Am. J. Vet. Res.* 2:165–166, 1941.

Jacobson, R. H., Worley, D. E., and Hawkins, W. W. Studies on pronghorn antelope (*Antilocapra americana*) as reservoirs of anaplasmosis in Montana. *J. Wildl. Dis.* 13:323–326, 1977.

Kreier, J. P., and Ristic, M. Anaplasmosis: VII. Experimental *Anaplasma ovis* infection in white-tailed deer (*Dama virginiana*). *Am. J. Vet. Res.* 24:567–572, 1963.

Kuttler, K. L. Combined treatment with a dithiosemicarbazone and oxytetracycline to eliminate *Anaplasma marginale* infections in splenectomized calves. *Res. Vet. Sci.* 13:536–539, 1972.

Kuttler, K. L., Graham, O. H., and Johnson, S. R. Apparent failure of *Boophilus annulatus* to transmit anaplasmosis to white-tailed deer (*Odocoileus virginianus*). *J. Parasitol.* 57:657–659, 1971.

Kuttler, K. L., Robinson, R. M., and Franklin, T. E. Serological response to *Anaplasma marginale* infection in splenectomized deer (*Odocoileus virginianus*) as measured by the complement-fixation and capillary-tube agglutination tests. *Proc. 5th Natl. Anaplasmosis Conf.* (U.S.A.), Stillwater, Okla., pp. 82–88, 1968.

Kuttler, K. L., Robinson, R. M., and Rogers, W. P. Exacerbation of latent erythrocytic infections in deer following splenectomy. *Can. J. Comp. Med. Vet. Sci.* 31:317–319, 1967.

Lestoquard, F. Transmission au buffle des piroplasmes du boeuf. Modifications subies par *Anaplasma marginale*. *Bull. Soc. Pathol. Exot.* 24:820–822, 1931.

Lignieres, J. La Vaccination des bovides centre l'anaplasmose. *Bull. Soc. Pathol. Exot.* 12:765–774, 1919.

Lohr, K. F., and Meyer, H. Game anaplasmosis: The isolation of *Anaplasma* organisms from antelope. *Z. Tropenmed. Parasitol.* 24:192–197, 1973.

Lohr, K. F., Ross, J. P. J., and Meyer, H. Detection in game of fluorescent and agglutination antibodies to intraerythrocytic organisms. *Z. Tropenmed. Parasitol.* 25:217–226, 1974.

McHardy, N., and Simpson, R. M. Imidocarb dipropionate therapy in Kenyan anaplasmosis and babesiosis. *Trop. Anim. Health Prod.* 6:63–70, 1974.

McMillan, B., and Bancroft, B. J. On the morphology of *Trypanosoma binneyi* Mackerras, 1959 from

the platypus *Ornithorhynchus anatinus*. *Int. J. Parasitol.* 4:441–442, 1974.

Neitz, W. O., Bovine anaplasmosis: The transmission of *Anaplasma marginale* to a black wildebeest (*Conochaetes gnu*). *Onderstepoort J. Vet. Sci. Anim. Ind.* 5:9–11, 1935.

———. Ovine anaplasmosis: The transmission of *Anaplasma ovis* and *Eperythrozoon ovis* to the blesbuck (*Damaliscus albifrons*). *Onderstepoort J. Vet. Sci. Animal Ind.* 13:9–16, 1939.

———. A consolidation of our knowledge of the transmission of tick-borne diseases. *Onderstepoort J. Vet. Res.* 27:115–163, 1956.

Neitz, W. O., and Du Toit, P. J. Bovine anaplasmosis: A method of obtaining pure strains of *Anaplasma marginale* and *Anaplasma centrale* by transmission through antelopes. *18th Rep. Div. Vet. Serv. Anim. Ind.*, Onderstepoort, Union of South Africa, p. 3–20, 1932.

Osebold, J. W., Christensen, J. F., Longhurst, W. M., and Rosen, M. N. Latent *Anaplasma marginale* infections in wild deer demonstrated by calf inoculation. *Cornell Vet.* 49:97–115, 1959.

Osebold, J. W., Douglas, J. R., and Christensen, J. F. Transmission of anaplasmosis to cattle by ticks obtained from deer. *Am. J. Vet. Res.* 23:21–23, 1962.

Peterson, K. J., Kistner, T. P., and Davis, H. E. Epizootiologic studies of anaplasmosis in Oregon mule deer. *J. Wildl. Dis.* 9:314–319, 1973.

Peterson, K. J., and Roby, T. O. Absence of *Anaplasma marginale* infection in American bison raised in an anaplasmosis endemic area. *J. Wildl. Dis.* 11:395–397, 1975.

Piercy, P. L. Transmission of anaplasmosis. *Ann. N.Y. Acad. Sci.* 64:40–48, 1956.

Renshaw, H. W., Vaughn, H. W., Magonigle, R. A., Davis, W. C., Stauber, E. H., and Frank, F. W. Evaluation of free-roaming mule deer as carriers of anaplasmosis in an area of Idaho where bovine anaplasmosis is enzootic. *J. Am. Vet. Med. Assoc.* 170:334–339, 1977.

Ristic, M. Anaplasmosis. *Ad. Vet. Sci.* 6:111–192, 1960.

Ristic, M., and Watrach, A. M. Anaplasmosis: VI. Studies and hypothesis concerning the cycle of development of the causative agent. *Am. J. Vet. Res.* 24:267–277, 1963.

Roberts, H. H., and Lancaster, J. L. Determining susceptibility of white-tailed deer to anaplasmosis. *Ark. Farm Res.* 12(Jan.–Feb):1, 1963.

Roby, T. O., and Mazzola, V. Elimination of the carrier state of bovine anaplasmosis with imidocarb. *Am. J. Vet. Res.* 33:1931–1933, 1972.

Smith, K., Brocklesby, D. W., Bland, P., Purnell, R. E., Brown, C. G. D. and Payne, R. C. The fine structure of intra-erythrocytic stages of *Theileria gorgonis* and a strain of *Anaplasma marginale* isolated from wildebeest (*Conochaetes taurinus*). *Z. Tropenmed. Parasitol.* 25:293–300, 1974.

Smith, T., and Kilborne, F. L. Investigations into the nature, causation and prevention of Texas or southern cattle fever. USDA, *BAI Bull.* 1, pp.1–301, 1893.

Splitter, E. J., Anthony, H. D., and Twiehaus, M. J. *Anaplasma ovis* in the United States: Experimental studies with sheep and goats. *Am. J. Vet. Res.* 17:487–491, 1956.

Splitter, E. J., Twiehaus, M. J., and Castro, E. R. Anaplasmosis in sheep in the United States. *J. Am. Vet. Med. Assoc.* 127:244–245, 1955.

Summers, W. A., and Gonzalez, L. L. Attempts to transmit bovine anaplasmosis to small laboratory animals. *Exp. Parasitol.* 16:57–63, 1965.

Swift, B. L., and Paumer, R. J. Vertical transmission of *Anaplasma marginale* in cattle. *Theriogenology* 6:515–521, 1976.

Theiler, A. *Anaplasma marginale* (gen. and spec. nov.): The marginal points in the blood of cattle suffering from a specific disease. *Govt. Rep. Vet. Bacteriol.*, 1908–1909, pp. 7–64. Transvaal, South Africa: Department of Agriculture, 1910.

Vaughn, H. W., Renshaw, H. W., and Frank, F. W. Survey of anaplasmosis in elk of the Clearwater National Forest (Idaho). *Am. J. Vet. Res.* 37:615–617, 1976.

45 *Eperythrozoonosis*

DUANE L. HOWE

Synonyms: **None.**

Eperythrozoonosis is a noncontagious infectious disease of rodents, ruminants, and swine. It is generally asymptomatic and is characterized by the occurrence of coccus-, ring-, and rod-shaped forms adhering to the red blood cells and free in the plasma.

HISTORY AND DISTRIBUTION. Eperythrozoonosis in sheep was first reported by Neitz et al. in South Africa in 1934. Two species of African antelopes have been found susceptible to experimental infection with *Eperythrozoon ovis*. In 1939 Neitz experimentally produced latent eperythrozoonosis in the blesbuck (*Damaliscus albifrons*), and in 1942 Enigk established a latent infection in an eland (*Taurotragus oryx*).

Naturally occurring latent eperythrozoonosis has been reported in deer on four different occasions, and once in North American elk. Osebold et al. (1959) observed eperythrozoonosis in Columbian black-tailed deer (*Odocoileus hemionus columbianus*). Kreier and Ristic (1963a) identified *E. ovis* in the white-tailed deer (*O. virginianus*); Howe et al. (1964) and Howe and Hepworth (1965) observed latent infections of unidentified eperythrozoa in mule deer (*O. h. hemionus*) and elk (*Cervus canadensis*); and Kuttler et al. (1967) found latent eperythrozoonosis in white-tailed deer in Texas.

Three species of *Eperythrozoon* have been reported from mice and voles on two continents. *Eperythrozoon dispar* was detected in the European vole (*Arvicola arvalis*) by Bruynoghe and Vassilaidis (1929) and in the American vole (*Microtus pennsylvanicus*) by Tyzzer and Weinman (1939). Tyzzer (1942) reported eperythrozoonosis due to *E. varians* in the mouse *Peromyscus maniculatus*). Both *E. dispar* and *E. varians* differ in morphology from *E. coccoides*, the common eperythrozoon of laboratory mice; and all three may be differentiated on the basis of host specificity.

Eperythrozoonosis apparently has a wide host and geographic distribution, although few investigations have been carried out to determine its occurrence in different geographic areas. It is likely to occur wherever suitable vectors are present.

ETIOLOGY. The classification of eperythrozoa has been the subject of some controversy, but they are now considered to be rickettsia and are included in the family Anaplasmataceae (Buchanan and Gibbons 1974). Eperythrozoa are small, coccoid, rod-shaped, circular, or ring-shaped and are often pleomorphic, the exact shape depending on the staining and viewing techniques used. They stain a bluish or violet color with Giemsa stain, showing no differentiation of nucleus and cytoplasm, and are gram-negative. The organisms occur both on the surface of the erythrocytes and free in the plasma (Fig. 45.1).

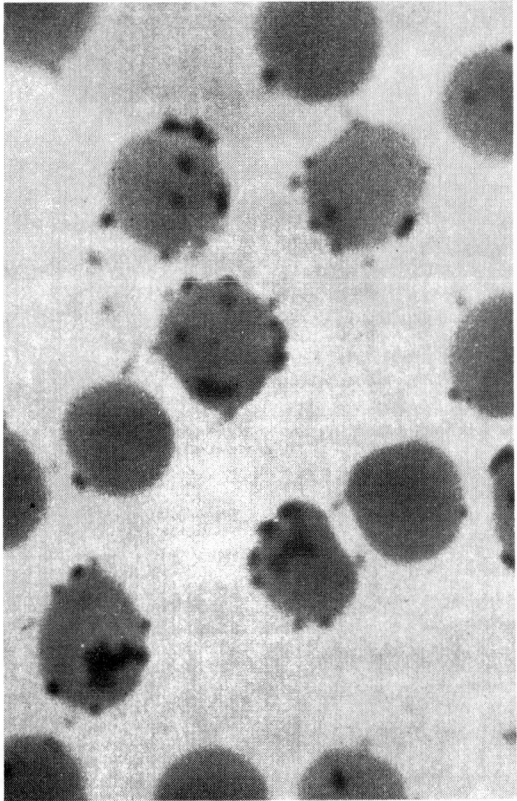

FIG. 45.1 *Eperythrozoon ovis:* Giemsa stain. ×3,200. (Photomicrograph courtesy J. P. Kreier.)

Eperythrozoon wenyoni occurs in the bovine and is considered nonpathogenic in that species. *Eperythrozoon suis* and *E. ovis*, on the other hand, may be pathogenic in their respective hosts, depending on the condition of the host and other factors not completely understood at the present time. Neither *E. wenyoni* nor *E. suis* have been reported from wildlife, and an attempt to establish *E. wenyoni* infection in a splenectomized deer was unsuccessful (Kreier and Ristic 1963b). *Eperythrozoon ovis* appears to be less host specific and is capable of infecting cattle, domestic sheep, and various species of wild ruminants.

Kreier and Ristic (1963b) employed the fluorescent antibody technique, phase microscopy, and electron microscopy as well as Giemsa-stained blood films in a thorough study of the morphology of *E. ovis* and *E. wenyoni*. The two organisms appeared morphologically similar, although *E. ovis* had a greater affinity for basophilic dye and appeared most commonly as rods or spheres near the periphery of red blood cells; whereas *E. wenyoni* stained less intensely and appeared most often as delicate ring structures.

In wet mounts viewed with the phase-contrast microscope, the eperythrozoa appeared as spheres; however, electron microscope preparations showed the organisms as oval rods and disk forms containing one or two granular masses (Fig. 45.2). The parasites occurred free in the plasma, on the surface of the red blood cells, and adjacent to the periphery of the cells. The eperythrozoa measured $0.3-0.4$ μ in diameter.

In ultrathin sections of parasitized red blood cells viewed with the electron microscope, the eperythrozoa appeared as ring structures resembling the *Anaplasma* initial body and were located in concavities that appeared to be eroded into the red blood cells by the parasites.

Neitz et al. (1934), in the initial description of *E. ovis* in Giemsa-stained blood films, primarily observed delicate ring structures $0.5-1.0$ μ in diameter along with frequent ovoid, rod, comma-shaped, dumbbell, and rounded triangle forms. They noted that the variations in shape appeared to be mechanical.

Eperythrozoon coccoides appears primarily as ring forms $0.5-1.4$ μ in diameter, averaging 0.7 μ (Bruynoghe and Vassilaidis 1929).

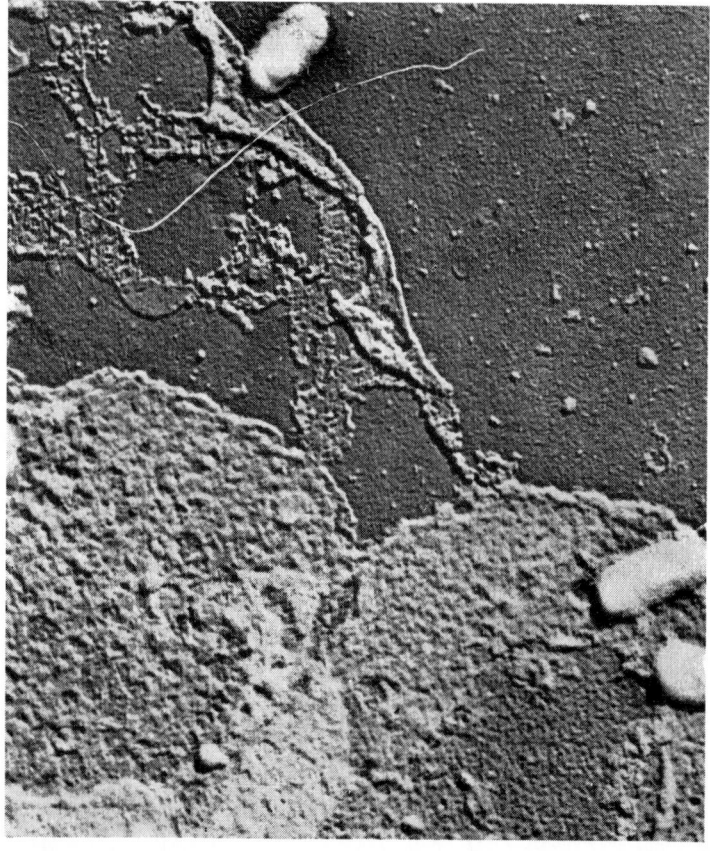

FIG.. **45.2** *Eperythrozoon wenyoni*. Granular bodies demonstrated by electron microscope shadow cast preparation. ×12,500. (Photomicrograph courtesy J. P. Kreier.)

Eperythrozoon varians occurs in a variety of forms, including cocci, rings, and rods, and is seen primarily in the plasma (Tyzzer 1942). *Eperythrozoon dispar* presents a large proportion of coccoid forms with few rings, measuring 0.5–0.7 μ in diameter (Tyzzer and Weinman 1939).

TRANSMISSION. Eperythrozoonosis is thought to be mechanically transmitted by arthropod vectors. Bruynoghe and Vassilaidis (1929) demonstrated that lice could transmit the disease in rodents, and presumably other external parasites are capable of effecting transmission. Experimentally the disease may be transmitted by the simple parenteral inoculation of infective blood into a susceptible host.

SIGNS AND PATHOLOGY. Due to the relative avirulence of *Eperythrozoon*, signs are rarely seen in normal animals. Splenectomy increases susceptibility, presumably as a result of the removal of an important part of the reticuloendothelial system which is responsible for the destruction of the parasites.

In experimental infections of splenectomized sheep, the incubation period is usually 1–2 weeks, but it may be longer in a natural exposure. A high fever signals the onset of parasitemia, and the eperythrozoa multiply rapidly until they outnumber the red blood cells by as much as 100 to 1. The parasitized erythrocytes are rapidly destroyed, and clinical anemia begins about a week after the first appearance of rickettsia.

If the infection becomes severe, a marked anemia results, manifested in the host by pale mucous membranes, rapid pulse and respiration, weakness, and collapse. Icterus may develop following destruction of large numbers of red blood cells. Postmortem lesions are limited to those associated with the anemia and include thin watery blood, pale mucous membranes, enlarged spleen, and icterus.

DIAGNOSIS. During the acute stage of infection, organisms may be demonstrated in Giemsa-stained blood films or by the use of fluorescein-labeled antibody. Complement-fixing antibodies are produced as a result of eperythrozoonosis and can be detected during the convalescent and premune stages of infection. A strong antigenic relationship exists between *E. ovis* and *E. wenyoni*, and these species cannot be differentiated by serologic methods. Weak cross-reactions also occur between *Eperythrozoon* and *Anaplasma* and can cause confusion in the serologic diagnosis of these diseases (Kreier and Ristic 1963b). Xenodiagnosis must be employed in the identification of the species of *Eperythrozoon*.

TREATMENT AND CONTROL. Neoarsphenamine and the tetracyclines are effective against early cases of eperythrozoonosis. Control is not considered important but may be accomplished by eliminating arthropod parasites that act as vectors.

REFERENCES

Bruynoghe, R., and Vassilaidis, P. Contribution a l'etude des *Eperythrozoaires coccoides*. *Ann. Parasitol.* 7:353–364, 1929.
Buchanan, R. E., and Gibbons, N. E. *Bergey's manual of determinative bacteriology*, 8th ed. Baltimore: Williams and Wilkins, 1974.
Enigk, K. Die Empfanglichkeit der Elenantilope fur *Anaplasma ovis* und *Eperythrozoon ovis*. *Dtsch. Tropenmend. Z.* 46:48–52, 1942.
Howe, D. L., and Hepworth, W. G. Anaplasmosis in big game animals: Tests on wild populations in Wyoming. *Am. J. Vet. Res.* 26:1114–1120, 1965.
Howe, D. L., Hepworth, W. G., Blunt, F., and Thomas, G. M. Anaplasmosis in big game animals: Experimental transmission and evaluation of serologic tests. *Am. J. Vet. Res.* 25:1271–1275, 1964.
Kreier, J. P., and Ristic, M. Anaplasmosis: VII. Experimental *Anaplasma ovis* infection in white-tailed deer (*Dama virginiana*). *Am. J. Vet. Res.* 24:567–572, 1963a.
———. Morphologic, antigenic, and pathogenic characteristics of *Eperythrozoon ovis* and *Eperythrozoon wenyoni*. *Am. J. Vet. Res.* 24:488–500, 1963b.
Kuttler, K. L., Robinson, R. M., and Rogers, W. P. Exacerbation of latent erythrocytic infections in deer following splenectomy. *Can. J. Comp. Med. Vet. Sci.* 31:317–319, 1967.
Neitz, W. O. Ovine anaplasmosis: The transmission of *Anaplasma ovis* and *Eperythrozoon ovis* to the blesbuck (*Damaliscus albifrons*). *Onderstepoort J. Vet. Sci. Anim. Ind.* 13:9–16, 1939.
Neitz, W. O., Alexander, R. A., and Du Toit, P. J. *Eperythrozoon ovis* (sp. nov.) infection in sheep. *Onderstepoort J. Vet. Sci. Anim. Ind.* 30:263–269, 1934.
Osebold, J. W., Christensen, J. F., Longhurst, W. M., and Rosen, M. N. Latent *Anaplasma marginale* infections in wild deer demonstrated by calf inoculation. *Cornell Vet.* 49:97–115, 1959.
Tyzzer, E. E. A comparative study of Grahamellae, Haemobartonellae and Eperythrozoa in small mammals. *Proc. Am. Phil. Soc.* 85:359–398, 1942.
Tyzzer, E. E., and Weinman, D. *Haemobartonella*, n.g. (*Bartonella* olim pro parte), *H. microti*, n.sp., of the field vole, *Microtus pennsylvanicus*. *Am. J. Hyg.* 30:141–157, 1939.

46 *Miscellaneous Bacterial Diseases*

DUANE L. HOWE

Vibriosis

Synonyms: **Vibrionic abortion.**

Vibriosis is an infectious disease of the genital tract of cattle and sheep. The disease is worldwide in distribution and in North America is especially prevalent in the Rocky Mountain area. It has been reported in North America among pronghorn antelope (*Antilocapra americana*).

ETIOLOGY AND TRANSMISSION. Vibriosis is caused by *Campylobacter fetus*, a pleomorphic, gram-negative rod, varying from a comma-shaped form in tissues and young cultures to filamentous forms in older cultures. Three subspecies (Buchanan and Gibbons 1974) are recognized: *C. f. fetus* (formerly *Vibrio fetus venerealis*), a pathogen of the bovine; *C. f. intestinalis* (formerly *V. f. intestinalis*), a pathogen of sheep; and *C. f. jejuni* (formerly *V. jejuni*), a normal intestinal inhabitant of cattle, sheep, swine, and other animals and birds.

Transmission is primarily by ingestion in sheep and by coitus in cattle. The mode of transmission in the pronghorn antelope is not known but is presumed to be by ingestion.

SIGNS. Ovine vibriosis is characterized by abortion late in gestation and by the birth of weak lambs. Infertility and abortion are the most common manifestations in cattle. It is a self-limiting infection in both species.

In antelope, vibriosis apparently causes either abortion in late gestation or an increased neonatal mortality.

PATHOLOGY. Trueblood and Post (1959) recovered *C. fetus* from five pregnant antelope taken from a herd in Wyoming with a history of poor reproduction. Isolations were made from blood, amniotic fluid, and fetal stomach contents. Oral inoculation of this isolate into pregnant domestic ewes resulted in abortions.

The antelope herd in question had suffered from declining fawn production or survival for several years. This may indicate greater sus-ceptibility among antelope than domestic stock in which the disease is self-limiting.

Pathologic changes in sheep are limited to the uterus and fetus. Edema and congestion of the uterine wall and fetal membranes occur, and the cotyledons may be swollen with gray areas of necrosis. The fetus may show subcutaneous edema, sanguineous fluid in body cavities, and necrotic foci on the liver (Jensen et al. 1961).

DIAGNOSIS AND CONTROL. Diagnosis is dependent on clinical signs, pathology, and the isolation and identification of the causative organism.

Prevention in antelope herds would presumably be aided by limiting contact between susceptible antelope and infected sheep. Streptomycin is the drug of choice in treating vibriosis. Effective vaccines are available for cattle and sheep but have not been tested in antelope.

Actinomycosis

Synonyms: **Lumpy jaw, poll evil, fistulous withers, suppurative mastitis.**

Actinomycosis is an infectious disease, usually of an insidious nature, characterized by suppurative granulomatous lesions occurring commonly in the mandibular region of deer, moose, pronghorn antelope, mountain sheep, cattle, domestic sheep, and muskrats. It also occurs in the soft tissues of other wild and domestic species and is worldwide in distribution.

ETIOLOGY. *Actinomyces* is a gram-positive, filamentous, anaerobic bacterium. It forms branched mycelia which break up into small coccoid or bacillary segments that function as conidia. The organisms commonly occur in the oral cavities of healthy animals, but their mode of entry into the tissues is not definitely known.

Actinomyces bovis is usually associated with lumpy jaw in wild and domestic ruminants. The typical bony tissue lesions may involve the maxilla, turbinate, or palatine bones but most commonly occur in the mandible. *Actinomyces bovis* is also associated with poll evil and fistulous withers in horses and suppurative mastitis in sows. Soft-tissue actinomycotic abcesses occurring in wild Canidae are also attributed to *A. bovis* (formerly *A. canis*).

SIGNS. Aside from the obvious swelling that develops from the osteitis or soft-tissue abscesses (Fig. 46.1), signs may include stertorous breathing caused by involvement of the turbinate bones and difficulty in prehension and mastication resulting from pain or mechanical interference from swellings in the jaw or tongue. Central nervous system signs have been seen in deer with brain involvement. Regional lymphadenopathy often occurs in carnivores with soft-tissue infections.

PATHOLOGY. Lumpy jaw is a rarefying osteitis affecting the mandible and occasionally the maxilla, palatine, and turbinate bones. The characteristic lump on the ventral aspect of the mandible results from a necrotizing infection and tissue reaction. Invasion of the bone by *A. bovis* is followed by a granulomatous infiltration and osteoporosis. Bone is destroyed by liquefaction necrosis and is replaced by a granulomatous mass interwoven with trabeculae of osteogenic tissue.

In soft tissues actinomycosis occurs as encapsulated abscesses containing thick, tenacious, yellow, nonodorous pus. A similar exudate occurs in fistulous tracts and granulomatous masses of lumpy jaw and other bone lesions. So-called sulfur granules, which resemble small grains of sand, are found in these actinomycotic lesions. If the granules are crushed and stained with Gram stain, the presence of gram-positive cocci, rods, filaments, and rosettes of radiating clubs and filaments may be demonstrated.

Dentoalveolar abscesses occur in Columbian black-tailed deer (*Odocoileus hemionus columbianus*) with the first molar of the lower arcade the most commonly affected, probably because of its early eruption and relatively fast wear (Cowan 1946). Actinomycosis of the jawbone has been reported in roe deer (*Capreolus capreolus*) in Germany (Bamberger 1952; Schiel 1937), chevreuils in France (Bouvier et al. 1962), and mule deer (*O. hemionus*) and white-tailed deer (*O. virginianus*) in the United States (Honess and Winter 1956).

Typical lumpy-jaw lesions are not uncom-

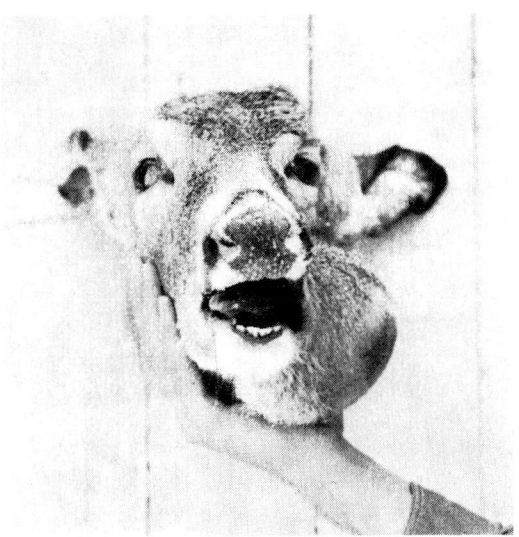

FIG. 46.1 Actinomycosis in a 4-year-old white-tailed deer. (Photo, D. O. Trainer.)

mon in bighorn sheep (*Ovis canadensis*) in Banff National Park, where the disease is considered a significant mortality factor. Transmission is thought to occur at mineral licks and water holes (Green 1949). Similar lesions are also commonly seen in an isolated herd of black mountain sheep, or stone sheep (*Ovis stonei*), in northern British Columbia (Blair 1906).

Actinomycoticlike lesions have been associated with food impaction and worn feet in older moose (*Alces alces*) in British Columbia (Ritcey and Edwards 1958).

Actinomyces bovis has also been associated with encephalitis in mule deer (Ryff 1953) and a fatal lumpy-jaw infection in muskrats (*Ondatra zibethica*) (Dozier 1943).

Actinomycosis in carnivores is an infection of the soft tissues, forming abscesses or extensive phlegmonous swellings with multiple fistulae. Regional lymph nodes become inflamed but do not suppurate (McGaughey 1952). The disease may occur as a purulent pleuritis in silver foxes (Eieland 1949).

DIAGNOSIS. Actinomycosis is recognized clinically on the basis of the typical bony enlargements of the jawbones of ruminants. Involvement of the turbinate or palatine bones may occur without causing external swellings, and in these cases the first signs may result from interference with breathing or mastication.

In soft-tissue actinomycosis, a tentative diagnosis may be based on the occurrence of the typical exudates. In the absence of these lesions, and in the case of a tentative diagnosis based on such lesions, confirmation must await the isolation and identification of the causative organism.

The typical sulfur granules occurring in actinomycotic lesions are also formed in soft-tissue lesions caused by *Actinobacillus*, and differentiation of the two must be made microscopically. Smears of crushed granules of *A. bovis* appear as branched gram-positive filaments, whereas those of *Actinobacillus* are gram-negative and uniformly rod shaped. In the absence of fresh tissues, Miller et al. (1975) used radiography to determine the presence and prevalence of actinomycosis in barren-ground caribou in Canada.

TREATMENT. In early cases, surgical extirpation and drainage of bone lesions plus potassium iodide given orally or sodium iodide given intravenously is effective treatment. Fistulas and abscesses should be curetted. Packing the wounds with tampons soaked in tincture of iodine after surgical intervention is of benefit.

Blackleg

Synonyms: **Black quarter, symptomatic anthrax.**

Blackleg is an acute febrile noncontagious infection of deer, cattle, sheep, and probably pronghorn antelope. It is characterized by sudden onset, fever, and emphysematous serohemorrhagic swellings in the subcutaneous tissues and heavy musculature. The disease is worldwide in distribution.

ETIOLOGY AND TRANSMISSION. Blackleg is caused by *Clostridium chauvei* (*feseri*), an anaerobic, gram-positive, spore-forming rod, and possibly by other closely related species. The organisms are commonly found in soil and in the intestinal tracts of animals. Infections may arise through contaminated wounds or may occur spontaneously from ingested spores.

SIGNS. Animals of all ages are susceptible to blackleg, but younger animals, 6 months to 2 years of age, generally have a more severe clinical response. The clinical course of disease is short and may not be noticed until an animal is found dead. Clinical signs are characterized by sudden onset—beginning with lameness, high fever and depression—followed by crepitant swellings on the shoulder, neck, back, or thigh. Death usually occurs 1–2 days after the onset of signs. In one deer a stiff, high-stepping gait was noted (Armstrong and MacNamee 1950).

PATHOLOGY. In cattle, postmortem lesions are typified by extensive subcutaneous emphysematous swellings, rapid putrefaction, oozing of frothy blood from body openings, and dry, dark-colored swollen musculature disrupted by gas bubbles in one or more areas of the body. The affected muscles appear spongy and have a sweetish odor. A subcutaneous hemorrhagic gaseous edema occurs over the affected muscles.

Typical hemorrhagic lesions in the musculature are sometimes absent or overlooked, especially when their occurrence is limited to the less obvious muscle groups. Fluids are often present in the peritoneal cavity and sometimes in the thoracic cavity and pericardial sac. The fluids may be blood tinged or dark brown in color.

The lesions noted in deer were rather typical of blackleg in cattle. With the exception of the spleen, the internal organs exhibited pronounced congestion and edema. Significant losses of white-tailed deer (*Odocoileus virginianus*) due to blackleg were reported by Armstrong and MacNamee (1950), but other reports of the disease in wildlife have been incidental and of a suggestive nature (Howe 1966; Trainer 1961).

DIAGNOSIS. A presumptive diagnosis may be made on signs and lesions, but the isolation and identification of the causative organism is necessary for a positive diagnosis and differentiation from malignant edema.

TREATMENT. Treatment is seldom effective unless begun in the very early stages of infection. Parenteral administration of large doses of penicillin or broad-spectrum antibiotics and antiserum have provided satisfactory treatment in domestic animals and captive deer.

CONTROL. Immunization with formolized whole cultures of *C. chauvei* is effective in preventing blackleg in domestic livestock. Appropriate environmental management, such as prompt disposal of carcasses infected with blackleg organisms to minimize contamination of soil with the spores, is also important in its control.

Malignant Edema

Synonyms: **Gas edema, gas phlegmon, braxy.**

Malignant edema is an acute nonconta-gious febrile disease of domestic and wild ru-minants, including deer and elk, characterized by spreading edematous and emphysematous swellings. Death usually results from toxemia in 1–4 days. The disease is worldwide in dis-tribution and occurs sporadically with low mor-bidity and high mortality.

ETIOLOGY AND TRANSMISSION. The causa-tive agent of malignant edema is *Clostridium septicum (C. septique, C. septicus, C. oedematis maligni, Bacillus oedematis maligni, Vibrion septique)*, an anaerobic, gram-positive, spore-forming rod. It is a common soil con-taminant, gaining entrance to the animal through breaks in the skin. Other species of clostridia may also be involved in gas gangrene infections in wildlife species (Howe 1965).

SIGNS. Because of the acute nature of malig-nant edema, clinical signs of the disease are not often evident in either domestic livestock or wild hoofed mammals. Hot, painful edematous swellings primarily involving the subcutaneous tissue occur around the site of a wound and spread to adjacent areas. The swellings later become cooler and less sensitive, and signs of toxemia soon develop. Emphysema may be de-tected around the wound in the later stages.

PATHOLOGY. Infected white-tailed deer (*Odo-coileus virginianus*) usually have edema of the skin and subcutis, as well as hemorrhagic em-physematous areas which appear light colored under the skin and between muscle layers of the extremities. A clear, straw-colored fluid may be found in the thoracic and abdominal cavities, and bloody fluids exude from the body openings. Internal organs appear edematous, the liver is dark colored, and the spleen is mushy and tar-like on the cut surface. Catarrhal enteritis has been observed (LeDune and Volkmar 1934; Post 1957).

Erosion of the lining of the rumen and upper small intestine has also been associated with malignant edema in white-tailed deer (McKenney 1938). This form of the disease more nearly resembles the condition of "braxy" reported in sheep in Norway, Iceland, and Scot-land.

A gas gangrene infection that closely re-sembles the condition described for deer has been observed in elk (*Cervus canadensis*). Young animals appear to be very susceptible and die a short time after exposure, with sub-cutaneous and intramuscular hemorrhage and edema, emphysematous swellings in the ex-tremities, and pale pink musculature. Internal organs are edematous, the blood is tarlike, and bloody fluids exude from body openings. Clos-tridia other than *C. septicum* have been asso-ciated with the disease in elk (Hepworth 1963; Howe 1965).

DIAGNOSIS AND TREATMENT. Diagnosis is based on signs and pathology, with isolation and identification of the causative organism necessary for a positive diagnosis. Parenteral administration of large doses of broad-spectrum antibiotics is effective against early infections. Since the clinical course is rapid, however, many animals will die before treatment can be administered.

CONTROL. Immunity may be conferred to do-mestic livestock and captive wild ruminants by vaccination with a whole-culture bacterin of *C. septicum*. Polyvalent bacterins are available that will give protection against both blackleg and malignant edema.

REFERENCES

Armstrong, H. L., and MacNamee, J. K. Blackleg in deer. *J. Am. Vet. Med. Assoc.* 117:212–214, 1950.

Bamberger, H. Seltines fall von aktinomykose bie rehwild. *Oesterr. Weidwerk* 17:170, 1952.

Blair, W. R. Actinomycosis in the black mountain sheep. *N.Y. Zool. Soc. Ann. Rep.* 11:132–141, 1906.

Bouvier, G., Burgisser, H., and Schneider, P. A. Ob-servations sur les maladies du gibier et des an-imaux sauvages faites en 1959 et 1960. *Schweiz. Arch. Tierheilk.* 104:440–450, 1962.

Buchanan, R. E., and Gibbons, N. E. eds. *Bergey's manual of determinative bacteriology,* 8th ed. Baltimore: Williams and Wilkins, 1974.

Cowan, I. McT. Parasites, disease, injuries and anomalies of the Columbian black-tailed deer. *Odocoileus hemionus columbianus* (Richardson), in British Columbia. *Can. J. Res.* 24(sec D):71–103, 1946.

Dozier, H. L. Occurrence of ringworm disease and lumpy jaw in the muskrat in Maryland. *J. Am. Vet. Med. Assoc.* 102:451–453, 1943.

Eieland, E. Et tilfelle av actinomycose (streptothri-cose) hos solvrev. *Nord. Vet. Med.* 1:395–402, 1949.

Green, H. U. *The bighorn sheep of Banff National Park.* Natl. Parks Hist. Sites Serv., Dev. Serv. Branch. Ottawa: Can. Dept. Res. Dev., 1949.

Hepworth, W. G. *Federal aid in wildlife restoration,* project FW-3-R-10, Wyoming Game and Fish Dept., Cheyenne, Wyo. p. 13, 1963.

Honess, R. F., and Winter, K. B. Diseases of wildlife in Wyoming. *Wyo. Game Fish Comm. Bull.* 9:21, 1956.

Howe, D. L. *Federal aid in wildlife restoration,* project FW-3-R-12, Wyoming Game and Fish Dept., Cheyenne, Wyo. pp. 14–15, 1965.

———. *Federal aid in wildlife restoration,* project FW-3-R-13, Wyoming Game and Fish Dept. Cheyenne, Wyo. p. 16, 1966.

Jensen, R., Metler, V. A., and Mollelo, J. A. Placental pathology of sheep with vibriosis. *Am. J. Vet. Res.* 22:169–185, 1961.

LeDune, E. K., and Volkmar, F. Malignant edema in deer. *Vet. Med.* 29:276–279, 1934.

McGaughey, C. A. Actinomycosis in carnivores: A review of the literature. *Br. Vet. J.* 108:89–92, 1952.

McKenney, F. D. Malignant edema in deer. *Trans.*

North Am. Wildl. Conf. 3:886–889, 1938.

Miller, F. W., Cawley, A. J., Choquette, L.P.E., and Broughton, E. Radiographic examination of mandibular lesions in barren-ground caribou. *J. Wildl. Dis.* 11:465–470, 1975.

Post, G. *Federal aid in wildlife restoration,* project FW-3-R-4, Wyoming Game and Fish Dept. Cheyenne, Wyo., pp. 5–6, 1957.

Ritcey, R. W., and Edwards, R. Y. Parasites and diseases of the Wells Gray moose herd. *J. Mammal.* 39:139–145, 1958.

Ryff, J. F. Encephalitis in a deer due to *Actinomyces bovis. J. Am. Vet. Med. Assoc.* 122:78–80, 1953.

Schiel, O. Ergebnisse der Wilduntersuchungen im Veterinar-Untersuchungsant Oppelnaus den Jahren, 1925 bis 1936. *Z. Hyg. Infectionskrankh.* 52:180–186, 1937.

Trainer, D. O. Diseases of the white-tailed deer (*Odocoileus virginianus*). Ph.D. thesis, University of Wisconsin, 1961.

Trueblood, M. S., and Post, G. Vibriosis as a factor in the reproduction of antelope (*Antilocapra americana*). *J. Am. Vet. Med. Assoc.* 134:562–564, 1959.

3 *Neoplastic Disease*

47 *Viral Tumors*

G. E. COSGROVE   L. D. FAY

Certain tumors of wildlife are apparently associated with infection by viral agents. In this chapter we include skin papillomas and fibromas of Artiodactyla, oral papillomatosis in the coyote and wolf, and lymphomas in several orders of mammals. The chapter on myxomatosis and related conditions elsewhere in this volume is also related to this subject. There are a number of rare or infrequently reported tumors which may prove to be of infectious origin which are not included here.

Skin Papillomas and Fibromas of Artiodactyla

Synonyms: **Warts, papillomas, fibromas, neurofibromas, fibrosarcomas.**

This subject was reviewed for the Cervidae by Fay in 1970 with a brief update confined to the white-tailed deer by Cosgrove et al. in 1979. No extensive revision to the earlier review is needed, but new information from recent reports, and extension of the species involved, is presented.

The lesions are hyperplastic, of viral etiology, and usually of self-limited duration without true neoplastic progression.

HISTORY. The review by Fay 1970 indicated the time sequence of case reports, mostly in deer, starting with 1925 and continuing sporadically until that time. Identification of the lesions varied but the stated characteristics of the skin growths were relatively uniform throughout. Shope (1955) and Shope et al. (1958) did considerable work on this condition and suggested the name "infectious cutaneous fibroma" as most appropriate. The recent review of the condition in white-tailed deer (Cosgrove et al. 1979) added later references which extended the reported range of the disease in the United States and Canada.

DISTRIBUTION. Skin tumors have a wide distribution in North American deer of all species

and subspecies. They are reported infrequently in moose, caribou, and pronghorn in North America and also in European and African hoofed game animals. There are also reports from zoological gardens.

The previous reviews give extensive tabulations of reports of White-tailed deer (*Odocoileus virginianus*). Of special note are the frequencies of 1.4% in about 3,000 deer in New York (Friend 1967) and of 1.3% of 1,065 deer in the southeastern United States (F. A. Hayes, personal communication, 1978).

As indicated in the previous reviews, the disease has been reported from mule deer and black-tailed deer (*Odocoileus hemionus*) in several areas of the North American West.

There have been occasional reports of the disease in moose (*Alces alces*) (Fay 1970) with an added report by Fyvie (1969) from Ontario.

From North America, skin tumors of this type have been reported from caribou (*Rangifer tarandus*) (Broughton et al. 1972) and from pronghorn (*Antilocapra americana*) (Honess and Winter 1956). In Europe the disease appears in various ungulate game animals, for example, red deer (*Cervus elaphus*) (Jennings 1968), roe deer (*Capreolus capreolus*) (Borg 1963), fallow deer (*Dama dama*) (Heidemann 1974), and chamois (*Rupicapra rupicapra*) (Wetzel and Rieck 1962), and in Africa in impala and giraffe (Karstad and Kaminjolo 1978). We did not review the European and African literature, but it seems reports are few and relatively recent from this area where game has been intensively studied for a long time.

ETIOLOGY. At least some of the skin tumors of Cervidae are now known to be caused by a papovavirus which is transmissible by cell-free filtrates or by tumor cell suspensions in contact with skin wounds (Allison 1965; Koller and Olson 1972; Shope et al. 1958; Tajima et al. 1968). Deer fibroma virus has been seen in the epithelial cell portion of the tumor by electron microscopy (Tajima et al. 1968). Viral particles characteristic of papovaviruses were demonstrated also in the papillomas of impala and giraffe (Karstad and Kaminjolo 1978). Apparently few cases are studied by modern virological techniques, and little is known about the etiologic agents in other wild artiodactyls.

TRANSMISSION. There has been little progress in this aspect since the earlier review. Direct contact, insect vectors, and mechanical injury remain as possibilities. The case report of ossifying fibromas of both ears following implantation of tags on a white-tailed deer suggests virus introduction during the procedure (Roscoe et al. 1975). There have been cross-transmission studies to other fibroma-papilloma-prone species, including cattle, which indicate virus specificity (Allison 1965; Koller and Olson 1972; Shope et al. 1958; Tajima et al. 1968).

PATHOGENESIS. It appears that the skin tumors rarely have important pathologic effects on the host or greatly influence health and survival. The tumors usually are localized at the attachment site and do not invade deeper structures. Frequently the animals are reported to be fat or in good condition even in cases with massive growths. Massive tumors about the head could interfere with vision or eating.

PATHOLOGY

Gross Pathology. These skin tumors are warty, raised, pigmented growths which may be single or multiple. In severe cases there are massive confluent areas especially on the head and neck. Individual tumors range from tiny to 22 mm or more. Small ones are rounded, nodular, and low, while larger ones are irregular, pedunculated, and even pendulous. Almost all are freely movable. The larger tumors often undergo breakdown and surface ulceration, bleed, and afford portals of entry for secondary infection. On incision the cut surface has a dense, pale, fibrous core covered with varying depths of dark pigmented surface epithelium which is rough and fissured. Two reports indicate the presence of related fibrotic nodules in the lungs (Koller and Olson 1971; Wadsworth 1954), and a more recent report indicates a degree of local invasiveness indicating sarcomatous malignancy (Elwell et al. 1977).

Histopathology. The epithelial surface of the fibromatous type of tumor is irregular, hyperpigmented, occasionally hyperplastic but not malignant in appearance. There may be foci of liquefaction and cell ballooning. The core and bulk of the tumor is usually composed of dense, irregular, rather mature connective tissue with mild to moderate vascularity. Some infarctive necrosis may occur with hemorrhage in the tissues and with an ulcerated and scabbed surface (Fay 1970; Shope et al. 1958). When lung nodules occur, they are solely of the fibromatous component with areas of calcification (Koller and Olson 1972; Wadsworth 1954). The epithelial surface of the grossly warty or papillomatous type is hyperplastic, folded, with irregular surface and basal irregularity. A gradation between the two histologic extremes involves chiefly the amount and hyperactivity of the squamous epithelium.

IMMUNITY. Fay 1970 mentioned observations indicating that the skin lesions tend to disappear without residual. This indicates that more animals in the herd have been infected than would be evident by casual observation of gross tumors. Antibodies against the papilloma virus develop and probably prevent further infection as well as leading to regression of the skin lesions (Olson et al. 1969).

TREATMENT AND CONTROL. No methods have been developed for treatment and control of this disease.

Oral Papillomatosis of Coyotes and Wolves

Synonyms: **None.**

This condition has been reported from coyotes (*Canis latrans*) in Texas and coyotes and wolves (*Canis lupus*) in western Canada. It resembles transmissible oral papilloma of dogs. Electron microscopy of lesions revealed a papovavirus.

HISTORY AND DISTRIBUTION. In 1966 and 1967 oral papillomatosis was diagnosed in three coyotes in Texas (Trainer et al. 1968). This was followed by a report of three cases from Canada which had occurred in the early 1950s and 1962 in Alberta and in 1969 in Saskatchewan (Broughton et al. 1970). Greig and Charlton (1973) reported a case in a coyote from Manitoba. Nellis (1973) reported five further cases in coyotes, and Samuel et al. (1978) reported ten in coyotes and two in wolves, all from Alberta.

ETIOLOGY AND TRANSMISSION. Each report indicated the morphologic similarity of the disease to oral papillomatosis of dogs, noted epithelial inclusion bodies, and in one case, transmission from coyote to beagle dogs was successful (Thomsen, J. J. cited in Samuel et al. 1978). Greig and Charlton (1973) and Samuel et al. (1978) found a papovavirus by electronmicroscopy on tissues from their cases.

PATHOGENESIS AND PATHOLOGY. All cases had extensive papillary tumor formation of the oral mucous membranes of lips and tongue, and deep into the throat. These were described as wartlike growths, dark, irregular, and confluent. They were extensive enough to interfere with feeding, although weight loss was not obvious in some of the affected coyotes. Histopathology was similar in all cases, with thickened and folded epidermis with fronds on thin fibrovascular stalks. Epithelial inclusion bodies were inconsistently seen.

IMMUNITY, TREATMENT, AND CONTROL. There is no known immunity, treatment, or control for this disease.

Lymphoma

Synonyms: **Lymphosarcoma, lymphoblastoma, lymphatic leukemia, lymphomatosis.**

Lymphomas comprise a spectrum of malignant neoplasms derived from cells of the lymphoid system manifested by massive proliferation and distribution, either localized or widespread, of the atypical cells. In certain instances, there is mounting evidence that the diseases are associated with virus infection or are contagious.

HISTORY AND DISTRIBUTION. Sporadic cases of lymphoma have been reported from wildlife (Garner and Schwartz 1969), including wild ungulates (Fay 1962; Hansen and Borg, 1966; Jennings 1968), hares and rabbits (Lopushinsky and Fay 1967), marine mammals (Larsen 1962; Stedham et al. 1977; R. K. Stroud, personal communication, 1978), and rodents (Gardner et al. 1973). The presence of lymphoma in zoo animals, some recently introduced from the wild, has also been reported (Effron et al. 1977; Griner 1971, 1975; Lombard and Witte 1959).

ETIOLOGY. Recent progress has been made

linking lymphoma of wildlife to infectious etiologic agents. Gardner et al. (1973) found murine-type C virus in much higher incidence in a population of wild house mice (*Mus musculus*) with a correspondingly higher incidence of lymphoma that was found in other nearby wild populations of *M. musculus*. *Herpesvirus sylvilagus* has been isolated as an indigenous virus in cottontails (*Sylvilagus floridanus*) with lymphoproliferative disease; it was productive of experimental lymphoproliferative disease as well as lymphoma in experimental rabbit hosts (Hinze 1971; Lewis and Hinze 1976). Viral etiology is suspected in a case of lymphoma in an infant fur seal (*Callorhinus ursinus*) where electron microscopy revealed possible virus inclusions in neoplastic cell cytoplasm (Stedham et al. 1977). R. K. Stroud (personal communication 1978) is studying another case in a harbor seal (*Phoca virulina*) for possible virus etiology. In the cases of lymphoma of two young harbor seals recently introduced to a zoo from the wild, some unsuccessful attempts were made to demonstrate viral etiology (Griner 1971).

TRANSMISSION AND EPIZOOTIOLOGY. The mode of transmission and the epizootiology of this condition are unknown.

PATHOLOGY

Gross Pathology. Case reports from various species of wildlife—white-tailed deer (Debbie and Friend 1967; Fay 1962), roe deer (Woodford 1966), hares and rabbits (Hinze 1971; Lopushinsky and Fay 1967), mice (Gardner et al. 1973), and seals (Griner 1971; K. Osborne and L. Cornell, personal communication, 1978; Stedham et al. 1977; Stroud, personal communication, 1978)—are quite similar. Widespread lymphadenopthy is consistent with variable involvement of a variety of other sites. The involved organs show pale, firm, but not hard, infiltrates usually in circumscribed nodules or tumorous aggregates.

Histopathology. The described cases in wildlife involve proliferations of cells of the lymphoid series with varying degrees of immaturity. Sometimes there is an element of histicytic cells. A widespread pattern of involvement is typical, infiltrating most hemopoietic tissues and, variably, other organs as well, with loss of normal histoarchitecture. The thymus, however, is not usually involved. In many of the cases, the abnormal cells enter the blood with resulting high white blood cell counts, and these

therefore represent lymphoblastic or lymphocytic leukemias.

DIAGNOSIS. Some cases come to attention because of impairment of the natural ability of
the animal to cope with life situations; others
are discovered by accident. Biopsy of tumor
nodules, examination of the blood for abnormal
cells, or necropsy and histopathology all give a
good chance of accurate diagnosis.

IMMUNITY, TREATMENT, AND CONTROL.
There is no known immunity, treatment, or
control for this disease.

REFERENCES

Allison, A. C. Viruses inducing skin tumors in animals. In A. J. Rook and G. S. Walton, eds.,
*Comparative physiology and pathology of the
skin*, pp. 665–684. Oxford: Blackwell, 1965.

Borg, K. Pathology and wildlife relationships: Research on wildlife diseases in Sweden with special reference to some pathological conditions,
e.g. tumours in roe deer. *Proc. 1st Int. Conf.
Wildl. Dis.*, New York, 1962, pp. 317–328, 1963.

Broughton, E., Gaesser, F. E., Carbyn, L. N, and
Choquette, L. P. E. Oral papillomatosis in the
coyote in Western Canada. *J. Wildl. Dis.*
6:180–181, 1970.

Broughton, E., Miller, F. L., Choquette, L. P. E. Cutaneous fibropapillomas in migratory barren-
ground caribou. *J. Wildl. Dis.* 8:138–140, 1972.

Cosgrove, G. E., Satterfield, L. C., and Nettles, V. C.
Neoplasia. In F. Hayes, and V. C. Nettles, eds.,
Diseases of white-tailed deer. Athens: University
of Georgia Press, 1980. (In press.)

Debbie, J. G., and Friend, M. Lymphosarcoma in
white-tailed deer. *Bull. Wildl. Dis. Assoc.*
3:38–39, 1967.

Effron, M., Griner, L., and Benirschke, K. Nature and
rate of neoplasia found in captive wild mammals,
birds, and reptiles at necropsy. *J. Natl. Cancer
Inst.* 59:185–198, 1977.

Elwell, M. R., Bruger, G. T., Moe, J. B., White, J. D.,
and Stookey, J. L. Fibrosarcoma in white-tailed
deer. *J. Wildl. Dis.* 13:297–299, 1977.

Fay, L. D. Neoplastic diseases of white-tailed deer.
Proc. 1st Natl. White-tailed Deer Dis. Symp.,
University of Georgia, Athens, pp 132–137,
1962.

———. Skin tumors of the Cervidae. In J. W. Davis,
L. H. Karstad, and D. O. Trainer, eds., *Infectious
diseases of wild mammals*, pp. 385–392. Ames:
Iowa State University Press, 1970.

Friend, M. Skin tumors in New York deer. *Bull.
Wildl. Dis. Assoc.* 3:102–104, 1967.

Fyvie, A. *Manual of common parasites, diseases and
anomalies of wildlife in Ontario*. Ontario: Dept.
of Lands and Forests, 1969.

Gardner, M. B., Henderson, B. E., Estes, J. D., Menck,

H., Parker, J. C., and Huebner, R. J. Unusually
high incidence of spontaneous lymphomas in
wild house mice. *J. Natl. Cancer Inst.*
50:1571–1579, 1973.

Garner, F. M., and Schwartz, L. W. Spontaneous
hematopoietic neoplasms of free-living and captive wild mammals. In C. H. Lingeman, and F.
M. Garner, eds., *Comparative morphology of
hematopoietic neoplasms*, Natl. Cancer Instit.
Monogr. 32, pp. 153–156. Washington, D.C.:
U. S. Government Printing Office, 1969.

Greig, A. S., and Charlton, K. M. Electron microscopy
of the virus of oral papillomatosis in the coyote.
J. Wildl. Dis. 9:359–361, 1973.

Griner, L. A. Malignant leukemic lymphoma in two
harbor seals (*Phoca vitulina geronimensis*). *Am.
J. Vet. Res.* 32:827–830, 1971.

———. Hematopoietic neoplasia in animals at the
San Diego Zoological Garden. In *Verg. 17th Int.
Symp. Uber die Erkankungen der Zootiere*, pp.
253–259. Berlin: Akademie-Verlag, 1975.

Hansen, H. J., and Borg, K. Leucosis in wild-living
ruminants. In G. Winqvist, ed., *Comparative
leukemia research*, vol. 6, pp. 221–225. New
York: Pergamon, 1966.

Heidemann, G. Papillomatose bei einem Damhirsch
(*Cervus dama* L. 1758). *Z. Jagdwiss.* 20:157–158,
1974.

Hinze, H. C. Induction of lymphoid hyperplasia and
lymphoma-like disease in rabbits by *Herpesvirus
sylvilagus*. *Int. J. Cancer* 8:514–522, 1971.

Honess, R. F., and Winter, K. B. Diseases of wildlife
in Wyoming. *Wyo. Game Fish Comm. Bull.*
9:279, 1956.

Jennings, A. R. Tumors of free-living wild mammals
and birds in Great Britain. *Symp. Zool. Soc.
Lond.* 24:273–287, 1968.

Karstad, L., and Kaminjolo, J. S. Skin papillomas in
an impala (*Aepyceros melampus*) and a giraffe
(*Giraffa camelopardalis*). *J. Wildl. Dis.* 14:
309–313, 1978.

Koller, L. D., and Olson, C. Pulmonary fibroblasto-
mas in a deer with cutaneous fibromatosis.
Cancer Res. 31:1371–1375, 1971.

———. Attempted transmission of warts from man,
cattle, and horses and of deer fibroma to selected
hosts. *J. Invest. Dermatol.* 58:366–368, 1972.

Larsen, S. A survey of postmortem findings in Pinni-
pedia autopsied during the 10 year period
1952–1961. *Nord. Vet. Med.* 14:150–160, 1962.

Lewis, H. S., and Hinze, H. C. Epidemiology of *Herpesvirus sylvilagus* infection in cottontail rabbits. *J. Wildl. Dis.* 12:482–485, 1976.

Lombard, L. S., and Witte, E. J. Frequency and types
of tumors in mammals and birds of the Philadelphia Zoological Garden. *Cancer Res.*
19:127–141, 1959.

Lopushinsky, T., and Fay, L. D. Some benign and
malignant neoplasms of Michigan cottontail
rabbits. *Bull. Wildl. Dis. Assoc.* 3:148–151, 1967.

Nellis, C. H. Prevalence of oral papilloma-like lesions
in coyotes in Alberta. *Can. J. Zool.* 51:900, 1973.

Olson, C., Gordon, D. E., Robb, M. G., and Lee, K. P.

Oncogenicity of bovine papilloma virus. *Arch. Environ. Health* 19:928–837, 1969.

Roscoe, D. E., Veikley, L. R., Mills, M., Jr., and Kinds, L. III. Debilitating ossifying fibromas of a white-tailed deer associated with ear tagging. *J. Wildl. Dis.* 11:62–65, 1975.

Samuel, W. M., Chalmers, G. A., and Geenson, J. R. Oral papillomatosis in coyotes (*Canis latrans*) and wolves (*Canis lupus*) of Alberta. *J. Wild. Dis.* 14:165, 1978.

Shope, R. E. Infectious fibroma of deer. *Proc. Soc. Exp. Biol. Med.* 88:533–535, 1955.

Shope, R. E., Mangold, R., McNamara, L. G., and Dumbell, K. R. An infectious cutaneous fibroma of the Virginia white-tailed deer (*Odocoileus virginianus*). *J. Exp. Med.* 108:797–802, 1958.

Stedham, M. S., Casey, H. W., and Keyes, M. C. Lymphosarcoma in an infant northern fur seal (*Callorhinus ursinus*). *J. Wildl. Dis.* 13:176–179, 1977.

Tajima, M., Gordon, D. E., and Olson, C. Electron microscopy of bovine papilloma and deer fibroma viruses. *Am. J. Vet. Res.* 29:1185–1194, 1968.

Trainer, D. O., Knowlton, F. F., Karstad, L. Oral papillomatosis in the coyote. *Bull. Wildl. Dis. Assoc.* 4:52–54, 1968.

Wadsworth, J. R. Fibrosarcoma in a deer. *J. Am. Vet. Med. Assoc.* 124:194, 1954.

Wetzel, R., and Rieck, W. *Krankheiten des Wildes.* Hamburg and Berlin: Verlag Paul Parey, 1962.

Woodford, M. Lymphosarcoma in a wild roe deer. *Vet. Rec.* 79:74, 1966.

Index